Nursing elderly people

To all our elders, and their friends,
who are the recipients of our care

Nursing
elderly people

Edited by

Sally J. Redfern BSc PhD RGN
Director, Nursing Research Unit, Department of Nursing Studies,
King's College, University of London, London

CHURCHILL LIVINGSTONE
EDINBURGH LONDON MELBOURNE NEW YORK AND TOKYO 1991

CHURCHILL LIVINGSTONE
Medical Division of Longman Group UK Limited

Distributed in the United States of America by Churchill
Livingstone Inc., 650 Avenue of the Americas, New York,
N. Y. 10011, and by associated companies, branches and
representatives throughout the world.

First edition 1986
Second edition 1991
   Reprinted 1992

ISBN 0-443-04138-5

British Library Cataloguing in Publication Data
Nursing elderly people. — 2nd. ed.
   1. Old persons. Nursing
   I. Redfern, Sally J.
   610.7365

Library of Congress Cataloging in Publication Data
Nursing elderly people/[edited by] Sally J. Redfern. — 2nd ed.
      p.   cm.
   Includes bibliographical references.
   Includes index.
   ISBN 0-443-04138-5
   1. Geriatric nursing.   I. Redfern, Sally J.
   [DNLM: 1. Geriatric Nursing.   WY 152 N974603]
RC954.N886   1991
610.73'65—dc20
DNLM/DLC
for Library of Congress   90-2583
                                                  CIP

The
publisher's
policy is to use
**paper manufactured
from sustainable forests**

Produced by Longman Singapore Publishers (Pte) Ltd.
Printed in Singapore.

Preface to the Second Edition

In this second edition of Nursing Elderly People we have retained the approach and format of the first edition, but have modified and expanded it considerably to take account of topics that were omitted in the first edition, and of recent developments in health care and in nursing that have had a major impact on the care of old people. Four new chapters have appeared, ten have been rewritten and nearly all the remainder have been substantially modified and updated. The four new chapters, Chapters 18, 23, 25 and 29 are included to fill substantial gaps in the first edition.

In Chapter 18, Ian Norman describes the extent of mental health problems in the elderly population and discusses the importance of thorough assessment and planning of individual care from the perspective of the multidisciplinary team. He advocates inclusion of a nursing contribution to a multidisciplinary problem-oriented record, rather than slavish adherence to the *nursing* process. In this way, the client is more likely to receive a co-ordinated package of care rather than fragmented care.

In Chapter 23, Miriam Bernard and Chris Phillipson look at self-care and health in old age. They highlight the increasing trend of old people to take more active control of their own health, and the subsequent development of self-help groups run by elders who have similar health and social concerns. This self-help trend requires nurses and other health workers to change their own attitudes, to encourage involvement of old people in their own care and to respond to health care demands that their clients increasingly will make. The out-

come is likely to be a substantial rise in the quality of life in old age.

Another gap that has been filled is Maggie Pearson's Chapter 25 on care of black and ethnic minority elders. She emphasizes the point that if black and ethnic minority communities have been 'invisible' in this country, then their elderly folk have been even more so. Her chapter covers the family circumstances, the living conditions, health and well-being of these people, and the failure of the services to meet their needs. The statutory services have much to learn from the growing number of self-help groups that have emerged in many local minority communities.

Chapter 29 by Sally Redfern, focuses on continuing care of old people in long-stay settings ranging from residential Homes to nursing Homes and hospital wards. For these elders who can no longer cope in their own homes, finding a Home that offers the required amount of autonomy, freedom and choice rather than restrictive 'people-processing' characteristics is the priority. Enterprising initiatives are growing, many initiated by nurses, but it will be a long time before all old people who face life in a long-stay setting will benefit.

The concluding chapters in Part 4 of the volume contain a good deal of material missing in the first edition. In Chapter 31, the section on old people from ethnic minorities has disappeared, since this topic now has its own chapter. In its place, we have expanded our discussion of ageism and have included a case study of an old lady who, we argue, was a victim of ageism yet whose story we have seen repeated in many different settings. In Chapter 32, we have retained the emphasis on the quality of living and of dying. The balance of rights and risks is considered and the importance of giving old people the chance to take risks, like everybody else does, is emphasized. The section on surgery for old people has been expanded to include the measures that could easily be, but tend not to be, taken to reduce the incidence of osteoporosis, particularly for elderly women.

Chapter 33 on the nurse's role in the care of old people has been substantially revised. We update the reader on some of the developments in nurse practitioner and clinical nurse specialist roles; and we move from a nursing process perspective, which was implicit in the first edition, to the current emphasis on individualized care and primary nursing. At the time of going to press, 'Project 2000' had received the green light and pilot schemes were being set up in new nursing education colleges throughout the country. Whether Project 2000 achieves its ambition, to produce a

new kind of nurse who can meet the health needs of our aged society in the 1990s and beyond, remains to be seen.

The illustration on the cover of the first edition shows two white-haired women engrossed in a game of pool. The setting could be anywhere, such as a hospital, a nursing Home, a club or a pub. For the second edition, we have chosen an equally stereotype-breaking picture, but this time, one depicting two elderly men engrossed in baking a cake. This picture is borrowed from Chapter 7, and as with the pool game, it could be in a hospital or community setting.

For this second edition my specific thanks go to my patient contributors, both old and new, and to Carolyn Dereky, Bee Ogilvie and Sylvia Berkovitz for their mastery of the word processor and their speed in production. Also, as before, to Beryl Bailey for her continued perfectionism in producing the Index.

London, 1990   S. J. R

Preface to the First Edition

Our attempt has been to combine the expertise of many people concerned with care of elderly people (nurses, social scientists, doctors and other specialists) into a comprehensive nursing textbook. We cover social, psychological and physiological aspects of ageing, the common nursing problems of elderly people, and provision of health care. Our approach is a warm-blooded, humanitarian one in which old people are seen as a precious 'commodity' who have wisdom and other positive contributions to make to society. This book will have been successful if it encourages its readers to value the old people they care for and to promote opportunities for well-being and psychological growth rather than helplessness and deterioration in their old age.

The intention has been to produce a text which is not overly parochial and which can cross cultural and geographical boundaries. The material on the organization of health care and provision of services, however (especially Part 3 and Part 4), necessarily emphasizes a British perspective, although much of it is appropriate to other western industrial countries.

We hope the book will be a key text for nurses specializing in the care of elderly people, which would include post-basic course students. In addition, since many student nurses will care for old people when they are qualified, either by choice or otherwise, this book should provide them with useful reference material. A truly comprehensive nursing textbook for the elderly might encourage more student nurses to choose to specialize in this field, particularly if they use the book during their basic training. The leadership might also include doctors joining departments of geriatric medicine and other members of the health care team, all of whom require some knowledge of nursing and the nurse's role. Above all, our aim is that the book will appeal to the socially aware nurse of post-industrial societies in which social problems such as ageing populations, mass unemployment and increased leisure time are of major concern, and in which ageism will take its place, along with sexism and racism, as an acknowledged discrimination issue.

The illustration on the cover of this book was chosen to reflect a positive view of old age. It shows two white-haired women who could be friends, engaged in a challenging activity not traditionally regarded as feminine. The activity is self-initiated, there are no health care workers in sight, and it could be located in a hospital or community setting. The exclusion of men from the picture is not deliberate, but it does illustrate the fact that most old people are women. This reason alone would dictate departure from convention and the use of the female gender throughout this book when referring to old people in the singular.

The book contains four parts. In *Part 1*, the focus is on what it means to be old and the changes which may occur as a result of ageing. Although the term 'aged' is used as a category to describe old people, it is inappropriate because 'ageing' and 'aged' are time-dependent concepts. A child 'ages' over time but is not classified as aged. Lumping all old people into a homogeneous, rigid category, although convenient, denies recognition of their individual differences. It also increases the risk of their being classified as a low status minority. This occurs with other groups, such as 'the disabled'. It is usual to distinguish between functional and chronological age, especially with reference to child development; we talk, for example, of the 'mental age' of a child. Similarly, not all old people are functionally, physiologically, psychologically and socially at the same point at the same age. The use of classifications such as 'retirement age' encourages misleading categorization. In practice the outcome is that 'old age' is often negatively regarded as a period of non-productivity and illness, when it can be, and often is, a time of positive experience, health and optimism, especially as a result of the technological, material and social advances in our society. In Chapter 1, Malcolm Johnson explores these ideas. The attitude held by society tends to demean old people and reflects the destructive stereotyping of ageism, not dissimilar to that experienced by women and black people. Problems of frailty do occur, but they vary according to people's life experiences, to variations in exposure.

In Chapter 2, Sally Robbins continues the discussion on the fallacy of ageist stereotyping. Some of the psychological theories of ageing are described as are the effects of changes in role and the impact of life events. The research evidence on changes in cognitive processes (intelligence, learning, memory, perception, etc.) which result from growing older does not always support the assumption of inevitable decline. People adjust to being old in different ways, and adjustment is a healthy lifetime process not confined to old age. Health care demands and health care itself would alter substantially if in both preventive and reactive medicine greater account were taken of old people's individuality.

Some of the physiological theories of ageing are summarized by Gerry Bennett in Chapter 3. He describes the physiological changes which occur with age and emphasizes the importance of distinguishing between changes which occur as a result of age alone and those which accompany diseases common in old people.

Part 2 contains 18 chapters and has a clinical emphasis, covering the nursing problems commonly experienced by old people. It takes a client-centred individualized approach and accep-

tance of the 'nursing process' is explicit in most of the chapters.

Communication and sensory deficit are central to Chapters 4, 5 and 6. In Chapter 4, Jill Macleod Clark explains the principal components of communication. She focuses on the nurse's role in assessing and meeting the needs of elderly patients with communication difficulties in general, but particularly those with speech impairment following a stroke. In Chapter 5, Katia Gilhome Herbst reminds us that to be old and deaf constitutes a double stigma as well as double handicap, and deafness is often associated with 'daftness' (incorrectly) and with depression (correctly). The prevalence of deafness is much higher than is generally believed and most old people have some hearing loss. Nurses have an important role in assessment of hearing loss, in improving communication with deaf old people, and in helping them take advantage of personal and environmental hearing aids. Bob Greenhalgh, in Chapter 6, notes that most people who are partially sighted or totally blind are elderly. He discusses assessment of visual ability, the factors which influence sight, and the nurse's contribution to the rehabilitation of old people with impaired sight.

Chapters 7 to 16 attend to essential human needs and functions which often present difficulties in old age. In Chapter 7, Amanda Stokes-Roberts discusses the importance to old people of maintaining their earlier activities and interests, and the factors which influence an old person's ability to keep occupied. Amanda identifies what can be done to keep old people in the environment of their choice and to enhance their well-being in institutions.

Mobility is the subject of Chapter 8, and Lynn Batehup and Amanda Squires discuss the prevalence of immobility of old people and the factors which affect their mobility. The specific mobility problems of people with certain pathologies (Parkinson's disease, hemiplegia, arthritis, amputation, falls) are described, and guidance is given on their management. The relative merits of stroke units on recovery of patients compared with conventional care are discussed. The subject of mobility continues in Chapter 9 on care of the foot. Foot problems tend to be given low priority, yet they cause so much pain and incapacity for old people and are relatively easy to prevent and to treat. Mike Hobday discusses the common problems and their management. There is much nurses can do to relieve an overstretched chiropody service.

Difficulty in breathing also limits mobility. In Chapter 10, Angela Heslop covers cardiovascular and respiratory fitness of old people, and the nursing management of people with breathing difficulties. Keeping fit with regular exercise is advocated for younger people. The right kind of exercise is equally important for old people, both in good and in poor health.

It is tempting, particularly for those living alone or with mobility problems, to eat unwisely. Sue Thomas, in Chapter 11, describes the risk factors which affect the nutritional status of old people, the prevalence of malnutrition, and the nutritional problems which occur. She gives guidance on how to help old people to eat properly and outlines the nutritional services available in the United Kingdom.

Old people find it embarrassing to talk about their bodily functions, particularly problems of elimination, and the prevalence of urinary incontinence is probably higher than that published. In Chapter 12, Christine Norton describes elimination needs and the assessment and management of people with defaecation and micturition difficulties. She discusses the controversy surrounding the emergence of the incontinence adviser into a nursing climate in which all nurses might regard themselves as specialists.

Deaths of old people from hypothermia frequently make headlines, and the recognition and management of hypothermia occupies a major part of Chapter 13. Michael Green urges that nurses and doctors should be vigilant for abnormally low and high body temperatures in old people, should be aware of those in the population at risk, and should become politically active in an effort to improve the financial and social circumstances of this vulnerable group.

With increasing numbers surviving into very old age, many more immobile old people are at risk from pressure sores. The prevention and management of pressure sores forms a major part of Sally Redfern's discussion in Chapter 14. As with incontinence, management of people with, or at risk of developing, pressure sores requires a multidisciplinary team approach, but these are areas in which nurses can take the lead.

Chapter 15 covers sleep and rest. We all need adequate sleep, yet the function of sleep continues to be debated. Morva Fordham discusses sleep patterns of old people compared with young, and the effects of different patterns on daytime behaviour. She describes the multiple causes of sleep problems of old people and emphasizes the nurse's role in assessing and managing these problems.

In Chapter 16, Christine Webb returns to the subject of stereotyping and prejudice, and discusses the widespread myth that old people, particularly women, are asexual. Sexual expression tends to be discouraged, particularly in institutions and for old people with disabilities. Nurses are in an ideal position to act as advocates in helping old people fulfil their need for self-respect, companionship, love and intimacy. Like sexuality, pain is a personal and private experience. In Chapter 17, Susan Gollop outlines the effect of ageing on the experience of pain. She focuses on the assessment of pain and the various ways in which the nurse can intervene in caring for an old person in pain.

Chapters 18 and 19 refer to the elderly mentally frail. Although dementia is common in the very old, it is not, as is often thought, synonymous with ageing, a point made clear by Julia Brooking in Chapter 18. Julia also clarifies the difference between dementia and confusion, and provides an optimistic approach to treatment and care of these frail old people. She goes on in Chapter 19 to discuss another common problem for old people, depression, and highlights its social, biological and psychological antecedents. Suicide and other so-called 'functional' disorders of old people are discussed briefly, and the approaches to care which are most helpful are identified. This should be useful material for nurses without specialized psychiatric training.

Old people consume nearly a third of the National Health Service drugs budget and this proportion is likely to increase. In Chapter 20, Jill David discusses both the value and the hazards of drug use for old people. Nurses have a crucial role in teaching patients about their drugs, in monitoring progress and reporting side-effects, and in preparing patients (or relatives) to administer their own drugs safely when discharged from hospital.

Part 2 ends with Chapter 21 by Jo Hockley on death and dying. She discusses the causes of death in the elderly and where people die. 'Natural' deaths seem to be much less common today, perhaps because few occur at home. Useful guidance is given on the management of problems often experienced by people who are dying, including care of relatives. Following this is a discussion of the merits of hospice care and a comment on euthanasia. The chapter ends with a poem written by a 90-year-old patient just before her death, which carries a message for all nurses — to ensure that patients do not die alone.

Part 3 examines the provision of care for elderly people and focuses mainly on a British perspective. Helen Evers' Chapter 22 is essential reading if we are to understand the organization of care for old people in this country. She outlines some of the characteristics of the elderly population and describes the historical development of health service provision, noting that needs and services seldom match well. Helen draws on research into the organization of nursing and highlights the perennial problems of this low status specialty, particularly those of long-term care. The arguments are strongly made for nurse-led long-term care units without the clinical atmosphere of the hospital, where old people who require little medical attention can live in a homely, personalized environment, and where the links with community nursing are strengthened. Long-term care is the focus of Chapter 23 in which Barbara Wade refers to research carried out with old people living in long-term geriatric wards and residential and private nursing Homes. The impression which emerges is one of inflexibility by the authorities and little choice for old people. Barbara advocates a 'supportive model' of care which would be appropriate to all settings and would give old people and their relatives the choice and freedom they seek.

Psychiatric care for elderly people has developed as a specialty more recently than geriatrics, and there is a serious shortfall of psychogeriatricians and specialist nurses. In Chapter 24, Julia Brooking identifies the facilities required for the elderly mentally frail, facilities which are not available for most of these old people. It is their families who are left with the major burden of care.

Virtually all hospital nurses care for old people, but, in Chapter 25, Pauline Fielding focuses on the variety of organization and facilities provided in geriatric units, and specifies the basic requirements of such units. Comprehensive assessment of an old person's level of independence is an essential prerequisite for successful nursing intervention, and planning for the patient's discharge from hospital should begin soon after admission. The important role that nurses working in geriatric units have is emphasized, in protecting the patients from the negative effects of an impersonal and institutionalized environment.

Although integration of hospital and community services for old people is an attractive proposition, separation of these services is the reality today. In Chapter 26, Fiona Ross describes the complexity and challenge for the nurse caring for old people at home, and she describes the organization of primary health care and social service provision in this country. She argues for development of the district nurse as the key worker for old people in the primary care team, responsible for preventive as well as therapeutic nursing. This would leave the health visitor free to continue to focus on child care.

In Chapter 27, Alison While describes the surveillance and health promotion and maintenance functions of health visitors, and agrees that, apart from the few who specialize in care of old people, most health visitors give priority to child care. She regards the health visitor as essential in maintaining the well-being of old people at home, and believes that rather than extending the role of the district nurse as advocated by Fiona Ross, health visitors should expand their clientèle to include all members of the family, i.e. old people as well as children. Alison While also gives us insight into the problems of growing old in inner-city areas, into the ageing experience of people from ethnic minorities, and into violence against old people.

In *Part 4*, Sally Redfern draws together issues

raised in earlier chapters and discusses others relevant to the care of old people. The focus in Chapter 28 is the elderly person, in Chapter 29 it is the elderly patient or client, and in Chapter 30 it is the nurse's role and health care provision for old people. Chapter 28 refers to some of the earlier discussions on the impact of an ageing population; it highlights the experiences that women, men and people of different ethnic origin have in being old, victims of discrimination and dependent on inadequate services. More positively, some aspects of 'successful ageing' are discussed, together with ways in which nurses can help old people to stay healthy.

Some of the major issues concerning the quality of living and of dying for the frail old person who needs short-term hospital care or continuing support are discussed in Chapter 29. We focus on communication with elderly patients or clients, on the organization of nursing in different institutional settings, and on surgery for old people. Striking a balance between allowing old people the rights to which any individual is entitled and avoiding unnecessary risk is a continuing theme, and is perhaps the key to high quality nursing. The theme continues in the discussion on the quality of dying in which the focus is the patient's right to refuse treatment, informed consent, and the care of dying people.

In discussion of the nurse's role, in Chapter 30, the main concerns are the debate about independent nurse practitioners and nurse education. An attempt has been made to give an overview of health care provision and to make recommendations for the future. In the final section we identify some of those areas in nursing elderly people which would benefit from further research. Nurses who examine their own practices, who continue to learn about nursing old people and who investigate nursing issues themselves, will ensure that the quality of nursing will improve and, with it, the quality of life for old people.

I am grateful to Dorothy Baker for writing the Foreword. She is a specialist and teacher on the nursing of elderly people, and an advocate for the elderly in her work as a member of a local Health Authority. Her research on the organization of nursing in geriatric wards is well known to the profession.

This book would not have been written without each contributor's commitment and patience. Many waited a long time between sending me their chapters and the final appearance in print. I am indebted to Churchill Livingstone, particularly to Ellen Green who put the idea to me in the first place, and to Sally Morris and Dinah Bagshaw who nursed me through all the stages of production. Specific thanks go to Pat Shipley who gave me much of her time in discussion of my ideas and her skill at constructive criticism, to Pam Coles, Joyce Hine, Doreen Newman and Christine Terrey for their high quality typing of this manuscript, and to Beryl Bailey for her indexing skills.

London, 1986   S. J. R.

Foreword to the First Edition

It would be unusual if nurses when asked of their work 'whose side are you on?' did not answer 'the side of the patient, of course.' And this answer would come not only from clinical nurses, since our nursing leaders also are much exercized about 'accountability', 'quality assurance', 'the nurse as the patients' advocate'. Elderly people tend not to be amongst the most privileged of patients, but we must assume that the generalized concern for 'the patient' does not exclude them.

If we are indeed on the side of the elderly patient, acting as her or his advocate, we will immediately recognize the complexity and delicacy of our work, and the depth of knowledge and understanding necessary for it. In this volume Sally Redfern and her fellow contributors have made a major contribution to that knowledge and understanding. They alert us to make the necessary meticulous assessment of each nursing situation, and, in co-operation with the patient, to construct an appropriate care plan.

In ideal circumstances the next steps — acting on the plan and evaluating its effectiveness — would proceed without obstacle. In practice, the necessary resources of time, competent assistance and equipment are not always available, and the plan, even if formulated, often cannot be carried out. Short cuts are taken, 'getting through the work' becomes the norm, and wider aims, such as helping the patient to become independent, are abandoned. There may even be pressures which result in the nurse suspending the rules which govern the normal civilities between adults. Through no fault of her own, the nurse finds herself involved in a standard of care which in no way reflects her ideals as 'the patient's advocate'. What now of 'quality assurance'?

A positive response to inadequate resources, arising from thoughts inspired by this book, might perhaps be considered. Rather than 'coping' and 'muddling through' in the time-honoured manner, the nurse might record those items on the care plan which she has not been able to carry out, and the consequences for the patient. This information could be passed to the nurse managers, thus providing them with valuable data to support their claims for resources, as well as assisting them in their endeavours to remain in close contact with what Stacey describes as 'the clinical coal face'. These insights could, in appropriate circumstances, be shared with the members of the Health Authority and the Community Health Council, to their great benefit.

Were such a practice adopted widely by nurses working with elderly patients, the precepts of this excellent book could both illuminate and ultimately change nursing practice. In any case, the book provides a stimulus for nurses to eliminate the gulf between the succession of fine sounding slogans about nursing and the reality of life on the ward or in the home of the frail and sick. The outcome may both bring comfort to the elderly and pose a challenge for those in highest authority, and for the nurse in between there is no escape from the question 'whose side are you on?'

Manchester, 1986   D. E. B.

Contributors

Lynn Batehup BSc MSc RGN DipN
Lecturer/Director, Nursing Development Unit, Dulwich Hospital, Camberwell Health Authority, London

Miriam Bernard BA PhD
Lecturer, Centre for Social Gerontology, University of Keele

Jill Macleod Clark PhD BSc RGN
Professor, Department of Nursing Studies, King's College, University of London

Tim R. Cullinan MD MSc MRCOG FFCM
Formerly Senior Lecturer in Environmental and Preventive Medicine, St Bartholomew's Hospital Medical College, London

Jill A. David BSc MSc RGN HV MIBiol
Manager, Holme Tower Marie Curie Home, Penarth, South Glamorgan

Helen K. Evers BSc MSc PhD
Researcher, Consultant and Partner, Salutis Partnership, Health and Social Care Research and Training, King's Norton, Birmingham

Pauline Fielding BSc PhD RGN
Manager, In-Patient Services, Whipps Cross Hospital, Waltham Forest Health Authority, Essex

Morva Fordham BSc MSc PhD RGN SCM RNT
Formerly Lecturer, Department of Nursing Studies, King's College, University of London

Christine Hanks BSc RGN SCM RNT
Senior Lecturer, Department of Nursing and Community Health Studies, Polytechnic of the South Bank, London

Rosamund A. Herbert BSc MSc RGN
Lecturer/Practitioner, Nursing Development Unit, Dulwich Hospital, Camberwell Health Authority, London

Katia Gilhome Herbst MA PhD
Policy Development Officer, The Mental Health Foundation, London

Mike Hobday BA FChS DPodM
Head, Division of Chiropody and Podiatric Medicine, School of Biological and Health Sciences, Polytechnic of Central London

Jo Hockley RGN SCM
Senior Nurse, Palliative Care Team, St Bartholomew's Hospital, London

Malcolm L. Johnson
Professor and Director, Department of Health and Social Welfare, The Open University, Milton Keynes

Ian J. Norman BA MSc RMN RNMH RGN RNT DipAppSocStud CQSW
Lecturer, Department of Nursing Studies, King's College, University of London

Christine Norton MA RGN
Professional Development Officer, Association of Continence Advisors, Disabled Living Foundation, London

Maggie Pearson MA PhD RGN
Lecturer in Medical Sociology, Department of General Practice, University of Liverpool

Chris Phillipson BA PhD
Professor, Centre for Social Gerontology,
University of Keele

Sally J. Redfern BSc PhD RGN
Director, Nursing Research Unit, Department
of Nursing Studies, King's College, University
of London

Sally E. Robbins BSc MPhil
Principal Clinical Psychologist, Maidstone
Hospital, Maidstone Health Authority,
Maidstone

Fiona Ross BSc PhD RGN NDNCert
Senior Lecturer in Primary Health Care
Nursing, Department of General Practice and
Primary Care, St George's Hospital Medical
School, London

Miriam Rowswell BSc MSc RGN DipN OncCert
Lecturer, Department of Nursing Studies,
King's College, University of London

Kate Seers BSc PhD RGN
Research Fellow, Psychology Unit, Royal Free
Hospital Medical School, London

Amanda Squires MSc Grad Dip Phys MCSP SRP
District Physiotherapist, Waltham Forest Health
Authority, Essex

Amanda Stokes-Roberts DipCOT SROT
District Training and Development Manager,
Wandsworth Health Authority, London

Susan Thomas SRD Dip HE
Formerly Dietician to the Geriatric Unit, St
James' Hospital, Balham, London

Barbara E Wade RGN BEd PhD
Director, Daphne Heald Research and
Development Unit, The Royal College of
Nursing, London

Christine Webb BA MSc PhD RGN RSCN RNT
Professor, Department of Nursing, University of
Manchester

Alison E. While BSc MSc PhD RGN HVCert
Senior Lecturer, Department of Nursing
Studies, King's College, University of London

Contents

PART 1.
Ageing and old age

1. The meaning of old age   3
   Malcolm L. Johnson

2. The psychology of human ageing   19
   Sally E. Robbins

3. The biology of human ageing   39
   Rosamund A. Herbert

PART 2.
Nursing elderly people: their needs, their resources and their problems of living

4. Communicating with elderly people   67
   Jill Macleod Clark

5. Hearing   79
   Katia Gilhome Herbst

6. Sight   91
   Tim Cullinan

7. Maintaining activities and interests   99
   Amanda Stokes-Roberts

8. Mobility   115
   Lynn Batehup, Amanda Squires

9. Care of the foot   147
   Mike C. Hobday

10. Breathing   157
    Christine M. Hanks

11. Eating and drinking   171
    Susan Thomas

12. Eliminating   185
    Christine Norton

13. Maintaining body temperature   199
    Rosamund A. Herbert, Miriam Rowswell

14. Maintaining healthy skin   221
    Sally J. Redfern

15. Sleep and rest   243
    Morva Fordham

16. Expressing sexuality   263
    Christine Webb

17. Pain and elderly people   273
    Kate Seers

18. Mental health problems of elderly people: assessment and planning   289
    Ian J. Norman

19. Confusional states and dementia   309
    Ian J. Norman

20. Depression in old age   341
    Ian J. Norman

21. Drugs and elderly people   373
    Jill A. David, Sally J. Redfern

22. Death and dying   391
    Jo Hockley

PART 3.
The organization of care for elderly people

23. Self-care and health in old age   405
    Miriam Bernard, Chris Phillipson

24. Care of the elderly sick in the UK 417
    Helen K. Evers

25. Care of black and ethnic minority
    elders 437
    Maggie Pearson

26. Health visiting and elderly people 449
    Alison E. While

27. Nursing old people in the community 465
    Fiona M. Ross

28. Nursing old people in hospital 485
    Pauline Fielding

29. Continuing care in long-stay settings 497
    Sally J. Redfern

30. Choice and flexibility in long-term care
    settings 519
    Barbara E. Wade

PART 4.
Care of elderly people: conclusions

31. The elderly person: the challenge of an aged
    society 531
    Sally J. Redfern

32. The elderly patient 549
    Sally J. Redfern

33. The nurse's role in the care of old
    people 567
    Sally J. Redfern

Index 583

Part 1

Ageing and old age

CHAPTER CONTENTS

The biology of ageing 4

Research on old age 5

Contribution to the pathology model 6

Life-history approaches 7
The importance of biography 8
Cohorts, generations and history 10

Health, retirement and work 12

Corporate consciousness and action 13

Recolonization of eldership 14

An ageist modern world 15

1

The meaning of old age

Malcolm L. Johnson

The process of ageing is classically depicted as one of constant and inexorable decline after reaching a peak of bodily function and efficiency around the end of the second decade of life. Moreover, the later years of life are conventionally seen as ones where pathologies of mind, body and social relationships take place. Indeed the period known as old age has been seen, until very recently, as one of withdrawal from the mainstream of life due to infirmity.

Elaborating on traditional presentations of ageing as an inexorable process of decline, modern medical science has created a pathology model of ageing which indicates declining function in all bodily systems. Also reflecting accounts in literature, history, biblical sources and folk lore, psychologists and psychiatrists have produced a body of data which they claim follows a decremental pattern. The advance of chronological age is said to produce a consistent erosion of capacity for memory, cognition, learning and creativity. In terms of psychological health, later life is associated with widespread confusional states, dementia and depression of epidemic proportions. Social scientists have made their own contributions to the prevailing picture by focusing on the poverty of retired people, their high consumption of health and social services and their 'burdensome' claim on social security budgets. Research has focused largely on the negative impact of retirement and its consequences for conjugal relationships, levels of morale and isolation from former social networks.

This chapter will attempt to reconcile this

sombre picture of the ageing process with some recent trends both in research and in the patterns of
behaviour to be observed amongst the increasingly
large numbers of people who are active in later
life. In doing this we will give some attention to
the life histories of individuals and the value of
biographical analysis in gaining a more authentic
picture of the social processes of ageing. It will also
be necessary to look briefly at the constraints
which limit the opportunities for elderly people to
fulfil their potential — thus helping to reinforce
the negative stereotypes of old age.

THE BIOLOGY OF AGEING

Later chapters (particularly Chapter 3) deal in detail with the physical changes which accompany
ageing processes. For present purposes it is
necessary only to indicate what the biological and
clinical sciences have to say about the human body
throughout the lifespan.

Accumulated evidence points fairly unequivocally to the declining efficiency of most bodily
systems with age. Once biological maturity has
been reached — between the ages of 15 and 25
years — the degenerative processes begin. In the
early stages the reductions in function are small,
but continue over time in an increasing and cumulative fashion. Rates of age-related degeneration
vary considerably. Moreover, the onset of decline
occurs at different points in the life-path for different parts of the body. Within individuals, the
variance from statistical norms will be influenced
by genetic inheritance, lifestyle and factors such as
obesity, diet, exercise and medical history.

This brief sketch of biological decline is indicative of the overall position. It offers a picture of
the human body as an organism which increases
in stature and efficiency during the first two decades of life, reaching its peak around the middle
of the third decade. From that point the speed of
decline is variable but inevitable. Amongst the intervening factors which can influence and even
arrest the pace of advancing physical inefficiency
are two broad categories of action. The first concerns the behaviour of individuals — their diet and

general lifestyle. The second is the increasing
capacity of medical science to treat, ameliorate or
cure those conditions which speed up the ageing
process or lead to premature death. With increased
capacity to manipulate these variables it has been
possible to increase dramatically the numbers of
people, in developed societies, who live a full
lifespan.

Yet, whilst biology conveys an uncompromizing
message of degeneration and medicine a complementary one of increasing illness associated with
age, there is a cross-current of evidence of a more
positive kind. Its effect is to offer the prospect of
a less pathological mode of growing old which
allows continuity of life experience and a wide
range of activity. The debate about how far modifications of personal conduct combined with good
medical care can create supernormal life expectancy and how far it can lead to a healthier
existence is now in full flow. After decades of negative findings and decrementalism, there has
arisen an antithetical concept of ageing with more
positive connotations. Perhaps best encapsulated
in the vigorously optimistic pages of Fries and
Crapo's (1981) volume *Vitality and Ageing: Implications of the Rectangular Curve*, the dialogue now
offers ageing as both an inexorable decline and as
a process capable of considerable manipulation.
The new debate claims that what have been previously considered as normal processes of ageing
can be considerably slowed down. Indeed the
image of the rectangular curve is offered as one
which reflects the impact of better health so that
the major maladies of adulthood are compressed
into a relatively short space of time immediately
prior to death. The survival curve will become rectangular rather than one of linear decline, after an
early peak.

The argument the book seeks to advance is that
the present upper limit for human longevity, of
about 115 years, is unlikely to be extended in the
foreseeable future, but that progress in health and
welfare will delay the onset of the most damaging
ailments of later life. It is contended that most of
the disabling conditions of old age are self-inflicted
(through alcohol, tobacco, poor diet, lack of exercise, etc.), or occur as a result of the way society
is organized in that it may cause ill health (en-

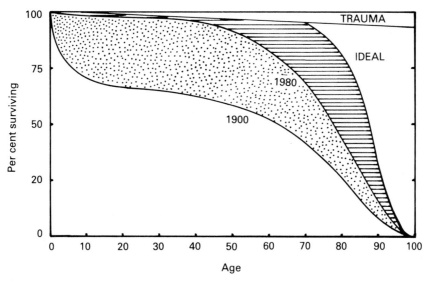

Fig. 1.1 The rectangular curve. *Source: Fries and Crapo (1981).*

vironmental pollution of various kinds) and fail to provide adequate health and welfare services. A remedy for these causes of illness lies in health education, political action and more positive personal behaviour. Were this approach to be adopted, the authors predict a general raising of health standards. Consequently, the chronic illnesses of insidious onset (cancers, rheumatism, degeneration of the heart and so on) will reach an acute stage later in life and concentrate themselves in a short period of perhaps three years prior to death. Thus the downward curve of survival would become more like a rectangle (Fig. 1.1).

Whilst the extension of life and health debate is being conducted in a somewhat value-laden manner, there is a growing body of scientific evidence for the more optimistic view which needs to be unravelled. Within governmental thinking, pressured by rising demand for medical services and the desire to reduce public spending, the focus of this new trend is on the behaviour of individuals. Smoking, diet, exercise, early medical consultation, prophylactic medication and changes in lifestyle are all the subject of health education programmes. The individual is seen to be responsible for his or her own health state and responsible for reducing claims on health resources. In parallel,

there is another view (to which we return later, Townsend 1981) which rejects the emphasis on personal conduct and urges changes at a different level, that is, in patterns of work, transport and social organization — social and political solutions which will make life safer for all.

RESEARCH ON OLD AGE

Studies of ageing and old age (gerontology) are no longer rare, as might have been claimed confidently as little as 20 years ago. But in the intervening period the growth of geriatric medicine, the expansion of academic and policy related research, along with changes in the demographic structure, have made later life more important and better understood. Having said this, it is essential to recognize that gerontology is still very youthful as a field of study. Much material has been gained through recent research which has aided our social and medical understanding of old age; but it remains largely confined to studies of the maladies which come with age.

CONTRIBUTION TO THE PATHOLOGY MODEL

The history of British research into old age over the past 100 years tends — as do contemporary studies — to be linked to the resolution of problems connected with the rising proportion of elderly people in the population and their absolute numbers. In 1881 people over the current retirement ages in England and Wales (65 for men and 60 for women) formed little more than 5% of the population. By the turn of the century it had risen to more than 6%. At the last published census in 1981 it had advanced strikingly to 17%, with the greatest expansion taking place in the 75 plus age groups.* A century ago, the great concerns brought to public attention by the growing school of social surveying reformers were with poverty, illnesses and institutional care of the aged. These culminated in the report of the Royal Commission on the Poor Law (1905–09), which laid down a blueprint for the welfare state, and more immediately led to the introduction of old age pensions.

During the next half century the interests put so firmly on the political agenda by the researches of Charles Booth (1902), Seebohm Rowntree (1901), Beatrice Webb (1926) and Bowley and Burnett Hurst (1912) remained fixed. As founders of the social survey method, they each contributed powerfully effective descriptions of the nature and extent of poverty, ill health and social breakdown. Their detailed statistical accounts provided evidence of a kind which circumscribed the everyday conditions of the artisan classes, including older people. Between them these pioneers had uncovered areas of ignorance so vast and forms of need so fundamental that few of their successors reached out beyond the territory they had defined. As a result, it became a commonplace that old age

for those from all but the most privileged classes was characterized by physical illness, poor nutrition, inadequate housing and fear of the pauper's death. Thus, whilst important basic scientific research proceeded slowly on the biological bases of ageing, the greatest efforts of medical research were to do with ill health both physical and mental. (Handbooks which attempt to provide syntheses of existing work tend to be a sound guide to the pattern and distribution of existing research. In gerontology, such a series of handbooks was published under the general editorship of James Birren (Binstock & Shanas 1976, Birren & Schaie 1977, Finch & Hayflick 1977). In 1981 a new series edited by Carl Eisdorfer, *Annual Review of Gerontology and Geriatrics*, appeared. The foci of attention remain in the clinical management and pathologies of later life; and the same is true of the leading *Journal of Gerontology*.)

This small but consistently growing body of knowledge provided a basis for Sheldon (1948) to complete his important study of old people in Wolverhampton early after the Second World War. In the resulting book he was able to provide a taxonomy of the sicknesses which were attributed to old age and to suggest ways in which these could be medically managed. Significantly, the studies which followed have been developments of specialist areas of his broad-ranging studies. Incontinence, falls, strokes, dementia, confusion and depression remain high in the profile of medical research.

Social scientists in Britain have always been fewer in number in the gerontological field, despite their work having had enormous impact both on the public consciousness and politically. They too have been preoccupied with the causes and consequences of poorer physical health and social deprivations which appear to follow retirement from work. After the major policy reforming studies at the turn of the century there was a lull in activity. The interwar years produced a very modest literature about the effects of retirement, but it has failed to leave any permanent mark.

The resurgence of interest in social welfare provision occasioned by the Second World War and the wartime planning for a welfare state served to refocus attention on old age. Beveridge's pension plan revived the debates of the first decade of the century about the quality of life after retirement (Macintyre 1977). Income, health and housing resumed their position at the head of the agenda — an agenda which has survived almost intact to the present day. But as empirical studies of life circumstances of old people began, they soon developed specialist orientations (Cole 1962, Townsend 1962, Brockington & Lempert 1966, Tunstall 1966). Apart from Peter Townsend's *The Family Life of Old People* (1957) there have been few notable studies which look at the subject in the round. In particular, research of a social and medical kind alike gave pride of place to studies of 'need'. As a result the enormous output of research which has been produced since the early 1950s has provided a highly detailed account of the structural characteristics of the retired population, the illnesses which are likely to afflict them, the sources of their income, the quality of their housing, their occupancy of hospital beds and consumption of general practitioner (family doctor) services, their need for social support services at home, the changes in family support which have necessitated increased public provision and the quality of institutional care. More recent work has turned to the effectiveness of social policy provision to meet the needs of elderly people, particularly as the rising (and ageing) of this sector of the population became apparent. Studies of geriatric care, old people's Homes and the whole range of domiciliary services, both statutory and voluntary, became increasingly common.

The pathology model of ageing can, of course, be extended too far, for studies within what is here called 'normal ageing' do exist. Psychologists, although equally afflicted by the desire to depict old age as a deviance from the arbitrary norms of early adulthood, have nonetheless done much to identify the general characteristics of retired populations. Yet until very recently their explanations of normal cognitive functioning, personality integration, memory retention and learning skills have served to reinforce the image of old age as a period of chronic decline. These studies have formed the mainstream of 'human growth and development' studies which map the whole life as a series of age related stages. Until the upsurge of 'lifespan' stud-

ies in the United States, influenced by the work of Goulet and Baltes (1970), Nesselroade and Reese (1973) and Baltes and Schaie (1973), the last stages of any publication or taught course on human development presented a picture of expected (and therefore normal) decline on all major parameters. Only in the past few years has this orthodoxy been firmly challenged, drawing strength from a close scrutiny of prior assumptions and inappropriate methodologies (Taub 1980). Thus, for example, it is now claimed that the view of decrements in memory function with age are in some measure due to the inappropriate nature of the tests (coming as they do from an earlier culture, old people find them meaningless) and the failure to recognize that as people grow into middle age and beyond they sift information more carefully and store only the essential, rather than whole chunks of undigested material (Labouvie-Vief 1982).

LIFE-HISTORY APPROACHES

Equally, there are shifts of interest to be observed across the social sciences. As the editor of an international and multidisciplinary journal, *Ageing and Society*, I receive and read over 100 articles a year, submitted for publication. The bulk remain in the mould outlined, but increasingly there is an awareness of the need to theorize, to examine the political economy of old age and to view old age as a particular product of a life lived (Taylor & Ford 1981, Townsend 1981, Walker 1981, Estes 1982).

It would be possible to further document and classify the output of age related research, but this would be as lengthy as it is unnecessary. Convincing evidence of the pathology orientation of studies in old age can be readily found in the series of annual publications produced by the Centre for Policy on Ageing (formerly National Corporation for the Care of Old People), entitled *Old Age: A Register of Social Research*. This annual compendium contains details of all the serious work being undertaken in the field. Each year an analysis is produced of the main subject areas and the percentage of projects under each heading. The volume for 1979/80 identified 165 studies under 40 headings. Of the headings themselves, only three could be said to be of a non–problem-centred kind; these contributed 8% to the total. Typical headings are labelled: rehabilitation, sheltered housing, information needs, mental disorder, residential care, etc.

Too much emphasis on these features of the body of research on ageing could lead to a misunderstanding of the purpose of drawing attention to them. There is no implication that this work is in any important sense bad, only that it is providing us with a distorted picture of later life which lacks congruence with my own studies and experience of work with older people. It has led both policy makers and the world at large to see old age as synonymous with sickness, poverty and mental decrepitude. The fact that these conditions do occur amongst the older members of our society is neither to be denied nor ignored. What is important, however, and a central proposition of this chapter, is to recognize that much of what professional observers and helpers see as pathological and problematic is not seen in that way by older people themselves.

For some years now I have been involved in both theoretical writing and empirical studies of social ageing, as well as in social policy issues in old age. Throughout this period I have been anxious to encourage researchers and analysts to take more account of how elderly people see and value their own lives, in particular in the context of their life-histories. In other places I have written at length about the relationship between life experience and the experience of old age. Inevitably, former lifestyle and practices are powerful and formative factors, not only in the material conditions of life in retirement, but also in the way it is perceived and interpreted. All too little account is taken of these factors in determining what society will do for its older members. Indeed I frequently use a metaphor which compares the social and medical pathologists with spectators in the arena at the end of a marathon race who see the runners enter for the last lap tired and bruised. They see their task as attending to relieving the weariness and the pain of the runners without ever asking how the race was run or what plans they may have for further racing.

THE IMPORTANCE OF BIOGRAPHY*

To suggest that by collecting biographical accounts of people's lives we will see a more dynamic and authentic picture is not to say that it solves all problems or that it has no drawbacks. Among the drawbacks are the ways researchers deal with personal stories and explanations of events which may be subject to poor recall, partial interpretation and internal contradiction. Such accounts are said not to be 'objective' or 'scientific'. But biographical studies of ageing do not take every statement from the teller as factually true. The student of biographies is concerned with the *meaning* of social events as seen through the eye of the self-observer. Like all observers, his or her view will be selective and subject to interpretation. This is obvious from any biography or autobiography you may read. But this very selection tells us much about the way individuals see themselves. In the case of older people it is possible to see the present as a product of the past even when interpretations they might put on particular events are suspect or facts are open to correction. For what emerges is a distillation of their view of themselves and what has happened to them, which has survived through life and will provide the basis for the future. It is the basis of their self-esteem and self-image.

Robert Butler (1963), whose book on old age in America won a Pulitzer Prize, has written of the significance of what he calls the life review. He argues that reminiscence is an integral part of human psychological health and an aspect which increases with age (and the amount of life to review). We have a constant need to reconstruct our self-images and personal histories in the light of recent and current happenings. Thus personal biographies are possessions which we all have and which we tend to keep in good repair, incorporating new material all the time. They provide the framework for so much decision making. This is

---

*Parts of this section are taken from Johnson (1979).

evident in the way people — especially older people — tell and retell stories about those parts of their lives which, in retrospect, were most important to them. For my own father, the Second World War and his six years as a gunner in Britain and Europe undoubtedly provided a high spot. The events and relationships of that period had a profound effect on his life.

Those who 'take' biographies from others always have a theme or themes which they want to pursue. As Stimson (1976) in explaining his biographical approach to drug users said:

The successful in this world provide us with suitable biographical accounts of their success. For some the success is explained as personal endeavour in a free society, for example the rags to riches career of a working-class boy who makes it to company director. For others, especially women, personal beauty is the way out of the slum. Yet other biographies show the early development of talent — the pop star whose parents always knew he would be successful by the way he handled his toy guitar as a child. (Stimson 1976, p. 1)

By taking a particular dimension of life such as work, sport, love life, etc., it is always essential to examine the developments (or career) of the chosen theme and the way in which it interacts with other continuing careers like marriage, relations with children and involvements in other major activities. A person's biography can be seen as the product of a number of separate but related careers moving along side by side and influencing each other, sometimes minimally, sometimes dramatically. The path — or career — of their health is an important influence on everyone's life.

It is in the very process of unfolding a biography that relationships can be most fruitfully observed. For there you see the whole and continuing nature of, say, the marital relationship or the employer/employee relationship. It is the history which gives meaning to the major events which may not otherwise come to notice. In the setting of later life such histories are vitally important. They provide the explanations which are needed when crises occur and professionals are deciding the future.

If the argument so far has been clear, it will be apparent that by seeing relations and relationships as continuing processes within personal histories,

we can see both the satisfactory and the problematic features of old age more clearly. Much of the literature in geriatrics, nursing, social work and other caring professions dealing with older people concerns itself with externally defined pathology. For example, the presence of severe chronic bronchitis, or persistent post-bereavement depression leading to self-neglect, can be seen as objectively observed states which require professional intervention. These crises are often 'life events' which may be misunderstood and misinterpreted if the processes which preceded them are not examined.

Robert Butler, who uses the biographical approach as a method in psychiatry, writes:

I have used the concept of the life review in my psychotherapeutic work with older persons. Life review therapy includes the taking of an extensive autobiography from the older person. . . . Use of family albums, scrapbooks and other memorabilia . . . evoke crucial memories, responses and understanding in patients. . . . Such life-review therapy can be conducted in a variety of settings from senior centers to nursing homes. Even relatively untrained persons can function as therapists by becoming "listeners" as older people recount their lives. (Butler 1975, p. 413)

Clearly, a great depth of understanding is not always required. But when a serious situation is perceived by the helper which might lead to radical changes in lifestyle for the older person (e.g. hospitalization or transfer to an old people's Home), then biographical knowledge becomes important. If helping means assisting others to achieve their own objectives (insofar as circumstances allow) then these objectives need to be uncovered. Unfortunately, they rarely lie on the surface and are often not articulated in response to direct questions of the 'Tell me what you want . . .' sort. My own experience is that the interviewer should be clear about the objectives of the interview and to be armed with key questions which will stimulate the right sort of reminiscence. Roy Fairchild (1977) talks about these questions as 'openers' and 'hookers'.

As Maggie Kuhn, the leader of the American Gray Panthers movement, says:

Old people ought to have a sense of history. They must be encouraged to review their own history, valuing their origins and past experiences. If we could stimulate life review, we could see what we have lived through and the ways in which we have coped and survived. (Hessel 1977, p. 30)

Just as many younger people are unclear about where they are going and what they want from life, so too are some older people. But experience of life-history interviewing shows that the process of exploration draws attention to the important features of that life and almost automatically raises questions about how those lost elements might be reconstructed (however imperfectly) in the changed circumstances of later life. For example, for many retired women who had no paid employment, the most satisfying part of their lives was when their children were at home. It may be that no acceptable substitute is available to meet that latent need, but if we were more concerned with meeting individual needs than dispensing the resources we have available (home helps, meals-on-wheels, old people's clubs, etc.) more solutions might emerge, like the fostering schemes whereby a family takes in an older person for a short time and provides a substitute and sympathetic family life.

Whilst manuals and textbooks are readily available to explain the taking of a medical history, diagnostic interviews or casework methods, there are few guides to biographical interviews. The ground rules are simple to understand though less easy to carry out. First, establish a clear interest in the interviewee for his or her own sake. Second, approach the interview without introducing the subject of the person's 'problem'. Third, express a real interest in her life and what she sees as its major themes and events. By listening hard and talking only as much as is needed to move the story on, the account will unfold and the 'problem' will fuse into a context which will give it meaning and possibly suggest some solutions. Paul Thompson's excellent book *The Voice of the Past* (1978) provides a helpful interview guide. Ken Plummer has provided a detailed manual in his *Documents of Life* (1983). At a simpler level Help the Aged's *Recall* (1981) pack is also valuable.

It is no longer necessary to defend the biographical approach as a technique. Its roots can be found, as Rosenmayr (1981) has reminded us, in the European tradition of sociology exemplified in such classic studies as *The Polish Peasant* (Thomas & Znaniecki 1927). In the literature of psychology, the study of the processes of life development goes back to Freud and Jung, taking a specific biographical form in the work of Erikson (1950). More recently, the biographical approach has been given impressive application in studies of middle age by Neugarten (1968) and Valliant (1977), amongst others. At the same time there has been increasing sociological attention to life-histories, particularly in relation to ageing and old age. In America, retrospective accounts in Glen Elder's (1974) *Children of the Great Depression* and in *Aging and the Life Course*, edited by Tamara Hareven (1981) are testimony to the confident and increasingly sophisticated analysis of whole or partial biographies. In France, Anne-Marie Guillemard's (1972) study of retirement has been followed by others in this form, amongst them Gaullier's (1982) researches on the redundancy experience of men in their fifties. The most widely read life-history studies of recent years have been Dan Levinson's (1978) *The Season of a Man's Life* and the linked volume of more dramatically depicted accounts, Gail Sheehy's (1974) best selling book *Passages*. Their success has served to legitimize an approach which has had to struggle for respectability, despite its long and honourable history. This may explain the dearth of such studies in Britain, where the prevailing views about suitable methodologies for the study of ageing processes have favoured more structured survey-based approaches.

COHORTS, GENERATIONS AND HISTORY

The essential argument for viewing ageing throughout the lifespan as a continuous and ever-changing process which takes different forms in each successive cohort, has already been made. But before going on to look at the practical issues which arise out of these shifting patterns we must give some attention to conceptual tools and the ways they are to be applied.

The notion of 'generation' as a description of biological and lineage relationships goes back into ancient history. It provides much of the organizing framework of Jewish history as recorded in the Old Testament and was an equally well-developed set of relationships in classical Greece. It served then as a system of age-grading which made possible the allocation of roles, relationships, economic tasks and patterns of authority. In modern Western societies the temporal aspects of generational differences have come to the fore. Social organization no longer rests on lineage, nor does it indicate any universal attribute of authority or status. Indeed, as we have already observed, the longer-lived generations are more likely to find themselves suffering from status deprivation than from celebration of their seniority. Within studies of ageing it has been common to avoid the wider applications of the term 'generation' and to confine attention to the social membership category which is formed by the different layers of family formation. In its looser usage, 'generation' can mean a group of individuals who share a common experience, such as 'the Second World War generation' or the group described by Glen Elder as the 'Children of the Great Depression'. The pioneering work of Leonard Cain (1967) used the term in this way. In writing of 'the new generation of elderly people' he was referring to a demographic cohort rather than a sociobiological category. To avoid confusion, and because it appears to be a more valuable device, attention here will be confined to age cohorts.

A cohort is constituted by the coincidence of the birth of its members within a specified time period. This is not to say that a cohort is merely an age group in the manner commonly adopted when presenting population based data in tabular form. The routine analysis of data by dividing subjects into 5 or 10 year age groups is one of the principal practical reasons why we have neglected the historical dimension in social science and medical empirical research. It leads to the comparison of arbitrary age segments in a way which assumes that any differences are attributable to age. It is the unconsidered use of that practice which leads to the age labelling this chapter is attempting to challenge.

What constitutes the organizing experience of a cohort which will allow its proper segregation (for analytical purposes) from the rest of a given population is a matter of historical judgment. It is a judgment which acknowledges the unifying influence of social structure on the experience of individuals. There is no opportunity here to elaborate the long-standing debate about the duality of ego and community in the lives of individuals which has consumed social scientists for many decades. Readers are referred to an excellent summary by Philip Abrams (1982), who also provides in his volume *Historical Sociology* a most coherent argument for the combining of historical and sociological analysis.

Abrams' concern is with the refinement of the notion of a 'sociological generation', but his argument is one which can equally serve the more specific subset — the cohort. He draws attention to the way in which human history, or what is sometimes called the tide of events, acts as a powerful force in shaping people's lives. These forces are part of the 'structure' within which lives are lived. They are capable of creating such a distinctive set of common experiences (as in wartime) that those who have shared in them are bound together in their thinking and their actions, by the events they shared. According to this approach, a sociological generation could include people drawn from a variety of age groups, and for this reason I choose to confine attention to age-based cohorts for use in relation to old age.

In considering the parameters of a cohort, it is essential to consider the pervading influences in the lives of those encompassed. Jane Synge (1981), in her study of Canadian family patterns of people born in the last decade of the nineteenth century and in the early part of the twentieth century, lays particular stress on the need to integrate personal and historical factors in family life for a group born in a specific and transitional historical phase. She continues:

In addition, data from these sources may also indicate whether characteristics that we currently associate with ageing may stem in part from the specific features of the early life experience of people now in their seventies and eighties.

Similarly, Martin Kohli et al (1983), in reporting a study of flexible retirement in Germany, observed how the arrangement of life experiences into age stages imposed severe limitations on people who were forced to take early retirement.

Historically, not only the chronological age at which the socially structured transitions in the life-course occur has changed, but the character of the temporal organisation itself.

He goes on to identify factors relevant to his sample of early retirees, which include

the development of an age-graded school system, of other age-graded systems of public rights and duties, the transformation from a demographic pattern of random experience to a pattern of predictable lifespan and the narrowing of the age for the "normative" events of the family cycle and work career.

Thus, in examining those who now fall into the groups called old, it is increasingly necessary to find demarcations of historical identity. My own markers in this process include the commencement of the First World War, the points at which universal education was extended, and — in relation to health and social welfare — the extent of adult working life completed before the full introduction of the welfare state in Britain (Phillipson 1982).

HEALTH, RETIREMENT AND WORK

In looking at those who are currently old, it is important not to treat the whole age span (say from 65 to 105) as forming a single group. Even more to the point, we should not presume that each new group of elders will be like the last. New cohorts bring new experiences, strengths and expectations.

In a book about her views on ageing, Maggie Kuhn (Hessel 1977), quotes a section from Alex Comfort's (1977) volume *A Good Age*, which summarizes the position well:

Unless we are old already, the next 'old people' will be us. Whether we go along with the treatment meted out to those who are now old depends on how far society can sell us the bill of goods it sold them — and it depends more upon that than upon any research. No pill or regimen known, or likely, could transform the latter years of life as fully as could a change in our vision of age and a militancy in attaining that change. (Comfort 1977, p. 13–14)

Attention on 'the active elderly' usually focuses on the retention of physical and psychological fitness to lead a life in much the same way as younger people. It implies being ambulant, capable of walking distances, carrying purchases, negotiating busy roads and coping with public transport; essentially the retention of functional capacities in dealing with what are known as activities of daily living. Clearly this is one of the interpretations which must be taken into account, for the decline in physical health and strength is a seriously limiting factor of older people. But the severe onset of these conditions is being kept at bay until later in the lifespan, and this, combined with a less hostile environment, could release a more creative phase during retirement.

So, in addition to functional health, we need to examine two other forms of increased activity which coincide with and are stimulated by a greater healthiness. The first might be termed 'corporate consciousness and action', the second the 'recolonization of eldership'.

Functional health in old age, it is well established, is highly correlated with previous lifestyle and status. Shanas and Maddox sum it up neatly when they say:

In general the lower the socioeconomic position of an individual, the higher the prevalence of disease and the higher the age-specific death rate. These commonly observed associations between socioeconomic position, illness and life expectancy have a complex explanation. Indices of socioeconomic position usually include measurements of income, occupation and education. Such factors, singly or in combination, are reflected in different styles of life and differential access to, and use of, health resources. For instance, low income, a manual occupation and minimal education generally predict a high incidence of disease and elevated death rates in all industrialised countries. (Shanas & Maddox 1976, p. 602)

The implication of these relationships is that middle-class people are more likely to survive into old age, whereas artisans whose work has been particularly arduous or dangerous to health die at earlier ages. In general this picture is supported by official data on mortality, resulting in a situation whereby those who do survive into retirement can expect to live to age 80 and beyond. Population projections indicate that, from 1986 until the end of the century, those aged 85 years and over will increase in numbers constantly and dramatically to 60% above the 1986 level. The consequences of more people living a full lifespan are mixed. They are expected to remain independent and living in the community for longer but in doing so will suffer the accumulated affects of chronic disease.

The detail of age-related health status is not an essential part of this chapter, but it has been necessary to lay the ground for our understanding of the extended period of physical and psychological well-being, sufficient to allow adequate social functioning. It can be simply but graphically illustrated by pointing to the rising average age of admission to old people's Homes. Ten years ago average admission age was in the lower seventies, with places being given on occasions to people still in their sixties. Now it is difficult for elderly people to gain admission to an old people's Home before their eightieth birthday.

As this group of 'old old' consolidates its position, changes in the social structure of the retired population as a whole will be taking place. There will be more people within it, at all ages, whose socioeconomic position is higher than that of previous cohorts, reflecting improvements in working conditions and the *embourgeoisement* (the growth of the middle classes) of mid-twentieth century Britain, with its better nutrition, housing and education. In sum, there will be more older people throughout the age ranges who have health sufficient to allow for full and active participation in society. These new cohorts will have experienced relative prosperity, support of the welfare state and the rise of consumerism. A new and more aggressive climate of expectation can be anticipated to replace the polite acquiescence and minimal expectations to which researchers and practitioners are currently accustomed. Cohort changes provide the key to many of the likely developments in the future. Life experience for groups of people of the same age group inevitably conditions their expectations and their responses to social and economic circumstances. Those who are currently over 70 years of age in Britain were mostly born in an Edwardian era which marked the end of Britain's dominance of world trade, an era which led directly to the First World War. The interwar

depression followed, being terminated by the 1939–45 war, which in turn brought several years of continuing hardship. Only in the 1950s, when this group of people were already moving towards the end of their working (employment) life, did prosperity of a pervasive kind emerge. This historical phase has therefore been one of privation followed by relative plenty, creating amongst those who are now old an understandable sense of comparative well-being.

Again drawing on my own life-history studies (Johnson 1982a) it is clear that relative deprivation is the linchpin of satisfaction or dissatisfaction in later life. For this generation, reference groups are principally themselves in the past and their own parents in retirement. Any objective assessment of living standards would give support to the view that Mark Abrams (1980) discovered, namely that the current cohort is comparatively well off and perceives itself as such. Yet for those who saw the welfare state constructed during their mid-life or earlier and particularly those who were young in the immediate post-war period, the comparison will have an increasingly negative effect. Current expectations of income in retirement are having to be radically revised, whilst projections about the costs of future financial support for the retired give little cause for optimism.

Frustration and unmet expectations may breed political reaction. In most of Europe there is a long way to go, but during the period under consideration here, the strong likelihood is that successive cohorts will not only be more highly motivated to take action, but their higher skills will facilitate an organized lobby of a kind as yet unknown in Britain. Their demand for opportunities to carry out work in its various forms is likely to become more insistent.

CORPORATE CONSCIOUSNESS AND ACTION*

Corporate consciousness and action can reasonably be predicted, then, as the response of the increas-

---

*The ideas in this section and the next were first reported in Johnson (1982b).

ingly articulate and socially skilful retired population. It will be a group which is less poor overall than its predecessors, as occupational pensions and home ownership supplement state support. Like its American counterpart it is likely to seek a better deal for retired people in everyday transactions where prejudice and commercial practice limit their opportunities. There are no immediate signs of a common consciousness emerging amongst older people in Britain. Certainly no political allegiance is observable yet. But there are signs of an increasing commercial recognition of retired people as a worthwhile market, especially in transport, holidays, domestic equipment and personal services. Banks, building societies, insurance companies, employers and the trade unions continue to exercise unremittingly ageist discrimination against retired people in a manner which may not be tolerated for much longer.

The American experience of increasing consciousness by elderly people of their common position arose out of their desire to challenge commercial interests and later to act as lobbyists in influencing government policy at state and federal level. Perhaps inevitably, those who became involved in organized activity to secure better treatment from those offering goods and services in the market-place were what Pratt (1976) in his book *The Gray Lobby* calls the 'slightly privileged'. In first pursuing preferential treatment amongst traders of all kinds, and then in the 1960s focusing more clearly on political influence, a number of influential national groups emerged. The largest and most durable of them are: The American Association of Retired Persons (AARP) and the National Retired Teachers Association (NRTA), which function in national affairs as one body; The National Council of Senior Citizens (NCSC), which was set up in the 1960s to campaign for Medicare, and then extended its interests, has a less middle-class membership than AARP; more cross-sectional in their membership and more campaigning in their approach than either of these are the Gray Panthers.

Together these mass-membership organizations (their combined membership is counted in millions) are able to act as foci for political reform within the United States and to influence state and federal policy directly. In recent years the US Senate passed legislation raising the compulsory retirement age for public employees to 70 years. Such a development is currently inconceivable in Britain because elderly people are not organized, nor do they appear to wish to be organized on their own behalf. But relative deprivation has proved to be the most powerful force for dissatisfaction in later life. It is likely to increase dramatically as those who expected a long and comfortable retirement find themselves in straitened circumstances because of inflation; also, governments may want to execute a backlash against retired people in favour of employed and unemployed younger people. Should these speculations come to pass, they could be the triggers for mass-membership organizations on the American model. If they do arise, these groups will undoubtedly seek re-entry into all the corners of social and economic life, to establish a respected place for old age.

RECOLONIZATION OF ELDERSHIP

Recolonization of eldership is an expression of this desire to re-enter the social world on equal or even positively discriminated terms. The phrase adopted here is not meant to denote the return to another golden age but takes eldership to mean recognition of and due respect for experience. At its core this 'recolonization' is about self-respect and mutual respect across generations. It requires society to make a more generous place for old age; but one which also allows greater opportunity for intergenerational support and cross-generational exchange.

In his study of early retirement in France, Xavier Gaullier (1982) depicts the post-war period of policy on old age as having gone through three phases. The first period he saw as the transformation of old age into retirement. The second, in the 1960s, was characterized by the transformation of old age into the third age (a period of leisure, autonomy and self-realization). In the latest stage, dating in France from about 1976, he sees the policy for old age as having become a policy on unemployment. Rising unemployment has brought about earlier and earlier enforced retirement (down to age 50 years in some parts of the country). Gaullier writes:

An individual is declared 'old' by authorities responsible for employment and rejected definitively from the job market uniquely on account of his age, regardless of his state of health, his biological or psychological ageing. . . . There is no longer a promotion of a way of life but rather the payment of allowances to the unemployed. . . . For a long time old-age policy favoured the social insertion of the elderly, the new policy brutally excludes them from social life. (Gaullier 1982)

These observations have a familiar ring not only in the British context, but in almost all the countries in Europe and North America, where economic recession has led uniformly to early retirement and redundancy, coupled with a reduction of services and monetary benefits. In this account the author attributes the crisis in old-age policy to weaknesses in the capitalist structure as well as to the political allegiance of governments to the 'working population'. Certainly, structural factors are pre-eminent in the situation. The restitution of France's third age conception is not likely to be achieved by individual effort. Yet to urge a return to conceptions of society which provide open access for older people to all its major arenas is simply to restate a tenet of human rights.

Within the reconstructed forms of eldership, there will need to be provision for a great diversity of lifestyles. Thus the most important reforming function to be performed would be the systematic removal of constraints on personal decision making. So the agenda might well include the removal of paternalistic practices amongst health and social welfare practitioners, housing managers and so on, who presently take significant decisions for older people with little or no real consultation. It is, then, a restoration of the civil rights which have become so eroded, as Alison Norman (1980) has reminded us. Her discussion on the balance between rights and risk is referred to in some detail in Chapter 32.

AN AGEIST MODERN WORLD

A picture has been created in this chapter of old age which is viewed as an illness and regarded as unproductive. Whilst attention has been drawn to many positive aspects of later life, the prevalent image in developed societies is one of bodily decline and reduced ability to be socially useful. Associated with these beliefs goes an attitude of mind which demeans elderly people. In many respects it resembles the negative stereotyping of women and of black people which we now know as sexism and racism. Ageism is an equivalent term.

Whilst it would be foolish to pretend that growing old is a period of endless vitality and growing excitement, it is important to draw to the fore the neglected positive features of old age. The whole truth about it is not to be found in the pathology models of the professionals or of the traditional researchers. A more balanced view will recognize that the later stage of life will be very different for people with different social statuses and personal experiences. It will incorporate a respect for individual life-histories and their formative influence on the character of old age. At the same time it will acknowledge the way society can minimize or extend the opportunities and satisfactions of being an elder. Even the language it uses about those who are old will be more thoughtful — less ageist. Perhaps we should begin by abandoning the word 'geriatrics' as a term to describe people and retain it for its only proper use: as a title for the practice of medicine on older people.

REFERENCES

Abrams M 1980 Beyond three score years and ten. Age Concern, Mitcham
Abrams P 1982 Historical sociology. Open Books, Shepton Mallet, Somerset
Age Concern 1976 Profiles of the elderly, Vols 1–8. Age Concern, Mitcham
Baltes P B, Shaie W (eds) 1973 Life-span developmental psychology: personality and socialization. Academic Press, New York

Birren J E, Schaie K W (eds) 1977 Handbook of the psychology of aging. Van Nostrand Reinhold, New York

Booth C 1902 Life and labour of the people of London. Macmillan, London

Bowley A L, Burnett Hurst A R 1912 Livelihood and poverty. London

Brockington F, Lempert S M 1966 The social needs of the over eighties. Manchester University Press

Brown E 1982 Older Americans' use of health maintenance organisations. Research on Aging 4 (June): 2

Butler R N 1963 The Life review: An interpretation of reminiscence in old age. Psychiatry 26: 1

Butler R N 1975 Why survive? Being old in America. Harper and Row, New York

Cain L D 1964 Life course and social structure. In: Faris R E L (ed) Handbook of modern sociology. Rand McNally, Chicago

Cain L D 1967 Age status and generational phenomena: the new old people in contemporary America. Gerontologist 7

Cole D 1962 The economic circumstances of old people. Occasional Papers on Social Administration. Bell, London

Comfort A 1977 A good age. Mitchell Beazley, London

Eisdorfer C (ed) 1981 Annual review of gerontology and geriatrics. Springer, New York

Elder G 1974 Children of the Great Depression. University of Chicago Press, Chicago

Erikson E 1950 Childhood and society. Norton, New York

Estes C 1982 Dominant and competing paradigms in gerontology. Ageing and Society 2 (July): 2

Fairchild R 1977 Life story conversations: diversions in a ministry of evangelistic calling. United Presbyterian Program Area on Evangelism, New York

Finch C D, Hayflick L (eds) 1977 Handbook of the biology of aging. Van Nostrand Reinhold, New York

Fries J F, Crapo L M 1981 Vitality and aging: implications of the rectangular curve. W H Freeman, San Francisco

Gaullier X 1982 Economic crisis and old age — old age policies in France. Ageing and Society 2 (July): 2

Goulet L R, Baltes P B (eds) 1970 Life-span developmental psychology: research and theory. Academic Press, New York

Guillemard A M 1972 La retraite — une mort sociale. Mouton la Haye, Paris

Hareven T K (ed) 1981 Aging and the life course. Guildford Press, New York

Haug M 1979 Doctors and older patients. Journal of Gerontology 34 (November): 6

Help the Aged 1981 Recall: a reminiscence guide. Help the Aged, London

Hessel D (ed) 1977 Maggie Kuhn on ageing. Westminster Press, Philadelphia

Johnson M L 1976 That was your life: A biographical approach to later life. In: Munnichs J M A, van den Heuval W J A (eds) Dependency and interdependency in old age. Martinus Nijhoff, The Hague

Johnson M L 1979 An ageing population: relations and relationships. Open University Press, Milton Keynes

Johnson M L 1982a The implications of greater activity in later life. In: Fogarty M (ed) Retirement policy, the next fifty years. Heinemann, London

Johnson M L 1982b Ageing, needs and nutrition — a study

of voluntary and statutory collaboration in community care for elderly people. Policy Studies Institute, London

Kohli M et al 1983 The social construction of ageing through work. Ageing and Society 3 (March): 1

Labouvie-Vief G, Blanchard-Fields F 1982 Cognitive ageing and psychological growth. Ageing and Society 2 (July): 2

Levinson D 1978 The seasons of a man's life. Knopf, New York

Macintyre S 1977 Old age as a social problem, some notes on the British experience. In: Dingwall R, et al (eds) Health care and health knowledge. Croom Helm, London

Nesselroade J R, Reese H W (eds) 1973 Life-span developmental psychology: methodological issues. Academic Press, New York

Neugarten B (ed) 1968 Middle age and ageing: a reader. University of Chicago Press, Chicago

Norman A 1980 Rights and risk. Centre for Policy on Ageing, London

Office of the Population Censuses and Surveys 1979 Population projections 1977–2017. Series pp 2 No 9. HMSO, London

Phillipson C 1982 Capitalism and the construction of old age. Macmillan, London

Plummer K 1983 Documents of life. Allen and Unwin, London

Pratt H J 1976 The gray lobby. University of Chicago Press, Chicago

Report of the Royal Commission on the Poor Law (1905–9) 1909 HMSO, London

Rosenmayr L 1981 Age, lifespan and biography. Ageing and Society 1 (March): 1

Rowntree B S 1901 Poverty: A study of town life. Macmillan, London

Russell L B 1981 An ageing population and the use of medical care. Medical Care 19 (June): 6

Shanas E, Maddox G 1976 Aging health and the organisation of health resources. In: Binstock R H, Shanas E (eds) Handbook of aging and the social sciences. Van Nostrand Reinhold, New York

Sheehy G 1974 Passages: predictable crises of adult life. Dutton, New York

Sheldon J H 1948 Social medicine of old age. Oxford University Press, Oxford

Stimson G 1976 Biography and retrospection: some problems in the study of life histories. Unpublished paper presented to the British Sociological Association Annual Conference

Synge J 1981 Cohort analysis in the planning and interpretation of research using life histories. In: Bertaux D (ed) Biography and society. Sage, Beverley Hills

Taub H A 1980 Life-span education: A need for research with meaningful prose. Educational Gerontology 5

Taylor R, Ford G 1981 Lifestyle and ageing. Ageing and Society 1 (November): 3

Thomas W I, Znaniecki F 1927 The Polish peasant in Europe and America (2 vols). Over Publications, New York

Thompson P 1978 The voice of the past: oral history. Oxford University Press, Oxford

Townsend P 1957 The family life of old people. Routledge and Kegan Paul, London

Townsend P 1962 Last refuge. Routledge and Kegan Paul, London

Townsend P 1981 The structured dependency of the elderly. Ageing and Society 1 (March): 1

Tunstall J 1966 Old and alone. Routledge and Kegan Paul, London

Valliant G E 1977 Adaptation to life. Little Brown, Boston

Walker A 1981 Towards a political economy of old age. Ageing and Society 1 (March): 1

Webb B 1926 My apprenticeship. Longman Green, London

CHAPTER CONTENTS

Introduction 19
Fundamental questions 20

Change 20
Role change 20
Individual change 21
Summary of changes 30

Adjustment 30
Two models of adjustment 30
Adjustment as a lifelong process 31

Adjustment to change 33
Summary of adjustment 34

The health service context 34
Informal assessment of psychological
functioning 34
Formal assessment 35
Interdisciplinary working 35
Individuality 36

Conclusions 36

2

The psychology of human ageing

Sally E. Robbins

INTRODUCTION

Psychologists divide the human lifespan into stages which correspond roughly with chronology: babyhood and infancy, 0–2 years; childhood, 2–12 years; adolescence, 12–18 years; adulthood, 18–65 years; and old age, 65+ years. There is a strong tendency within developmental psychology to concentrate on the first two or three of these stages, breaking them down into tiny subsections and tracing minute changes in behaviour, whilst leaving the last two stages of adulthood and old age largely unexplored. Old age is regarded as starting at around 60 or 65. When we talk about ageing we are usually referring to a process which involves people in this age group. It is as though those of us who are under 65 are immune to the phenomenon of ageing. Alongside the lack of exploration of developmental stages in old age goes a tendency to make simple generalizations about 'the elderly', mostly of a gloomy and derogatory nature.

In recent years there has been some increase of interest in adult development. Levinson (1978) outlined the 'seasons of a man's life' from the novice phase in the early twenties through to the late adult transition in the early sixties, and Kubler-Ross (1975) outlines five stages of the dying process. However, to date we have no accepted way of dividing either adulthood or old age into developmental stages. A tentative classification for old age might include three stages: the young active group, 65–75 years; the older retired group; and the aged survivors, 85+ years. In this chapter, through drawing on information from a wider group, I shall be concentrating mainly on those aged between about 65 and 85 years, our information on the 'aged survivors' being at present quite sparse.

FUNDAMENTAL QUESTIONS

There are three fundamental points to be examined:

1. Change. What psychological changes do we see as part of the ageing process?
2. Adjustment. How do people adjust to the changes involved in ageing?
3. Context. How do questions of psychological change and adjustment relate to the Health Service context?

We will examine each of these questions in turn.

CHANGE

The question of changes which are related to the ageing process will be dealt with in two main sections, the first summarizing the role changes which accompany old age and the second looking at changes in psychological functioning of the individual person.

ROLE CHANGE
Life events

The attainment of old age by a large proportion of the population is a relatively recent phenomenon. The current elderly population are often the first in their family to face the life events of later life. Some of these events are simply by-products of living a long life, such as multiple bereavements; however, many others are dictated by contemporary cultural patterns. The attainment of 'retirement age', qualification for pensions and concessions, and, for many old people, changes in housing are examples of culturally determined role changes in Western industrialized countries in the late 20th century. Life events of this sort constitute stresses whatever the quality of the change

(Gunderson & Rahe 1974) and both bereavement and retirement are clearly linked to subsequent illness and death (Murray Parkes 1975). The impact of the life event of retirement is aptly illustrated by a quote from Adela Irskine's chapter in *The Challenge of a Long Life* (Pincus 1981).

It was as if the structure of my life had collapsed — almost like being hit by a physical blow . . . after the first fine careless rapture, the feeling: God! What have I done? (p. 143)

Effects of role changes

Western retirement encourages the shedding of responsibilities and the acceptance of a more dependent lifestyle. The lower social and economic status that ensues leads to a lowering of expectations of the elderly person and by the elderly person. The role changes of later life, together with individual and social adjustments to them, can easily act in a cyclical manner, with burdens removed and progressively less expected of old folk until their value as contributors to society is both restricted and weakened. The negative effects that no longer being needed have on elderly people are emphasized by Lily Pincus (1981) in her examination of the challenge of a long life.

It is generally assumed that the sociological and physical signs of decline of the elderly are paralleled by a psychological deterioration. This view is consistently reinforced by the media, and when individuals are thus induced to say 'my mind is not as sharp as it was' or 'it's too much for me to think about at my age' we usually find ourselves nodding tacit agreement, albeit sympathetically. To be old is to accept the role of the incompetent. We demonstrate this attitude whenever we unthinkingly help old folk without considering whether they actually want or need special care. Interestingly, self-reports of generalized memory impairment correlate experimentally with depression (Rabbitt 1988), and this is also a common finding in clinical practice.

The cultural stereotype

The cultural stereotype of old age in contemporary Britain commonly runs along these lines: great achievements occur relatively early in life, mostly in the teens, twenties and thirties, and the picture thereafter is one of steady decline. This belief is strongly implicated in the so-called 'mid-life crisis' experienced by people in their 40s and 50s. In old age we are expected to become either nice old ladies and charming old gentlemen, or awkward old biddies and dirty old men. The individual character is lost and devalued regardless of whether the positive or the negative stereotype is applied.

The cultural stereotype is not without factual support. Scientific advances have largely been made by young people. Marconi transmitted the first radio signals at 21 and Bell made the first telephone at the age of 29. Lehman (1953) looked at the achievements of great chemists in relation to chronological age and reported that their peak of productive output occurred between the ages of 30 and 34 years. Whatever the balance of evidence behind the expectation of decline and impairment in old age, the effect of the stereotype when internalized by elderly folk may well be that of a self-fulfilling prophecy. It is difficult to maintain motivation and concentration on psychological tasks when you and everyone else around you believes that all old people become mentally frail and demented, and so when someone asks you to do a test you do badly — just as everyone expected.

The experience of ageing

Current literature suggests that the actual experience of ageing can be quite different from the stereotype. Most adults feel younger than their chronological age anyway and this feeling increases with advancing age. Kastenbaum et al (1972) investigated the concepts of personal and interpersonal age with the help of 75 people aged between 20 and 69. They concluded that personal age, that is the age a person feels, is so distinct from chronological age that gross errors are likely to occur whenever the two are confused. This classification of 'ages' is supported by Barak (1987) who found, moreover, that in his sample of 500 women the discrepancy between their chronological and their ideal age gave a measure of self-esteem. Several recent descriptions of the process of ageing based on

self reports suggest that the long accepted image of merciful retirement matching encroaching feebleness of mind and body may be far from correct (Blythe 1979, Pincus 1981, Stott 1981). These authors emphasize in particular the great differences which exist between individual experiences of ageing. They suggest that enormous variability in the ageing process is inevitable considering the diversity of life experiences and personal circumstances among elderly people.

INDIVIDUAL CHANGE

This section will attempt a summary of the information currently available regarding the changes in individual psychology which occur with the ageing process. After outlining the experimental data in this area, the methodological questions which are raised by the data will be examined.

Experimental evidence

The research data on individual change during ageing are summarized under six headings — intelligence, learning and memory, problem solving, perception, sex differences and personality. (Table 2.1 summarizes the evidence). During these summaries the terms *cross-sectional* and *longitudinal* will often be used to describe experiments. A cross-sectional study involves taking measures from different groups of subjects at the same time. In a longitudinal study the same subjects are tested repeatedly over time.

Intelligence

Much of our basic information on intelligence and ageing comes from studies using the Wechsler Adult Intelligence Scale (WAIS). Wechsler (1944) reported the findings from his standardization of the WAIS as showing a peak in intellectual capacity in the mid to late twenties. The test was standardized on approximately 2000 men and women who ranged in age between 16 and over 75 years. A cross-sectional design was used. This result was similar to that found in the earlier standardization studies for the Wechsler–Bellevue scale in which the highest scoring group was the

Table 2.1 Summary of experimental evidence of change in cognitive abilities

Studies suggestive of cognitive decline with ageing	Studies suggestive of preservation of cognition with ageing
Wechsler (1944), Eisdorfer and Wilkie (1973)	Bayley and Oden (1955)*, Owens (1966)*, Savage et al (1973)* — Intelligence/General ability
Blum et al (1972)*— Speeded psychomotor tests	
Cunningham et al (1975) — Fluid intelligence	Terman and Oden (1959)*— Concept mastery
Gilbert (1941) — Learning and memory	Gilbert (1973),* Green (1969)*— Verbal ability
Monge and Hultsch (1971) — Paired associate memory	Schonfield and Robertson (1966), Rabbitt (1988) — Memory
Eisdorfer et al (1963) — Serial learning	Savage et al (1973)* — Verbal and perceptual motor learning
Canestrari (1966)— Learning verbal associates	Harwood and Naylor — Learning German (Huppert 1982)
Talland (1965) — Immediate memory under stress	
Craik (1968) — Supraspan memory	
Schonfield and Robertson (1966) — Free recall	
Young (1966), Heglin (1956) — Problem solving	Wetherick (1964), Smith (1967) — Problem solving
Bromley (1957) — Abstract thinking	
Goldfarb (1941) — Complex reaction time	
Rabbitt (1965, 1981) — Ignoring irrelevent information	

*Longitudinal studies

early twenties. It was thought by many that this intellectual peak paralleled the acquisition of biological maturity and that the subsequent decline in intellectual capacity mirrored the physical decline seen in later life. Following the standardization studies, the assumption of intellectual decline with age was built into the WAIS norms. Apart from its use in research work, the WAIS is by far the most popular test of intellectual ability in adults in clinical settings.

The WAIS is composed of two sets of subtests, one measuring verbal ability and one measuring performance, or spatial ability. The effects of age on test score were particularly marked in four of the five performance subtests of the WAIS: block design, object assembly, digit symbol and picture arrangement. These subtests are all timed. These findings led Wechsler to classify the subtests into two categories as far as ageing effects were concerned. One group, known as 'hold' tests, showed little difference between the young and old subjects whilst the other group, known as 'don't hold' tests, were more poorly done by older subjects. The two categories both contain two verbal and two performance subtests. The two groups could be used to calculate a 'deterioration quotient'. For this, scores on the 'hold' tests were compared with scores on the 'don't hold' tests and the relationship interpreted in relation to that expected in a person of that age.

The discovery that certain tests showed more age effects than others has led some to draw a parallel with the idea of fluid and crystallized intelligence. This conceptualization of intellectual ability is particularly linked with Cattell (1963). Fluid intelligence is thought to reflect a person's basic potential to acquire new ideas and adapt to new situations, and is thought to stem from qualities inherent in the central nervous system. By contrast, the term crystallized intelligence was used to denote learned intellectual skills based on cultural and environmental experience. It seems logical that tests which reflect accumulated experience might show little decrement with advanced age, and might even show an increasing score. The vocabulary subtest of the WAIS is often cited as a possible example of a test reflecting this crystallized intelligence. The tests which show more of an age effect might reflect a more ephemeral fluid ability which ebbs as ageing progresses. If fluid intelligence does indeed decline more rapidly than crystallized intelligence, one would expect correlations between measures of the two to be higher in young subjects than in old ones. Cunningham et al (1975) confirmed this in a cross-sectional comparison using the WAIS vocabulary subtest to measure crystallized intelligence and Raven's progressive matrices to measure fluid intelligence. So far, then, studies suggestive of some decline in intellect during ageing have been noted. Not all studies agree with this. In 1959 Terman and Oden reported on a follow-up study involving a large group of especially gifted people in their early forties. Their subjects consistently showed a higher score on the concept mastery test than when tested 12 years before. Bayley and Oden (1955) had also reported increasing levels of intellectual ability between the ages of 20 and 50. In another longitudinal study 96 men were tested using the army alpha test at the age of 50 and again 11 years later. There were no significant differences between scores at the different ages. On retesting 31 years after the original there was a pattern of increasing ability (Owens 1966). Blum et al (1972) tested people aged between 60 and 93. They reported that only a timed and speeded psychomotor test showed any decline up to the age of 74. After that age all their tests showed some slight average decrements, but the variance between subjects increased markedly and some people's scores improved with age. Savage et al (1973) studied a group of elderly people in Newcastle over a seven-year period. Many of those studied were over 75 years old. The group of primary interest here is those who lived in the community, of whom there were 190. Savage et al reported no change in the overall intelligence quotient (IQ). Performance IQ improved whilst verbal IQ declined a little, a pattern opposite to that reported by Wechsler. This study, however, cannot be seen as conclusive, and certainly extensive recent work by Rabbitt and his associates supports the idea that performance tends to decline whilst verbal abilities are preserved in old age (Rabbitt 1988). Many subjects died during the seven-year period. Those who lived to be tested throughout may comprise a special 'survivor' group. However, further longitudinal studies do give some support to these findings of limited decline. Both Gilbert (1973) and Green (1969) reported no decline in verbal abilities in advanced old age in selected groups. In a 10-year longitudinal study, Eisdorfer and Wilkie (1973) found a small statistically significant decline in abilities in their 60–70 years age group, and a slightly larger decline in the 70–80 years age group. Furthermore, they suggest that the changes are too tiny to be of any practical significance. Finally, Schaie and Strother (1968), using a mixed cross-sectional and longitudinal design, confirmed that purely cross-sectional data exaggerates age-related changes, except where speed is of prime importance. In conclusion then it seems that generalized intellectual decline is not a universal and inevitable part of growing old.

Learning and memory

In an early study Gilbert (1941) demonstrated a decline in performance with age on a variety of tasks of learning and memory. A large body of the experimental literature since that time would support this.

The decrement found by Gilbert was particularly noticeable in a paired associate task, when a series of paired stimuli are to be remembered. Later studies suggest that the time period between pairs was particularly important. Older people did badly when there was little time to produce an answer (Monge & Hultsch 1971). This also seems to be true of serial learning tasks, in which a series of individual items is presented for memorization (Eisdorfer et al 1963). There is some evidence that older people are more affected by established linguistic habits since they apparently find learning new associations for words of high associative strength particularly difficult (Canestrari 1966).

The term immediate memory refers to a memory mechanism which registers incoming information and keeps it for a few seconds. Immediate memory appears to be little affected by ageing according to the results of memory span experiments. Only under conditions of very high task difficulty, for instance when required both to respond in conditions of interference and to search and match incoming material with remembered items, does the immediate memory of elderly subjects appear less efficient than that of their juniors (Talland 1965).

When memory span is exceeded, that is when material is stored for more than a few seconds or when a great deal of material is presented, age effects are often found (Craik 1968). Much research in this area has concentrated on finding the locus of the age-related deficit, and it seems that in many instances the problem lies in the retrieval stage of memory. Schonfield and Robertson (1966) used a free recall task with five age groups from the twenties to sixties. Free recall means that subjects may remember material in any order once the information has been presented. There was a clear relationship between age and performance for the recall task, with the older subjects scoring poorly. However, when a recognition task was used, in which the correct answers were chosen from among distractors, the age factor had no effect.

As with the intelligence studies, not all the experimental evidence is indicative of age-related decline. A study of learning ability was included in Savage et al's (1973) longitudinal study in Newcastle. They used both a verbal and a perceptual motor test of learning and found no real evidence of declining ability. Rabbitt's cross-sectional studies of over 6000 people aged from 50 to 96 show very little memory change until the 70s at least. Thereafter he reports slight but progressive changes (Rabbitt 1988). Similarly, experiments which focus on ability to retain newly learned information suggest that there is little or no age effect, particularly if the material is fully learned initially. Huppert (1982) quotes an Australian study by Harwood and Naylor to illustrate the potential learning capacity of the old. After 80 people aged 63–91 were given weekly German lessons for three months, more than half passed an exam which schoolchildren normally attempt after three years' tuition. It is interesting to note that the elderly people themselves were amazed at their ability.

Problem solving

The expectation of poor problem-solving ability among old people is logical given that there are many tasks of this sort in intelligence tests, and of course much research suggests poorer intelligence test performance in old age. Young (1966) compared an 'old' 45–76 years age group with a 'young' 29–45 years age group on a complicated problem-solving task. The groups did not differ on intelligence, but the older group performed less well in problem solving. Conversely, Wetherick (1964) found that his most difficult problem-

solving task was best solved by older people. He also suggested that they gained most from test experience, in terms of improving from problem to problem. Subjects were matched in overall intelligence. Later experiments suggest that, as well as intelligence, memory factors and the degree of abstractness of the task used can affect problem-solving performance. It may be that some reported age effects are due to these factors rather than an overall age-related deficit in problem-solving ability per se. The evidence we have to date suggests that elderly people are best able to solve problems when the information given is both concrete and personally relevant. It seems that older people use concrete methods to solve problems more often than abstract principles (Bromley 1957). This may well be linked to educational experience. Elderly people are also reported to adhere to tried and trusted methods rather than use new and more efficient problem-solving methods. If a series of problems is given, all solvable by the same method, and then a problem which could be solved using a more simple method is interpolated, it is often found that the older subject is more likely to stick to the inefficient method than is the young subject (Heglin 1956). However, it seems once again that other factors are also important. Smith (1967) produced different results in a very similar experiment and concluded that factors other than age were probably influencing the results. She felt that level of intelligence was probably the most important influence.

Rabbitt (1977) set out to test whether elderly people truly had difficulty in changing their problem-solving method, or whether such findings related to more complex problems in integrating and organizing information. He found his data supported the latter hypothesis; his older subjects accumulated more redundant information and thus put a greater strain on their memory capacity and reduced their problem-solving efficiency.

Perception

The stereotype of perception in the aged person is one of dulled senses — Shakespeare's 'sans eyes . . . sans everything'. In this short summary we will examine this point with particular reference to speed of response and the effect of irrelevant information.

A wide variety of experimental studies have reported a slower reaction time in elderly subjects than in younger people. This is often explained as being due to perceptual deficits. In fact, experiments focusing on perceptual sensitivity show only a minimal loss between average young and old people (Birren & Botwinick 1955). The slight differences found in simple reaction time are disproportionately increased as the task becomes more complex (Goldfarb 1941). It seems that it is the decision process and the associative aspects of the task which make for the disproportionate effect (Birren & Botwinick 1955). Similarly, Salthouse (1985) considers that slowing of information processing may be the most general cognitive change shown by elderly people. Further investigation of this effect shows that the older person can react as quickly as the young in many instances but that when there is time to review the situation the old person tends to respond more slowly. Some of the slowness appears to be a behavioural preference rather than a deficit per se, and practice can often lead to major reductions in the discrepancy between the times recorded by old and young subjects. (Rabbitt 1980, 1982)

A tendency to be adversely affected by irrelevant information is reported to be a perceptual concomitant of old age (Rabbitt 1965, 1981a). Rabbitt shows that elderly people in general find it difficult to ignore irrelevant information, probably because they tend to process smaller 'chunks' of information at a time. He goes on to relate this to practical issues affecting old people, suggesting that they may find group conversations particularly difficult to follow and that they are disadvantaged in reading. Schonfield (1974) thinks there may be even greater practical effects. He suggests that roadside advertising may adversely effect the elderly car-driver, and that more effort should be made to shield old people from surplus information whenever a task requiring great concentration is in hand.

Sex differences

The differential survival rates of the sexes have been well documented and publicized, but it is more rare to find reliable reports of sex differences in psychological processes. For the purpose of this summary only a few specific examples of sex differences in ageing will be examined.

Britton and Britton (1972) reported that in women survival itself appeared related to personality characteristics. Women who were more involved, active and satisfied, lived longer than their less engaged colleagues. Personality and survival did not appear to be associated for men. Savage et al (1977) reported a variety of sex differences in personality in their Newcastle sample. The men scored more highly on 'ego strength', while the women were more tense, sensitive, insecure and overprotected. With regard to self-image, the women showed more conflict and contradiction between their basic identity, self-acceptance and behavioural functioning than did the men. Differential ageing patterns are suggested by a problem-solving experiment employing subjects of both sexes aged between 41 and 76 years (Young 1971). The younger subjects showed the customary pattern of males being superior to females on the task, but for subjects aged 60 or more, the pattern was reversed. Although this could be simply a reflection of the different generations involved the author speculated that the males showed more decline in ability with age than the females, and that this might be related to physiological changes, particularly in cerebral circulation.

Personality

Part of the popular stereotype of personality in old age is an expectation that the old will be self-opinionated, unwilling to change and possibly boring. Rabbitt (1981b and 1988) suggests that some of these 'personality traits' or their related 'social skills deficits' may in fact be adaptations to the secondary effects on cognition of deafness. As seen above in 'The cultural stereotype', grannies and grandpas are supposed to be benign and contented or irascible and depressed. To fit the culturally accepted mores one must lose drive and ambition with age and one's interest in sex must fade rapidly (see Chapter 16). In this section we will examine some studies of measurable personality characteristics and old age, both cross-sectional and longitudinal.

Schaie and Marquette (1972) reviewed the current literature on personality and ageing. Reported personality differences between old and young included increases with age in introversion and cautiousness, and decreases in need for achievement, heterosexuality, responsivity, and psychopathology. However, many studies of the aged using personality assessment actually find a remarkable similarity in personality between the old and the younger age groups with whom they are compared. This, of course, says nothing about how introverted, cautious etc. they are.

Botwinick (1973) considers reports of increased cautiousness and rigidity in the aged to be of particular importance, and this is echoed throughout much of the literature. He cites a variety of evidence suggesting that elderly subjects are more likely to 'play safe' than their juniors, but it is evident that the increased cautiousness so often reported as an ageing effect is a far from unitary phenomenon. The same verbal label is employed for a great variety of personality characteristics displayed in many different experimental studies. Furthermore, there is clear evidence from Edwards and Vine (1963) that differences in a personality measure of cautiousness between age groups can be caused by differences in intellectual ability. Chown (1962) thinks the same is true of reported increases in 'rigidity' in old age. Intellectual factors can force people into dealing inadequately with complex situations whatever their basic personality. Once again experiments on 'rigidity' are very varied in nature though purporting to examine the same personality trait.

An American study of 87 men aged 55 to 84 years attempted to look at personality and adjustment before and after retirement and also to delineate personality types in the aged (Reichard et al 1962). The methods used included intensive interviews, ratings and psychological tests. The results suggested that a critical period of adjustment occurred shortly before retirement during which the men were agitated about the problems and implications of retirement. There was no one way of reacting to the problems presented. Reichard et al outlined five styles of personality found in their group: 'constructiveness' involving self-awareness, flexibility and general satisfaction; 'dependency' reflecting a passive and unambitious style of life; 'defensiveness' which involved being habit-bound, compulsively active and emotionally over-controlled; 'hostility' which is summarized as an aggressive and competitive style; and 'self hate', a strategy adopted by a few men, which was composed of a self-critical, depressed and pessimistic mode of living.

A more recent study included an analysis of personality in a larger investigation of memory and ageing (Botwinick & Storandt 1974). The experimenters felt that the subject group was a little better educated and of higher social class than the norm. They concluded that their group showed no relation between age and life satisfaction, and only a negligible link between sense of control over life and age. The female subjects also completed both a scale measuring depression and a general personality test. There was a slight tendency towards more depression in older subjects, but no age effects at all in the personality test.

As with the studies of intellectual ability, it is important to consider information gathered from longitudinal research as well as the cross-sectional data summarized above. In 1972 Britton and Britton reported the results of a nine-year study carried out in a village in Pennsylvania. They included a broad assessment of activity, health, attitudes, relationships, life satisfaction and conformity, and studied a group of 146 people aged 65 years and above. Most of those studied had sought and found continuity and consistency in their lives, but there were individual patterns showing both continuity and change in personality. The effects of external events were complex. It seemed that outside factors were filtered through the individual's personality system and had both indirect and at times multidirectional effects. Britton and Britton felt that on average the quality of personality adjustment declined, but that individuals separately showed patterns of improving personality adjustment as well as of declining.

An English longitudinal study by Savage et al (1977) sampled 82 subjects living in the community. They agreed with Botwinick and Storandt's (1974) cross-sectional survey in reporting no relation between life satisfaction and age. However, Savage et al are more unusual in reporting a number of other areas in which old people scored differently from the adult norms. On the general personality measure their subjects were more reticent, introspective, silent, reserved and detached than the norm. They showed cautiousness in their emotional expression, were shy, felt inferior, and were critical and uncompromising. There was also a higher level of emotional instability than was expected. An assessment of self-concept revealed the group were decisive and definite about themselves, and felt a strong sense of moral worth and of worth within their families. Although these subjects were rather defensive, their self-esteem was quite high and they were not particularly self-critical.

Methodological issues

The research summarized above gives some credence to the popular idea that ageing involves a psychological decline, and more especially an intellectual decline. In science, as in current affairs, there is a tendency to report the bad news and the spectacular differences rather than the intriguing similarities. Certainly a great deal of the experimental literature is of this sort.

Occasionally in the summary we have seen that a supposed 'ageing effect' is later explained by another factor. In order to have confidence in an experimental finding we need to be sure that the effect reported cannot be attributed to any other factor. Moreover, we have to feel that we can generalize from the particular experiment to elderly people at large, or at least to a reasonable subsection of them, if the information given by an experiment is to hold any practical importance. In many experiments on ageing there are flaws in the methodology which reduce our confidence in one or other of these points. We will examine these methodological points briefly in the two sections which follow.

Alternative influences on results

Many studies employ a cross-sectional method in which people of different ages are compared with each other on particular experimental variables. This is true of many of the early intelligence studies. When this method is used, the differences between subjects include not only their chronological age but also their life experiences such as education, nutrition and social climate. These other factors are known as cohort effects, and the results reported may be due to obsolescence in the context of a rapidly changing environment rather than true ageing effects. Thus it might be argued that for an individual growing up in the socially precarious environment of the 1930s the development of a cautious or prudent approach to life was adaptive. Figure 2.1 illustrates how cohort effects can appear to show decline when successive generations score better and cross-sectional methods are used.

Unfortunately, simply using a longitudinal method, in which groups are followed as they age, does not correct mistakes completely. Each group is subject to particular environmental influences and these may interact with ageing effects to produce spurious results. It is only when successive groups are studied over time that a true picture of the ageing process can begin to emerge.

Factors within the test situation itself are also influential. Younger people have generally had more exposure to the scientific setting and are more familiar with modern test methods than their elders. This general experience may well benefit them not only in doing the tasks presented but also in alleviating some of their test anxiety. High anxiety tends to have an adverse effect on performance. Test situations involve taking risks, particularly when time pressure is included. When the experimental conditions specifically require risky behaviour it seems that old people are as efficient as the young, but given a choice the older subject often performs more cautiously, often at the expense of lost marks. Commonly on tests our speed increases at the expense of mistakes. It seems that old people often prefer doing tasks thoroughly and carefully rather than rushing and risking more errors. A third matter for consider-

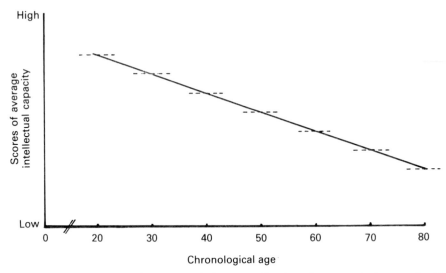

Fig. 2.1 Cohort effects in cross-sectional data: —— typical cross-sectional results; ------ cohort scores for each 10-year period.

ation in the test situation involves the attitudes of both the subjects and the experimenters. Since we know from general psychology that expectation of failure can depress performance and that experimenter characteristics affect results, it seems reasonable to suspect that using young experimenters, often steeped in the decline literature, may bias results.

The materials used in experiments are of concern since they were often originally designed for a young age group. If it is possible that they include cohort effects then their application across age ranges is suspect. Many tests used appear petty and irrelevant. Gardner and Monge (1977) investigated the use of 'adult relevant' tests and found that whilst school-related tests were more poorly done by subjects in their sixties and seventies the adult relevant tests showed no such age decline.

A final group of influences on results involve factors inherent in the subject group. We have already noted that basic characteristics such as intelligence or educational experience can contaminate results. However, more subtle effects may also be involved. People generally show a drop in mental ability in the year before they die (Reimanis & Green 1971). Given that a substantial proportion of subjects in elderly groups may be near to death when tested, results can be biased

towards a decline effect. Furthermore, undiscovered physical problems which are more common for elderly subjects, such as high blood pressure, may lead to an underestimate of average ability levels among the healthy (Wilkie & Eisdorfer 1971).

Problems of generalizability

One of the more striking facts about psychological experiments using older subjects is the range of ability levels they show. Typically the variance in an older group is much greater than in a young adult group, and indeed the variance may be far larger than the so-called age effect. Rabbitt (1981b) quotes a group of 1800 subjects doing reaction time and memory tests who showed a mean decrease in scores of only 20% between the 50 year olds and those aged over 80, but had an increase of 160% in the variance of their scores. Figure 2.2 shows a typical pattern of results.

Given that average scores are often quoted and attempts are made to draw conclusions about individuals from them, the variability is often lost. Schaie (1973) presented data from a 14-year study which showed increasing, decreasing and stable trends in performance in individual subjects. He

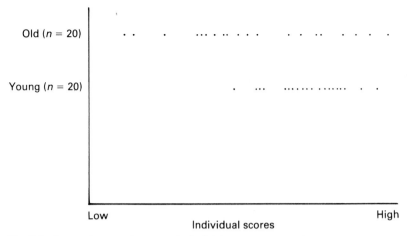

Fig. 2.2 Age and range of scores—typical data.

suggests that the large range of scores often obtained from the elderly is due to varied patterns of ageing together with diverse life experiences. In sum, 'the elderly' are not a homogeneous group, and yet we frequently discuss them and plan for them as if they were.

A second common mistake regarding generalizability involves the tendency to deduce a lifelong process from the measurement of two separate groups of subjects. Generally it is assumed that subjects who are midway in age between the groups studied will be midway in function, and that a trend based on the two measured groups can be expected to continue beyond the age range covered in the experiment. Figure 2.3 illustrates that mistakes may well arise from this.

Along with this mistake is the problem of thinking of 'young' and 'old' as entities. Since both these terms are relative, in different experiments they may mean very different things. A 60-year-old is young in comparison with a person of 75 but old in relation to a teenager. Often it is not stated what 'young' or 'old' means.

It is common to draw general conclusions about

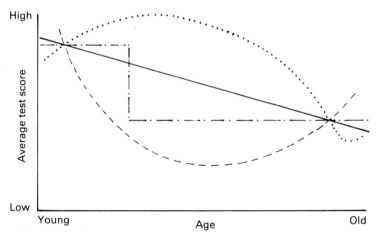

Fig. 2.3 Interpretation from two groups of data: — — commonly deduced 'trend'; — . — .; . . . . .; ----- other logical possibilities.

aspects of psychological functioning which strictly speaking are far removed from the actual experimental basis. This is particularly true in problem-solving and intelligence studies. This lack of accuracy should be studiously avoided, particularly in the field of intelligence where the work such as Guilford's (1956) suggests that intelligence is a very diverse set of abilities. Moreover we have no evidence that maturation has an equal effect on all aspects of ability.

A final consideration when generalizing from research involves the characteristics of the subjects themselves. The sample groups used must be comparable both to each other and to those to whom we wish to apply the results. If a very aged group is involved can it be seen as representative or is it rather a peculiar group of 'survivors'? In longitudinal studies we need also to consider what conclusions may be drawn when some subjects die before completing the study.

SUMMARY OF CHANGES

Support for the cultural stereotype of psychological decline in old age is at best equivocal. Many of the changes commonly thought of as part of the ageing process are by-products of role changes. These changes are imposed upon elderly people either by external events such as retirement or bereavement, or by the cultural mores to which they are expected to conform. It seems that people's individual reactions to these changes are extremely varied. Much of the experimental literature is suggestive of a cognitive decline in ageing (see Table 2.1) but some studies do not agree with this conclusion. Much of the research which supports the decline hypothesis is cross-sectional whereas the longitudinal studies often report no decline, or much more subtle effects. A variety of methodological issues are relevant to the consideration of the experimental data. Some personality studies suggest that negative personality traits are more common in old age, but again much of the literature supports the idea that personality is largely independent of age.

The most commonly cited change in function in old age centres on speed of information processing. Rabbitt (1982) considers that the individual's

capacity for self-optimization is reduced as a consequence of a gradual loss of flexibility in controlling cognitive performance. Effectively he is talking about a feedback loop in which reduced speed in information processing leads to increased memory load, which in turn reduces performance efficiency, which slows information processing, and so on . . . . The age at which these processes begin to change, as well as the individual's ability to compensate, varies, with more able people having much less of a decline. He relates this control system model to many observed changes in function in old age, noting in his 1981b paper that old people show changes in gait which are due to inefficient monitoring and feedback from environmental conditions well before changes which are due to physiological decline. In his 1987 Myers Lecture (Rabbitt 1988) he talks with some eloquence of the complex interactions involved in these changes.

ADJUSTMENT

The issue of how people adjust to the changes involved in ageing will be examined in three parts. The first section will contrast two popular models of ageing. In the second section, adjustment will be considered in terms of the individual's lifespan, and finally personal adjustment to change will be examined.

TWO MODELS OF ADJUSTMENT

There are two well-known models proposed to explain the general processes of psychological adjustment which are associated with ageing. The two are particularly concerned with successful adjustment in retirement. The most striking aspect of the models is that they have quite different implications for practical work with elderly people.

Disengagement

The most widely known model of adjustment in ageing was proposed by Cumming and Henry (1961) and is known as *disengagement theory*. The theory states that a process of mutual disengagement occurs during ageing in which both the individual person and the society in which that person lives withdraw from each other. To remain psychologically healthy and satisfied the elderly person retreats from the responsibilities and involvements which characterized middle life. Society in turn withdraws from the individual by decreasing the demands made upon the person and by policies linked to chronological age such as enforced retirement. An example of this might be a factory worker who after retirement from work also curtails the social activities which are linked with ex-workmates. These ideas were based on a study carried out in Kansas City in 1955 which involved 172 people aged 50–70 years and 107 aged 70–90 years. The subjects were interviewed regarding their activities, general health, welfare and interactions. People who do not disengage, the theory implies, are likely to become frustrated and possibly depressed. It is acknowledged that not all people disengage at the same time. One experimental prediction from disengagement theory might be that feelings of control over life would wane with advancing age, but this has not been born out by personality studies. The practical implications of this model, if adopted, would be enormous. To encourage disengagement would be to discourage active involvement, and in particular to discourage the initiation of new involvements in old age.

Activity

The main alternative model to disengagement theory, *activity theory*, suggests that, on the contrary, successful ageing occurs when new or modified channels for a person's energies are found to replace pre-existing activities, and the attitudes and activities of middle age are preserved as long as possible. Ageing may thus be characterized as a struggle to remain middle-aged. This model is associated with Havighurst (1963). Pre-existing activities may be curtailed when society withdraws through retirement, or when the individual disengages because of factors such as ill health. An example of this might be the avid squash player who turns to golf when squash becomes too physically taxing. The activity model predicts that the frustrated, depressed old people will be those who have been unable both to preserve the activities of younger days and to find alternative outlets. Some support for these ideas comes from Britton and Britton (1972), who reported that women who survived best through the nine years of their study tended to be those who scored highly on measures of activity involvement and satisfaction.

These two contrasting theories have interesting parallels in the Health Service. Units which specialize in the care of old people usually pay lip service at least to activity theory, but often the day-to-day workings of a such units are more akin to those associated with disengagement theory.

ADJUSTMENT AS A LIFELONG PROCESS

An alternative way of viewing the adjustments made in later life, and the success or otherwise of these, is to look at the life-course overall. All the major psychological theories have developmental implications which lead to predictions about adjustment in old age but few have articulated these in any depth. Erikson (1950) provides a contrast to this trend. He described eight stages of the life-span each of which was concerned with a particular issue of psychological development. Thus the earlier stages include 'identity versus role confusion', which he thought of as an adolescent concern, and the issue of 'intimacy versus isolation' which he saw as central to development in young adulthood. The stages were seen as successive, each building on the structure constructed in earlier stages. The final stage was that linked to old age. Erikson described this stage as focusing on the issue of 'ego integrity versus despair'. A state of ego integrity is achieved if the person on reflecting on her past life feels that life has been right and meaningful. Despair is the outcome if life is seen as having been useless, wrong, or pointless. A fear of death is often linked with this despair.

Lily Pincus (1981) says that the crucial aspect of this process is the question of whether the world is different because the person has been in it. An integral part of the process is an attempt to survey and summarize one's life, looking back to past events and trying to make sense of it as a whole. The idea that an important part of the psychological 'work' of old age occurs via a life review was taken up by Butler (1963). He noted the strong tendency for old people to reminisce. He also noted that old people often enjoy this while their juniors often discourage it as 'living in the past'. Butler proposed that it was through activities like reminiscence that people worked on their life review, and so came to terms with the meaning of their life and with their own mortality. Since his pioneering work the idea of promoting reminiscence among elderly people has become common practice in the caring professions, though the links between the practice and the underlying theory have often been lost. Thornton and Brotchie (1987) sound a note of caution on the belief in an age-specific, therapeutic reminiscence process.

The theme of a lifelong developmental process is echoed by Buhler (1961), and by Neugarten (1964) in her *continuity theory*. This suggests that individuals attempt to preserve pre-existing lifestyles and preferences. Ageing is thus characterized as a battle to preserve habits and preferences already established in earlier years.

Lily Pincus (1981) takes a similar view in reviewing her own 83 years of life and when discussing case material from others. She sets out to examine what it is in an individual's life-history that determines his or her experience of old age. Factors such as one's experience of loss, family context, dependency, and relationships are seen as being crucial.

A contrasting conceptualization of successful ageing can be gleaned from Maslow's (1968) work on 'self-actualization'. This state of 'full humanness' was achievable, he thought, when lesser human needs, for food, dominance, love etc. had been met and superseded. Self-actualizing people were devoting their lives to what Maslow calls 'being' values; that is, ultimate intrinsic values such as truth, beauty, and simplicity. He thought that it took time and the development of exceptional personal maturity to attain self-actualization and so only middle-aged and old people could be seen as having done so; indeed

Maslow thought it was impossible for most people to satisfy and transcend their 'lower' needs. Perhaps, then, the satisfied and successful old people are those who have transcended lesser matters and are self-actualizing. This idea certainly gains support from a survey by Mary Spain which is quoted by Lily Pincus (1981). Two thirds of 300 people aged 80–100 replied to her letter asking about their beliefs. Of these 200 people, only one mentioned her age in the reply. The rest were absorbed in issues outside themselves which gave meaning to their lives.

A number of alternative ways of understanding the ageing process have come from work in social psychology. The emphasis in these is on the interaction between ageing persons and the society around them. *Symbolic interactionism*, associated with Mead (1934), stresses language as allowing humans to live in both a symbolic and a physical world. The outcome of ageing is thus produced by the reciprocal relationship between the individual and the social environment, mediated by language. This idea is extended, in *exchange theory*, by concentrating on ageing as a social exchange (Dowd 1980). Individuals attempt to maximize gains and to minimize costs in their social interactions. As the older person's power diminishes her range of potential interactions, and the types of roles she can lead, decrease until finally only compliance is left. An alternative sociopsychological theory concentrates on the old as a deviant group. *Labelling theory* suggests that the old, like other deviant groups, are prey to stereotyping and hostility from the rest of society. This view of ageing draws on Berger and Berger's (1976) *theory of deviance*, which stresses the effect of labelling of groups as different from the norm. Elderly people are thus seen as a deviant group in society. Some sociologists take this further and view old people as a minority group. By contrast, *age stratification theory* takes a more gentle view of the identification of the old as a specific group. It stresses the existence of a variety of age status groups, e.g. teenagers. The meaning of each age group is defined by society, which has mechanisms for the allocation of roles to different groups, and people experience transition as they pass from group to group. Using this theory, then, we have the possibility of defining and changing society's ways of assigning roles to the old, and we can examine, and perhaps think of changing the ways in which the transition to old age is made.

ADJUSTMENT TO CHANGE

The broader issues of adjustment to change are probably best considered in relation to the major life changes of later life such as retirement, bereavement and death. The coping processes used determine to what extent changes are seen as gains or losses. Life events seem to be interpreted in relation to individual personality and life experience (Britton & Britton 1972). If adjustment is seen as a lifelong process, then successful adjustment to retirement rests on past experience of work and on the meaning of work to the individual. Similarly, bereavement reactions will be largely determined by the person's past experience of loss and by their relationship with the dead person.

Retirement

In recent years there has been a growing concern with preparation for retirement (Stott 1981). Such preparation involves both the practical aspects of sorting out financial matters and making decisions about where to live, and the psychological preparation for vast increases in leisure time and the loss of external time structure. Elwell and Maltbie–Crannell (1981) suggest that the role loss involved in retirement be considered as a stressor affecting both coping resources and life satisfaction. The study by Reichard et al (1962) found that a critical period of adjustment preceded the retirement date. Mary Stott points out that our retirement date is one of the few major decisions about life over which most of us have absolutely no influence. Kerckhoff (1964) looked at expectations and reactions to retirement among 108 husband and wife pairs in the United States. Most looked forward to the event, especially subjects from the middle and working classes, but few made definite plans. Once retired, the men experienced greater improvements than their wives. Those who had been retired more than five years tended to respond to Kerckhoff's questions more negatively. The hus-

bands especially wished they had retired later. In terms of income group there was a positive association between income level and tendency to plan for retirement, and between income level and the likelihood of a positive experience of retirement.

Bereavement

Bereavement is not, as is so often assumed, an experience peculiar to the old, but it is, of course, a more common experience as one outlives friends and relatives. Murray Parkes (1975) identified definite stages through which the bereaved adult of any age passes. He says the first stage of numbness leads on to a period of pining. This is followed by a stage of depression before recovery ensues. It is likely that the modern Western tendency to reduce the ritual of death and to discourage active mourning interferes with the process. Mourning is often treated as if it were a weakness or a self–indulgence. Mary Stott describes the feelings which result on the death of a beloved spouse as not only 'loneliness of the most devastating kind, but a wilderness of pain and desolation impossible to imagine beforehand or to protect oneself against'. (Stott 1981, p. 68)

In a development from Murray Parkes' seminal work, Worden (1983) outlines four tasks of mourning: accepting the reality of the loss, experiencing the pain of grief, adjusting to an environment in which the deceased is missing, and withdrawing emotional energy and reinvesting it in another relationship. He points out, with some delicacy, some of the problems which arise when people tackle these difficult tasks.

Death

Elisabeth Kubler-Ross (1975) describes the process of coming to terms with death as the final stage of growth. This thesis is similar to that of Erikson outlined earlier. Kubler-Ross identifies five stages of psychological adjustment which can be observed in the dying: denial, anger and guilt, bargaining, depression, and acceptance. A parallel is drawn with other life changes. Abandoning old habits and finding new ways of living is seen as a form of dying and regrowth. From this one might expect to observe similar stages as people adjust to the changes of ageing, but as yet we have only anecdotal evidence to support this.

SUMMARY OF ADJUSTMENT

There is no universally accepted model of adjustment in old age. The two best-known models are contradictory. Perhaps this lack of agreement is a reflection of the enormous variability referred to earlier in this chapter. Objectively the life events of old age are characterized by loss but the subjective experience appears to depend on personal style. Some common stages of adjustment to bereavement and death can be outlined but beyond this the individual's personality and experience is the key to understanding the adjustment process.

THE HEALTH SERVICE CONTEXT

In coming into contact with the health services the elderly person becomes in some sense abnormal — either physically, socially or psychologically. Our primary concern as health care workers must be first to determine what has brought the person into contact with us. What has changed so as to bring her to our attention? Sometimes the main factor is a physical or social change which can be pinpointed. The focus of intervention is often determined by this. For example, the elderly person has broken a leg this morning, or the forgetful elderly person functioned well with the help of her spouse but the crisis has been precipitated by the spouse's death, or the usual home help is on leave and the eccentric person refuses to eat food provided by others. Sometimes the crucial change involved is in the patient's psychological functioning or in the interaction between this and other aspects of her condition.

The initial assessment of what has changed often shows us where we should aim our therapeutic efforts, particularly when the client appears to have multiple problems some of which are chronic and incurable. Sometimes we can effect useful changes in other areas too, but the focus for intervention needs to be carefully considered in the light of the client's personal needs, preferences and aims.

In this section we will examine first the informal and formal assessment of psychological functioning, and the application of this to decision-making within the multidisciplinary context, before moving on to review the implications for the care of elderly people and of the individuality they show.

INFORMAL ASSESSMENT OF PSYCHOLOGICAL FUNCTIONING

Whatever the patient's general condition, her mental functioning must always be noted. Physical and mental functioning will always interact and sometimes the indirect effects are considerable. This is amply illustrated by studies on the use of analgesics and recovery from surgery (Melzack 1973). Roughly speaking, the informal psychological assessment can be summarized in three simple questions:

1. To what extent is the client in touch with what is happening around her?
2. How does the client relate to other people?
3. Can the person learn and use new information (e.g. faces, names, the way around the ward) when regular events happen?

These factors should be considered in a context which is personal for each client and which again can be summarized into two areas:

a. Are physical factors affecting mental functioning? This can be crucial for patients in confusional states, depression and anxiety. We need to consider how good the patient's senses are. With regard to learning new information, we need to consider how readily available the information is.
b. What was she like in earlier life?

These factors should be continually monitored by all those in contact with the patient, and should be considered in the planning of interventions and, if appropriate, of future placement. The Health Service often considers these points intermittently and disjointedly, and we are usually woefully unaware of the person's past life and character. The positive as well as the negative factors must be recorded. At times the fact that a person is particularly easy-going and sociable, for example, is the single most important fact about them. This may be crucial in obtaining and maintaining a place in an old people's Home or in ensuring that neighbours continue to support the person at home. The introduction of individualized patient care in this country should provide a more structured and consistent assessment of this sort.

In the course of this informal assessment we should be sensitive to the effects we ourselves are having. The change of role into patient or long-term patient may elicit particular responses. Institutionalization can result when people are admitted to hospital for more than a few days. Thus our own actions may have caused some of the withdrawal or dependency displayed by patients. We should be aware of the extent that our actions and our health service regime disrupts this or interferes with normal routines. These observations must be taken into account when considering a person's abilities and difficulties. Particular areas of importance, especially any problems, will need a more detailed assessment, and usually a formal gathering of data is necessary.

FORMAL ASSESSMENT

The most common formal assessment of psychological functioning required of a nurse is that of keeping precise records of some aspect of behaviour. The object of this may be to establish the pattern of existing behaviour before an intervention is applied. Such a record is known as a baseline. The formal recording of baseline data allows the precise effects of any intervention to be determined. Formal assessment may alternatively aim to determine the exact nature of the behaviour, to determine the quantity of that behaviour, to investigate the possibility that there may be a subtle pattern to the behaviour, or to determine the context of behaviour, that is what precedes it, whether it is environmentally linked, and what follows it. Nurses are also often required to fill out checklists or questionnaires about patient behaviour, or perhaps to complete a standardized assessment such as the Clifton Assessment Procedures

for the Elderly (CAPE, Pattie & Gilleard, 1979). The CAPE consists of a cognitive assessment scale and a behavioural rating scale, each of which indicates the dependency grade of the patient. The areas assessed include information and orientation, mental ability, psychomotor ability, physical disability, communication difficulties, apathy and social disturbance. There is also a shortened survey form. The object of these assessments is to obtain a precise measure of specified aspects of psychological functioning. Sometimes when more than one person is taking measures it is necessary to run a check on how the people involved vary in the way they take measurements, and perhaps to standardize further the way in which it is done. These procedures make the conclusions drawn more reliable. Some tests have rigid instructions to follow and contain information on how other comparable clients score. These so-called standardized tests allow the individual to be compared with an appropriate reference group.

A detailed nursing assessment of old people with dementia, confusion and depression is described in Chapters 18, 19 and 20.

INTERDISCIPLINARY WORKING

The data thus gathered will contribute to the planning and implementation of nursing care. Commonly though, it is in an interdisciplinary context that overall decisions are made. The contribution of each member is part of the group decision-making process. Clear presentation of the information gathered advances not only the management of a particular patient but also the understanding of the working team as a whole regarding elderly people and their problems.

The team decision will usually be implemented by the team so that the nurse may be cast as therapist, researcher, or counsellor in turn in the management of patients with psychological difficulties. Many teams have tried to avoid the old institutional practices by instituting keyworker systems and sharing decision-making. Some have tried to deny the realities of professional training and have varied responsibilities in an attempt to achieve 'equality'. In order to maximize her effectiveness in such a team, the nurse should focus clearly on her own abilities and limitations as well as being sensitive to those of her colleagues.

INDIVIDUALITY

A recurrent theme of this chapter has been the great variability shown by elderly people in all aspects of psychological functioning. Their expectations, needs and coping skills are impossible to summarize meaningfully. Institutions work through standardization and routine, and the Health Service is no exception to this. Even with the growing trend toward community work, encouraged by the 'rising tide' of people over 65 years of age, we carry institutional practices and standardization into people's homes with unfortunate effects.

The influence of this chapter should be to encourage the struggle towards reconciling the needs and rights of the individual old person with the system in which we work. The exploration of how far one can encourage individuality and personal expression in hospital wards without major interference with health care needs far more attention. The introduction of more personal possessions in hospitals, choice of meals, and flexible visiting times is part of this movement but we will have to go a great deal further to match the variability of our client group. Remember it is only really in the last decade that practices in children's wards have become more flexible and more in keeping with the psychological make-up of the clients. Let us hope the next ten years will see a similar revolution in wards for old people.

In addition to these changes, another area for development concerns how to foster healthy adaptive processes in individual clients. More encouragement of active mourning, and of reminiscence, and the growth of the hospice movement for terminal care indicate that this development is beginning. We need further to consider how best to help people keep in touch with events in their own lives and in the outside world. Greater involvement of the family and of the informal network of carers, such as friends and neighbours, is an invaluable part of this (Pottle 1984). The use of reality orientation, reminiscence, and validation techniques to help people keep in touch with life

and personhood is another essential element (Holden & Woods 1982, Norris & Abu El Eileh 1982, Feil 1982).

CONCLUSIONS

This chapter has examined (a) the experimental evidence on the changes which accompany ageing, both of role and of individual psychology, and (b) the adjustments which occur during later life. We have seen in this review how limited a contribution these make to the working context. However, geriatric services would be radically changed if the meagre applications which do spring from the psychological studies were put into practice. A synthesis of how our knowledge of the psychology of ageing relates to the health service context has been attempted.

Our health care reflects the cultural stereotype of an inevitable and uniform psychological decline in ageing just the same as the rest of our society. Our institutions are geared to uniformity and standardization. It is time to discard the ridiculous stereotype, to embrace the individuality of ageing, and to change our practices accordingly.

REFERENCES

Barak B 1987 Cognitive age: a new multidimensional approach to measuring age identity. International Journal of Aging and Human Development 25: 109–128
Bayley N, Oden M H 1955 The maintenance of intellectual ability in gifted adults. Journal of Gerontology 10: 91–107
Berger P L 1976 Sociology: a biographical approach. Penguin, Harmondsworth
Birren J E 1963 Psychophysiological relations. In: Birren J E (ed) Human aging (USPHS Publ 986). US Public Health Service, Washington DC
Birren J E, Botwinick J 1955 Age differences in finger, jaw and foot reaction time to auditory stimuli. Journal of Gerontology 10: 429–432
Blum J E, Fosshage J L, Jarvick L F 1972 Intellectual changes and sex differences in octogenarians: A twenty year longitudinal study of aging. Developmental Psychology 7: 178–187
Blythe R 1979 The view in winter — reflections on old age. Penguin, Harmondsworth
Botwinick J 1973 Aging and behaviour. Springer, New York

Botwinick J, Storandt M 1974 Memory, related functions and age. Charles C Thomas, Springfield, Illinois

Britton J H, Britton J O 1972 Personality changes in aging: a longitudinal study of community residents. Springer, New York

Bromley D B 1957 Some effects of age on the quality of intellectual output. Journal of Gerontology 12: 318–323

Buhler C 1961 Meaningful living in mature years. In: Kleemeier R W (ed) Aging and leisure. Oxford, New York

Butler R N 1963 The life review: an interpretation of reminiscence in the aged. Psychiatry 26: 65–76

Canestrari R E 1966 The effects of commonality on paired associate learning in two age groups. Journal of Genetic Psychology 108: 3–7

Cattell R B 1963 Theory of fluid and crystallized intelligence: a critical experiment. Journal of Education Psychology 54: 1–22

Chown S M 1962 Rigidity and age. In: Tibbitts C, Donahue W (eds) Social and psychological aspects of aging. Columbia University Press, New York

Craik F I M 1968 Short-term memory and the aging process. In: Talland G A (ed) Human aging and behavior. Academic Press, New York

Cumming E, Henry W E 1961 Growing old: the process of disengagement. Basic Books, New York

Cunningham W R, Clayton V, Overton W 1975 Fluid and crystallized intelligence in young adulthood and old age. Journal of Gerontology 30: 53–55

Dowd J 1980 Stratification amongst the aged. Brooks-Cole, Monterey, California

Edwards A E, Vine D B 1963 Personality changes with age: their dependency on concomitant intellectual decline. Journal of Gerontology 18: 182–184

Eisdorfer C, Axelrod S, Wilkie F 1963 Stimulus exposure time as a factor in serial learning in an aged sample. Journal of Abnormal and Social Psychology 67: 594–600

Eisdorfer C, Wilkie F 1973 Intellectual changes with advancing age In: Jarvick L F, Eisdorfer C, Blum J E (eds) Intellectual functioning in adults. Springer, New York, p 21–29

Elwell F, Maltbie-Crannell A D 1981 The impact of role loss upon coping resources and life satisfaction of the elderly. Journal of Gerontology 36: 223–232

Erikson E H 1950 Childhood and society. Hogarth Press, London

Feil N 1982 Validation — The Feil method. Edward Feil Productions, Cleveland

Gardner E F, Monge R H 1977 Adult age differences in cognitive abilities and education background. Experimental Ageing Research 3: 337–383

Gilbert J G 1941 Memory loss in senescence. Journal of Abnormal and Social Psychology 36: 73–86

Gilbert J G 1973 Thirty five year old follow up study of intellectual functioning. Journal of Gerontology 28: 68–72

Goldfarb W 1941 An investigation of reaction time in older adults and its relationship to certain observed mental test patterns. Contributions to Education no 831. Teachers College, Columbia University, New York

Green R F 1969 Age–intelligence relationship between ages sixteen and sixty-four: a rising trend. Developmental Psychology 1: 618–627

Guilford J P 1956 The structure of intellect. Psychological Bulletin 53: 267–293

Gunderson E K E, Rahe R H (eds) 1974 Life stress and illness, Charles C Thomas, Springfield, Illinois

Havighurst R J 1963 Successful aging. In: Williams R H, Tibbitts C, Donahue W (eds) Processes of aging, vol 1. Atherton Press, New York

Heglin H J 1956 Problem solving set in different age groups. Gerontology 11: 310–317

Holden U P, Woods R T 1982 Reality orientation: psychological approaches to the 'confused' elderly. Churchill Livingstone, London

Huppert F A 1982 Does mental function decline with age? Geriatric Medicine 12: 32–35

Kastenbaum R, Derbin V, Sabatini P, Artt S 1972 The ages of me: toward personal and interpersonal definitions of aging. Aging and Human Development 3: 197–211

Kerckhoff A C 1964 Husband-wife expectations and reactions to retirement. Journal of Gerontology 19: 510–516

Kubler-Ross E 1975 Death. The final stage of growth Prentice Hall, London

Lehman H C 1953 Age and achievement. Oxford University Press

Levinson D J 1978 The seasons of a man's life. Ballantine, New York

Maslow A H 1968 Towards a psychology of being. 2nd edn. Van Nostrand, New York

Mead G C (ed) 1934 Mind, self, and society. University of Chicago Press, Chicago

Melzack R 1973 The puzzle of pain. Penguin, Harmondsworth

Monge R H, Hultsch D 1971 Paired-associate learning as a function of adult age and the length of the anticipation and inspection intervals. Journal of Gerontology 26: 157–162

Murray Parkes C 1975 Bereavement: studies of grief in adult life. Pelican Books, Harmondsworth

Neugarten B L 1964 Personality in middle and late life. Atherton Press, New York

Norris A D, Abu El Eileh M 1982 Reminiscing — a therapy for both elderly patients and their staff. Nursing Times 78: 1368–1369

Owens W A 1966 Age and mental abilities: a second adult follow up. Journal of Education Psychology 57: 311–325

Pattie A H, Gilleard C J 1979 Manual of the Clifton assessment procedures for the elderly (CAPE). Hodder and Stoughton, Sevenoaks, Kent

Pincus L 1981 The challenge of a long life. Faber, London

Pottle S M 1984 Developing a network oriented service for the elderly and their carers. In: Treacher A, Carpenter J (eds) Using family therapy. Blackwell, Oxford

Rabbitt P M A 1965 An age decrement in the ability to ignore irrelevant information. Journal of Gerontology 20: 233–238

Rabbitt P M A 1977 Changes in problem-solving ability in old age. In: Birren J E, Schaie K W (eds) Handbook of the psychology of aging. Van Nostrand Reinhold, Cincinnati, Ohio

Rabbitt P M A 1980 A fresh look at changes in reaction times in old age. In: Stein D (ed) The psychobiology of ageing: problems and perspectives. Elsevier/North Holland, New York

Rabbitt P M A 1981a Talking to the old. New Society 140–141

Rabbitt P M A 1981b Cognitive psychology needs models

for change in performance in old age. In: Long J, Baddeley A (eds) Attention and performance IX. Lawrence Erlbaum Associates, Hillsdale, N J

Rabbitt P M A 1982 How do old people know what to do next? In: Craik F M, Trehub S (eds) Ageing and cognitive processes. Plenum Press, New York

Rabbitt P M A 1988 Social psychology, neurosciences and cognitive psychology need each other; (and gerontology needs all three of them) The Psychologist: Bulletin of the British Psychological Society 12: 500–506

Reichard S, Livson F, Peterson P G 1962 Aging and personality: a study of eighty-seven older men. Wiley, New York

Reimanis G, Green R F 1971 Imminence of death and intellectual decrement in the ageing. Developmental Psychology 5: 270–272

Salthouse T 1985 A theory of cognitive ageing. Springer, Berlin

Savage R D, Britton P G, Bolton N, Hall E H 1973 Intellectual functioning in the aged. Methuen, London

Savage R D, Gaber L B, Britton P G, Bolton N, Cooper A 1977 Personality and adjustment in the aged. Academic Press, London

Schaie K W 1973 Methodological problems in descriptive developmental research on adulthood and ageing. In: Nesselroade J R, Reese H W (eds) Lifespan developmental psychology: methodology. Academic Press, New York

Schaie K W, Marquette B 1972 Personality in maturity and old age. In: Dreger R M (ed) Multivariate personality research: contributions to the understanding of personality in honour of Raymond B Cattell. Clautors, Louisiana

Schaie K W, Strother C R 1968 A cross-sequential study of age changes in cognitive behaviour. Psychological Bulletin 70: 671–680

Schonfield D 1974 Translations in gerontology — from lab to life: utilising information. American Psychologist 796–800

Schonfield D, Robertson B 1966 Memory storage and aging. Canadian Journal of Psychology 20: 228–236

Smith D K 1967 The Einstellung effect in relation to the variables of age and training. Dissertation Abstracts 27B: 4115

Stott M 1981 Ageing for beginners. Blackwell, Oxford

Talland G A 1965 Three estimates of the word span and their stability over the adult years. Quarterly Journal of Experimental Psychology 17: 301–307

Terman L W, Oden M H 1959 The gifted group at midlife: thirty five years follow up of the superior child. Genetic studies of genius, vol. 5 Stanford University Press, Stanford, California

Thornton S, Brotchie J 1987 Reminiscence: a critical review of the empirical literature. British Journal of Clinical Psychology 26: 93–111

Wechsler D 1944 The measurement of adult intelligence, 3rd edn. Williams and Wilkins, Baltimore

Wetherick N E 1964 A comparison of the problem solving ability of young, middle-aged and old subjects. Gerontologia 9: 164–178

Wilkie F, Eisdorfer C 1971 Intelligence and blood pressure in the aged. Science 172: 959–962

Worden J W 1983 Grief counselling and grief therapy. Tavistock Publications, London

Young M L 1966 Problem-solving performance in two age groups. Journal of Gerontology 21: 505–509

Young M L 1971 Age and sex differences in problem solving. Journal of Gerontology 26: 330–336

CHAPTER CONTENTS

The study of human ageing 41

Maintenance of homeostasis in elderly people 42
Functional reserve within systems 43
Flexibility and adaptability 44
Physical capacity 44

Functional changes with ageing 45
Nutrition and gastrointestinal tract 45
The immune system 47
The endocrine system 48
The respiratory and cardiovascular systems 50
The nervous system 51
The special senses 52
The skin 53
Supporting tissues 55
The reproductive system 56

Theories of ageing 56
The free radical theory of ageing 58
The disposable soma theory of ageing 59

Health and disease in elderly people 60

3

The biology of human ageing

Rosamund A. Herbert

Research into the biology of human ageing has in the past always seemed to emphasize the loss or deterioration of function as a person gets older, and so most of us tend to have a pessimistic view of ageing. Ageing is often seen as synonymous with reduced biological efficiency. However, we can adopt a more positive approach, since evidently the majority of older people function very adequately in a biological sense and so this negative view of biological ageing is unwarranted.

Undoubtedly, with the passage of time over the adult period, profound changes in appearance and function do occur in all organisms, including humans. However, what tends to be forgotten is that these changes result from the combined influences of lifestyle, nutrition, state of physical fitness and disease, all of which are superimposed on what is commonly referred to as the ageing process. The health of an individual from a physiological viewpoint, whatever her age, ultimately depends on the efficient functioning of the individual cells and tissues in all systems of the body. Many factors are acknowledged as influencing one's health: diet, exercise, personal habits (e.g. smoking) and psychosocial factors all play an important role in determining one's state of health at any age — 8, 18 or 80! The ageing process is a continual process during life (not just in the latter stages of life) and is a reflection of numerous exogenous and endogenous factors and related medical, social and inherent characteristics.

Another issue that is widely debated is what is meant by 'normal ageing'. One of the most obvious findings in gerontology is the enormous variability between individuals, even if they are of a similar chronological age. For instance, one finds some 70 year olds able to run a marathon or to windsurf, whilst others are hardly able to perform the daily activities of living. Acknowledging this variability is important, as it makes generalizations about an elderly person's capabilities virtually impossible. The explanation for this variability is, as discussed above; many factors influence the ageing process.

There is a strong association between the length of life of parents and that of their offspring and this again reflects the combination of genetic, lifestyle and environmental factors. There is a genetic component to ageing; studies comparing identical and non-identical twins show that age of death is closer in identical twins. Also, the consistent sex difference of longevity, with females living longer than males, is further indication of genetic influences. Gerontologists now also recognize the importance that variations in lifestyle, such as diet, patterns of activity and smoking have on health status and lifespan. Similarly, socioeconomic factors are relevant, as are disease-related factors such as exposure to infectious diseases.

For all these reasons chronological age is a relatively weak indicator of physiological age. The enormous variability, or heterogeneity as it is often referred to, is one issue that complicates discussion of normal ageing and also makes research into the study of human ageing more problematic. In order to be able to make any meaningful comments about the biological ageing process, researchers need to study large numbers of people. The realization of the extent of variability within human ageing has also led to further clarification of what is meant by 'old'. For instance: 65–75 might be referred to as young old age/elderly; 75–85 as middle old age/old; and 85+ as old old age/very old.

Another problem in discussing normal ageing is the difficulty in determining whether any changes observed in people are in fact due to ageing itself or due to a disease process superimposed upon ageing. In an attempt to overcome this, Strehler (1962), an American gerontologist, proposed that any physiological phenomenon must meet four criteria before it can be unequivocally stated to be a component of the overall ageing process: the

change must be shown to be *universal* (identifiable in all members of a species), *intrinsic* (occurring from within the organism), *progressive* and *deleterious*. This last factor is controversial, but these are useful criteria to consider when considering changes observed in older people; for example, loss of hearing caused by shingles or an ototoxic drug is not an age-related change, whereas loss of hearing due to age-related decline in sensory nerve cells in the auditory pathway is.

Some physiological changes that are observed in older people are simply due to the fact that they have become less fit. We are aware that if we reduce our habitual activity levels for some reason — maybe illness, bedrest, temporary injury, or apathy — then our physical capabilities are reduced. However, we can build up our fitness again and this cycle applies to the elderly too. Thus Strehler's criteria that change must be progressive and universal before it can be classified as an age change can be helpful in distinguishing the cause of change — in this example, change is due to the individual's deconditioning or just becoming less fit, rather than to an intrinsic change.

Thus, in many ways the term 'normal ageing' has limitations. Rowe and Kahn (1987) have suggested an alternative: namely, 'usual and successful' rather than 'normal' ageing. As Rowe and Kahn point out, the use of the term 'normal' in this context neglects the heterogeneity of older people in the non-diseased group and also implies that the changes are harmless or without risk; we tend to think of 'normal' as somehow natural and therefore beyond purposeful modification. Accordingly, Rowe and Kahn describe people who age successfully as those having minimal physiological loss when compared with the average of their younger counterparts, i.e. those broadly successful in physiological terms (the marathon runners would certainly be in this category). People who show typical non-pathological age-linked losses demonstrate usual ageing. Together, 'successful' and 'usual' define the heterogeneous category of 'normal' (i.e. non-diseased) in any age group. This approach is most constructive, particularly with regard to health promotion for the elderly: the aim would be to move people from the usual age category 'up' into the successful ageing group.

THE STUDY OF HUMAN AGEING

Knowledge and understanding about the biology of ageing has been gained from many different areas of research, although biological gerontology is still in its early stages. Much work is done studying the changes of ageing cells in cultures — isolated groups of cells, e.g. fibroblasts, artificially grown 'in vitro' (literally, in glass). Research on ageing animals, from rats to primates, attempts to gain knowledge from suitable animal models; often, this information is extrapolated into an analogy with humans. There are obvious inadequacies with cell cultures and animal studies in telling us about human ageing, but they still are invaluable in increasing general understanding of the ageing process.

In addition to animal studies, many studies are performed on people across a wide age range and the findings for different age groups are then compared. Since the 1950s two main approaches have been used to study human ageing, namely cross-sectional and longitudinal studies. Both approaches have their own particular limitations but information gained from these two methods together has given us considerable knowledge about human ageing.

Cross-sectional studies involve taking a sample of people in any one population at one time from a wide age range (e.g. 20, 40, 60, 80 year olds) and assessing their physiological function to look for changes that seem to occur with increasing age. Much of the early work in the 1950s and 1960s was done using this approach and produced findings that indicated a deterioration in function. Using this approach it is impossible to control for variables like nutrition and lifestyle that are known to influence the ageing process. The problem of looking at different age groups and directly comparing their responses is that people from different age decades have lived through very different circumstances, e.g. wars, economic depression, food shortages, access to health and medical care. If these factors affect the variable under consideration (this is called the 'cohort effect'), differences in average values may wrongly be ascribed to ageing.

To avoid some of the pitfalls and limitations of cross-sectional studies, longitudinal studies have been set up — for instance, the Baltimore Longitudinal Study of Ageing (BLSA) and Duke studies started in the 1950s. The advantage that longitudinal studies have is that they follow the same individuals over a long time-span. These are obviously very costly studies to run and so there are relatively few undertaken; often, financial constraints lead to their discontinuation, e.g. the Duke study was discontinued in the 1970s whilst BLSA still continues. This approach also requires researchers with altruistic tendencies; unlike studies on rats, where ageing changes occur in a period of 2–3 years, studies on human ageing may not yield results within the working life of the researchers.

Longitudinal studies are not without their problems, too, which must be considered when assessing the significance of the results. For example, the sample for BLSA until 1978 was only made up of male subjects (which, given the fact that females live longer than males, is somewhat inappropriate). Also, the fact that the subjects participating must be interested and motivated enough to take part in a longitudinal programme involving considerable commitment on their part often leads to a sample biased towards higher social classes and those with a particular sympathy for research. The BLSA does have an excess of subjects with better-than-average educational backgrounds and socioeconomic status.

The inference drawn from averages based on cross-sectional studies that functions generally decline over the entire adult lifespan was contradicted by longitudinal studies: for example, a substantial number of subjects aged 65 and over showed no decline in health status or intellectual function and some actually showed improvement in health over a number of years (Maddox & Douglass 1974). Even subjects who had substantial impairment of physical functioning, EEG abnormalities, cardiovascular disease or impairment in vision and hearing, often remained active in the community, living fairly mobile and independent lives.

Longitudinal observations have shown that the rate of change with age for some variables observed in individual subjects did not differ significantly from the mean rates derived from analysis of cross-sectional observations. On the other hand, many individuals followed patterns of ageing that could never have been identified from cross-sectional data alone. For example, many subjects experienced periods of 5–10 years during which their kidney function showed no sign of change, whilst the average curve (from cross-sectional data) was declining. In a few individuals, kidney function actually improved over a 10-year interval when average values were falling. Conversely, there were some people whose decrement was greater than that predicted from cross-sectional studies (Shock 1985).

It is often difficult to find human subjects for research and some of the early studies on human ageing used a population that was easy to access, namely institutionalized elderly people. These people were obviously not representative of the 'normal' elderly population. Using samples like this may have been one reason for the skewing of research findings towards decrements in function. Again because of very real practical of constraints, studies were often carried out on small samples of elderly people and the variability of individuals makes meaningful interpretation often very difficult. Perhaps it is easy to see why ageing research results sometimes seem contradictory. Rigorous attention to methodology is essential. It is much easier to study ageing in rats than in humans!

The general conclusion from longitudinal studies is that relatively few individuals follow the pattern of age changes predicted from averages based on measurements made on different subjects. Chronological age itself is a poor predictor of performance and ageing is so highly individualized that average curves give only a rough approximation of patterns of ageing followed by individuals. Gerontologists now appreciate the importance of lifestyle in the ageing process, but very little is understood about how critical events such as retirement, onset of pathology, loss of mobility and death of a spouse actually affect performance.

So different methods for studying ageing all contribute to our understanding, but they have their own advantages and disadvantages; by critically combining data from a variety of sources, a fuller picture of the biology of ageing can be gained.

MAINTENANCE OF HOMEOSTASIS IN ELDERLY PEOPLE

In the study of human ageing there is a tendency to compartmentalize, considering changes in single systems within the body (e.g. blood glucose control or kidney function) without thinking of the function of the individual as a whole. However, it is whole body function that matters ultimately, i.e. can the individual manage an independent life? From a physiological viewpoint, the health of a person depends on the efficient functioning of the individual cells and tissues in all systems of the body, i.e. on maintaining the stability of the internal environment. The maintenance of this steady state (despite variations in both internal and external environments), or homeostasis, involves a complex series of physiological and biochemical changes and responses and almost all organs and systems in the body participate in this process, albeit to different degrees.

Is homeostasis maintained in the elderly? The simple answer is yes, since most older people are able to live a normal independent life, and most processes in the body appear to function adequately under basal or resting conditions. However, it is true to say that most physiological processes in the body become less effective under certain circumstances with increasing age and it is generally accepted that with ageing there is a decline in the functional competence of the individual. This decline in function may be due in part to the progressive loss of functioning body cells — i.e. there is a gradual loss of body tissue in many systems with age. The age-related deficits that exist are apparent only when the body or system is physiologically stressed, e.g. by illness, strenuous exercise, or exposure to extreme environmental temperatures. So, values for body temperature, blood glucose, and so on do not change significantly under resting conditions but if these values are increased for some reason, changes are often greater in older people than younger ones and more time is required to return the parameter back to its original value.

Elderly people do become more susceptible to disturbance of fluid and electrolyte balance. Reflexes that maintain blood pressure when going from lying to standing positions become less efficient and some elderly people are prone to develop postural hypotension (this is probably one of the factors associated with an increase in the incidence of falls in the elderly). Liver and renal function is less efficient and so metabolism and excretion of drugs are altered, and drugs can accumulate in the body more easily and reach toxic levels.

Therefore, disorders of homeostasis with age can be considered to arise not by virtue of changes in equilibrium levels, but in the efficiency with which these steady states can be re-established once displacement has occurred. This is sometimes described as a decline in the adaptive ability of the body to cope with changes or stress imposed. Thus, homeostasis is still maintained, but with increasing difficulty as the years pass by.

FUNCTIONAL RESERVE WITHIN SYSTEMS

It is characteristic of many biological systems that each has a certain amount of 'spare capacity' or functional reserve. An obvious example is that we can manage perfectly well with one kidney although we are born with two. This is an important concept because it relates to the decline in function shown by researchers to occur with ageing; because of this reserve a decline in function may proceed for many years without lowering the functional capacity below that required for homeostasis (Fig. 3.1). It is only when the functional capacity can no longer meet homeostasic needs that failure becomes evident (Johnson 1985). So system failure occurs only when the spare capacity or functional reserves are depleted below the levels required for homeostasis — and this may happen only after years of continual loss of function.

An example of this is coronary arteriosclerosis (the thickening and loss of elasticity of the arterial

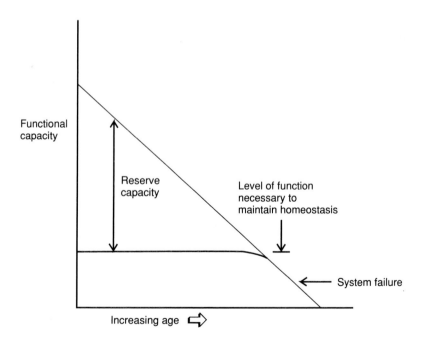

Fig. 3.1 System failure occures only when functional reserve is depleted and homeostatic needs can no longer be met.

walls) which begins in childhood and in many individuals is well advanced by the age of 30. This steady loss of coronary vessel function usually goes unnoticed because there is still an adequate perfusion of the myocardium — in other words, because there is no effect on homeostatic function.

FLEXIBILITY AND ADAPTABILITY

Another complicating factor in studying homeostasis is that the decline in function of the various systems of the body is not uniform, and some aspects do not appear to deteriorate to any great extent. For instance, velocity of nerve conduction does not decline very much, whereas muscle strength does show a measurable decline in function.

The complexities of looking at homeostasis are illustrated by a study by Rodeheffer et al (1984), who looked at cardiac function under resting and exercise conditions in fit subjects ranging in age from 26 to 79. It has been widely stated in the literature that cardiac output (the output of the heart per minute) decreases with increasing age. However, Rodeheffer et al found that resting cardiac output in these fit subjects was not age-related and that with exercise there was no age-related decline in cardiac output even at high levels of exercise. There were, however, differences in the way the young and elderly subjects achieved the increased cardiac output under exercise stress. Cardiac output can be increased by increasing either or both the heart rate and stroke volume (the amount of blood ejected per beat by the ventricle). The young subjects achieved the improved cardiac output primarily by increasing the heart rate, whereas the elderly people, whose maximum achievable heart rate had decreased with age, achieved the increase primarily by increasing the stroke volume.

This study demonstrates a key feature of the body's response to ageing: there is considerable inherent flexibility and adaptability of the physiological processes in the body, so that if one organ or system is compromised (or perhaps has 'aged' more), then other systems and mechanisms can take over to compensate. This adaptability is seen in many circumstances.

PHYSICAL CAPACITY

One aspect of ageing that is often very obvious is a decline in the physical capacities affecting exercise, agility and mobility. These depend on co-ordination between many systems in the body; for example, muscles, joints, the cardiovascular and respiratory systems, balance, neural factors and 'skill' all affect the ability to perform physical activity. Often in elderly people (this is again a generalization!) you can see a decline in fitness, stamina and muscle strength. Some of these changes are due to the ageing process itself and some are due to the harmful or negative effects of inactivity. There are ageing changes in joints, cartilage and collagen, and an increase in osteoporosis and a decline in the number of muscle cells, which could account for some of the observed changes. The cardiovascular system is not thought to be the limiting factor normally, and certainly skill factors are retained and can often compensate for the decline in strength. Structural and functional changes in the respiratory system seem to be important in restricting severe exercise and certainly the psychological factors of decreased confidence, self-esteem and motivation probably account for some of the decline (Young 1986).

Aniansson et al (1980) looked at simpler movements, including activities of living, rather than at exercise capacity per se. They investigated, for instance, manual dexterity (e.g. putting a plug in a socket or a key in a lock), aspects of hygiene and dressing activities, ability to get up from a stool, function in the kitchen (e.g. lifting objects onto shelves, pouring water from a jug), dialling numbers on a phone, stepping onto a platform on a bus and the most comfortable walking speed across pedestrian crossings. Studies like these, evaluating activities of living, can form the basis for recommendations to create an environment that is adapted to the needs of elderly people — an environment that would provide, among other things, strategically placed handrails, well-designed furniture and pedestrian 'walk' signals that would give elderly people enough time to cross the road.

By the time they are in their 80s, the maximum contraction that many elderly people can generate in their quadriceps (thigh muscles) is just enough to get up from a chair without using their arms; if they use their arms to help push up, then they need less strength in their quadriceps. The classic 'armless chair' is the toilet — this is why handrails, etc. are so useful for some elderly people.

Once at this stage the ageing changes then greatly interfere with the ability to lead a normal independent life. This brings us back to the point discussed earlier about maintaining activity levels in older people. So often with the change in lifestyle that accompanies advancing age, physical activity in general declines and cardiorespiratory and muscular systems in particular become 'deconditioned'. Physical deconditioning will accentuate age-related declines in performance, particularly in response to physiological stress. So appropriate activity and exercise (be it simply standing to do the washing up, walking upstairs to the toilet or hill-walking in the Lake District) should be encouraged for all elderly people; there is still likely to be an overall decline in capacity but it will be less if the individual is fitter. (This is a message to all of us who have a tendency to 'do things' for older people, thinking we are helping them; we may not be helping at all).

FUNCTIONAL CHANGES WITH AGEING

The last section emphasized the importance of considering the interrelationships between ageing in the various systems in the body as a whole. It is still valuable to consider more discrete individual systems too, provided the reader remembers that a decline in function may not mean impaired homeostasis (see Functional Reserve within Systems, p. 43). A detailed and comprehensive review of ageing changes is beyond the scope of this chapter. However, the discussion below selects some important aspects for further consideration.

NUTRITION AND GASTROINTESTINAL TRACT

One of the earliest findings in experimental gerontology was that food restriction significantly increased the length of life of rats; this was work done by Clive McCay and colleagues in the 1930s (McCay et al 1935), and these findings have been repeatedly confirmed. The relationship of nutrition to the ageing process in humans is complex. The role of nutrition in maintaining normal body function and also in prevention of negative changes is well accepted now. In McCay's work, dietary restriction prolonged the life of rats — in many instances, because of the delayed onset of chronic diseases — and was accompanied by better retention of many physiological functions. With any experiments on laboratory-kept animals one must keep in mind the fact that controlled laboratory conditions bear little relation to normal situations in the wild, where the animals would hunt for food and get exercise

As already seen, there is a progressive decline throughout adult life in many physiological functions which are accompanied by changes in body composition (Fig. 3.2) and in metabolism of nutrients. There is little evidence relating human

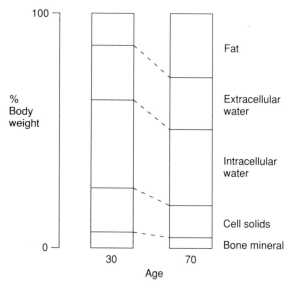

Fig. 3.2 Approximate changes in body composition with ageing. (Individual variations are large.)

nutrition to these fundamental changes, except with regard to the role of diet in the development of osteoporosis. Many dietary factors (calcium, phosphorus, vitamin D both from the diet and skin, protein, fluoride and fibre) are implicated in determining the extent of osteoporotic bone loss, as is the extent of weight-bearing use.

It is well established that food intake diminishes with age, but little is directly known about the nutrient requirements of the elderly and whether the reduced intakes of elderly people fall below desirable levels. The study by McGandy et al (1966), which looked at the reduction in energy intake with age, showed that there was a reduction in basal metabolic rate (approximately 200 kcal) which parallels the decline in lean body mass resulting mainly from a reduced muscle mass. The reduction in energy intake is also due to a much larger decline in physical activity undertaken by elderly people (400 kcal reduction in energy expenditure). Exton-Smith (1980), in a study of 70–80 year olds, showed a more rapid reduction in energy intake in later years due to disabilities limiting the physical activity of the ageing person. Studies of energy intakes of nursing Home patients, whose immobility is often considerable, confirm this.

As a consequence of this decreased energy requirement, energy intake (i.e. the amount of food eaten) throughout adult life declines, and so the essential nutrients present in the energy source (food) are liable to be eaten in smaller amounts by the ageing individual. Studies have shown varying results; McGandy et al (1966), for example, only found a slight reduction in intakes of iron, thiamine, riboflavin and niacin, and no reduction in intake of calcium, vitamin A and ascorbic acid as age increased. However, other studies looking at elderly people from less privileged groups (Exton-Smith & Stanton 1965) have shown that intakes of all nutrients underwent extensive reductions during the period of 70–80 years of age.

However, it is not known whether this reduced intake brings the older person to levels below the levels of adequacy. The specific recommended dietary allowances (RDAs) are just not known for the elderly. Do the needs of elderly people for individual nutrients become less, remain the same, or possibly even increase, from factors such as

malabsorption? This again underlies the desirability of remaining physically active into old age, with the double advantage of maintaining energy expenditure and physical fitness.

There are many changes in the gastrointestinal tract, some of which are briefly described below. However, despite all these changes, the function of the gut is usually adequate. This is another illustration of there being reserve capacity within biological systems, so that loss of function does not necessarily impair function.

In the oral cavity, dental decay and gum recession can lead to inadequate dentition. Salivary flow, too, is reduced in individuals after the age of 50. Atrophic gastritis, reducing gastric secretion, is common in elderly people but there is debate as to whether this is a pathological process. In the small intestine the villi shorten and become broader which significantly reduces the surface area for absorption; but there is no evidence that absorption of major nutrients is impaired in a healthy older person. Amino acid absorption does not appear to be impaired although lipid absorption is reduced. The liver is reduced in size and weight and in the number of hepatocytes, which leads to some reduced storage capacity and function. The digestive functions of the pancreas are well conserved. In the colon there is atrophy of mucosa and muscle layers leading to reduced and weaker peristaltic action. There is an increased incidence of diverticulae and reduced elasticity of the rectal wall, which gives a reduced maximal tolerance to faeces.

Throughout the gut and associated organs (liver, pancreas, etc.) there is a reduction in perfusion and a reduction in the co-ordination of the enteric nerve reflexes which co-ordinate events in the gut. Despite all these changes, function in 'healthy' elderly people remains adequate. Constipation is a frequent occurrence in old age and has a multifactorial aetiology: loss of muscle tone and motor activity in the colon, a low-fibre diet, reduced mobility, a rise in the threshold of stimulation for initiation of defaecation reflexes and damage by laxative abuse all contribute.

Malnutrition does occur in elderly people and its causes are wide ranging — from ignorance regarding the need for a balanced diet, to social isolation, poverty which restricts the range of food available to some old people, mental disorders such as confusion, excessive intake of alcohol and use of therapeutic drugs which can interfere with nutrient utilization, as well as changes in the gastrointestinal tract itself.

THE IMMUNE SYSTEM

It is well established that there is a general decline in immunocompetence with ageing (Hausman & Weksler 1985), which could be an important contributor to senescence and to the development of chronic diseases and disorders. The evidence of a role for the immune system in ageing is more convincing for the diseases of old age rather than for the normal processes of ageing. As immunological efficiency decreases, there is an increased incidence of infections, autoimmune diseases and cancer. However, some theories suggest that normal ageing is the consequence of a developing immunodeficiency; these are attractive theories since they imply that the process might then be potentially accessible to manipulation!

The immune system, which is distributed throughout the body and interacts with all other systems, provides a vital aspect of defence of the internal environment. The immune system recognizes foreign molecules (antigens) and acts to immobilize, neutralize or destroy them. When it operates effectively, this system protects the body from a wide variety of infectious agents as well as from abnormal body cells. When it fails, malfunctions or is disabled, some of the most devastating diseases, such as cancer, rheumatoid arthritis and AIDS may result.

Humoral and cell-mediated immunity are the two main components of a functioning immune system and the responsiveness of both decline with increasing age. With ageing, lymphoid tissue is lost from the thymus, spleen, lymph nodes and bone marrow. Present evidence suggests that the major change in the system is in the T-cells or T-lymphocytes that mature in the thymus gland. T-cells are the non–antibody producing lymphocytes that constitute the cell-mediated arm of immunity. These T-cells directly attack and lyse body cells infected by viruses or other intracellular parasites, cancer cells and foreign grafts, and release chemical mediators that enhance the inflammatory response or help to activate lymphocytes or macrophages. Changes in the B-cells which are responsible for the humoral response (i.e. by circulating antibodies) are smaller and often secondary to changes in T-cell-population.

The involution of the thymus gland during the first half of life may explain the altered formation and function of the immune system observed during the second half of life. The thymus gland is at its maximum size at sexual maturity and after puberty its size decreases; by the age of 45–50 only 5–10% of the cellular mass of the thymus remains. The concentration of thymic hormones in the serum begins to decline between the ages of 20–30 and thymic hormones can no longer be detected after 60 years of age (Lewis et al 1978). The thymus is the site of differentiation of immature lymphocytes from the bone marrow; the lymphocytes then enter the cortex of the thymus gland and eventually become T-lymphocytes.

The level of natural antibodies also decreases with age and there is an increase in auto-antibodies (i.e. antibodies which react against an antigenic component of the individual's own tissues). Auto-antibodies to nucleic acids (e.g. DNA, RNA), smooth muscle, mitochondria, lymphocytes, gastric parietal cells, immunoglobulins and thyroglobulin have all been found with increased frequency in old people.

Almost all studies show a decline in the antibody response with age. Abundant evidence exists to show how the immune system changes with age. To summarize, cell-mediated and humoral immune response to foreign antigens decreases whilst response to autologous (belonging to the same organism) antigens increases. The changes are undoubtedly complex, and one problem is that age-associated changes in the immune system do not always distinguish between an immune system impaired by age (i.e. an ageing change itself) and an immune system compromised by the environment within an elderly host (i.e. a consequence of other ageing changes within the individual). Environmental factors known to influence immune competence include disease, nutrition and exposure to ionising radiation.

The possible relationship between nutrition and immunity in the elderly is interesting. It is known that both undernutrition and overnutrition suppress immune responses in the body. Chandra and colleagues have studied the effects of dietary intake, nutritional status and risk of infection in old age (Chandra & Puri 1985); they argue that impairment of the immune response is not an inevitable part of ageing, as some elderly people are as immunocompetent as young people. Chandra and colleagues have demonstrated that both nutritional supplementation and regular moderate exercise can positively influence immune competence. Also, the duration of illness in those elderly people taking nutritional supplementation was reduced, i.e. people taking supplements were ill for a shorter time.

THE ENDOCRINE SYSTEM

The endocrine system plays a central role in many of the body's regulatory and adaptive responses. Some of the early work gave conflicting information on age-related changes in endocrine function; as with other systems in the body, there are many complicating factors or influences that need to be taken into consideration. For instance, disease, medications, smoking, alcohol, diet, exercise, percentage body fat, social factors and methodological factors can all influence hormone levels and so make it difficult to say whether any changes observed are due to ageing or reflect alterations in some other parameter. At one time the thyroid gland was thought to be implicated in ageing since some of the features of hypothyroidism are similar to observations in ageing (e.g. drying of skin, loss of hair); however, the capacity to maintain a euthyroid ('normal') state continues during ageing in many elderly people despite some changes in overall secretion and metabolism, and there is no significant change in plasma thyroid hormone levels.

Studies on the endocrine system now extend beyond simple measurement of blood hormone levels under different physiological stresses, since it is appreciated that the plasma levels of a particular hormone depend upon many factors, for instance secretion of regulatory hormones, transport around the body, binding with receptors on target cells

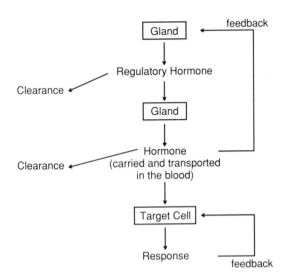

Fig. 3.3 The sequence of hormone action and regulation. Clearance refers to removal from the blood, and feedback is usually negative.

and the clearance of the hormones from the blood. Figure 3.3 shows some of these stages.

Many of the endocrine glands do seem to decrease in weight and to develop a patchy atrophic appearance accompanied by vascular changes and fibrosis. Basal (resting) hormonal levels are generally not influenced by age, but some elderly people have reduced serum levels of the most active forms, e.g. renin, aldosterone, T3 and, in men, an androgen known as dihydroepiandrosterone. There does seem to be a decline in the secretion rate of many hormones with advancing age, but at the same time as there is a reduced clearance rate from the circulation — the net result being 'normal' hormone levels. Thus the body seems to retain the capacity to adjust hormone secretion in order to maintain stable plasma levels of hormones.

A range of effects are apparent in the endocrine system with ageing. For instance, there is no major impact of ageing on some important endocrine functions, e.g. the reserve capacity to secrete cortisol appears unchanged with advancing age. However, growth hormone secretion is reduced in certain situations; in particular, there is a decline in its normal secretion during sleep.

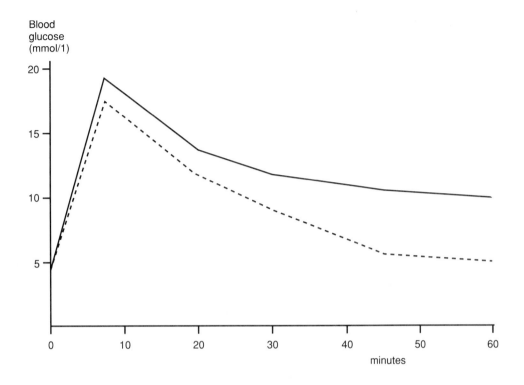

Fig. 3.4 Effect of glucose administration on young and elderly subjects.

—————— age 60 – 70 years

- - - - age 20 – 30 years

On the other hand, ageing may mimic a disorder with a major morbidity. For instance, carbohydrate intolerance leads to a progressive increase in blood glucose levels with ageing; although this may share certain common mechanisms or clinical complications, it can be distinguished from clinical diabetes. What may be happening is that ageing is eroding the physiological reserve of the endocrine systems; this may in turn be related to the expression of disease or the increased mortality known to be associated with certain other stresses, e.g. burns and surgery, in advancing age. The sympatho-adrenal system is a modifier of much of the endocrine system and ageing appears to be associated with an enhanced sympathetic response (see The Nervous System, p. 51). This may in turn influence other endocrine functions such as carbohydrate tolerance.

The age-related impairment in the capacity to maintain carbohydrate homeostasis after a glucose challenge, e.g. in a glucose tolerance test, has been known for years (Davidson 1979). Some clinical studies indicate a very slight age-related increase after maturity in fasting blood glucose levels in healthy people, but the most striking change is the elevation in blood glucose levels after oral or intravenous glucose loads (Fig. 3.4). This age-related impairment in glucose metabolism is less marked but still present after very careful screening for factors such as diet, lack of exercise and increased adiposity that influence blood glucose metabolism. Ageing does seem to be associated with marked insulin resistance, possibly due to loss of insulin receptors, but the precise mechanisms for insulin insensitivity with ageing are still unknown. There also seems to be a marked impairment in the ability to dispose of glucose with increasing age. So there is some genuine impairment of glucose utilization with age, partly due to explainable changes but possibly also from ageing changes. There is also evidence that some of the well-known ageing changes are linked with high levels of glucose in the body; there is a similarity between tissue changes in diabetes and in ageing, e.g. senile cataracts, joint stiffness and atherosclerosis (Furth & Harding 1989). This is discussed further under Theories of Ageing, p. 56.

THE RESPIRATORY AND CARDIOVASCULAR SYSTEMS

The respiratory and cardiovascular systems work together to ensure that an adequate supply of oxygen is delivered to the tissues and that carbon dioxide is removed from the body. The cardiovascular system also has a more general role in transporting heat and substances such as nutrients, hormones and waste products around the body.

A variety of structural changes occur in the thorax and lung with ageing and have an adverse effect on function (see also Ch. 10). For example, there are changes in lung volume and capacity that result in a reduced surface area being available for gas exchange, e.g. the fraction of lung volume occupied by the airways increases at the expense of alveolar space and the alveoli become smaller. The lung tissue seems to lose its elasticity due primarily to stiffening changes in the collagen. More muscular work is required to move air in and out of the lungs, due to the stiffening of ribs and other joints in the thorax and the structural changes in the lung tissue.

One of the main defence mechanisms in the lungs to protect against inhaled particulate matter is sometimes described as the 'mucociliary escalator'. This depends on particles being trapped in the layer of mucus lining the larger airways, after which the mucus is 'wafted' up to the larynx by beating movements of the cilia (hair-like projections) situated on the bronchial epithelium. With ageing, cilia are lost from the airways and the 'vigour' of the remaining cilia is reduced. Thus

the mucus escalator is less effective in removing debris. Macrophages that form the last line of defence 'further down' the airways at the alveolar levels also become less efficient. These changes partly account for the increased incidence of respiratory infections in the elderly.

Thus there is an age-related loss of respiratory function. The loss of function is substantially greater in smokers than in non-smokers and some return in function does occur if smokers give up; this is a strong reason for advising cessation of smoking at any age, but particularly for older people, when a decline in respiratory function can already be compromising.

The study of ageing changes in the cardiovascular system has been dogged by methodological problems. It is difficult to get a 'coronary-artery-disease-free' population for study so that ageing changes rather than disease-induced changes can be investigated. It is also particularly important when comparing the cardiovascular function of young and older subjects to ensure that the level of physical conditioning or fitness is similar in subjects of all ages; heart rate, blood pressure and other cardiorespiratory parameters vary substantially according to the amount of physical activity normally undertaken.

The notion that there is a substantial obligatory decline in cardiovascular function at rest is not supported by the research. It has been shown that in subjects living independent (i.e. non-institutional) lives, cardiac output (i.e. heart rate and stroke volume) is not markedly affected by age (see Rodeheffer et al's (1984) work discussed earlier). However, there are changes in the various components of the cardiovascular system. The heart and blood vessels are highly dependent for their normal function on the physical properties of connective tissue and muscle, namely distensibility, contractitility and elasticity, and these alter with ageing. Heart weight, as a fraction of body weight, tends to increase slightly. Sometimes a mild left ventricular hypertrophy develops as an adaptive response to the changes in aortic compliance that occurs (due to changes in collagen in blood vessel walls). There is a change in the character of the connective tissue matrix which leads to some stiffness of the myocardium. Despite some loss of cells in the sinoatrial node of the heart, the pacemaker function seems unimpaired.

The blood vessels undergo changes with ageing, too. There are major structural alterations in the arteries due to an increase in collagen and smooth muscle which leads to increased arterial stiffness and reduced compliance with increasing age. As elsewhere in the body, collagen tends to become cross-linked and calcium is deposited in the framework. Veins become increasingly tortuous, the walls become weaker due to loss of elastic tissue and varicosities occur in veins subjected to high pressure. The basement membrane of the capillary endothelium becomes thicker and the fenestrations (windows) of the endothelium become fewer. These changes in the capillary structure in association with the increased density of ground substance of connective tissues impairs the diffusion of gases and nutrients to and from the cells.

The work done by the heart tends to reduce slightly with age, whilst the total peripheral resistance increases at a rate of approximately 1% per year from the age of 40 onwards (Kenney 1989). Thus, there is a tendency for perfusion of the organs in the body to be reduced, although the extent of this reduction varies considerably. Blood flow to the kidneys is reduced by up to 50% and there are also large decreases in the splanchnic and cutaneous circulations. Cerebral blood flow is thought to reduce by 20%. Changes in resting blood flow to the myocardium and skeletal muscle is less marked; however, the ability to increase blood flow to these tissues when required, e.g. following tissue hypoxia, is reduced in older people.

Many of the factors mentioned above would be expected to increase arterial pressure. Both longitudinal and cross-sectional studies have shown an increase in systolic pressure with age with a smaller rate of increase in the diastolic pressure. In the very old, diastolic pressure may fall. There is debate, however, as to whether this increase in blood pressure is an inevitable consequence of normal healthy ageing. Individuals who live in isolated, primitive societies do not show an increase in blood pressure as they age, nor do chronic psychiatric patients who grow old in a protected institutional environment (Kenney 1989). It may well be that the age-related rise in pressure is a consequence of other factors such as diet and social stresses.

As discussed earlier, some early research showed a reduced ability of the cardiovascular system to adapt to stress or exercise with increasing age, but the extent of the changes have been exaggerated due to effects of deconditioning and undiagnosed coronary artery disease; physical endurance of many older people is much greater than some earlier studies indicated. There is a true age-related decline in the maximum heart rate that can be achieved with age and the decline seems to be approximately linear. Several equations are used to predict this decline, but one that is widely accepted was proposed by Astrand and Rodahl (1977):

$$\text{Maximum heart rate} = 210 - (0.65 \times \text{age}).$$

So, for a person aged 75, it would be approximately 162.

The decline in achievable maximum heart rate has been suggested to be due to a change in the number of β-adrenergic receptors, a reduced release of neurotransmitters or changes in the sinoatrial node. Some studies put forward a strong case to suggest that there is a diminished target organ responsiveness to β-adrenergic stimulation and that this could be a key mechanism for the age-related differences in many facets of the stress response (Lakatta 1983).

THE NERVOUS SYSTEM

The general picture of the ageing nervous system is of declining efficiency although, as with other systems, function is maintained. There are enormous inconsistencies in research findings on the ageing brain, often due to methodological problems. Some of the losses or decrements observed in the central nervous system (CNS) may in fact reflect an age-dependent decline in the need or use of certain circuits. Brain weight and volume have been shown to decline with age (this seems to occur more rapidly after the age of 60), but in carefully screened mentally normal older individuals these declines are probably not significant. Some investigators have reported neuronal loss in selected layers and regions of the ageing human cortex, but not in most brain stem structures (where the vital centres that control functions such as heart rate, blood pressure and respiration are located). Neurofibrillary tangles and senile plaques are seen in the brains of aged normal people and patients with neuropathology (Chapter 19). Results are available which support almost any type of age-dependent change in CNS circuitry — loss of synapses, increases, or no change at all! Synaptic growth and remodelling probably occurs well into old age and can repair small injuries or 'nicks' in brain circuitry.

As mentioned previously, cerebral blood flow does decrease with age, but adequate oxygen delivery is maintained as oxygen extraction from the blood is increased (more oxygen is released from the haemoglobin). The vertebral arteries that deliver blood to the brain tend to become tortuous with ageing due to changes in the vertebrae and intervertebral discs and may become kinked with movements of the neck. This can lead to transient ischaemic attacks to which many old people are prone.

There are changes in patterns of neurotransmission with changes in synthesis, storage and release of neurotransmitters. Changes in the metabolism of neurotransmitters can have profound effects on both behavioural and regulatory systems. The cholinergic system has been studied because of its involvement in memory and disorders such as Parkinsonism and Alzheimer's disease. Alzheimer's-type dementia is discussed in detail in Chapter 19. There is also reduced velocity of conduction of nerve impulses with age. Some of the reflexes, e.g. Achilles tendon reflex, are depressed and reaction time is longer by about 30% (i.e. slower reactions) in old subjects: some of this deterioration is due to nerve changes, but some to a reduction in muscle power and stiffer joints.

The autonomic nervous system is clearly affected by age in humans (Collins et al 1980). Autonomic dysfunctions are implicated in many pathophysiological changes of age, including postural hypotension, impaired thermoregulation and gastrointestinal function, urinary incontinence and impaired penile erection in men. It is not known whether these changes stem from central control (i.e. within the brain) or from a lower level.

A relatively consistent picture of sympathetic activity has begun to emerge, showing that plasma noradrenaline levels increase in ageing humans. It is not resolved as yet as to whether this is due to release of more noradrenaline or whether clearance (removal from the blood) of noradrenaline is reduced (this type of 'shift' in metabolism was discussed also under The Endocrine System, p. 48). Thus plasma noradrenaline appears to rise more readily in response to most stimuli, seems to require longer periods to return to its baseline and may well exhibit higher baseline levels.

In contrast to this trend toward increased activity of the sympathetic nervous system, many tissues and organs themselves seem to become less responsive to sympathetic stimulation with ageing. For instance, blood pressure and cardiovascular responses to stimuli such as tilting, standing or exercise, which test the function of sympathetic reflexes, are often significantly reduced with ageing. The whole area is complex, since not all tissues become less responsive with age, and the extent of decline varies among individuals. The decrease in cardiac responsiveness with age is also probably due to a decrease in sensitivity to adrenergic stimulation.

Although less is known about the parasympathetic nervous system, age-correlated impairments are also reported in this system. Thus, substantial alterations in autonomic function occur during ageing; these changes are likely to play an important role in the decline of normal physiological homeostasis.

THE SPECIAL SENSES

Hearing is at its most efficient in both acuity (clearness) and range of perceived frequencies at age 10 and it becomes gradually impaired with advancing age. There is a particular decline in sensitivity for higher frequencies and this loss contributes significantly to difficulty in understanding speech. There are changes in all parts of the ear. The tympanic membrane becomes more rigid and there is an increased rigidity of the bones in the middle ear along with some loss of muscle fibres. In the inner ear there are changes in the

Reissner's and basilar membranes and a significant loss of hair cells in the Organ of Corti. It has also been shown that there is a gradual loss of ganglion cells and fibres of the auditory nerve and that neurons are lost throughout the auditory pathway in the brain. The auditory orientating reflex, i.e. the location of sounds, becomes slower and less accurate with age, contributing perhaps to the confusion that some older people show when in a three- or four-way conversation. It is no wonder, with all these changes, that there is a marked hearing loss with age: presbyacusis is the term used for these changes.

Vision is affected by age, too. There is a loss of retro-orbital fat around the eye, which leads to recession of the eye; loss of elastic tissue of the eyebrow and upper lid can lead to ptosis and occlusion of the upper visual field, whilst loss of elastic tissue in the lower lid may allow the lid to fall forwards, separating the lid from the eye and interfering with the normal drainage of tears. Tear production also diminishes, which can lead to dry eyes. The cornea and conjunctiva become thinner. The diameter of the pupil is at a maximum in early teens and gets smaller to a minimum around the age of 60. Changes in the fibrous network of the iris fixes the pupil at this small size and substantially impairs the amount of light admitted. This leads to a rise in the threshold for light perception and an increase in the level of illumination necessary for reading. An arcus senilis (a white ring encircling about 1 mm within the corneal margin) is a corneal degeneration that is often apparent, but does not itself damage sight.

Presbyopia, the loss of ability to accommodate for near vision, is well known, and is essentially due to loss of flexibility of the lens, making it is unable to adapt its shape appropriately and so focus the image on the retina properly. The lens continues to grow throughout life by laying down new cells on the surface of the lens; consequently the lens gets thicker with increasing age. The near point (the distance from the eye at which print can be read) begins to recede; at the age of 20 it is about 10 cm from the eye, but by the age of 70 is about 100 cm. This explains the common experience of having to hold books further and further away in order to be able to read them.

Receptors are lost from the retina, mainly the rods of the peripheral retina, and this reduces the size of the visual field. There are minor losses of receptors at the fovea (the area of clearest vision), which leads to loss of visual acuity. The chemical processes of vision involving photochemical pigments become impaired, so that adaptation to dark/light conditions occurs more slowly and to a lesser extent.

The sense of taste and smell undergo deteriorative changes, too. The taste papillae on the tongue degenerate and the number of taste buds is reduced. Some reports have shown a reduction by two thirds in the number of taste buds between childhood and age 80. Loss of taste sensation is also exacerbated by a reduced saliva flow and reduced content of amylase, which starts the digestive process. This can lead to the pleasure of eating being diminished with possible nutritional consequences. A decrease in taste sensation may also result in excessive sugar and salt being used, which is undesirable. Also, the sense of taste acts as a protective mechanism and this too is diminished.

Maintenance of balance relies on an integration of responses from the visual system, the vestibular system in the inner ear and from proprioceptors in muscles and joints. Older people require greater angular movements in the joints for proprioceptor perception to be achieved. The increased sway seen when elderly people stand still with their eyes closed demonstrates the reduced efficiency of vestibular and proprioceptor systems.

THE SKIN

All tissues in the skin, including the hair, undergo regressive changes and although there is no 'skin failure' as such with ageing, old skin can and does impair the quality of life.

Very little is known about the changes that occur in the hair, despite grey hair being one of the most obvious signs of ageing. Paradoxically, the hair on the head thins but there is an increase in hairs in the nose, ears and eyebrows. Scalp hair growth rate decreases, with noticeable thinning past the age of 65; most people over 40 have some greying of the hair. The tendency to go grey is inherited, as is baldness.

The structure of the skin is altered with ageing. The epidermis flattens because of the loss of papillae; the papillae are responsible for the undulating contour (rather like egg boxes!) which ensures good adhesion between the layers of the skin. This loss of papillae reduces the strength of attachment between the dermis and epidermis. Consequently, a shearing force produced say, during poor lifting techniques, will more readily peel off the epidermis in ageing skin; this is one of the contributing factors to the predisposition of elderly individuals to develop pressure sores (see Chapter 14). The precise cause of the 'wrinkle', one of the most telltale signs of ageing, is still unexplained, but is probably due to some changes in the collagen and elastin components of the dermis. Figure 3.5 shows the difference between young and old skin.

Throughout the skin are a large number of nerve endings that are sensitive to temperature, pain, touch, and pressure, and some of these nerve endings are affected by age. Observations suggest that pain and thermal sensation are diminished and this increased threshold of pain sensation means that some elderly people are less capable of sensing danger, for instance hot surfaces, and may not act appropriately. Tactile sensitivity diminishes with age as well. In the very old, sensitivity to pain seems to increase again and it has been suggested that this is due to the excessive thinning of the skin which allows a greater number of nerve endings to be stimulated.

There is regression and disorganization of small blood vessels and capillaries in the skin and as this will reduce the supply of fluid, nutrients, etc. to the skin it may account for thinning hair and reduced sweating. This degeneration of the small vessels is almost certainly an intrinsic age change and progresses relentlessly even in protected skin. Topical therapy, where drugs are absorbed into the body via the skin, may not be as effective in elderly people as it is in younger people due to these changes in the microcirculation. The changes in the connective tissue in the dermis result in a loss of support for the cutaneous vessels, leading

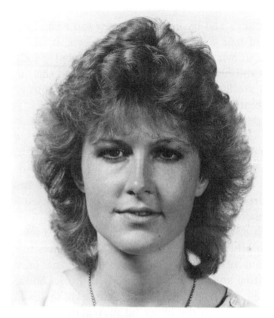

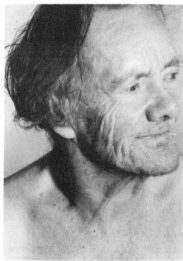

Fig. 3.5 Young and old skin.

to increased fragility and the easy or spontaneous bruising often seen in elderly people.

The acute inflammatory reactions in the skin are reduced in elderly people and this again leads to a decrease in obvious danger signals. Surgical experience clearly shows that even the very old (beyond 85) can effectively repair extensive wounds, but on the whole, the wounds do take longer to heal. The tensile strength of 5-day wounds is considerably reduced in elderly people and collagen deposition slower (Sandblum et al 1953). This is important to remember when caring for old people after surgery. Wound dehiscence is more common in the elderly. With regard to more superficial wounds, re-epithelialization takes twice as long for 75 year olds as it does for 25 year olds (Orentreich & Selmanowitz 1969). As usual, there is considerable variation amongst elderly people with respect to ageing and changes in the skin.

SUPPORTING TISSUES

Connective tissue, cartilage and bone are the three major supporting tissues of the body, and changes in these tissues are widespread with ageing. Connective tissue has two major components: the ground substance, which consists of mucopolysaccharides in the form of a hydrated gel, and fibrous proteins (collagen, elastin and reticular fibres). With age there is an increased density of fibres, meaning that the volume occupied by the ground substance is reduced. The gel also becomes less hydrated. Consequently, the diffusion of material through the connective tissue is impaired and mobility of cells (e.g. macrophages) is reduced. These changes threaten both the nutrition of cells and the repair processes. The collagen fibres increase in size and number and cross-linkage occurs between fibres and so the collagen becomes more stable. The elastic fibres also undergo cross-linkage and become more rigid.

The normal elastic properties of cartilage are lost, too, as it loses water and fibres are deposited. The increased fibre density in connective tissue and cartilage provide a 'mesh' for the deposition of calcium and this accounts for the increased calcification seen with ageing.

Connective tissue is widespread — it is found just about everywhere in the body and so the changes in connective tissue affect every part of the body. As we have already seen, skin loses its elasticity and becomes wrinkled, the lungs lose their elastic recoil and the costal cartilages become increasingly rigid, making breathing harder, and joints in the body become stiffened by the increase in fibrous tissue. The loss of hydration in the cartilage in the intervertebral discs leads to compaction of the vertebrae and shrinkage in stature. The cardiovascular system, which depends to a great extent on the properties of distensibility and elasticity, is adversely affected: the chambers of the heart become less distensible; there is reduced contractility; the valves of the heart become stiffer; and the elastic arteries become more rigid.

Bone tends to lose mineral as it ages — this process is known as osteoporosis. The bone tends to erode from within whilst deposition occurs at a slower rate on the outer surface. Thus, the external diameter of the bone increases, but the walls become thinner. This thinning of the cortex of the long bones weakens them and fractures can occur even under slight loads.

The loss of bone mass is greater in women than in men. Longitudinal studies, starting just before the subjects reached menopause, found that the rate of loss of bone is most rapid within 5–10 years after the menopause and after that there is a fall in the rate of loss (Johnston et al 1979). There are many factors involved in this bone loss, including the size of the initial bone mass, which depends on genetic factors, the individual's sex, the amount of physical activity undertaken, and nutritional factors in early life. Girls at the age of 18 have a 20% lower bone mass in relation to body weight than males. Thus females start off with less bone; together with the rapid loss after the age of 50, this means that there is likely to be a higher prevalence of osteoporosis in older women.

It is not oestrogen deficiency alone that determines post-menopausal osteoporosis. Several other hormones are believed to be involved, namely parathyroid hormone, vitamin D, calcium and possibly also progesterone and corticosteroids. Oestrogen deficiency may accelerate bone loss by increasing the sensitivity of bone to the resorbing (breakdown) action of parathyroid hormone, which leads to an increase in calcium released from the bone and increased renal excretion of calcium. Hormone replacement therapy measurably decreases bone loss by suppressing bone turnover.

Calcium and vitamin D play a role in determining age-related bone loss. Calcium absorption from the gut may fall with age and vitamin D levels are sometimes low. Low vitamin D levels are believed to be due primarily to a lack of exposure to sunlight, limiting vitamin D synthesis in the skin and leading to a further decrement in calcium absorption. Whether calcium intake is inadequate in older women is debatable but inadequate intake could at least be part of the cause of post-menopausal bone loss.

The more sedentary lifestyle (or periods of immobility) common among elderly people certainly does contribute to bone loss, i.e. disuse leads to atrophy of the bone. There is significant bone loss from the vertebrae in both sexes, but this is more marked in females and leads to increased spinal curvatures. Shortening of the cervical vertebrae can also lead to kinking of the vertebral arteries — a contributing factor in transient ischaemic attacks experienced by some old people.

THE REPRODUCTIVE SYSTEM

The reproductive organs in both sexes undergo many age-related changes which are similar to those occurring in other organs and tissues. The function of the reproductive organs is greatly influenced by a hierarchy of hormones from the hypothalamus, anterior pituitary and the gonads (ovaries and testes) and many changes are influenced by these hormones.

Females have a more or less abrupt end to their reproductive lifespan with the menopause occurring at an average age of 50–51 years. It is often difficult to study the decline in reproductive capacity in women due to the widespread use of contraceptive devices and decreased frequency of intercourse. From the age of 30 onwards, ovarian weight decreases, the amount of connective tissue increases and perfusion diminishes. There is a reduction in the number of follicles that undergo normal growth and development. Women have lower fertility and a higher rate of miscarriage in the years before onset of the menopause.

The other reproductive organs undergo changes mainly due to a decrease in the quantity of female hormones. The uterus atrophies and shrinks to a small proportion of its premenopausal size. The vagina becomes smaller in length and diameter; the protective cornified layer of epithelium can be lost and the glandular secretions that are under the influence of the ovarian hormones are often inadequate. This can lead to reduced lubrication during intercourse and cause dyspareunia. The alterations in vaginal secretions lead to changes in the vaginal flora leading to symptoms of vaginitis which can progress to ulceration and bleeding. Breast tissue atrophies and relaxation of ligaments and loss of muscle tone occur.

Men do not show the same sharp cut-off in reproductive function: reduction in reproductive capacity seems to be a more gradual process, and some men retain full reproductive capacity into extreme old age. In the testes sperm production continues into old age, but the rate of spermatogenesis slows down and there is an increase in the number of abnormal sperm. Testosterone and androgen secretions from the Leydig cells in the testes diminish, although the extent of decline varies.

The prostate gland shows many different histological, biochemical and functional changes with ageing, resulting in an enlargement of the gland. This is known as benign prostatic hypertrophy and is present to some extent in all men. Connective tissue accumulates and this leads to the familiar problems with micturition so common among older men — namely frequency, urgency and a poor stream of urine. The changes in the prostate gland are related to alterations in the sex hormone levels of ageing men, but the precise role of the hormones is not clear. Changes also occur in other male reproductive organs: the capacity of seminal vesicles decrease and sclerotic changes occur in the erectile tissue in the penis.

THEORIES OF AGEING

Why does ageing occur and what causes ageing are questions that have fascinated people for years. Much of the early interest in the ageing process was directed at finding the 'elixir' of life and ways of increasing longevity. However, in some respects, relatively little is known even now about these fundamental questions.

Many different theories (it has been suggested more than 200!) have been proposed in an attempt to explain ageing; some of the theories can be grouped together since they incorporate similar approaches. For example, some theories have looked at the genetics of ageing and these can be linked with evolutionary aspects. Some researchers have investigated changes in whole body function or in one particular system, whilst others have concentrated on changes in cell structure and function. More recently, interest has been directed at the molecular basis of ageing. Fortunately, many of the theories about ageing are not mutually exclusive — they just seek to explain ageing in a different way.

As discussed earlier, knowledge about the biology of ageing has come from many different sources — from cell-culture work, from studies using animals as models for human ageing, or from investigations of conditions with some features similar to those of ageing, e.g. Progeria and Down's syndrome (see below). Mathematical models and predictions based on accepted biological principles have also been proposed. It is not possible in a chapter of this nature to consider or do justice to all the theories of ageing; however, a few interesting issues will be considered briefly.

It is an attractive proposition to look for one single explanation for all features of ageing; however, research to date has not suggested that there is a unitary cause of ageing or indeed that all cells and tissues age in the same way. It is likely that different tissues in an animal not only age at different rates but also age for different reasons. Each ageing individual may have a mix of changes and/or impairments at the cellular or tissue level and these together contribute to the common manifestations of ageing.

Some classic work with human fibroblasts (immature connective tissue cells) was done by Hayflick and colleagues (1985). Hayflick showed that normal animal cells have a fixity of lifespan that indicates a kind of genetic programme of ageing in the cell — a programme that could underlie ageing of the whole body. Healthy cells taken from a human fetus divide normally enough in culture if supplied with food and a place to grow, but they divide only 50 times or thereabouts. Cells from a short-lived species were shown to double less often than cells from longer-lived species. Hayflick originally proposed that there was a finite predetermined number of times that a cell could replicate even under the most favourable conditions. (This is not the case for cancer cells — these abnormal cells seem to become immortal and have an infinite lifespan.) However, in the light of more recent work it now seems likely that although normal cells do have a finite capacity for replication this limit is very rarely reached in vivo (i.e. in the body). Hayflick himself now suggests that other functional problems occur prior to the cessation of capacity to divide, i.e. before the normal cells have reached their maximum proliferative capacity (Hayflick 1985).

It has been suggested that evolutionary pressures would lead to a programmed ageing of species and it has even been proposed that there are genes that determine ageing, i.e. genes that in one way or another programme for ageing. Certainly heredity plays a part as we know from familial data, and from studies on identical twins (who have exactly the same genetic make-up). Some human genetic disorders display features of accelerated ageing; Down's syndrome, for example, shows many signs and symptoms that resemble accelerated ageing. Individuals with Down's have an extra chromosome 21 and it has been proposed that gene dosage, i.e. the amount of genetic material, may play a role in ageing processes. Studies on families of patients with Alzheimer's disease have revealed an excessive incidence of relatives with trisomy 21.

In contrast to the idea that ageing is pre-programmed, there are 'error' theories which suggest that function carries on until some 'catastrophe' occurs and only then is normal function lost. This might occur suddenly or as a result of wear and tear, or of, simply, an accumulation of different minor deteriorations. For instance, one small error in the long chain of reactions during protein synthesis would produce an imperfect structural protein or enzyme which in turn might interfere with cell function. The evidence is against this approach at present; some enzymes do show signs of ageing and protein synthesis does slow down, but it is by no means universal and there are many instances of normal biochemical processes in the body at all ages. In fact, dozens of functional changes are seen in ageing cells and some of these may lead to a loss of 'normal' cell function and play a role in the expression of ageing — but are they a cause or a result of ageing? Failure in part of the immune system has also been implicated in the aetiology of ageing.

Various theories have been concerned with changes in DNA. Some work suggests that with ageing there is a failure of the cell's ability to repair damaged DNA or that random genetic damage accumulates despite the existence of repair processes (which are themselves imperfect) in the cell. Any accumulation of errors in protein synthesis would result in abnormal proteins and these are found in ageing cells. There may also be a failure to remove abnormal proteins. One theory along these lines links the changes seen in proteins in diabetic people with those seen in ageing individuals, as in both instances there is an accumulation of glycosylated proteins (these are proteins that have become associated with glucose). For example, glycosylated proteins are thought to be implicated in the development of cataracts and atherosclerosis. Thus the changes in diabetic people are rather like premature ageing effects (Furth & Harding 1989).

Another cluster of ageing theories relates to the accumulation of cross-linkages in macromolecules. As we have already seen, collagen changes with age; it becomes much stiffer and loses its usual properties due to an increase in cross-linkages. Cross-linking of some cellular macromolecules, e.g. proteins and lipids, produces fluorescent chemical compounds, collectively called age pigments or lipofuscin. (These age pigments are not the same as the common changes in skin pigmentation seen with advancing age.) Age pigments seem to accumulate particularly in cardiac muscle and the nervous system. The role of these pigments is disputed, although it is accepted that they are a good indicator of 'degree' of ageing; regardless of its function, lipofuscin accumulation is used as an index of physiological ageing. It has been suggested that age pigment accumulation may impair cell function although there is no direct evidence for this. These substances may result

from the correction of free radical damage (see below).

THE FREE RADICAL THEORY OF AGEING

All the theories mentioned above beg the question of what actually causes the changes in ageing. The free radical theory of ageing, first discussed by Harman (1956) and developed considerably by a number of gerontologists since then, attempts to overcome this issue; it proposes that free radicals are central agents in producing changes at tissue, cellular and sub-cellular levels. Free radicals are produced normally during some metabolic processes in the body. Free radicals are highly reactive unstable molecules due to the presence of an unpaired electron; this results in a large increase in free energy which allows them to attack adjacent molecules. According to the theory, free radicals damage important biological molecules and accumulation of this damage leads to the decline in function seen with ageing. The superoxide molecule, an excited form of oxygen, is one such free radical.

Organisms have evolved enzymes (e.g. superoxide dismutase and catalase) and non-enzymatic systems (e.g. vitamins C and E) for scavenging free radicals and destroying potentially harmful products before further damage can occur. Normally, any superoxide radicals that form during metabolism are inactivated by superoxide dismutase found naturally in the cells. Enzymes like these seem to have evolved specifically to help to protect important substances in the cells; thus if there is a defect in these protective mechanisms, oxidative damage could result. According to the theory, accumulated damage due to free radicals leads to an age-related decrease in function.

Membrane lipids both on the cell surface and within the cells in organelle membranes seem to be particularly vulnerable to free radical attack. The damage caused can take many forms, e.g. it can cause cross-linkage in collagen, nucleic acids, proteins and membrane phospholipids. If this occurs the normal function of the molecule is impaired. It is known that when these molecules are attacked in this way fluorescent pigments are produced; hence the link with the so-called 'age pigments'.

It has been known for some time that irradiation also causes life shortening and seems to lead to an increased incidence of age changes. Whether changes due to radiation are the same as 'normal' ageing changes is a matter of some debate; life shortening induced by ionizing radiation or mutagenic compounds appears to differ both quantitatively and qualitatively from the normal process of ageing. However, it does seem that the harmful effects of radiation are also due to the formation of free radicals. Thus free radical reactions are suggested to be the cause of many degenerative changes in ageing cells.

A major attraction of the free radical theory is that it makes ageing potentially treatable: chemical antioxidants should be able to prevent this oxidative damage to important molecules. Vitamins C and E are examples of chemical antioxidants which are capable of interrupting free radical reactions. When this theory was first proposed, it did in fact lead to substantial sales of vitamins E and C; this may be the reason why the theory has become so popular! Some animal experiments have suggested that antioxidants do extend the lifespan, but others have shown no effect on the rate of ageing or on lifespan. However, there is no evidence in humans for these vitamins having any direct benefit.

THE DISPOSABLE SOMA THEORY OF AGEING

Kirkwood and Holliday (1986) suggest two theoretical approaches that may be taken in explaining the evolution of ageing: namely, that ageing can be said to be either adaptive or non-adaptive. The former approach implies that ageing is a beneficial trait in its own right and 'good' for the species. For example, ageing prevents overcrowding and promotes evolutionary change through the generations with turnover of genetic material. But if ageing is adaptive, i.e. is such a good thing, it is strange that it is rarely seen in wild populations. Another difficulty with the idea is that ageing is

clearly disadvantageous to the individual, although possibly beneficial to the species.

The non-adaptive theories are currently favoured by some gerontologists (remember, theories do go in and out of vogue!). In these theories ageing is said to occur because natural selection is either unable to prevent the deterioration of old organisms or it is a by-product of selection for other adaptive qualities. Ageing is thus detrimental or at best neutral, and so its evolution must be explained indirectly.

One non-adaptive theory considers the alleged exhaustion of physiological energy reserves; this looks at the association between the rate of living and longevity — those with a high rate having a shorter lifespan. There are known to be specific instances where sexual activity hastens senescence; in the drosophilia fruit fly, for example, copulation and egg-laying shorten life. There is no evidence to support this theory in humans!

Kirkwood and Holliday have proposed a nonadaptive theory along these lines which they have called the 'disposable soma theory' (Fig. 3.6). In this theory an organism is considered rather like a 'black box' which takes up energy from the environment in the form of nutrients and then transforms this energy into progeny (offspring). However, in order to maintain life part of the energy input must be allocated to and used for normal maintenance and repair of the nonreproductive bodily tissue (i.e. the soma). Maintenance and repair includes prevention and removal of DNA damage, protein synthesis, breakdown of defective or unwanted molecules, wound healing, immune responses and so on. In this theory the more energy the organism allocates to somatic maintenance the less is available for reproduction and vice versa; hence the name, disposable soma theory. In other words, there is a trade-off between normal maintenance and repair, and reproduction. So a balance must be struck between the competing benefits of living longer (by allocating resources to cope with random damage) or reproducing at a greater rate.

Kirkwood and Holliday have demonstrated mathematical support for this theory; they also suggest that it explains some of the special features

ORGANISM

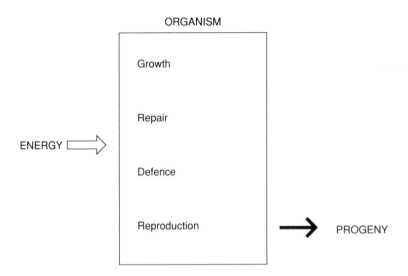

Fig. 3.6 The disposable soma theory of ageing.

of human ageing that are not generally seen in other animals; survival well into the post-reproductive period, the menopause and the slow development of children are predominately human phenomena. Something similar to the menopause may be seen in some primates but it does not exist in lower animals.

Humans certainly do have a significant expectation of survival into the senescent phase or post-reproductive phase of their lifespan. The complex social behaviour seen in human society affords significant protection against environmental hazards, but at the cost of greatly delaying maturation and prolonging the dependence of children on parents. As a female grows older, the hazards of further pregnancies increases and beyond the age of 40–50 it may be more advantageous for a woman to cease to reproduce whilst she is bringing up her children (i.e. to direct energy towards maintenance and repair). Thus the advent of the menopause is 'good' since it stops fertility and allows energy to be directed towards maintenance and repair and so extend the lifespan.

Part of the attractiveness of this theory is that it allows other theories to be incorporated; for in-

stance, ideas that postulate particular kinds of somatic damage as the cause of ageing. Thus, damage by free radicals, somatic mutation, errors in protein synthesis, macromolecular cross-linkage and so on could all be included. It could also encompass the idea that senescence is due to wear and tear — not because wear and tear is inevitable, but because it arises as the indirect result of optimizing the balance between somatic maintenance and repair with reproduction.

As the above discussion shows, many of the theories of ageing are not mutually exclusive — some can indeed be integrated. In the final analysis, ageing is likely to be a combination of programmed (genetic) and random ageing processes.

HEALTH AND DISEASE IN ELDERLY PEOPLE

Promotion of physical health in later life requires attention to exactly the same factors as at any age — for instance, regular exercise, a balanced diet and a 'healthy' lifestyle (e.g. avoiding smoking and so on).

The importance of maintaining regular activity is often not stressed. As discussed earlier in the chapter, it is often difficult to sort out the effects of disuse, i.e. physical deconditioning, from those of ageing; as a consequence, old age is often considered to be synonymous with disability, but there is much evidence to dispute this. The amount of physical activity undertaken can be low for many reasons; genuine disability, disease, lack of knowledge about the benefits of exercise, a desire to 'take it easy', lack of appropriate facilities, and lack of companionship for exercise are just a few possibilities.

However, the evidence of research studies is very convincing — even a minimal amount of regular physical activity has a significant effect on aspects of health. For instance, undertaking the 'right' exercise can have a positive effect on bone mass, maintain joint flexibility, reduce joint stiffness, improve balance and increase muscle tone. Emes (1979) conducted a study on 24 elderly people (15 women and 9 men). These subjects, with an average age of 77, participated regularly in an exercise programme at a drop-in centre. The group participated in light exercise of gradually increasing intensity three times a week for 12 weeks. Significant weight loss occurred, with the men losing more than the women. Both resting and exercise heart rate declined, as did systolic and diastolic blood pressures. Balance whilst standing on one foot was also improved. Buskirk (1985) gives an excellent review of the role of exercise in health maintenance and longevity.

It has been suggested that active older people adopt a lifestyle that promotes overall health through proper sleeping habits, regular meals, moderate alcohol consumption, maintenance of normal weight and abstinence from smoking. Such a lifestyle has also been associated with increased longevity.

The results of participation in a physical conditioning regime are measurable in people at any age — at least up to the time that senescence makes exercise most difficult. Obviously not every elderly person is in a position to be active in the sense of going for a walk or going swimming , but knitting,

sitting in a chair and doing ankle exercises, walking to the toilet or the telephone may be appropriate 'exercise' to encourage in other instances.

Certainly, the functional alterations brought about by regular exercise blunt the downward trends commonly associated with ageing. Perhaps educational efforts are required to counter the rather negative perceptions among many elderly people of the desirability of physical activity. One great disservice we can do to an older person, even if for the best of intentions, is to reduce the amount of physical activity undertaken; it may be as little as stopping her standing up at the sink to wash up, or going to fetch something for her to save her the effort. It does not bear thinking what regimes of inactivity we inflict on old people in many care settings. No wonder that elderly people when discharged after a stay in hospital have difficulty in coping — whilst in hospital they have lost so much of their fitness. It may be simplistic, but if you don't use it, you lose it! The type of exercise that is encouraged will obviously depend on the individual's capabilities, but generally, rhythmic exercise involving the use of a large muscle mass is recommended; walking is perhaps the ideal activity.

Whilst aiming to optimize an individual's physical health, it is perhaps unrealistic to refer only to 'healthy' elderly people; the interaction between ageing and disease is complex, with a continuum between 'normal' ageing changes and pathology or disease. At one end of the spectrum there are instances where there is no interaction between ageing and disease (as in skin cancer for example), whilst at the other extreme the changes that occur with age actually represent or mimic disease, e.g. an altered glucose tolerance, or the development of cataracts. Some physiological changes that occur with ageing can increase the likelihood or severity of disease; normal ageing is associated with a decline in pulmonary function, for instance, and this together with reduced efficiency of the immune system may mean that a respiratory tract infection could lead to a marked loss of lung function. The same infection in a younger person may not have such a debilitating effect.

Multiple pathology is also common in older people. Here the decline in function within several systems might interact to increase the likelihood of a problem; for example, the higher incidence of falls in the elderly almost certainly is due to a combination of factors — increased postural sway and poor balance, postural hypotension, poor sight and reduced muscle strength might all make a contribution.

Some physiological changes that are aspects of normal ageing clearly have adverse clinical consequences. For instance, the menopause is 'normal' but increases the risk of osteoporosis; similarly, the endocrine changes in men that result in benign prostatic hypertrophy frequently lead to urinary tract problems. Thus, some normal age-related changes certainly increase the risk or likelihood of health problems. To add further to the complexities, the presentation of the disease or problem may also be altered in elderly people; consider, for example, the classic painless myocardial infarction, or the reduction in elevation of temperature with infections in older people.

This chapter has considered some of the important aspects of the biology of human ageing and the implications of these physiological changes. Clearly, the changes observed in ageing are not all as 'bad' as they are often portrayed; quite the opposite: most elderly people, in a biological sense, cope very adequately. What must be remembered is the enormous variability amongst older people; what is normal for one 80-year-old might be quite inappropriate for another. Similarly, there are ways of promoting or optimizing the physical capacities of an old person, just as there are for a younger individual.

REFERENCES

Aniansson A, Rundgren A, Sperling L 1980 Evaluation of functional capacity in activities of daily living in 70 year old men and women. Scandinavian Journal of Rehabilitation Medicine 12: 145–154
Astrand P, Rodahl K 1977 Textbook of work physiology. McGraw-Hill, New York
Buskirk E R 1985 Health maintenance and longevity: exercise. In: Finch C E, Schneider E L (eds) Handbook of the biology of ageing, 2nd edn. Van Nostrand Reinhold, New York

Chandra R K, Puri S 1985 Nutritional support improves antibody response to influenza virus vaccine in the elderly. British Medical Journal 291: 705–706
Collins K J, Exton-Smith A N, James M H, Oliver D J 1980 Functional changes in autonomic nervous responses with ageing. Age and Ageing 9: 17–24
Davidson M B 1979 The effect of ageing on carbohydrate metabolism: a review of the English literature and a practical approach to the diagnosis of diabetes mellitus in the elderly. Metabolism 28: 688–705
Emes C G 1979 The effects of a regular program of light exercise on seniors. Journal of Sports Medicine 19: 185–190
Exton-Smith A N 1980 Nutritional status: diagnosis and prevention of malnutrition. In: Exton-Smith A N, Caird F I (eds) Metabolic and nutritional disorders in the elderly. John Wright, Bristol
Exton-Smith A N, Stanton B R 1965 Report of an investigation onto the diets of elderly women living alone. King Edward's Hospital Fund, London
Furth A, Harding J 1989 Why sugar is bad for you. New Scientist Sept. 23: 44–47
Harman D 1956 Ageing: a theory based on the free radical and radiation chemistry. Journal of Gerontology 11: 298–300
Hausman P B, Weksler M E 1985 Changes in the immune response with age. In: Finch C E, Schneider E L (eds) Handbook of the biology of ageing, 2nd edn. Van Nostrand Reinhold, New York
Hayflick L 1985 The cell biology of ageing. Clinical Geriatric Medicine 1: 15–27
Johnston C C, Norton J A, Khairi R A, Longscope C 1979 Age-related bone loss. In: Barzel U S (ed) Osteoporosis II. Grune and Stratton, New York
Johnson H A 1985 Relations between normal ageing and disease. Raven Press, New York
Kenney R A 1989 Physiology of ageing: a synopsis, 2nd edn. Year Book Medical Publishers, Chicago
Kirkwood T B L, Holliday R 1986 Ageing as a consequence of natural selection. In: Bittles A H, Collins K J (eds) The biology of human ageing. Cambridge University Press, Cambridge
Lakatta E G 1983 Determinants of cardiovascular performance: modification due to ageing. Journal of Chronic Disease 36: 15–30
Lewis V M, Twomey J J, Bealmear P, Goldstein G, Good R A 1978 Age, thymic involution and circulating thymic hormone activity. Journal of Clinical Endocrinology and Metabolism 47: 145–150
Maddox G L, Douglass G B 1974 Ageing and individual differences: a longitudinal analysis of social, psychological and physiological indicators. Journal of Gerontology 29: 555–563
McCay C M, Crowell M F, Maynard L A 1935 The effect of retarded growth upon the length of life span and upon the ultimate body size. Journal of Nutrition 10: 63–79
McGandy R B, Barrows C M, Spanias A, Meredith A, Stone J L, Norns A 1966 Nutrient intakes and energy expenditure in men of different ages. Journal of Gerontology 21: 551–558
Orentreich N, Selmanowitz V J 1969 Levels of biological functions with ageing. Trans Academic Science Series B 31: 992–1012

Rodeheffer R J, Gerstenblich G et al 1984 Exercise cardiac output is maintained with advancing age in healthy human subjects: cardiac dilatation and increased stroke volume compensate for a diminished heart rate. Circulation 69: 203–213

Rowe J, Kahn R 1987 Human ageing — usual and successful. Science 237: 143–149

Sandblum P H, Peterson P, Muren A 1953 Determination of the tensile strength of healing wounds as a clinical test. Acta Chir. Scandinavia 105: 252–257

Shock N 1985 Longitudinal studies of ageing in humans. In: Finch C E, Schneider E L (eds) Handbook of the biology of ageing, 2nd edn. Van Nostrand Reinhold, New York

Strehler B L 1962 Time, cells and ageing. Academic Press, New York

Young A 1986 Exercise physiology in geriatric practice. Acta Med. Scand. supplement 711: 227–232

Part 2

Nursing elderly people: their needs, their resources and their problems of living

CHAPTER CONTENTS

Elements of communication 67

The communication needs of elderly people 68
Communication skills needed to assess and meet
the needs of elderly patients 68

**Reasons for communication problems of elderly
people** 70
Problems caused by visual impairment 70
Problems caused by hearing impairment 71
Problems caused by sensory deprivation 72
Problems of disorientation and confusion 73
Problems caused by speech impairment 73
Communication difficulties caused by stroke 74

Conclusion 77

4

Communicating with elderly people

Jill Macleod Clark

It is ironic that in old age, when people have more time to communicate for pleasure, they often develop problems which make communication more difficult. The desire to communicate is a central human drive and the need for communication usually increases in situations of stress and uncertainty.

For many elderly people, the experience of becoming a patient is an extremely stressful, often frightening event. However, several research reports have highlighted the fact that nurses spend only a small proportion of their time actually communicating with their elderly patients (Stockwell 1972, Norton et al 1975, Wells 1980) and it is essential for nurses to develop the skills necessary to communicate as well as possible with such patients. This chapter begins with an overview of the elements of verbal and non-verbal communication which mesh together to produce successful interaction skills. This is followed by a description of some of the most common communication difficulties that elderly people may have to cope with. These difficulties are discussed in the context of the most appropriate ways to assess them, and where possible, to overcome them.

ELEMENTS OF COMMUNICATION

Communication between human beings involves a meshing of verbal and non-verbal behaviours. The principal components of communication include:

- Verbal communication — the words that are spoken or written
- Intonational communication — the stress, pitch and intensity which give words extra meaning
- Paralinguistic communication — laughter, crying, coughs and spluttering
- Non-verbal (kinetic) communication — body and facial movements.

Non-verbal communication is particularly important when caring for elderly people (Burnside 1981, Hardiman et al 1979). There are many elements of non-verbal behaviour, including facial expression derived from movements of the eyes, eyebrows and mouth; eye contact and gaze, head movements such as nods; gestures of hands, head, shoulders; posture which can indicate attitudes and emotional states; proximity and body contact and touch. It is the flexibility of non-verbal communication which makes it so valuable in communication with old people. If speech, hearing or sight is limited then skilful use of non-verbal communication, particularly touch, can ensure that patients are aware that they are being cared for. Observation of the patient's use of non-verbal behaviours can also be vital to the accurate assessment of physical and psychological needs.

THE COMMUNICATION NEEDS OF ELDERLY PEOPLE

The communication needs of elderly people will not necessarily differ from those of any individual in hospital (Fig. 4.1). It is often felt that old people are lonely and therefore have special needs for social contact. However, they may also be used to their own company and can find the public life of

1. The need for social contact and interaction
2. The need for explanation, confirmation
3. The need for advice, education, support
4. The need for comfort and reassurance

Fig. 4.1 Patients' communication needs.

a hospital, nursing Home or residential Home confusing and disturbing.

The nurse's primary role is to become skilled at recognizing and assessing the extent of each patient's needs for different types of communication and to plan care appropriately. For some old people, the need for social contact can be met simply through the knowledge that others are around them. They do not necessarily require conversation. For others, their main need is for someone to talk to (or often for someone to listen to them).

In order to assess a patient's needs and to communicate effectively it is essential that nurses have the appropriate skills.

COMMUNICATION SKILLS NEEDED TO ASSESS AND MEET THE NEEDS OF ELDERLY PATIENTS

The communication skills listed in Figure 4.2 are essential prerequisites for effective assessment of and communication with elderly people. By observing, listening and attending to what the patient says and does (the patient's verbal and non-verbal communication) the nurse will be able to build up a picture of the patient as an individual. Active listening will also help the nurse to recognize and respond to the patient's direct questions and, more importantly, to their indirect questions, statements or cues. Macleod Clark (1981) found that 80% of surgical patients' requests for information are indirect or subtle, and this may be even higher for old people who can be diffident and unsure of themselves. The skill of asking questions appropriately is essential if a patient's needs are to be assessed accurately. If the intention is to explore how someone is really feeling, then 'open' questions will be most useful. However, if the patient has difficulty in speaking or hearing then simple 'closed' questions requiring a Yes or No answer may be the most appropriate. Old people tire easily and may have a limited memory span, and so it is vital to choose the right moment to give important instructions or information. It is also a good idea to repeat the information and, possibly, to write it down, using short sentences, and avoiding jargon.

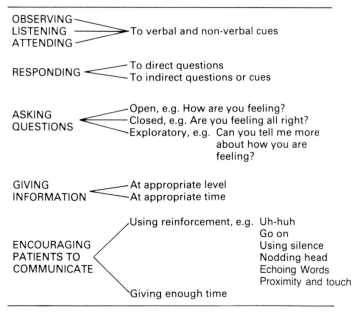

Fig. 4.2 Some communication skills necessary for assessing patients' needs.

Unfortunately, research evidence suggests that nurses may not always use these verbal communication skills in practice. Walton and Macleod Clark (1986) found that nurses caring for elderly patients who had suffered a stroke often asked multiple questions, did not wait for patients to respond and gave too much complex information at any one time. Similarly, Jones and Van Amelsvoort Jones (1986) describe the limitations of communication between nurses and their elderly patients, and Wells (1980) identified a pattern of infrequent and routinized verbal interaction between nurses and patients in geriatric wards, with nurses showing a general lack of communication skills.

One of the most valuable communication skills is that of being able to encourage other people to talk. Many old people become withdrawn and may need a great deal of encouragement to talk freely. Using reinforcement strategies such as saying 'When?', 'Go on', 'I see', will always help the patient to carry on talking. Nodding your head and repeating important words back to the patient are also very effective. The skill of staying silent and giving time for an elderly person to think and answer will also facilitate communication.

Non-verbal communication skills are specially important when caring for elderly people. These skills include the ability to listen actively and to remain silent when appropriate. The use of eye contact and maintaining a positive facial expression is also vital. It is also necessary to be able to assess accurately the degree of proximity that is appropriate for each interaction. Most important of all, perhaps, is the skilled use of physical contact and touch. There is substantial evidence to support the view that not only do human beings have a basic need for physical contact but that this need increases at times of stress (Goodykoontz 1979).

However, research has demonstrated that elderly patients in hospitals are often deprived of such physical contact and touch during this time of great potential stress (Barnett 1972, Watson 1975). A more recent study by Le May and Redfern (1989) suggests that the majority of touch occurring between nurses and elderly patients is instrumental in nature, i.e. it is related to a practical task. Only 10% of the touch recorded could be described as expressive, i.e. fulfilling an emotional function rather than practical purpose. Other research has shown the positive effect that increased physical contact can have on the well-being of elderly patients. For example, Seaman (1982) demonstrated that touch can result in an increase in verbal interaction and can also act as a calming influence. Ernst and Shaw (1980) also suggested that nurses who use touch frequently are liked more by patients and are perceived as being helpful and ready to listen. Copstead (1980) and Langland and Panicucci (1982) found that increased touch from nurses resulted in an overall increase in communication between those nurses and their patients.

The importance of non-verbal communication in general and the use of touch in particular cannot be over-emphasized when considering the nursing care of elderly patients. For many older people the need for non-verbal communication and physical contact will be even greater than the need for verbal communication. Warmth, empathy and caring can all be transmitted effectively through the appropriate use of non-verbal skills even when the patient's own ability to communicate is impaired. The reality is that, for many older people, communication does become difficult for a variety of physical and psychological reasons (Gravell 1988). The challenge of helping patients to cope with and overcome these difficulties can only be confronted successfully if the nurse has the necessary verbal and non-verbal communication skills.

REASONS FOR COMMUNICATION PROBLEMS OF ELDERLY PEOPLE

The process of ageing is accompanied by degeneration of neuronal tissue in the central nervous system, although whether these changes occur as a result of ageing itself or of pathology is not altogether clear (see Chapter 3). In consequence, the reactions of elderly people become slower. Sensory inputs are reduced and this is particularly noticeable in relation to the special senses of vision and

hearing. When sight and hearing are impaired, then communication becomes more difficult.

Other factors also create problems and these include the increase in sensory and social deprivation that often occurs in old age. Elderly people can be confused and disoriented and many develop speech difficulties. Such difficulties are often related to diseases such as Parkinsonism, or pathology such as cerebral vascular accidents and atheroma.

PROBLEMS CAUSED BY VISUAL IMPAIRMENT

With the passage of time, the power of visual accommodation diminishes and there can be particular difficulty with accommodating to darkness. Presbyopia, or farsightedness, is an almost universal phenomenon so that nearly all elderly people require glasses for seeing things that are nearby. Problems of sight are discussed in Chapter 6.

Assessing patients' visual acuity and overcoming problems

Since the majority of elderly patients will have some limitations of vision it is necessary for the nurse to establish the extent of disability and to try to compensate for this where possible.

All patients (or their relatives) should be asked about their sight and the use of spectacles. Many old people do not have their eyes tested regularly and as a consequence their prescription lenses may not be effective. If you suspect that the patient's glasses are ineffective and if the patient is in hospital for any length of time an attempt should be made to get her sight retested and new lenses prescribed. If the patient does wear glasses she should be encouraged to wear them at the times when she would normally wear them at home. They should also be checked to make sure they are clean.

- When communicating with patients with poor vision it is essential to introduce yourself before you speak because the patient may not be aware of your presence.
- Sit or stand in a position which suits the patient best.

- Do not sit or stand too close. This can be uncomfortable for old people whose eyes cannot focus or accommodate to very near objects.
- Non-verbal communication is vital, especially touch and the use of clear intonation.
- Try to keep the patient's environment as consistent and familiar as possible.

PROBLEMS CAUSED BY HEARING IMPAIRMENT

The incidence of deafness increases with age and, as discussed in detail in Chapter 5, 60% of people over 70 years are deaf (Gilhome Herbst & Humphrey 1981). Hearing is a vital means of orientation, giving information on proximity and distance. However, degeneration of this sense (presbyacusis) is also an inevitable concomitant of ageing. Cochlear problems include diminished hearing and tinnitus while vestibular problems result in disturbance of balance. Irreversible physiological changes to the hearing mechanism typically begin sometime after the age of 30 years, with a gradual loss of acuity for high-frequency sound. This loss steadily increases and gradually encroaches upon lower sound frequencies and both ears are usually affected at much the same rate.

Old people often complain that they are unable to 'understand' rather than not being able to hear, and this difficulty in discrimination is usually experienced initially when the environment is noisy or when speech is rapid. As the ageing ear becomes incapable of reacting to higher sound frequencies, the perceived quality of sound also changes. Since increase in loudness cannot compensate for missing sounds, hearing aids may be of limited use. With progressive inability to hear various speech sounds, the total speech flow becomes less intelligible. Lip-reading (or speech reading) may be the only practical form of help available but if hearing loss is accompanied by impaired vision then lip-reading will have limited value.

It is easy to understand why acquired hearing loss is often strongly associated with feelings of depression and isolation. It is hard to feel 'part of things' when you cannot hear well or understand.

Coping with hearing problems

Many people feel that the answer to deafness is to provide a hearing aid. However, it is clear that a hearing aid is not the ultimate answer for every elderly person who is hard of hearing. When there is high-frequency hearing loss the aid will do very little to help discrimination of sounds — it merely amplifies sound. It is important for nurses to remember that hearing aids amplify all sounds in the vicinity, not just speech. Many patients cannot and should not tolerate their aids being switched on permanently.

Elderly patients often seem to have difficulties with their aids. Practical difficulties can arise as a result of the patient's poor vision, when they are unable to set the aid appropriately or insert it correctly. Poor memory can result in the patient forgetting which ear takes the aid, forgetting to turn it off or on as appropriate, forgetting to change the battery, forgetting the right settings and getting the old and new batteries mixed up. Deficiencies in manual dexterity, caused, for example, by arthritis, can result in difficulty in manipulating and inserting the aid and in changing the batteries. As a consequence elderly deaf people require a good deal of sensitive and practical assistance from the nurses who care for them. These issues are discussed in greater detail in Chapter 5.

Since hearing loss does affect the majority of elderly patients, all nurses looking after old people should routinely assess their patients' hearing and plan care to facilitate communication. There are many practical steps that can be taken to recognize the extent of deafness and these include:

- Observation of the patient's behaviour with nurses, with other patients and with visitors.
- Observation of the patient's response to noises, particularly loud noises, in the environment.
- Observation of the patient when in conversation with you:

  Does the patient appear withdrawn?
  Does the patient seem inattentive?
  Does the patient appear to respond with inappropriate irritation or anger when spoken to?

How does the patient respond to you touching her?

Does the patient move in response to your change of position?

Does she have difficulty in following instructions?

Does she ask for things to be repeated or say 'What?', 'Pardon?', etc. frequently?

Does she tend to turn one ear towards you?

Is her voice monotonous, unusually loud or soft?

- If the answer to any of the above questions is Yes, then it is likely that your patient has some degree of hearing impairment. Having established this, it is necessary to make sure that any hearing aid is working, worn and switched on. In the absence of a suitable aid, arrangements should be made for a hearing assessment to be done.

If the patient is deaf, the extent of the deafness should be documented clearly in the patient's care plan. If a hearing aid is available, this should also be documented. It is essential that everyone involved with the patient knows that he or she is hard of hearing.

Whatever the extent of deafness, all communication with the patient must be carefully planned. Various strategies to improve communication are suggested in Chapter 5, such as always sitting or standing where the patient can see you and your lips, and making sure the patient has his or her glasses on before you speak. Other important points to remember are:

- Try to avoid the distraction of extra noises by going to a quiet room or corner.
- Turn off the television or radio before speaking.
- Ensure the hearing aid, if it exists, is switched on and working.
- Write down important messages.
- Repeat your message if you do not think you have been understood.
- Give your patient time to think about what you say and respond to it.
- Ask simple, clear questions.
- Use short sentences.

PROBLEMS CAUSED BY SENSORY DEPRIVATION

Many elderly people lead isolated and lonely lives, with 45% of women and 17% of men living alone (Office of Population Censuses and Surveys 1982). Some elderly people live in circumstances which could be described as seriously deprived, in the sense that their environment is restricted to a level of dull monotony. The combination of environmental monotony and reduced sensory acuity can result in old people being assessed inappropriately as confused or demented.

It has been demonstrated that sensory deprivation tends to exaggerate existing personality traits and can distort perceptions of shape, size, colour and time (Vernon et al 1961). Emotional changes can also occur, such as increased boredom, restlessness, irritability, anxiety and panic (Soloman et al 1961). In extreme circumstances marked behaviour changes can take place, such as hallucinations, delusions, and confusion of sleeping and waking states. Hebb (1949) demonstrated that monotony produces a disruption of the capacity to learn and the ability to think and in the absence of adequate stimulation the brain functions less efficiently.

Once the problem of sensory deprivation has been recognized it is often possible to produce a good response by increasing stimulation in the environment. However, stimulation should be introduced gradually since rapid increases can result in emotional outbursts (Lambert & Lambert 1979) and an apparently negative reaction to attempts to make life more interesting. It is important for nurses to be aware of this reaction and assess each patient's needs for stimulation individually and to pace the introduction of stimulation accordingly. It has been found that sensorily deprived patients respond best initially to gentle and consistent stimulation such as touching, stroking and being talked to quietly (Wolanin & Phillips 1981).

For the institutionalized, privacy and space can become inaccessible luxuries. Roberts (1973) suggests that old people work hard to maintain a sense of personal space using strategies such as accumulating clutter, props or significant personal items and by showing possessiveness. Nurses can respect and facilitate this need in a number of ways. These include moving slowly into private space or private thought, encouraging the collection of personal items, avoiding transferring the patient to another bed or room unless requested, and not moving any personal items without permission.

PROBLEMS OF DISORIENTATION AND CONFUSION

If a man does not keep pace with his companions perhaps it is because he hears a different drummer. Let him step to the music which he hears, however measured or far away (Thoreau 1845, p. 285).

Confusion occurs when present reality is distorted but the term is easily misplaced when applied to patients. It can often be the nurse who is confused. When patients are confused it is important to identify the source of confusion.

Distortion of time perception

Keeping track of time requires an individual's attention and interest and these are easily diverted by physiological factors or psychological stress. This disordered time perception is often the first aspect of disorientation to be manifest, with patients being unclear about 'real' time. Being unclear about time puts the individual out of step with the rest of the world. Reality orientation in this case can be attempted by developing a regular daily routine and providing cues in the form of clocks, cards, calendars and name boards (Conroy 1977).

Distortion of place perception

This type of perceptual disorientation usually occurs following a physical change of environment such as moving from one house to another, or from a house to a nursing Home or even from one room to another. Patients who are disoriented in this way will often try to fit events or characteristics of the new location to their old way of life.

Often there is confusion about time and place and when this happens elderly people can slip into the familiarity and security of the distant past: 'My mother is cooking dinner.' It can be very frustrating and distressing when patients persistently claim they are in a different place or call for someone who is not there (as often as not, someone who is dead). Arguing with the patient does not work and it is important to try to increase orientation. This can be attempted in the following ways:

1. Assess the patient's needs for stimulation, remembering that too much may cause stress and too little facilitates the delusion.
2. Make frequent visits to the patient, introducing yourself each time and explaining what you want to do.
3. Try to find objects that provide comfort and security, such as pictures and photographs.
4. Use cards or labels to identify important items, such as clothes, spectacles, etc.

Old age brings an inevitable decrease in physical mobility and the resulting immobility can also have an effect on mental alertness. Petrov and Vlahlijska (1972) found that groups of elderly residents in nursing Homes were able to think and verbalize more clearly and coherently after taking part in exercise groups. This may be a strategy which could be used effectively in other settings to increase the effectiveness of reality orientation programmes. Confusion in elderly people is discussed in detail in Chapter 19.

PROBLEMS CAUSED BY SPEECH IMPAIRMENT

Speech can be impaired in elderly people for a variety of reasons. Sometimes the impairment is a result of serious pathology, but there are a number of simple and practical interventions that can improve speech.

Unclear speech can be related to severe hearing loss, and if this deafness has been previously unrecognized then improving hearing will also improve speech. Another common cause of speech difficulty in the elderly is that of ill-fitting or absent dentures. Speech is inevitably more difficult in the absence of teeth, and dentures which do not fit adequately can cause a variety of speech peculiarities. One old lady was quite impossible to understand until it was discovered that she had to keep her tongue on the roof of her mouth all the time she was speaking in order to keep her top denture in place.

Another common cause of speech problems in elderly people is confusion or disorientation. This can be exacerbated by distraction and noise in the environment, especially from televisions and radios. Such distractions make it impossible for confused old people to concentrate and their speech may become disjointed and inappropriate. Those for whom English is not their first language have added difficulties. There is a tendency for them to revert to their native language, certainly in terms of their thoughts (Cumming & Henry 1961) and this can make verbal communication more problematic.

One of the most difficult problems is that related to the inherent isolation and social withdrawal of many old people. They quite simply get out of the habit of talking and communicating and it can take some time for them to become used to a more public existence. It has been suggested that those who have spent many years alone may also have forgotten the 'rules' of social interaction, especially in terms of when to speak and what to speak about (Panicucci et al 1968).

Speech problems can also occur as a result of pathology or disease such as cerebral atrophy, atheroma, Parkinsonism or stroke. Patients who have suffered from a stroke can present a special challenge in terms of coping with or overcoming the communication problems that occur.

COMMUNICATION DIFFICULTIES CAUSED BY STROKE

The incidence of stroke, or cerebrovascular accident, rises steadily with age, affecting approximately three persons in every 1000 of those aged under 65 years, eight persons in every 1000 of those aged between 65 and 74 years, and 25 persons in every 1000 of those aged over 75 years. The sexes appear to be equally affected (Harris et al 1971).

For most of the many thousands of elderly patients who suffer a stroke, communication becomes a major problem. It has been estimated that over two thirds of those suffering from a right-sided hemiplegia will have a significant degree of speech impairment. A similar proportion of those suffering from a left-sided hemiplegia will suffer from more obscure but equally distressing communication difficulties. As Smith (1967) says: 'Loss of control over one side of the body is a disaster, loss of the ability to communicate is a catastrophe.'

Difficulty with communication can be aggravated by a variety of factors such as sensory or perceptual decrements, intellectual changes, impaired memory span, reduced ability to concentrate, fatigue, emotional lability and apathy. For the stroke patient and his or her family, an overwhelming concern is whether the stroke victim will be able to communicate again (Jenning 1981).

Stroke patients depend upon nurses in the immediate post-stroke period for all aspects of care and support (Christo 1978). The potential role that nurses have for helping and encouraging these patients to cope with their communication difficulties cannot be overestimated. The pathology underlying speech and communication difficulties after strokes is complex. The terminology used is confusing and the explanations for different types of disability is still a matter of some debate (Licht 1975). However, the communication problems that a stroke patient has to cope with are determined by the size and site of the cerebrovascular accident, and the side on which weakness is manifested.

Right-sided hemiplegia

A lesion occurring in the left hemisphere of the brain may result in a right-sided hemiplegia and, very commonly, a degree of speech loss or impairment. The terms most frequently used to describe this impairment are as follows:

1. Dysarthria. This term is used to describe disorders of articulation where the mechanisms which produce sounds and speech are faulty. Dysarthria is thus a speech impairment resulting from a disruption of the neuromuscular control of speech. The degree of dysarthria can range from slight slurring of the speech to total inability to articulate any sounds.

2. Aphasia. Strictly interpreted this term means complete absence of speech but it is frequently used instead of the term dysphasia.

3. Dysphasia. This term encompasses any degree of impaired or partial loss of speech ability. As most people have left hemisphere dominance, strokes in the left side of the brain are most likely to produce dysphasia. It is believed that lesions in different parts of the cortex disturb speech in certain ways. The most common classification is that of:

a. Broca's aphasia (motor or expressive dysphasia). Broca's area lies close to the motor cortex and a lesion in this area is said to result in an inability to translate speech concepts into meaningful articulated sounds. Speech is often limited initially to one or two words and the patient may say the opposite to what is meant. Emotional expressions or expletives may be unaffected. If the lesion is restricted completely to Broca's area then comprehension is thought to be unimpaired.

b. Wernicke's aphasia (sensory or receptive dysphasia). Wernicke's area lies in the auditory cortex (the left superior temporal gyrus) and lesions in this region are said to impair the comprehension of speech, so that the meaning of words received in the auditory cortex is not understood. If such lesions are localized then the production of speech is unimpaired and the patient will produce speech which is fluent and rhythmic but whose content is abnormal. This is because the patient is unaware of the words being used and in severe cases may only produce a stream of meaningless words.

c. Global aphasia or global dysphasia. This label is given to speech disorders where there appear to be deficits in terms of expression and reception of words. This situation is thought to occur when there is an extensive lesion in the patient's dominant cerebral hemisphere involving both frontal and temporal lobes.

It has been suggested that most patients suffering from dysphasia have expressive and receptive deficits (Karis & Harenstein 1976) and there is a continuing controversy about the theory of localized lesions (Gonzalez 1977). This controversy highlights the importance of assessing each individual patient's speech impairment or difficulty. In summary, the patient who has suffered a left hemisphere stroke and whose speech has been affected is likely to have some or all of the following problems: poor speech, impaired word recognition, impaired word retention and recall, difficulties in articulation, impaired comprehension. Although speech is poor and may initially be absent, it is probable that overall intellectual activity and mentation are generally quite good.

Left-sided hemiplegia

A lesion occurring in the right hemisphere of the brain may result in a left-sided hemiplegia with no obvious speech loss or impairment. However, this does not mean that the stroke patient with a left-sided paralysis will not have any problems with communication. Paradoxically, these patients are often able to express themselves well and no intellectual damage is apparent. In reality the disruption to their sensorimotor, conceptual and spatial abilities can be very severe and cause more difficulties in communication and rehabilitation than the lack of speech.

Patients with a left-sided paralysis can suffer from a disturbance in body image, spatial judgment, time judgment, impaired drawing and writing and mathematical ability, and an inability to understand the written word. All these problems inhibit communication and such patients are often labelled as 'difficult', particularly since they seem to be unaware of the mistakes that they have made.

It is clear that in order to help patients who have suffered a stroke, wherever the lesion is sited, nurses must develop the skills and strategies which will encourage and facilitate communication.

Physical rehabilitation is a crucial part of eventual recovery in terms of communication. Efforts to encourage the patient to chew and swallow food efficiently will result in an increased ability to articulate sounds and words.

Patients must be encouraged to utilize all auditory, visual, tactile and emotional inputs. Some language problems are common to most dysphasic patients and these problems include a very limited vocabulary (maybe restricted to emotional speech only), reduced verbal memory span, grammatical and semantic confusions, varying degrees of ability to understand written as well as spoken words and, of course, varying degrees of difficulty in writing.

Guidelines for communicating with stroke patients

- Ensure that you have obtained the patient's attention before speaking.
- Ensure that the patient can see and hear you.
- Tell the patient you are trying to help her to speak.
- Speak directly to the patient, talking clearly and slowly but with normal intonation and phrasing.
- Use simple sentence structure, incorporating one idea at a time.
- Commands can be given in single words, e.g. watch, listen, wait, swallow.
- Repeat key words, rephrase if necessary.
- Do not shout.
- Label important items, e.g. cup, glass, spectacles.
- Ask simple closed questions so that the patient can answer with one word, e.g. 'Would you like tea or coffee?'
- If the patient cannot answer Yes or No, try to devise a gesture or sign language for these words, e.g. thumbs up for Yes and thumbs down for No.
- Do not push your patient too hard; learn to pick up signs of distress such as perseveration (meaningless repetition of a word or act), loss of concentration, eye blinking, irritability and sweating.
- Do not underestimate the patient's comprehension or potential capacity to communicate.
- Avoid distractions, especially noise.
- Give enough time for the patient to respond.
- Find out what interests the patient (from relatives or visitors if necessary) and talk about these things.
- Promote 'ritual' communication. Familiar phrases reduce stress and improve performance.
- Involve relatives and friends in all stages of care and teach them to help the patient communicate.
- Use alternative methods of communication such as communication boards, written instructions, picture cards, etc. Encourage patients to use the unaffected hand for writing or drawing.

People who have recovered from a stroke are very consistent in their descriptions of the problems and frustrations they suffered. Nearly all these problems focus upon aspects of communication. Ritchie (1978) wrote a compelling and comprehensive account of the difficulties and frustrations encountered as a patient recovering from a stroke. Ritchie's experience mirrors that of many others in the same situation. Skelly (1975) compiled an overview of the problems described by 50 stroke patients who were able to identify the following common complaints related to aspects of communication:

- Their ability to comprehend what was said was reached sooner than those caring for them realized.
- Input was too fast and too dense with nurses and doctors speaking too quickly and with too much complexity.
- Not enough time was given for patients to try to reply to questions, etc.
- Noise level was generally too high and made the patients feel irritable.
- They felt there were too many people to interact with.
- They were not told what was happening and speech difficulties were not discussed with them by nurses or doctors, only by speech therapists if and when they saw one.

This list of complaints emphasizes the importance of communication with all patients who have speech problems or indeed any difficulty in communicating with others. The responsibility for initiating appropriate care and encouraging and maximizing communication with such patients lies squarely with the nurse. It is nurses who spend most time with patients and who are in a position to give the most consistent help and support.

It has been demonstrated that early encouragement with communication results in better levels of speech recovery after stroke (Leutenegger 1975), and it is essential that encouragement with communication is seen as an active part of the nursing care plan in the immediate post-stroke period. Once a clear plan or strategy has been designed then all those involved with care can provide consistent and regular support and teaching. Concerned relatives or friends of the patient should be included in all activities which encourage the redevelopment of communication ability.

Aronson (1983) has demonstrated that speech and language therapy in the immediate post-stroke period produces significant improvements in speech rehabilitation. The speech therapist obviously has an important role to play in the rehabilitation of speech-impaired stroke patients. However, the service provided in most National Health Service hospitals is limited and often does not continue after discharge from hospital (Bailey 1983). It is therefore the nurse who must act as the co-ordinator of this aspect of care for stroke patients.

CONCLUSION

This chapter has covered a range of issues which can result in problems of communication for elderly people. Impairment in the ability to communicate can be viewed as possibly the greatest burden of all for old people. Diminution of visual and auditory acuity will limit the reception of both spoken and written information. Changes in tongue, jaw and lip movements combined with cerebral degeneration or disease will impair expressive function. Such changes will reduce elderly people's ability to express needs and emotions and to understand the world about them. This will inevitably lead to problems of social adjustment, which in turn can lead to withdrawal and isolation. The nurse's role is paramount in assessing the extent of any impairment and in planning care so as to minimize isolation and withdrawal and maximize the patient's ability to communicate.

REFERENCES

Aronson A 1983 Aphasia therapy on trial. Proceedings of First European Conference on Research in Rehabilitation. Edinburgh

Bailey S 1983 The response of general practitioners to the problems and rehabilitation of stroke patients with communication handicaps. Proceedings of First European Conference on Research in Rehabilitation. Edinburgh

Barnett K 1972 A survey of the current utilisation of touch by health team personnel with hospitalised patients. International Journal of Nursing Studies 9: 195–209

Burnside I 1981 Nursing and the aged. McGraw Hill, New York

Christo S 1978 Nursing approach to adult aphasia. Canadian Nurse 74(7): 34–39

Conroy C 1977 Reality orientation: a basic technique for patients suffering from memory loss and confusion. British Journal of Occupational Therapy 40(10): 250–251

Copstead L 1980 Effect of touch on self-appraisal and interaction appraisal for permanently institutionalised older adults. Journal of Gerontological Nursing 6(12): 747–752

Cumming E, Henry W 1961 Growing old. Basic Books, New York

Ernst P, Shaw J 1980 Touching is not taboo. Geriatric Nursing 1(3): 193–195

Gilhome Herbst K R, Humphrey C H 1981 Prevalence of hearing impairment in the elderly living at home. Journal of Royal College of General Practitioners 31: 155–160

Gonzalez D E 1977 Receptive-expressive aphasia. Does it really exist? Journal of Neurosurgical Nursing 9(3): 122–3

Goodykoontz L 1979 Touch: attitudes and practice. Nursing Forum 18(10): 4–17

Gravell R E 1988 Communication problems in elderly people. Croom Helm, London

Hardiman C, Holbrook A, Hedrick D 1979 Non-verbal communication systems for the severely handicapped geriatric patient. Gerontologist 19(1): 96–101

Harris A, Cox E, Smith C 1971 The handicapped and impaired in Great Britain. Part 1. Office of Population Censuses and Surveys. HMSO, London

Hebb P O 1949 The organisation of behaviour. Wiley, New York

Jenning S 1981 Back to basics. Communicating with your aphasic patients. Journal of Practical Nursing 31: 22–23

Jones D, Van Amelsvoort Jones G 1986 Communication patterns between nursing staff and the ethnic elderly in a long-term care facility. Journal of Advanced Nursing 11: 265–272

Karis B, Harenstein K 1976 Localisation of speech parameters by brain scan. Neurology 26: 226–230

Lambert V, Lambert C 1979 The impact of physical illness and related mental health concepts. Prentice Hall, Englewood Cliffs, NJ

Langland R, Panicucci C 1982 Effect of touch on communication with elderly confused patients. Journal of Gerontological Nursing 8(3): 152–155

Le May A, Redfern S 1989 Touch and elderly people. In: Wilson Barnett J, Robinson S (eds) Directions in nursing research. Scutari Press, London

Leutenegger R 1975 Patient care and rehabilitation of the communication impaired adults. Charles C Thomas, Springfield, Illinois

Licht S 1975 Stroke and its rehabilitation. Waverly Press, Baltimore

Macleod Clark J 1981 Nurse patient communication. Nursing Times 77(1): 12–18

Norton D, McLaren R, Exton-Smith A N 1975 An investigation of geriatric nursing problems in hospital. (Reprint.) Churchill-Livingstone, Edinburgh

Office of Population Censuses and Surveys 1982 General household survey for 1980. HMSO, London

Paniccuci C, Paul B, Symonds J, Tambellini J 1968 Expanded speech and self-pacing in communication with the aged. ANA clinical sessions. Century Croft, New York

Petrov I, Vlahlijska L 1972 Cultural therapy in old people's homes. Gerontologist 12: 429

Ritchie D 1978 Stroke: a diary of recovery. In: Carver V, Liddiard P (eds) An ageing population. Hodder & Stoughton with Open University Press, Sevenoaks, Kent

Roberts S 1972 Territoriality: space and the aged patient in intensive care units. In: Burnside I (ed) Psychosocial nursing care of the aged. McGraw-Hill, New York

Seaman L 1982 Affective nursing touch. Geriatric Nursing 3: 162–164

Skelly M 1975 Aphasic patients talk back. American Journal of Nursing 77(7): 1140–1144

Smith G W 1967 Care of the patient with a stroke. A handbook for the patient's family and nurse. Springer, New York

Solomon P et al 1961 (ed) Sensory deprivation. Harvard University Press, Cambridge, Mass

Stockwell F 1972 The unpopular patient. Royal College of Nursing, London

Thoreau H 1845 From Walden XVIII. Conclusion. (Reprinted 1946.) Dodmead, New York

Travis L E (ed) 1971 Handbook of speech pathology and audiology. Appleton, New York

Vernon J et al 1961 The effect of human isolation on some perceptual and motor skills. In: Soloman P et al (eds) Sensory deprivation. Harvard University Press, Cambridge, Mass

Walton L, Macleod Clark J 1986 Making contact. Nursing Times 82(33): 28–32

Watson W 1975 The meanings of touch: geriatric nursing. Journal of Communication 25(3): 104–112

Wells T 1980 Problems in geriatric nursing care. Churchill-Livingstone, Edinburgh

Wolanin M, Phillips L 1981 Confusion: prevention and care. Mosby, St Louis

CHAPTER CONTENTS

The stigma of deafness 79

Prevalence of deafness 81

Deafness and social theories of ageing 82

Assessment of hearing loss 83

Rehabilitation 83
Improving communication 83
Wearing a hearing aid 84
Other services available 86

The consequences of deafness 88

5

Hearing

Katia Gilhome Herbst

The stigma of deafness

One of the great tragedies of deafness is that it is traditionally accepted as a suitable subject for music-hall jokes and is therefore not taken seriously. Indeed, when in 1953 Barker and his colleagues published their now famous study on jokes about handicaps, deafness was reported as being the third most joked-about physical defect. It came third after 'having an unattractive face' and 'fatness' (Barker et al 1953). Note, for example, that much of the humour of 'Steptoe and Son' on television was derived from Steptoe's deafness.

In addition, deafness is generally accepted as a hoax disorder. It is often understood to be aggressive behaviour, with overtones of deliberate withholding of communication ('Old Mrs So-and-So seems to hear only when, and what, she wants to'). Hence that well-known saying, 'None so deaf as those who will not hear'. The implication is that the deaf could manage if only they pulled up their socks. No parallel proverb exists which accuses the blind of peeping when they particularly want to see. Furthermore, it would be considered very poor taste to laugh at a blind woman because she bumped into things. But not so with deafness.

What is it that is so special about deafness? Why are attitudes to deafness so negative?

It is important to consider this quite seriously since nurses, doctors and their elderly patients are all members of our society and, to that extent, will tend to hold prevailing attitudes to the disorder. Recent research by the author and colleagues has indicated that negative attitudes to deafness, coupled with a very hazy idea of the true psycho-social implications of the disorder, inhibit demand for deafness-specific services by the elderly deaf themselves and inhibit referral to other services by the general practitioner or nurse (Humphrey et al 1981, Gilhome Herbst 1982a).

There are many factors which contribute to prevailing negative attitudes to deafness. These are too varied and wide ranging to be discussed thoroughly here, but have been the subject of a review paper by the author (Gilhome Herbst 1982b).

The fundamental problem with deafness, which puzzled the ancient Greeks (Aristotle, *History of Animals* Bk IV, 9) and still puzzles the general public today (Bunting 1981), is that it is very difficult to distinguish between the symptoms of deafness and those of some types of mental disorders (particularly defects of reason). These symptoms — indistinct speech, not answering when spoken to, answering inappropriately or out of context, pitching the voice incorrectly — often encourage people to talk to and treat hearing-impaired people as if their cognitive abilities were also impaired. Regrettably, deafness has in consequence become a disorder to be ashamed of: 'I felt as if I were living in a twilight world. Deafness seemed a badge of shame.' (Jack Ashley, MP, 1973).

The second problem is that one cannot see deafness. It has to be volunteered by the handicapped person if it is to be known. It can be, and more frequently than not is, hidden. Hiding one's deafness is undoubtedly detrimental for both the hearing-impaired person and those with whom she wishes to communicate. The normally hearing person may not realize what the cause of the communication problem is and jump to his or her own conclusions. At the same time he or she will, in all probability, feel ill at ease, frustrated, finally resigned and even embarrassed. Unfortunately, we tend to laugh at things that embarrass us.

Our work has shown that such responses are well perceived by the deaf of all ages, but particularly by the elderly who are most sensitive to being considered 'senile' (Gilhome Herbst 1983). It is the embarrassment and the sense of shame and stigma that prevent people from announcing what the problem is. Such feelings apparently affect people from all walks of life. Beethoven suffered terribly: 'Yet I could not bring myself to say to people, "Speak up; shout, for I am deaf" . . . . Oh, I cannot do it' (Beethoven 1802).

The third crucial reason for the general dislike of deafness is undoubtedly its popularly accepted, and well-founded, association with ageing. Intuitively we all 'know' that many elderly people are deaf. This knowledge has been used by playwrights and novelists throughout the centuries when depicting old age. It is much more strongly associated with ageing than is poor sight. Regrettably, it is often used in an allegorical sense to represent a breakdown in meaningful communication with the world.

Thus people will often resist any acceptance that they might be deaf for as long as possible — in part because they do not wish to be seen to be suffering from an age-related disorder and in part because they do not wish to be mistaken as being of unsound mind.

Thus we have a disability which is stigmatized in its own right and associated very closely with two other 'conditions' which are equally stigmatized: mental disorder and old age. Indeed, in our ageist society, it could be argued that much of the dislike of deafness is derived from its very synonymity with old age and its attendant frailties. To admit to deafness is tantamount to admitting to being old and of unsound mind, although the common belief that deafness is associated with confusion and dementia, is not supported if the effect of age is eliminated (Gilhome Herbst & Humphrey 1980). It is this stereotypical fusion between deafness and old age that is probably the root cause of the neglect in reporting and treating the disorder.

Being deaf does make elderly people feel differently about themselves. They say that deafness makes them 'feel closed in', 'feel inferior', 'get frustrated or depressed', 'tend to evade other people'. These sentiments express the feeling of personal degradation associated with being deaf (Gilhome Herbst 1983).

Yet another problem is the patchy auditory performance so typical of acquired deafness (particularly in the elderly) whereby, apparently for no reason, conversations and words (names in particular) are clearly understood. This, of course, fuels the none-so-deaf-as-those-who-will-not-hear school of thought. Interestingly enough, the very (apparently freak) conditions in which improved hearing occurs in this way are those which those who live and work with old people should foster.

PREVALENCE OF DEAFNESS

Denial of deafness by young and old alike has been noted since early times by psychologists and researchers (Menninger 1924, Wilkins 1948, Gregory 1961, Townsend & Wedderburn 1965, Nguyens 1984). It has generally been assumed that the stigma of being deaf was the prime factor behind this denial. It is a major force to contend with and one that has been ill understood. For doctors and nurses who are responsible for setting in motion rehabilitation and care of deafness of the elderly, probably the central problem will be to detect the deafness in the first place. Some discussion now of the probable prevalence of deafness in old age, and how estimates of the prevalence have been arrived at, will expose the scale, and importance, of the problem of denial.

Estimates of hearing loss of the elderly have traditionally been undertaken in order to establish the probable numbers of elderly people likely to require hearing aids under the National Health Service. Thus we are talking about a level of bilateral impairment that would, by convention, be deemed to require amplification from a hearing aid.

Community studies of the elderly which have included questions concerning hearing loss are numerous. A review of 15 such studies by the author confirmed the conventionally held belief that between 30% and 40% of all persons of retirement age are hearing impaired to the extent that they would benefit from amplification (Gilhome Herbst & Humphrey 1981, Gilhome Herbst 1983). All these studies assess the presence of hearing loss either by asking the elderly person some questions associated with their hearing (Sheldon 1948, Harris 1962, Kay et al 1964, Brockington & Lempert 1966, Abrams 1978) or by the assessment of the clinician or interviewer (Stockport County Council 1958, Williamson et al 1964, Sheard 1971, Cumbria County Council 1973).

Until recently, these estimates, whilst accepted as being of questionable validity (Rawson 1973, Haggard et al 1981), were still used by the Department of Health when considering rehabilitation services for hearing impaired people (DHSS 1977). In 1981, preliminary results from the National Study on Hearing (NSH) (Haggard et al 1981) cast doubt upon them. The NSH sent a postal questionnaire to a random sample of 11 740 adults aged 17 years and over, asking them about their hearing. From this, a stratified sub-sample of 759 persons attended clinics for otological and audiometric investigations (Davis 1983). By extrapolating from Davis's work, one can see that the NSH suggests that some 55% of all persons aged 75 years and over will report some hearing impairment of sufficient severity to merit amplification by a hearing aid. Davis admits that the method used in the NSH probably led to an under-representation of those aged 75 years and over living at home.

A wide-ranging and thorough review of the literature reveals no estimates of prevalence of deafness of the elderly based upon thorough audiometric assessments of old people living at home other than the work of the present author (Gilhome Herbst & Humphrey 1981). In this study (inter alia) the prevalence of hearing impairment in a community sample of the elderly aged 70 years and over was assessed using pure-tone audiometry. 'Deafness' was defined as an average loss over the speech frequencies at 1 kHz, 2 kHz and 4 kHz of 35 dB* or more in the better ear. The proportion found to be 'deaf' was 60%. A statistically significant association between increas-

---

*Sound frequency, or pitch, is expressed in numbers of vibrations (cycles) per second. By convention these vibrations (cycles) are called Hertz. kHz means thousands of cycles of sound per second. Output of sound is measured in decibels (dB). By convention, hearing loss is measured in terms of the output (dB) necessary for sounds at certain pitches (kHz) to be heard.

ing age and the incidence and severity of deafness was also found (Gilhome Herbst & Humphrey 1981), such that of all those aged

70 yrs+ 60% were deaf
75 yrs+ 69% were deaf
80 yrs+ 82% were deaf
85 yrs+ 84% were deaf

In addition, a further 14% of the sample were found to have a unilateral loss of 35 dB or more. Under auroscopic examination, wax in both ears was observed in 25% of the sample. The presence of wax was not significantly related to deafness.

The findings of that study challenge conventionally held assumptions about the prevalence of hearing impairment in old age, which until very recently have resulted in the scale of the disorder being considerably underestimated, in both professional and official thinking. The results of the National Study on Hearing confirm these findings (Haggard et al 1981). It is of particular interest to the present discussion on the problems of detecting deafness to note that, in that same study, the conventional kind of question 'Do you think you are at all deaf?' (as used in all other studies which attempted to estimate the prevalence of deafness by questionnaire techniques) yielded similar results (Gilhome Herbst & Humphrey 1981). This is displayed on Table 5.1 The discrepancy in the results is important. It shows the discrepancy between 'true' impairment and the number of elderly persons who either do not notice that they have a hearing problem or who wish to hide it. Whilst to some extent this discrepancy may be due to genuine ignorance of the fact, it is likely that deliberate denial of the problem was present. Those studies which provide results of the prevalence of deafness based upon the clinician's or researchers' assessments provide results which are

equally at odds with those based upon audiometric findings as are those based on self-estimate.

It is very difficult for the general practitioner, nurse and caring others to recognize the disorder when it is not volunteered by the patient. This is, first, because the very high prevalence of deafness amongst elderly people renders it almost synonymous with old age, and secondly because its major effects — namely impoverished communication and a subsequent tendency to withdraw from social intercourse — may too readily be mistaken for so-called 'normal ageing'.

In our study, of those elderly people found to be significantly bilaterally hearing impaired, 26% refused to accept any suggestion that they might be hearing impaired despite the evidence of their audiograms. The mean dB loss of this group was 43.9 dB in the better ear. A further 25% admitted to the interviewer that they knew that they had a hearing loss but had never mentioned this to their doctor. The mean dB loss of this group was 51.9 dB in the better ear. Thus over half the deaf elderly population under investigation had never mentioned their deafness to their general practitioner (Humphrey et al 1981). Yet, as a group, they were substantially impaired. This gives some indication of the size of the problem facing doctors and nurses.

DEAFNESS AND SOCIAL THEORIES OF AGEING

An awareness of the synonymity of deafness and ageing can provide some useful insight into social theories of ageing (see Ch. 2), particularly into Cumming and Henry's disengagement theory (Cumming & Henry 1961). This theory strives to explain the observed phenomenon of social withdrawal which may often accompany advancing years. It suggests that ageing people naturally and voluntarily withdraw from being too involved with others, thus also diminishing their emotional investment in personal relationships. It also suggests that the elderly are generally satisfied with comparatively casual, superficial social contacts and proposes that this diminution in social involvement

Table 5.1 Estimates of prevalence of deafness in an elderly person (N = 253).

	Age in years			
	70+	75+	80+	85+
Based on self-estimate	38%	39%	54%	69%
Based on pure-tone audiometry	60%	69%	82%	84%

is convenient for the young — society being content to release its elderly from the normal demands of responsibility and accountability. The emphasis is on this being a 'natural' and 'mutual' process and one to be condoned and promulgated. Such a theory seems to draw directly, if unwittingly, on the effects of deafness as a communication interrupter. Deafness supports, or at least explains, the observed phenomenon of mutual release, or should one say breakdown, in communication between young and old. Consequently, from a disengagement perspective, deafness can be seen as a normal and natural part of ageing which may not therefore demand attention.

The opposing view, sometimes known as the activity or continuity approach to explaining the observed social changes that accompany old age, is that the diminishing world of the older person is largely societally constructed and reinforced. It suggests that in fact people continue throughout their lifespan with very much the same social and emotional requirements (e.g. Abrams 1979) and that it is therefore a fallacy that older people are content with less because they are old and physically less robust.

Thus the very recent interest in the social implications of deafness in ageing goes hand in hand with the widespread rejection of disengagement. Indeed there is a general antagonism to the acceptance of any of the disorders of ageing as unalterable and inexorable. Deafness must now be seen as another physical disorder requiring treatment and care for which our understanding of the social and psychological implications of the disorder is a necessary prerequisite.

ASSESSMENT OF HEARING LOSS

One certainty results from our research — when a person complains of hearing loss they are very likely to be correct in their assessment and should be encouraged, before time is lost, to make use of appropriate services. In our study, such people were substantially bilaterally impaired with average loss of between 56.3 and 69.5 dB in the better ear (Humphrey et al 1981).

Certain very simple strategies may help to disclose poor hearing amongst those who do not volunteer it (though severity of loss is difficult to judge). The two best are speaking in a normal voice to the patient with the back turned and simultaneously, or in addition, asking unexpected questions or questions that may be slightly out of context. These are rough-and-ready techniques and no more to be firmly relied upon than are the simple techniques used by health visitors when testing infants. Our own work has shown that with care and regular calibration of the audiometer, simple pure-tone audiometry can successfully and accurately be carried out in a non-clinical setting by suitably trained staff.

REHABILITATION

IMPROVING COMMUNICATION

The following conditions and strategies will improve communication with an elderly person who is hearing impaired:

- Ensure that light is on the face (of the speaker) so that the whole face, and in particular the lips, are clearly seen.
- Improve visual acuity, by encouraging the elderly person to wear her spectacles — it will help her to lip-read and in consequence to understand speech better.
- Ensure that the face of the speaker is not obscured (by hands) or distorted (by eating or smoking).
- Ensure that the elderly person is concentrating on what is to be said and is not doing something else which may distract her.
- Talk clearly, and enunciate clearly. If the voice is raised, be sure not to shout as this both distorts the mouth and face (which can be interpreted as aggressive behaviour).
- Shouting can cause pain. It is characteristic of sensorineural deafness (which is the kind of deafness most frequently associated with ageing) that the transition from hearing little or nothing, to hearing sounds very loudly

(called recruitment) is abnormally abrupt. Pain is caused by over-boosting those frequencies which are not impaired.

- Use familiar words and phrases. This reduces guess-work.
- Use words in context — single words repeated again and again with no clues offered will be more difficult to 'hear'.
- Talk slowly.
- Talk with kindness and sympathy. The tone of the voice will be understood even if the words are not (remember that children understand tone well before they understand language. Even animals understand tone).
- All people perform best in an atmosphere of sympathy. It is crucial to reduce stress on the part of both hearing impaired and normally hearing people. When difficulties arise, try to laugh.

WEARING A HEARING AID

Researchers have found that the earlier a person is referred for a hearing aid the more likely they are to learn to benefit from and continue using their aid (Pedersen et al 1974) well into advanced age (Gilhome Herbst 1983). Those elderly people who do have aids (who represent a minority of the elderly deaf) have been found to use their aids about as frequently as do people of employment age (Humphrey et al 1981). Poor hearing aid usage is not specific to the elderly, though their reasons for poor usage may be different from those of younger people (Brooks 1989). It is, rather, a sad reflection on the state of hearing aid services in this country and the complex nature of sensorineural deafness.

It is unfortunate that sensorineural deafness, which characterizes hearing impairment in old age, is progressive, associated with recruitment and tinnitus and lends itself but grudgingly to amelioration with the use of a hearing aid. Nonetheless, for a substantial number of persons, even the elderly, some benefit is to be derived from wearing an aid and it should be tried. Furthermore, access to other services — from volunteers, the hearing therapist and even the social worker for the deaf — is often to be found through referral from the hearing aid clinic. Domiciliary visits from the hearing aid clinic are available and crucial for the very old and frail amongst whom deafness is most prevalent.

It seems probable that nurses and general practitioners take a rather similar view to that of old people, and indeed society at large, about the inevitability of deafness in old age and the futility of attempting much in the way of rehabilitation. Ironically, to some extent they are being realistic in doubting the value of the rehabilitative service for elderly people in the present circumstances. The problem is circular as long as, for the reasons discussed above, elderly people tend either to defer demand for aids indefinitely or at least postpone it for as long as possible; the majority who do come forward, therefore, are liable to be very old, very frail and almost 'stone deaf' (Brooks 1979, Ward et al 1979). It has been suggested (Alberti 1977) that attempting to initiate aural rehabilitation with such subjects is largely a waste of time. Rumour of the failure of rehabilitative measures when undertaken with the very deaf and very old may well contribute one further reason for the elderly deaf not to bother to come forward in time to benefit from rehabilitation. It certainly lowers morale within the hearing aid service. A strong case is therefore made for the encouragement of early intervention and an improvement in the service available (Haggard & Armstrong-Bednall 1984).

Indeed, the NHS hearing aid service has improved dramatically since the behind-the-ear (BE) programme (BE10 series) was introduced in 1974 with the BE11 model (Fig. 5.1). The B10 series provides medium power behind-the-ear aids. There are now seven aids in the BE10 series: the BE11, BE14, BE15, BE16, BE17, BE18 and BE19. The BE14 and BE15 do not have forward-facing microphones — all the others do. Otherwise there is little difference in performance among the aids. The main reason for such a choice of aids in this series is the purchasing policy of the Department of Health, which tries to ensure that it does not depend on a single manufacturer to supply all NHS aids (Johnson 1981).

The BE30 series of high power, high gain aids is intended for patients who are unable to use the

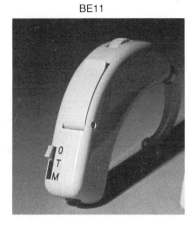
BE11

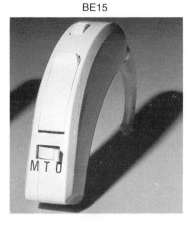
BE15

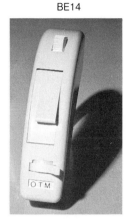
BE14

Fig. 5.1 Behind-the-ear hearing aids: BE10 series. BE11 BE15 BE14

BE10 series because of insufficient output (Fig. 5.2). It is also intended for those persons who can only use the BE10 series when set at maximum output. There are now five models in this range — the BE31 to the BE35. Only the BE31 does not have a forward-facing microphone. Aids in this series have been available since December 1980.

A further series, the BE50 series of aids, was launched in the spring of 1982. The three aids in this series are more powerful still than the BE30 series. Figure 5.3 shows examples of this series.

With the introduction of the BE50 series, the programme of development is seen to be at an end, although thought is being given to still further types of aids with more facilities. This does not exclude the planned updating of obsolescent mod-els, but it does mean that the Department of Health is sufficiently confident that NHS aids will be of a wide enough range to fit all types and degrees of hearing loss now that all restrictions on the supply of commercial aids through the NHS have been lifted. As from 1 July 1980, health authorities have been empowered, at their own discretion, to make arrangements for the supply of commercial models to patients of any age who have exceptional medical need and for whom a standard NHS aid is not satisfactory. As a temporary measure the Department of Health made arrangements for private sector hearing aids to be available under the NHS for persons who would

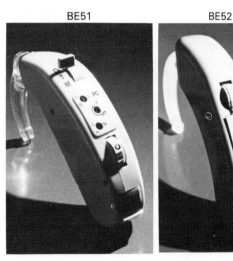
BE51 BE52

Fig. 5.2 Behind-the-ear hearing aids: BE30 series. BE31 BE32

Fig. 5.3 Behind-the-ear hearing aids: BE50 series. BE51 BE52

BW61   BW81

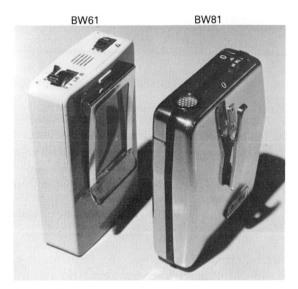

Fig. 5.4 Body-worn hearing aids: BW60 and BW80 series. BW61 BW81

normally be deemed to benefit from the new BE50 series.

The old body-worn Medrescos (OL56, OL58, OL66), which were the only hearing aids available under the NHS until November 1974, are being replaced by new body-worn aids under the BW60 and BW80 series (Fig. 5.4). The range of body-worn aids available under the NHS will be kept up-to-date by the introduction of new aids when necessary. Both series are intended for patients with very severe hearing losses who need high power and high gain particularly in the lower frequencies. Bone conduction fittings are available with both the BW60 and the BW80 series.

Ear moulds, batteries, leads and all servicing and repairs to hearing aids have always been and still are offered free of charge under the NHS. Hospital nurses often do not realize that these items can be obtained from the audiometric department and hearing therapist. Acoustic aids (non-electric), the descendants of the old-fashioned ear-trumpet, are particularly useful where patients find it difficult or impossible to handle sophisticated hearing aids. They are available to the hearing impaired on the recommendation of an ear, nose and throat consultant in exactly the same way as are electric hearing aids and

are particularly useful for very frail elderly or disabled persons. They are also particularly valuable for all professionals working with elderly people, and it is wise to keep one on the ward.

There are three types of non-electric aids available: the OL340 'Banjo' telescopic plastic ear-trumpet; the OL370 plastic ear-trumpet (otherwise known as the London Horn); the OL38001 conversation tube with a swivel joint ear-piece (Johnson 1981). The ear-trumpet is simply held to the ear by the hearing impaired person. The conversation tube fits directly into the ear of the hearing impaired person — the other end is held to the lips of the speaker, thus enabling high levels of sound to be delivered. A recent review of the acoustic gain which can be obtained from these aids suggests that there is considerable potential for development of these so-called old-fashioned aids (Grover 1977).

Various non-electric instruments (speaking tubes, lorgnettes and ear trumpets) are also available for purchase from P C Werth Ltd* who are suppliers to the NHS. The cost of these vary from £25 to £120 and nurses are recommended to try them out before purchasing.

P C Werth also produce an 'electric lorgnette' (Fig. 5.5); the earphone is simply held against the listener's ear and the volume can be adjusted by the nurse or doctor using a small rotary control. It is either microphone or induction driven.

Other communicators are available from the commercial sector. Inter-Tan UK Ltd, produce a very useful stereo listener — catalogue no. 33–1093 currently retailing at £14.95 (see Fig. 5.6). It is designed to be used whenever extra sound amplification is needed and would be particularly valuable in a surgery or hospital outpatient setting. Headphones or an earpiece are not supplied with the stereo listener, so it is necessary to purchase these separately. Almost any type of popular headphone should fit it.

OTHER SERVICES AVAILABLE

There may be many circumstances where environ-

---

* P C Werth Ltd, Audiology House, 95 Nightingale Lane, London SE12 8SP.

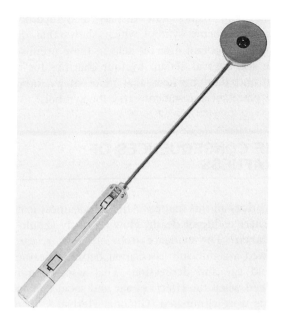

Fig. 5.5 Electric lorgnette.

mental aids and adaptations to the home are far more, or just as, relevant to the elderly person. People often will buy them, but if funds are a problem, statutory provisions for deaf and hard-of-hearing persons can be made. These are to be found in Section 2 of the Chronically Sick and Disabled Persons (CSDP) Act 1970, and are con-solidated in the Disabled Persons Act, 1986. Local authorities can provide: alarm bells or light systems to enable hard-of-hearing persons to know when a caller is at the door; special attachments for radio and television so that volume can be raised to an adequate level for the hard-of-hearing without disturbing other★; assistance to travel to club meetings and lip-reading classes and assistance with fees for such classes; assistance in obtaining special attachments for the telephone including an amplifier or extra head set where necessary.★

Sections 4, 7 and 8 of the CSDP Act require local authorities to wire all public and recreational halls with a loop system for the convenience of hearing aid wearers and to put up signs to show that this service is available.

★ The Royal National Institute for the Deaf (RNID) publishes several booklets offering advice on the purchase and installation of these aids as well as NHS and privately purchased hearing aids.

★ British Telecom publishes a well-illustrated booklet entitled: British Telecom's guide to equipment and services for disabled customers — 1988 (British Telecom. Action for Disabled Customers, Nov. 1987), in which telephone aids produced by the GPO and for purchase by local authorities under the Disabled Persons Act, 1986 are laid out. However, availability of devices is patchy throughout the country.

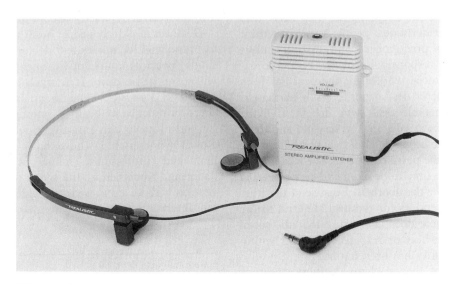

Fig. 5.6 Stereo listener and headphones

Nowhere is it specified who should be the responsible officer for ascertaining need for environmental aids. By convention this task has always been performed either by social workers, occupational therapists, or other local authority personnel. Where a hearing therapist is in post at the hearing aid clinic, this task may be carried out by her or him. The actual level of provision of aids for the deaf under Section 2 of the CSDP Act is extremely difficult to ascertain from national returns.

Although hearing aids have been available free under the NHS since its inception, a substantial number of elderly hearing impaired people do not know of this service (for example, as many as a third of a sample of elderly deaf people under study by the author and colleagues were ignorant of the free service (Humphrey et al 1981)). Ignorance of the service must inevitably dampen the reporting of deafness to the general practitioner. Steps can be taken by doctors to advertise the existence of the service.

Patients (and relatives) should be encouraged to try NHS hearing aids before embarking on the very expensive and often hazardous purchase of hearing aids from the private sector. However, if such action is preferred, the RNID offers a free service to the general public on how to set about buying a hearing aid.

The situation is far worse as regards environmental aids and adaptations. A truly tiny proportion of elderly deaf people know that these exist. General practitioners and district nurses have a central responsibility in this regard to ensure that the social worker for the deaf has been notified of elderly deaf patients — in particular, the most vulnerable deaf, who are those living alone. As has been said, for the very old and those living alone, environmental aids may be far more relevant than the personal hearing aid which must be worn all the time to be of any value for hearing the telephone or the doorbell. Because of the fragmentation of services for the deaf, referral to the hearing aid clinic does not ensure that the social worker for the deaf or responsible officer within the local authority has been notified.

Awareness of the problems deafness causes is slowly gaining public attention. Many shops, offices and banks now display a Sympathetic Hearing Scheme symbol which shows that deaf people can obtain discreet help in these premises. The scheme was set up by four charities for the deaf and they are keen that more shops, offices and places of amusement carry the symbol.*

THE CONSEQUENCES OF DEAFNESS

Why does all this matter? After all, deafness is not a matter of life or death. How seriously should it be taken? The evidence from our own research showed a significant association between deafness in old age and depression. This association remained when the effects of age and socioeconomic status were eliminated (Gilhome Herbst & Humphrey 1980). In addition, a significant overall association was found between deafness and low socioeconomic status, advanced age, poor health, reduced out-of-doors activity owing to fears of managing with poor hearing, loss of friends and loss of enjoyment of life. Indeed there was sufficient evidence to support the notion that deafness in old age is strongly associated with isolation, but not necessarily loneliness, and an artificially imposed loss of personal autonomy and physical independence. These associations were not necessarily perceived by elderly people themselves.

Deafness of elderly people poses many challenging problems for nurses and doctors. There is no single foolproof course of treatment to adopt that will solve the problem. It is largely a social malady caused by a physical impairment. In addition, the sheer prevalence of deafness amongst the elderly (hitherto known only intuitively) which renders it almost synonymous with ageing in both the popular and professional mind, is undoubtedly daunting. Nonetheless, the scope for early intervention with an aid is evidently wide and the scope for intervention with environmental aids even

---

* More information on the scheme can be obtained from the Sympathetic Hearing Scheme, 7/11 Armstrong Road, London W3 7JL.

wider. Regrettably, disinterest by physicians is reflected in the disinterest of nurses and paramedical staff and ignorance of the extent of the problem suppresses interest at policy level. Of all health care staff, the primary health care team holds the crucial role in the rehabilitation of the elderly deaf.

REFERENCES

Abrams M 1978 Beyond three score and ten. Age Concern Research Publications, Mitcham
Abrams M 1979 Transitions in middle and later life. Paper presented to the British Society of Social and Behavioural Gerontology, Keble College, University of Oxford
Alberti P W 1977 Hearing aids and aural rehabilitation. Journal of Otolaryngology 6: suppl no 4
Ashley J 1973 Journey into silence. Bodley Head, London
Barker R G, Wright B A, Myerson L, Gonick M R 1953 Adjustment to physical handicap and illness: a survey of the social psychology of physique and disability, 2nd edn. Social Science Research Council, Bulletin 55, New York
Beethoven L 1802 Heiligenstadt document. Stadtbibliothek, Hamburg
Berry G 1933 The psychology of progressive deafness. Journal of the American Medical Association 101: 1599–1603
Brockington F, Lempert S M 1966 The social needs of the over-80s. Manchester University Press
Brooks D N 1979 Hearing aid candidates — some relevant features. British Journal of Audiology 13: 81–84
Brooks D N 1989 The effect of attitude on benefit obtained from hearing aids. British Journal of Audiology, 23: 3–11
Bunting C 1981 Public attitudes to deafness. Social Survey of the Office of Population Censuses and Surveys. HMSO, London
Cumbria County Council 1973 Survey of the handicapped and impaired and elderly over seventy-five in Cumberland. Cumbria County Council
Cumming E, Henry H E 1961 Growing old: the process of disengagement. Basic Books, New York
Davis A 1983 Epidemiology of hearing disorders. In: Hinchcliffe R (ed) Medicine in old age — hearing and balance. Churchill Livingstone, Edinburgh
Department of Health and Social Security ACSHIP 1977 Report of a sub-committee appointed to consider the role of social services in the care of the deaf of all ages. Advisory Committee on Services for Hearing Impaired People, London
Gilhome Herbst K R 1982a Some social implications of acquired deafness in ageing. In: Taylor R, Gilmore A J J (eds) Current trends in British gerontology. Gower Press, London

Gilhome Herbst K R 1982b Social attitudes to hearing loss in the elderly. In: Creber A (ed) Barriers to communication: a national seminar on acquired hearing loss in elderly people. Beth Johnson Foundation, Keele University
Gilhome Herbst K R 1983 Psycho-social consequences of disorders of hearing in the elderly. In: Hinchcliffe R (ed) Medicine in old age — hearing and balance. Churchill Livingstone, Edinburgh
Gilhome Herbst K R, Humphrey C M 1980 Hearing impairment and mental state in the elderly living at home. British Medical Journal 280: 903–905
Gilhome Herbst K R, Humphrey C M 1981 Prevalence of hearing impairment in the elderly living at home. Journal of the Royal College of General Practitioners 31: 155–160
Gregory P 1961 Deafness and public responsibility. Occasional Papers on Social Administration no. 7, Codicote Press, Welwyn
Grover B C 1977 A note on acoustic aids. British Journal of Audiology 11: 75–76
Haggard M, Armstrong-Bednall G 1984 Requirements of structure and resource for an adequate audiology service in the post-Griffiths health service. British Journal of Audiology 18: 183–194
Haggard M, Gatehouse S, Davis A 1981 The high prevalence of hearing disorders and its implications for services in the UK. British Journal of Audiology 15: 241–251
Harris A 1962 The social survey. Health and welfare of older people in Lewisham. Central Office of Information, London
Humphrey C M, Gilhome Herbst K R, Faruqi S 1981 Some characteristics of the hearing impaired elderly who do not present themselves for rehabilitation. British Journal of Audiology 15: 25–30
Johnson J A 1981 National Health Service hearing aids. Hearing 36(1): 8–13
Kay D W K, Beamish P, Roth M 1964 Old age mental disorders in Newcastle upon Tyne. I: A study of prevalence. British Journal of Psychiatry 110: 146–158
Menninger K A 1924 The mental effects of deafness. Psychoanalytic Review 11: 144–155
Nguyens M 1984 Denial and follow-up as predictors of outcome among elderly clients screened in a hearing outreach program. Unpublished doctoral dissertation. California School of Professional Psychology, Berkeley
Pedersen B, Frankner B, Terkildsen K 1974 A prospective study of adult Danish hearing aid users. Scandinavian Audiology 3: 107–111
Rawson A 1973 Deafness: report of a departmental enquiry into the promotion of research. DHSS, HMSO, London
Sheard A V 1971 Survey of the elderly in Scunthorpe. Public Health London 85: 208–218
Sheldon J H 1948 The social medicine of old age. Report of an enquiry in Wolverhampton. Oxford University Press, London
Stockport County Council 1958 Report on the survey of the aged in Stockport. Stockport County Council
Thomas A J, Gilhome Herbst K R 1980 Social and psychological implications of acquired deafness for adults of employment age. British Journal of Audiology 14: 76–85
Townsend P, Wedderburn D 1965 The aged in the welfare state. Occasional Papers on Social Administration no. 14, G Bell, London

Ward P R, Gowers J I, Morgan D C 1979 Problems with handling the BE10 series hearing aids among elderly people. British Journal of Audiology 13(1): 31–36

Wilkins L T 1948 The social survey. Survey of the prevalence of deafness in the population of England, Scotland and Wales. Central Office of Information, London

Williamson J, Stokoe I H, Gray S et al 1964 Old people at home: their unreported needs. Lancet 1: 1117–1120

CHAPTER CONTENTS

Prevalence of sight difficulties among elderly people 92

Assessment of sight 92

Causes of visual loss in old age 93
Cataract 93
Macular degeneration 94
Glaucoma 94
Diabetic retinopathy 95

Light, contrast, size, colour 95
Lamps and bulbs 96
Contrast and colour 96
Size 97

Seeking help 97

Statutory and voluntary help 97
Statutory 97
Voluntary 98

6

Sight

Tim R. Cullinan

To the elderly person assumptions about sight are as dangerous, and as depersonalizing, as assumptions about anything else. But they are easily made — from childhood we have grown up with stereotypes about 'blind' people, often reaching back into our own fantasies and fairy-tales. For most of us there are few occasions to challenge our misconceptions until we are brought face-to-face with them, either in our own later lives or in caring for some other who needs a good deal more than our prejudices. The scramble to readjust invites confusion, yet so much can be done, without specialist knowledge, if the problem is approached simply and with confidence. The key person, as so often, is the nurse, or the relative, or the friend, who knows best what an elderly person wants most to do or is willing to take the sensitive steps to find out. What is least helpful is to believe that eyes and sight are a 'no-go' area to be handled only by specialists; though knowing when to seek their help, and how to make the best use of it, is essential.

Some assumptions may, of course, be shared by the elderly person: 'Nurses are not concerned with sight — that is for opticians and special doctors'; 'I can't expect to see well, I'm getting old'; 'My eyes are failing, I must avoid strong light'; 'I can see very well. It's my friend who is blind, but then she is older than I am' — and there are plenty more. It takes patience and sensitivity to get behind these protective beliefs and to discover what things an elderly person wants to be able to see to do, or is most fearful of being unable to do — and then, together, to seek ways of achieving them.

But in the end the approach is far more effective and long-lasting than trying to achieve a predetermined level of measurable visual acuity and believing everything will be simple after that. Such is the pattern of our society, and of the professionalization of knowledge, that unless the initial steps are taken by close carers, most elderly people will go without the help they need (Cullinan 1986).

PREVALENCE OF SIGHT DIFFICULTIES AMONG ELDERLY PEOPLE

In the average Health District of about 200 000 people, with average age spread, there are about 1000 living at home who have difficulty in seeing enough to manage the ordinary affairs of daily living (Knight & Warren 1978). Three quarters (750) of these may be in their retirement years and one half (500) over the age of seventy five. A little over half of all those with sight difficulties may already be registered as 'blind' or 'partially sighted' and so known to Social Services. However, the situation is very variable over England and Wales (Brennan & Knox 1973), though everywhere there is a fair number of elderly people living at home who are not registered, yet who see so badly that they would certainly qualify to become so (Graham et al 1968).

For about half the 750 or so, poor sight will be the only major disability they have (Cullinan 1977). If this is so, they are usually happy to discuss it freely and are likely to have had some help for it, though this may well need reviewing. If, on the other hand, they have some other major disability, perhaps arthritis or heart disease, it is likely that their sight problems will pass unnoticed — even if they have been inpatients in a general hospital (Fenton et al 1975). That is why it is so important not to be fearful of introducing the subject.

It is also worth remembering that the great majority of elderly people with poor sight have entered their retirement years with good vision — or, rather, with no more than the presbyopia which begins to affect us all as we pass through our 40s. So the slow onset of sight-limiting disease occurs at a time when we find it increasingly difficult to do anything about it; visits to the optician become ever rarer and more difficult and the doctor — perhaps the nurse — seems interested only in our arthritis or other major disability. Self-image, suppression, denial, stigma, all play a part, and a great deal of unnecessary suffering results.

ASSESSMENT OF SIGHT

It is simplest to consider the idea of 'sight' in two components: visual acuity, or what the eye and its nervous pathway is optically and neurologically capable of doing, and visual ability, or what is actually being achieved with that acuity. The first, of course, is much the easiest to measure and is the basis of most well-known sight tests — both distance (the Snellen chart) and near vision tests. It is quite possible to administer these tests with hand-held cards in a 'patient's' own home, with results comparable to the optician's, but the approach to them, and the path from them, should be through visual ability. Several sets of questions have been suggested, and have been validated (Harris 1971), as surrogates for acuity testing, but they are more suited to surveys than to individuals; it is much better to start talking about sight difficulties and then to focus on where the major problems lie. Remember that many elderly people value, and need, their near vision (to sew, read, etc.) more than distance vision — very few elderly people are housebound because of sight difficulties alone.

For distance vision, eye charts scaled down for use at 3 metres (10 feet) are best; few elderly people live in rooms large enough for the standard 6-metre card. The subject should be sitting comfortably, in a good overhead light, looking straight ahead. Make sure she has on whatever glasses have been prescribed, if any, for general, not reading, use, and that they have clean lenses. Hold the test card, tilted slightly forward to reduce glare, at 3 metres from the subject's eyes and test each eye separately. The subject can hold a piece of paper or card over the other eye; she should read down from the top of the test card and the smallest line of letters read without a mistake after two tries can be taken as the functional visual acuity for that eye.

For the testing of near vision, reading cards are available with print in different sizes from N36 down to N2. Again a good light, this time from over the shoulder, reading glasses if available, clean lenses and comfort are needed, but the subject can hold the test card at any distance she likes. If she can read N5, she can read anything; if N8, most of a well-printed newspaper; if N12, the headlines only. So if you have no test card, a newspaper may be a good substitute so long as it is printed black on white and has a good typeface.

In general, anyone with a distance vision, adequately corrected by glasses, of less than 6/18 in either eye has almost certainly got a sight-threatening disease and should have specialist opinion. If distance vision is between 6/9 and 6/18 and/or near vision no better than N12, and no assessment has been made by an ophthalmic optician within the last two years, a visit is well worthwhile. If there is any substantial disease the optician will spot it; if not, he may be able to improve vision substantially with appropriate corrective lenses.

A third component of sight is the field of vision; there are several diseases common in old age that affect the visual field, but many elderly people will not realize that they have field loss, at least in one eye, until it has progressed a long way. As a single symptom, it is not common. It can be roughly tested (again for each eye separately) by asking the subject to fix and stare into the eye of the tester at about two feet, face to face; the tester, returning the compliment, brings a lighted pen torch or coloured hat pin slowly into the space between their two faces from each side in turn and then from top and bottom. She notes where she first sees the object and when the patient does. If, on repeated testing, a field defect is suspected a specialist opinion is essential.

CAUSES OF VISUAL LOSS IN OLD AGE

The physiological changes in the eyes that accompany age have been briefly described in Chapter 3 of this book. The whole effect is to reduce the intensity of light that reaches the retina, and to scatter it; and for the retina itself, including the macula most particularly, to lose some of its exquisite powers of discrimination. Yet, at its worst, none of these physiological processes is truly disabling, given adequate lighting, contrast and lens correction; it is only when degenerative or other disease intervenes that sight becomes seriously compromised. The difficulty for many elderly people is, of course, that lighting, contrast and correction are often far from adequate, so that physiological processes alone can lead to disability.

CATARACT

Cataract is the most common eye disease of old age. Ederer (1977, 1978) found in the Framingham Eye Study that 20% of all people between 65 and 74 years of age with a corrected visual acuity of 6/9 or less had a discernable cataract in at least one eye; the proportion closer to 50% between the ages of 75 and 84. Most elderly people with cataracts are not troubled by them; the condition often remains static or only very slowly progressive and does not compromise sight to any degree. But if they do progress, objects in the middle of the field of vision become progressively blurred and colours are dull; as Dobree and Boulter (1982) put it, 'the house always seems to need decorating'. Most commonly the cataract occupies the nucleus of the lens, cutting off the visual path to the sensitive macula where fine discrimination occurs. But if, less often, the cataract is in the anterior part of the lens, glare may be a particular problem as the light reaching the lens is shattered and bright light, which may be helpful to a nuclear cataract, makes matters worse. This is why, as Gilkes (1979) remarks, some old ladies say they see better with their hats on. Many people, even with fairly advanced cataract, find going out and getting about the house not too difficult because they are using their peripheral fields to avoid bumping into things.

The only effective cure for cataract is operative but this is much less tiresome for an elderly person than it used to be. The old (aphakic) spectacle lenses that were used to replace the eye's removed lens until recently, were ugly, cumbersome, heavy and, being very strong, gave only a very narrow field of undistorted vision. Many elderly people found themselves unable to cope, especially as object sizes were often different to each eye, and gave up wearing them. But with modern intraocular lens implants the whole business is much better, and the eye has usually settled down to its newly found powers within a month or so. Unfortunately the backlog of people needing the operation is very long (London Health Planning Consortium 1980).

MACULAR DEGENERATION

This slowly progressive degenerative disease of the macula makes its biggest contribution to poor sight after the age of 75 years though in the Framingham study 10% of those between 65 and 74 years were found to have at least the early changes associated with it. Essentially, ageing pigment cells put out deposits of debris which lift them from the membrane on which they lie and so compromise their blood supply. The vessels, too, may leak or bleed and in this case the disease is usually much more rapidly progressive. The earliest symptom may be an increasing difficulty in distinguishing small objects and doing fine tasks but because the other eye comes to the rescue nothing may be noticed until it, too, becomes affected or the fine object is lost altogether in the first affected eye. Dobree and Boulter (1982) describe the progress of symptoms over five years — the first being a distortion of straight lines so that shelves and picture rails appear to have kinks. When the whole of central vision has been lost there is also a deal of distortion in the peripheral vision that remains, but, as with cataracts, the 'patient' can often still get about. Perhaps 10%–15% of people who have no macular function in one eye will eventually lose the macular function of the other as well; and 60%–70% of people with macular degener-

ation will be reduced to 'registerable blindness' within five years of the onset of visual disability (Lovie-Kitchen et al 1982).

There is no satisfactory cure for macular degeneration but recent studies have suggested that in many cases that have not progressed too far, photocoagulation may at least arrest further deterioration. Whatever the prognosis, a full specialist assessment is indicated.

GLAUCOMA

Glaucoma occurs when the pressure inside the eyeball rises above normal and begins to affect the blood supply to the retina and optic nerve. There are two main types of glaucoma — 'open angle' and 'closed angle', the angle being the gutter, between the front surface of the iris and the cornea, where the intraocular fluid drains away to the main circulation. In the open angle type the gutter itself remains open but the fine pores of the trabecula through which the fluid filters become gradually inadequate to filter it fast enough. This usually happens slowly over many years until gradually the pressure builds up, often to levels above 30 mmHg, bulging the optic nerve head, and compromising its blood supply. The earliest effect on sight is a patchy loss of visual field but because it is only partial and initially affects only one eye, and distance vision at that, it frequently passes unnoticed until a late stage is reached and the macula itself is affected.

The closed angle type, in which a gradually thickening lens may have pushed the iris into an unusually narrow gutter, may have a much more acute onset when, for instance, the lens is suddenly dilated (in darkness or in anger). Intense pain, or headache and vomiting is experienced with increasing visual disturbance; the eye looks red and congested and the pupil widely dilated. This is a medical emergency because complete blindness may result and it must not be mistaken for an attack of migraine. More often a recurrent, subacute pattern emerges with mild discomfort, haziness of vision and distortion in colours; this picture is much commoner in some tropical countries than in England, and especially so among people from the West Indies, particularly women.

Again, if glaucoma is suspected, specialist assessment is needed because operative correction, if done early enough, saves sight.

On the whole, glaucoma appears a decade or so earlier than the other major eye diseases of advancing years — in the 50s and 60s; even after 75 not more than 8% of people have the appearances suggestive of it, and fewer still any visual disability. Nevertheless, it has a strongly familial pattern and any elderly person who knows of a history of the condition in her family should be 'screened' for the disease even if she has no symptoms.

DIABETIC RETINOPATHY

This is not the most common of the major sight-threatening diseases in old age, but it should be the most predictable. It is the commonest cause of new sight loss in middle age and all patients with diagnosed diabetes should have at least an annual check on their eyes, with ophthalmoscopy. There are two main types of diabetic retinopathy — proliferative and background retinopathy. The first is more often associated with younger diabetic patients dependent on insulin (Keen & Jarret 1981); the second occurs with all types of diabetes. In the proliferative type there is a progressive growth of weak new vessels from the retinal arteries and veins onto the inner (vitreous) surface of the retina and these are liable to rupture. This usually occurs slowly so that clots have time to organize, but sudden bleeding and rapid sight loss can occur. In the background type small micro-aneurysms are formed, particularly near the macula; these too can leak, producing small haemorrhages and collections of plasma which, over time, deposit fat exudates and compromise retinal function.

Symptoms depend on where the bleeds occur or the exudates are deposited; if on the macula, loss of central vision will be an early feature and usually not pass unnoticed. But if most of the lesions are in the peripheral retina the disease can be quite extensive before anything much is noticed by an elderly person; patchy field loss in one eye is not easy to detect. About 40% of elderly diabetic patients in whom background retinopathy is discovered may suffer moderate or severe sight loss within five years. There is plausible evidence that the progress of diabetic retinopathy in younger adult life and childhood is related to disease control (Keen & Jarrett 1981), but whether this extends to elderly people is less certain.

These are the principal causes of new sight loss in old age. Most of them allow an elderly person to navigate reasonably well but spoil her central vision; the supermarket aisle is manageable, but when it comes to paying at the check-out the problems may be overwhelming. Sudden loss of visual field (hemianopia) can sometimes occur following a stroke if it affects the posterior cerebral arteries; but in any case every patient recovering from a 'stroke' deserves a full eye assessment because she will need all her faculties to make the best recovery.

LIGHT, CONTRAST, SIZE, COLOUR

Good sight needs good light, good contrast and adequate size and as the eye becomes older it becomes less and less able to make up for deficiencies. Because of changes in the cornea, the lens and the retina itself, the elderly eye needs three times as much light as the younger eye to achieve the same resolution. Add to this the extra dimming of an early cataract or the atrophy of macular degeneration and it is not hard to imagine how unsuited to good vision are the surroundings of many elderly people.

Cullinan et al (1979) showed that, in the homes of 56 elderly people attending a special low-vision clinic, ambient (overhead) lighting was woefully inadequate in almost every case; three quarters had less than 25% of the lighting available in the clinic. For near vision tasks, reading lamps were hardly any better — not more than a quarter came near the hospital standards. Yet improvements were very easy to make using a 60-watt bulb alone, and in almost half the cases improved the visual acuity of the patients by at least one line of the Snellen chart or one print size on the reading card.

The problem is that the environment in which elderly people live has too often grown old with them. Unpainted walls, old-fashioned dark colours and woodstains, dirty half-closed curtains, heavy old lampshades out of easy reach and the ever-present fear of the electricity bill all make for a dim environment, limiting the powers of remaining sight. Each of these factors is worth examining separately to see what can be done.

LAMPS AND BULBS

The common filament bulb is a woefully inefficient provider of light. It converts a very great deal of available energy into heat and gives out no more than 12 lumens of light for every watt burned; yet this is in a wide colour band and so allows for good colour discrimination. The yellow sodium vapour low-pressure bulbs such as are used on motorways are far more efficient (giving out at least ten times the light for each watt), but are restricted to the red-yellow end of the spectrum, thus cutting out many of the light rays that elderly people find most useful. The domestic fluorescent tube manages about 90 lumens per watt and is much cooler than the filament bulb — but elderly people dislike its start-up time, and it is difficult for them to change. Its life is greatly lengthened if it is left on all the time — some 7500 burning hours, but this may be halved if it is switched on and off hourly. New high pressure (long life) sodium bulbs have been introduced for domestic use which give off a much broader light spectrum; these are cool and are cheap to use but are at present expensive to buy (about £5–£6 each) and, like all gas bulbs, have a warming-up time.

Perhaps the most important feature is the position of the light source — over the shoulder for reading, but not so close as to be uncomfortably hot, overhead for ambient lighting, but not so as to throw shadows on a work surface or difficult stairs. Avoid if possible a concentrated light with relative darkness beyond it; accommodation becomes much slower with age and walking about should be as easy as possible.

This applies to television as well; the intensity of light from a back-lit television screen is greater than most people ever experience in other domestic situations, so to watch it in near darkness can be dangerous. For ambient lighting, it is worth remembering that merely lowering the central light fixture is much more effective, and cheaper, than putting in a higher wattage bulb — halving the distance of a light source increases illumination by four times.

For daylight hours a favourite chair in the best achievable lighting situation, both natural and artificial, is better than a series of options with the ever-present danger of trailing wires and small lamps knocked off tables. And for both near vision and ambient lighting a 60-watt bulb, properly placed, is usually adequate and does not give off too much heat. The difference between burning a 60-watt and a 40-watt bulb for eight hours each day for one month is about £1.

CONTRAST AND COLOUR

It is astounding what poor use is still made of contrast and colour in the designing of modern interiors and public areas. Grey concrete protrusions, invisible glass doors, monochromatic stairs, white electric switches against white walls — no colour codes for elderly eyes, and precious little joy for younger ones. If our modern designers can do no better, it is scarcely surprising that the interior of people's homes is often so bad. Yet almost all the things we need for daily living are available in contrasting colours, and together an elderly person and a caring nurse can have a great deal of fun exploring the possibilities. Gradually, coloured crockery can come to replace the white-on-white so often found, cooking utensils with brightly coloured handles can be introduced, and brighter, more visible versions of familiar objects, such as knitting needles, scissors, and spectacle cases can be discovered. So long as the effort is collaborative, the possibilities are endless. It is worth remembering that a coloured object on a white surface is preferable to a white object on a dark surface; a bright surface reflects 70%–80% of the light falling on it, a dark one not more than 20%. Negotiating a change in the decoration of walls, the colour of curtains, the position of furniture takes a little more doing because of familiarity and associations. But elderly people are often a lot more resilient to change than younger people give them credit for.

SIZE

For distance vision, size can always be increased by moving closer; elderly people without substantial eye disease seldom have difficulty watching television or negotiating furniture, even if they need lens correction and haven't got it. For the majority, though, near vision tasks without spectacles are almost impossible simply because many objects are too small to be discerned at the longer focal length of the ageing lens. There are many devices, some simple, some complicated, for making smaller objects appear bigger even after the limits of the ordinary spectacle lens have been reached (see below); but there are also many opportunities to buy objects with bigger handles, bigger letters, bigger instructions, and bigger faces. None of these things need specialist knowledge; all one needs is imagination, courage and perhaps a little wit. The Disabled Living Foundation (380–384 Harrow Road, London, W9 2HU. Telephone: 01 289 6111) has an excellent demonstration kitchen for poorly sighted people.

SEEKING HELP

In understanding and helping with these things, the nurse has already moved an elderly person a long way towards a well sighted vivid world. But it may be that more is needed and that the nurse is in the best position to suspect that substantial disease is present or that an elderly person needs more help than she has recently had.

Ophthalmic opticians not only test sight and prescribe corrective lenses; they also have a statutory duty to refer patients for further care when they detect, or suspect, a sight-threatening or other disease. Thus, if an elderly person is found by an ophthalmic optician to have a visual defect that cannot be adequately corrected by a spectacle lens, or an abnormality that cannot be treated inside the general ophthalmic services, or to need re-examining within six months, she will be referred to the family doctor who almost always refers on for specialist advice. While it is incumbent on both ophthalmic opticians and on ophthalmic medical practitioners to perform a good eye test, many will also add an examination for the early signs of disease, especially where good acuity cannot be achieved. Such an examination should include tonometry, for intraocular pressure, and a field test and ophthalmoscopy with dilated pupils. But if a nurse notices sudden deterioration in vision, especially in a patient with a known eye disease, specialist help is needed.

Although presbyopia does progress steadily throughout the later years of life and presbyopic (reading) lenses do need changing periodically, it seems to slow down with advancing years so that an eye test every 2–3 years in the 50s and 60s can reasonably be extended to 4–5 years in the 70s and 80s if all is otherwise well. But, as has been said, patients with known diabetes and a family history of glaucoma should be examined yearly.

STATUTORY AND VOLUNTARY HELP

STATUTORY

To become registered as blind in Britain a person must be 'so blind as to be unable to perform any work for which eyesight is essential' — a definition essentially unchanged since 1920 and much more suited to younger people than the elderly. In practice, anyone who cannot read even the top line of the optician's (Snellen) chart qualifies. Registration is always by way of assessment by a specialist ophthalmologist, who notifies the local Social Services, where the register is kept.

Benefits of registration include: increased tax allowances, a special blind pension, reduced rates for council house tenants, reduced, or even free, travel in many parts of the United Kingdom, a reduced television licence, tuition in Braille or Moon, and the use of a long cane. There is also access to the Talking Book service. The fiscal benefits are obviously of help but not many elderly people are able to learn Braille or Moon. About 120 000 people are at present registered as 'blind' in England and Wales, three quarters of them over the age of 70 years. There is also a register for the partially sighted. There is no statutory definition of 'partial sight' and no financial benefits to being registered, but it may give easier access to local social service provision. Unfortunately, many of the social workers specially trained to help 'blind' and 'partially sighted' people have lost that specialist role.

VOLUNTARY

Most parts of England and Wales have a local association for the 'blind' and many of these are now prepared to extend their help to those who are not officially registered. Addresses are available from the Royal National Institute for the Blind (224–228 Great Portland Street, London, W1N 6AA. Telephone: 071 388 1266) which is the central national body. Although it, too, concentrates on those registered as 'blind' — in activities such as publishing, stimulating research, running residential Homes and training establishments, etc. — many of its excellent productions may be of great help to elderly people with poor sight. Among the most useful may be Hints for Blind Housewives, and Useful Articles Sold in Shops or by Mail Order.

Almost all major public libraries now have a section of large print books and the range of what is available is rapidly expanding. The British Talking Book Service (Mount Pleasant, Alperton, Wembley, Middlesex HAO 1RR. Telephone: 01 903 6666) is available free to those registered as 'blind' or, by small annual subscription, to others. A letter from a general practitioner (family doctor), or ophthalmic optician is needed. The In Touch programme on BBC is already well known; many local radio stations are also taking up the challenge on behalf of poorly sighted people.

REFERENCES

Brennan M E, Knox F C 1973 An investigation into the purpose, accuracy and effective use of the blind register in England. British Journal of Preventive and Social Medicine 27: 154–59

Cullinan T R 1977 The epidemiology of visual disability: studies of visually disabled people. University of Kent Health Services Research Unit, Report No 28

Cullinan T R 1986 Visual disability in the elderly. Croom Helm, London

Cullinan T, Silver J, Gould E, Irvine D 1979 Visual disability and home lighting. Lancet 1: 642–644

Dobree J, Boulter E 1982 Blindness and visual handicap: the facts. Oxford University Press, New York

Ederer F 1977, 1978 The Framingham eye study: blindness. American Association of Workers for the Blind, Inc. Annual, Washington DC.

Fenton P, Arnold R, Wilkins P 1975 Evaluation of vision in slow stream wards. Age and Ageing 4: 43

Gilkes M 1979 Eyes run on light. British Medical Journal 1: 1681–1683

Graham P A, Wallace J, Welsby E, Grace H J 1968 Evaluation of postal detection of registerable blindness. British Journal of Preventive and Social Medicine 22: 238

Harris A et al 1971 Handicapped and impaired in Great Britain. Office of Population Censuses and Surveys, London

Keen M, Jarrett J 1981 Complications in diabetes. Arnold, London

Knight R, Warren R D 1978 Physically disabled people living at home: a study of numbers and needs. Reports on Health and Social Subjects no 13. HMSO London

London Health Planning Consortium 1980 Report on the Study Group on Ophthalmology Services in the North Thames Regions

Lovie-Kitchen J et al 1982 Senile macular degeneration: the effects and management. Department of Optometry, Queensland Institute of Technology, Brisbane

CHAPTER HEADING

The need to maintain activities and interests 99

Factors influencing the elderly person's ability to keep occupied 100
Time factors 100
Physical factors 100
Psychological factors 101
Cultural and religious factors 101
Climatic and environmental factors 102
Economic factors 104

What can be done 104
Keeping old people in the environment of their choice 104
Encouraging and enhancing well-being in institutions 107

7

Maintaining activities and interests

Amanda Stokes-Roberts

THE NEED TO MAINTAIN ACTIVITIES AND INTERESTS

People are living longer and are being forced to retire before they are ready to give up paid work. It is so important for society to develop an awareness of the difficulties associated with enforced leisure, and how it can best give constructive help. Life does not end at retirement but certain adjustments have to be made. All elderly people have certain needs which must be fulfilled in order to maintain a satisfactory quality of life. These might include physical and emotional health, adequate income and accommodation, congenial friends and neighbours with whom to enjoy absorbing interests, and an adequate personal philosophy of life. Those who have something to live for, a positive outlook on life and who maintain some level of continuity with their past, despite all the other changes associated with old age, seem to be the most successful at managing their old age. Interestingly, with the looming workforce crisis of the 1990s, society is once more looking to the potential of older workers. The skills and experience which elderly people possess are likely to regain their value; attitudes, of necessity, change.

To withdraw from life because one cannot adjust is a loss for the individual and for society. Boredom, depression and isolation may be symptoms of withdrawal, as is an apparent apathy when activity is reinstated. It is a great mistake, however, to think that because an elderly person is not obviously doing something she is doing nothing.

Silent reminiscence is important, as will be discussed later in this chapter, and so is the need for peace, quiet and solitude. Bromley (1974) observed that, with advancing age, activities selected by individuals show a trend towards spectatorship (such as watching television) rather than participation and that they are self-paced (for example, gardening, reading).

In spite of the potential for a change in attitudes towards older people, many elderly people nevertheless see ageing in terms of failure, as do younger people in our society. The maintenance of activities and interests provides opportunities for achievement which can improve an old person's confidence and self-esteem, and can preserve her identity and individuality.

FACTORS INFLUENCING THE ELDERLY PERSON'S ABILITY TO KEEP OCCUPIED

TIME FACTORS

For some, retirement can be a new beginning, a chance to indulge in activities and hobbies for which there has previously been too little time. For others it is like a life sentence. The value of planning and preparing for retirement is well documented and the increase in pre-retirement courses reflects a recognition of their role in assisting people to adjust to this period of their lives. Work such as that done by the Centre for Health and Retirement Education reinforces the fact that there is often a great capacity to achieve a positive and fulfilling lifestyle which may go unrecognized. As well as retirement from work there may be a change in family obligations. For example, many couples today have over 15 years to enjoy together after the marriage of their last child.

For those who have never had 'spare time', learning how to develop a new routine and the constructive use of the time they now have is especially important. Some old people use activities as a method to pass time and avoid loneliness. They need help, for this is an indication of a lack of adjustment to the circumstances in which they

find themselves. Time in retirement is rarely all leisure since daily chores still have to be done, and these may be much the same as those done before the issue of the old age pension. Education and recreational activities may now become priorities, with campaigns such as 'Age Well' (1988) run by Age Concern and the Health Education Authority being set up to facilitate and enable elderly people and those working with them to plan and develop a wide range of health promotion activities. The most notable worldwide contribution to the practice of education for elderly people is probably the University of the Third Age. For both these examples the self-help principle is uppermost. There are many opportunities to explore new areas of involvement, such as participating in community work, and it is frequently just a trigger that is required to set an individual off on the right track.

PHYSICAL FACTORS

For elderly people, good health affects quality of life and the degree of independence and ability to pursue a range of activities just as it does for other groups in society. Whilst we must acknowledge the increased frailty of those over the age of 75 years, assumptions should not be made that all these individuals will become dependent. Problems with mobility are particularly likely to affect the ability of elderly people to participate in leisure activities (Glyn-Jones 1975). Disability resulting from acute and chronic conditions will affect an individual's ability to perform any task. It is often a struggle just to cope with the activities of daily living, let alone indulge in other interests. For those with chronic conditions the knowledge that they will never get better may be very hard to come to terms with. Their self-confidence is low, an element reinforced by repeated failure, and they may, for good reason, be extremely difficult to motivate.

Blind and deaf people have special problems, primarily of communication. They may lack appropriate aids and not have had any expert advice. Those around them may be unaware of how to make the most of their other abilities. For blind people (see Ch. 6), mobility — especially in unfamiliar surroundings — is difficult and disorientating; it may be less frightening to stay at home. For deaf people (see Ch. 5), verbal communication may be almost impossible, and misinterpretation and ignorance by others may contribute to their isolation. Similarly, an incontinent person (see Ch. 12) might prefer to withdraw from human relationships than face possible rejection, avoidance, pity or ridicule (Kastenbaum 1979). These reactions are evoked by many other physical problems as well.

PSYCHOLOGICAL FACTORS

The capacity of old people to learn is underestimated, by elderly people themselves as well as by those around them. Many left school early, to go to work or to war, and apparently lack the background to attempt new tasks in retirement. For those elderly people motivated to do so, the provision of appropriate opportunities and support may demonstrate that they are in fact more than capable of achieving their potential in whatever area(s) they choose.

Any visual, auditory or sensory impairment will affect a person's ability to write, speak and gesticulate in some way or another. Communication skills are often taken for granted and problems in this area are rarely easily solved. Anyone who has tried to talk to a person with dysphasia, dysarthria or articulatory dyspraxia knows the frustration involved not only for the listener but also for the person who is struggling to communicate. Many give up and withdraw. People vary in their degree of articulateness and this will influence their ability to participate with confidence in activities. Nonverbal clues, such as an uneasy posture, may provide important information in these instances. Jill Macleod Clark in Chapter 4 discusses communication in more detail.

The outgoing, affable person who joins in and enjoys activities is welcome in any circle; the introverted, socially unskilled one less so. In a study of ageing and personality, Reichard et al (1962) identified five personality types: the first three types — the 'rocking chair' passive person, the 'armoured', vigorous, physically and socially active person, and the 'mature', well-adjusted person — had all adapted to their role in society;

the other two types — the 'angry' and the 'self-haters' — demonstrated a maladaptive pattern to ageing and were lonely and depressed as a result. Although this study was limited to men, on an intuitive basis it seems equally applicable to women.

A person who has a flexible and adaptable temperament and who is willing to seek out new areas that will give her satisfaction, will probably get more out of life than the passive individual who waits for events to happen. Some of those who have successfully adjusted to old age seem to be able to accept help when necessary, but others do not. Brought up in an era of self-help when the state did not provide either financially or practically, they find turning to bureaucratic establishments for help unpalatable and depressing. The next generations of our society, however, have changing expectations and this is likely to be reflected in differing attitudes towards service providers in the future, consumer choice being very much to the fore.

The majority of elderly people feel that others are concerned about them and see themselves as exceptions to a generally dreary picture. An important part of their activity is getting out and about, the most frequent reasons being to shop and visit friends. Many, given the chance, would have stayed on at work. These attitudes of old people are important considerations for those involved with their care (Age Concern 1974).

Old habits die hard, which is why preparation for retirement is so vital. Loss and bereavement increase with age; friends, family, health and belongings are all affected. The changes wrought by their loss can be devastating and disruptive. Kastenbaum (1979) describes a sense of panic and disintegration that an old person sometimes feels, and one of the outward manifestations may be a lack of motivation towards joining in activities and interests.

CULTURAL AND RELIGIOUS FACTORS

Certain expectations and beliefs concerning elderly people are prevalent. The popular image of physical frailty, mental ineptitude, inflexibility, dependency and non-productivity is very deeply entrenched.

Old age is viewed as a negative period preceding death, an approach described by Butler (1974) as 'ageism'. However, some of the men who dominate world politics and some very well-known musicians are good examples of another side to old age which contrasts vividly with the picture of the 80-year-old demented person in a long-stay ward. It is not surprising that the ambivalent attitude of society toward elderly people makes them so reluctant to ask for any form of assistance.

In certain cultures the elders are regarded as the head of the family whose role is to pass on historical information, customs and wisdom to the younger folk. In Britain this no longer occurs, and for elderly people belonging to ethnic minorities the insecurity of a new environment and the remoteness of the family left behind in the country of origin are additional problems. Norman (1985) in her book *Triple Jeopardy* describes how for them the problems of growing old are compounded by special difficulties, such as unfamiliar language and a very different way of life. They also suffer from discrimination and prejudice at the hands of the host community. These factors all contribute to their problems of survival, not to mention the difficulties involved in maintaining their activities and interests. Getting help is equally difficult, since not only have they little or no knowledge of the services available but they frequently are unknown to health and social workers (see Ch. 25).

The lifestyle of old people belonging to ethnic minorities is, to a large extent, dictated by their religion, just as it is for many old people in Western cultures. The spiritual and social support to be gained through contact with the church should not be underestimated. An Age Concern survey (1974) found that over 40% of those they questioned had some interest in, or contact with, the church. Religion may or may not have provided continuity throughout life, but in old age it may give special security and comfort. Beliefs, especially with regard to taboo subjects, can have an inhibitory effect on elderly people's ability to conduct their affairs as they would wish. Old folk on the whole are not afraid of death, whereas those around them often are. The process of coming to terms with life and accepting the prospect of death is often discouraged by younger relatives, friends and health workers, when what the old person really needs is support, understanding, and discussion of an inevitable and fairly imminent part of life.

Another subject considered to be taboo is sex. Comfort (1974) put the problem in a nutshell:

Old folks stop having sex for the same reasons they stop riding a bicycle — general infirmity, thinking it looks ridiculous, no bicycle — and of these reasons the greatest is the social image of the dirty old man and the asexual, undesirable older woman.

The attitudes of society inhibit expression of sexual desires even though such desires may remain as strong as ever. The intimacy of those who have shared a long life of joys and sorrows is both precious and life affirming and should be respected as much as they are for the young. Expressing sexuality is discussed in more detail by Christine Webb in Chapter 16 of this volume.

There exist many stereotypes concerning the activities and interests which old people can enjoy. Men apparently have no interest in self-expressive activities such as dancing, painting and cooking, and women only enjoy those concerned with homemaking. Figure 7.1, however, contradicts this stereotype. Members of the upper classes, having been managers and executives, belong to clubs and bridge circles, whilst those from the working classes, the skilled, semi-skilled and manual workers, play bingo and go to the pub. These are exaggerated examples, but give an idea of the generalizations that tend to be made.

Studies have shown that home-centred activities tend to revolve around cooking, housework, gardening, radio and television (Tunstall 1966). Those most commonly undertaken outside the home include shopping, visiting friends or going out for the day (Age Concern 1974). The social and economic background of an individual does have a tremendous influence on the activities and interests pursued. Each person's interests should be considered individually in order that maximum fulfilment and satisfaction can be achieved.

CLIMATIC AND ENVIRONMENTAL FACTORS

Winter heralds a period of decreased activity, the cold and damp slow both function and motivation.

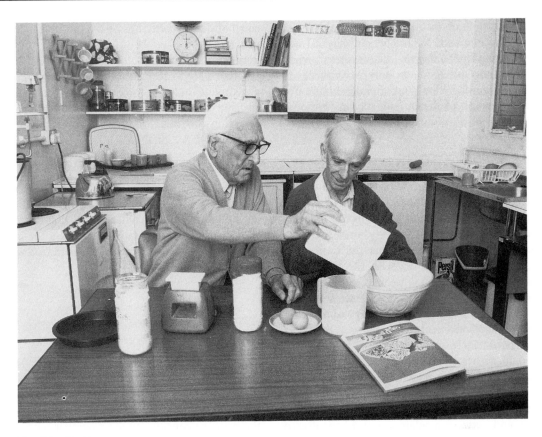

Fig. 7.1 Cooking.

The risk of falling is higher and the potential danger of venturing out after dark is a greater problem than in the summer. Most of the elderly people who visit relatives or who travel for social and recreational purposes use public transport. Those in rural areas are particularly vulnerable because services are unreliable and infrequent. Some 40% of journeys made by elderly people are for shopping (Age Concern 1978) but the reduction of public transport in many areas has put access to public facilities out of reach for many people. Local shops are decreasing in number and are often expensive, and the advent of Super Centres with their enormous areas render many elderly shoppers overwhelmed and exhausted.

Public facilities are rarely designed to suit elderly users. Steps instead of ramps, few handrails, poor lighting, lack of seating and toilet facilities, and little chance of assistance make any trip a daunting prospect. Fortunately, society is gradually becoming aware of the needs of elderly and disabled people, and many local authorities now issue information guides which pinpoint suitable facilities.

The problems that can be created by an institutional environment are probably even greater. In physical terms, facilities may be less than ideal: high beds, toilets with difficult access, unsuitable chairs, no lift, etc. The psychological effects of living in an institution may be even more traumatic. The stripping of individuality and status which occurs when an elderly person enters an institution is well documented (e.g. Goffman 1961). The loss of role, personal belongings, support of family and friends and a sense of personal control over one's life all contribute to a feeling of insecurity and isolation. A strange environment and a new routine can be extremely disorientating, their constraints leaving little time or inclination for the pursuit of activities and interests. Such a person may subside rapidly into a state of 'learned helplessness', when the motivation to carry out any activity, even though capable of it, has gone (Schulz 1980). For further discussion of life in long-stay institutions, see Chapter 29.

ECONOMIC FACTORS

Although pensions today may be supplemented by income from odd jobs, private investment or savings, they are frequently the sole source of income. Walker (1986) found that poverty among elderly people is still widespread and that the basic state pension, although increasing with the rate of inflation, is not rising quickly enough to ensure that the incomes of elderly people keep pace with that of the rest of the population. An old person's main outgoings are usually rent, food and fuel, the latter being a particularly difficult expense to bear. No old person wishes to add to the financial burdens of her family but she may feel she has nowhere else to turn.

There is considerable lack of knowledge about benefits and services available, and when offered these are too often accepted reluctantly, or refused as charity. Old people are frequently confused and worried about their future financial status and only with more effective targeting of resources by, for example, Local Authority Welfare Rights Units, will the most vulnerable section of the population be helped to lead as full a life as possible in the community. When it comes to priorities, food and warmth take precedence over recreational activities. Hendricks and Hendricks (1977) provide a comprehensive discussion of the myths and realities of ageing in modern mass societies.

WHAT CAN BE DONE

KEEPING OLD PEOPLE IN THE ENVIRONMENT OF THEIR CHOICE

Assessment of function

The ability of an elderly person to perform per-

sonal and daily activities of living often means the difference between being independent or dependent. Information should, where possible, be substantiated by careful observation and practical assessment, because sometimes old people are unrealistic about their capabilities. The purpose of assessing functional abilities is to establish which activities of personal care a person is able to perform; to assess how that ability, if necessary, can be improved; and to decide the best methods to use in order to achieve their maximum potential (Turner 1987). As well as the physical ability of an individual, psychological and social functioning should also be assessed, preferably by the use of a standardized instrument acceptable to all professional groups.

Mobility

This is the area of physical function that is likely to have the most effect on an old person's ability to cope, and is covered in detail in Chapter 8. Transfers, sitting, standing and walking safely are the primary considerations. Together with physiotherapists, decisions are made as to what, if any, aids (walking-stick, walking-frame, etc.) are most likely to achieve maximum mobility. An integral part of treatment and advice on mobility is the assessment of the environment, with particular reference to such details as the height of chair, bed and toilet, floor coverings, stairs and steps. Adaptations to existing equipment, such as chair, bed and toilet 'raises' and rails can be invaluable for old people who have difficulties, as can the employment of new methods.

Wheelchairs can give a chairbound old person considerable mobility. They can be self-propelled (manual or electric) or attendant-propelled. Careful assessment is necessary to ensure that the wheelchair suits both the mental and physical capacity of the individual and the environment in which she lives. Many models are available either on prescription or by private purchase. A full description of all hand-propelled chairs available on prescription is given in a Department of Health and Social Security handbook (1982).

Eating and drinking

These are often the first activities in which a disabled person can achieve independence. When assessing, it is necessary to consider the effects of muscle weakness, tremor, spasm, lack of co-ordination and any chewing or swallowing difficulties. An awareness of factors such as positioning and table heights is essential. For some, specially designed or adapted cutlery or crockery may be necessary. More detailed information on this subject can be found in Wilshere (1987).

Dressing and grooming

These activities should be assessed as soon as possible. Abilities here can boost patients' morale and enable them to look and feel normal. Undressing is easier than dressing and attention should be given to individual sequence, the way a person has dressed for the last few decades. There are often severe problems and much patience and practice may be required before a patient achieves independence. Clothing adaptations should only be attempted when all other techniques and methods have been tried. On the whole, it is better to buy loose fitting, front fastening, easily laundered clothes. Maximum independence may be possible but unrealistic, especially when there is a wife or husband who always helps. In order for confidence and self-esteem to develop, it is essential that an old person be encouraged to take pride in his or her appearance, by paying special attention to the care of hair, teeth and nails, and by encouraging the old person to shave regularly, or use make-up, if done so in the past.

Toilet management

For many elderly people in hospital being able to use the toilet is crucial for attaining personal independence and for fulfilling the requirements for resettlement. The hospital environment may be responsible for an old person's incontinence (see Ch. 12). Sometimes easy practical solutions can be found, for example toilet raises, rails at the side of the toilet, or simply advice on easily managed clothing. Night-time management should also be assessed; a commode at the side of the bed, or a urinal may be of help. For those alone at home with a toilet outside or one that is otherwise inaccessible, a chemical commode may be of use. Further details are to be found in Wilshere (1985).

Personal hygiene

Some old people live in properties that do not have bathrooms, and which also lack hot water. This may mean they have to boil kettles in order to wash, which presents additional problems. Those who do have the facilities may find bathing a difficult and strenuous process even with aids or the assistance of a bath attendant. Nevertheless, cleanliness and thorough washing should always be encouraged, and a shower might be easier than a bath.

Domestic tasks

These may include house-cleaning, meal preparation, cooking and serving, laundry, budgeting and shopping. Assessment of the old person's ability must be realistic and undertaken with knowledge of a patient's home situation, such as the help available (family, home help or meals-on-wheels). The kitchen is usually the area that causes most concern to relatives because of the risks involved, such as lighting gas cookers or carrying boiling water. It is also an area where the assessment of certain patients, such as those who are blind or partially sighted, can effectively be undertaken only in their home. Much practice may be needed to reinforce retraining, or to encourage the learning of new methods. A publication from the Disabled Living Foundation which provides comprehensive information and advice is *Kitchen Sense for Disabled or Elderly People* (Foott et al 1975).

Communication

A proportion of the patients being assessed will have communication difficulties of one sort or another. In conjunction with the speech therapist, the occupational therapist should be able to provide assistance with speech, hearing, reading and writing, and give advice on appropriate equipment. Additional information may be found in Wilshere (1987).

Assessment of home conditions

Once the assessment of a patient's function is complete, it is essential to have first-hand experience of that person in her own home, where several areas can be assessed. Home visits are usually done by an occupational therapist who may take a student nurse along. Sometimes the physiotherapist or social worker will come too and a representative from the community services might attend. Useful information may also be obtained if a domiciliary visit has been carried out prior to admission by the geriatrician.

The primary area to be assessed is the patient's physical capacity to cope with the accommodation and furniture, and the suitability of these in relation to the short and long-term consequences of the patient's disability. General mobility and transfers, and a person's ability to cope with the environment, for example plugs and heating, are assessed. Potential hazards such as loose carpets and poor lighting are also examined. Observations of what, if any, equipment/adaptations have been or could be provided to enable a patient to manage are also made. The most commonly supplied equipment is that to raise chair, bed and toilet and there is frequently a need for rails. Help from outside agencies such as the gas or electricity boards may be required.

What does the patient think about her home environment? Is she well oriented? Does she feel able to cope? All these demonstrate a person's attitude and the level of adjustment to her condition.

It is important to assess the level of physical and psychological support that exists as well as that which would be required to get the patient home from hospital. Social services, such as meals-on-wheels, friends, neighbours, day centres, church and voluntary bodies all come into this category. It is important also to identify the attitudes of the family and neighbours to having the old person at home, and the services that may be involved. Those people directly concerned may require counselling and reassurance, and to know that help is available. Those less directly concerned, for

example families who live some distance away, may feel guilty, and should be given the opportunity to discuss their feelings with someone who knows the patient well.

Once the home visit has been done, considerable liaison is necessary in order to plan and co-ordinate future care and resettlement. The importance of thorough and detailed communication between all those involved cannot be overstated. Many discharges from hospital have failed as a result of poor organization, and it is always the elderly person who suffers.

Services and equipment available

The services provided vary tremendously from area to area, and there is considerable confusion as to which organization is responsible for a particular service. The local social services department of the local authority should know whom to contact. This department is usually responsible for the major support services, for example meals-on-wheels, home help, laundry services and chiropody. They also run social clubs, day centres and luncheon clubs and help with transport facilities, as well as providing aids and adaptations to the home. Other services, such as the district nurses, are provided by the health authority. They may also be involved with medical loans and the supply of some equipment and gadgets.

Many elderly people rely on help from voluntary sources such as Good Neighbour schemes, Women's Royal Voluntary Service, and local schools and church organizations. These services give tremendous back-up support to those provided by the state. There are several national organizations which can be called upon for advice or assistance, such as Age Concern, Help the Aged, Royal National Institute for the Blind and the British Red Cross Society.

Booklets focusing on the needs of elderly people are produced by several areas giving a guide to local facilities; these should help increase awareness of the assistance that is available. There are many aids to daily living which can be borrowed, bought or made. The demand is such that many large chemists and stores stock a range of specialist aids and equipment, and items that were once provided for the disabled are now available as convenience items; for example one-handed whisks and non-slip bowls. It is worth remembering, however, that old people often abandon their aids once they return to their own homes as they revert to their old habits. It is therefore essential that the use of anything new is carefully taught and its value reinforced by all those involved with the care of that person.

Occupational therapists can advise on the use of aids as well as on adaptations to the home, such as stair rails and larger items of equipment like hoists and stair lifts. These may require liaison with housing and other social services departments. In his book, *Designing for the Disabled*, Selwyn Goldsmith (1976) gives detailed descriptions of those aspects that require attention.

The primary objective for the elderly person is to get home as soon as possible with minimum disruption to her environment. Counselling and reassurance of friends and relatives, and demonstration by the old person of her capabilities is vital if she is to manage at home. Many old people discharged from hospital fail to cope because of the anxiety of the carers, which affects the confidence of the patient. A level of risk has to be accepted, and absolute guarantees cannot be given.

Evidence exists (Cloke 1983) which highlights the stress involved in caring for elderly relatives, and the fact that elderly people themselves may be at risk of ill-treatment (see Chapter 26 by Alison While for further discussion of elderly abuse). The support, in both physical and psychological terms, and advice given to carers by all members of the multidisciplinary team is becoming increasingly important. A useful practical approach to the frustrations and difficulties of caring for elderly and confused people at home may be found in the book 'The 36 Hour Day' (Mace & Rabins 1985). The need for thorough co-ordination of effective support services on discharge from hospital should also be recognized as a high priority.

ENCOURAGING AND ENHANCING WELL-BEING IN INSTITUTIONS

The majority of people working in institutions underestimate the abilities of frail elderly people.

The attitudes of staff to their patients are probably one of the most important factors to consider in regard to the patient's well-being and quality of life. Millard and Smith (1981) found that lack of personal belongings increased the likelihood of an elderly person being perceived in a negative way. If a person is approached as being less able than others, it is likely that the more decrepit aspects of her behaviour will be reinforced. As mentioned earlier, elderly people need to take a positive attitude to their lives and so do the staff who tend them. Showing an interest in an old person as an individual and reinforcing the positive aspects of her abilities can do much for her self-esteem and confidence. Pride in personal appearance and the opportunity for choice about which clothes to wear, facilities to use, activities to pursue, etc. are most important.

Activities

Isolation and disorientation are common problems for people in institutions, and the use of individual and group activities can be of great benefit as well as enhancing a sense of well-being and satisfaction. The renewal of old and exploration of new interests and hobbies should be an integral part of institutional life. McCormack and Whitehead (1981), in their study of long-stay patients, found that engagement levels were consistently higher when activities were provided, with group activities on the whole being more successful than individual activities. They concluded that patients' engagement levels are usually low, not because they lacked ability, but because they are not given the opportunity or encouragement to participate in any activity.

When doing any activity, it is important to remember certain points which will affect the level of engagement and participation of those involved. Activities should be purposeful and enjoyable. No one will do something they see as pointless or join in for the sake of doing something. Wherever possible, use should be made of any previous experience and the activity tailored to the ability of the participant. There should be opportunities for choice, and patients should never be forced to join in an activity since this is likely to elicit an angry

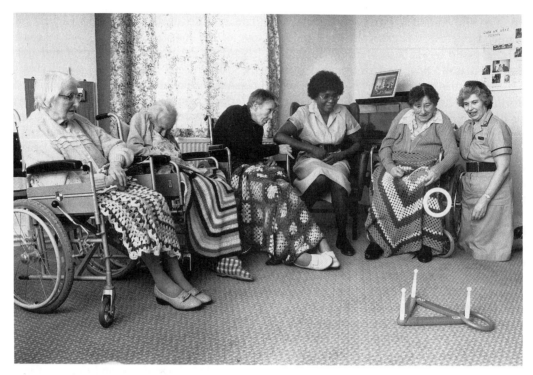

Fig. 7.2 Ward games.

response or further depress someone who is already withdrawn. Encourage them to watch, however, and curiosity will often win the day. Old people frequently find groups threatening; it takes time for them to relax in such a setting, and initially their concentration will be low.

Thorough planning and preparation of an activity, as described by Bender et al (1987), is essential; if disorganized, the participants will neither co-operate nor concentrate. Consideration must be given to environmental factors, staffing, types of patients and the activity itself. The venue for the group, such as dayroom, ward, occupational therapy department, and the amount of space available will affect the choice of activity. The suitability of furniture also requires assessment, and factors that may act as distractors, such as television, should be avoided. The number of staff available will affect the activity that is done, as some require much higher staff/patient ratios than others. A great deal of enthusiasm and resilience is necessary, and it is important that the

quality of the teaching is as high as possible. The patients themselves need both encouragement and support, and not all activities will suit all patients. In order to avoid increasing their sense of failure an activity should be offered to those who will get the most enjoyment out of it and who will cope fairly well with the task. Some patients need a lot of help in order to achieve success, but it is important to give them the opportunity. There is a tremendous range of activities which can be used in original or adapted form. There are those provided by specialists, such as art and music therapists and local authority teachers, and many others which may be provided by occupational therapists, physiotherapists and voluntary helpers.

More recently, the role of Activity Nurses has been developed. Together with other members of the multidisciplinary team they ensure that activities are provided on a regular rather than ad hoc basis, thereby providing a continuous level of stimulation for both individuals and groups. Traditional activities such as knitting, embroidery and woodwork remain much in evidence as well as a wide variety of new ideas such as those described by Hamill and Oliver (1980).

Occupational therapists together with other specialists provide many other types of activities which aim to be physically, socially and educationally stimulating as well as to assist orientation. Many good examples are cited by Comins et al (1983) and Cornish (1983). Exercises and games are popular, the enjoyment of the participants is evident, and the opportunity to 'let off steam' especially during team games appears to be most welcome (Fig. 7.2). Powell (1974) showed exercise to be beneficial for the cognitive and behavioural capacities of the aged. For this reason, Salter and Salter (1975) emphasized recreational activities involving exercise in their study of the effects of an individualized activity programme on elderly patients. The use of music and movement has proved invaluable in many institutions, not only for the physical benefits achieved but also for the sheer pleasure that is created. Copple (1983) gives striking evidence to support the work of Mary Bagot Stock who instigated a scientifically graded and recreational exercise system involving a rhythmic musical accompaniment. Although this particular project was community based, it could apply equally well in institutions.

The elderly people in hospital are frequently withdrawn and isolated. The stimulation of social interaction is therefore most important. Table games, sing-alongs, gardening, bingo, quizzes and discussions are a few examples (Fig. 7.3). Many activities used to this end also have features which are instructive. In the book *Care of the Long-Stay Elderly Patient* (Denham 1983) the potential of occupations such as poetry, art and music are explored (Fig. 7.4). They provide:

the opportunity to be, to act, to express, to manipulate, to rehearse, to listen, to participate, to practise, to perform. In such circumstances the patient is not the object of attention, the dependent one, but is to an increasing extent, the chooser, the mover, the doer (Jones 1983, p. 126).

The value of music and art as 'therapy' has in the past been underestimated since both have been regarded as mere entertainment. But many of the problems of old age such as adjustment, physical handicap, lethargy, apathy, loneliness and depression, can in part, at least, be alleviated by the use of these activities.

Another form of stimulation which can have

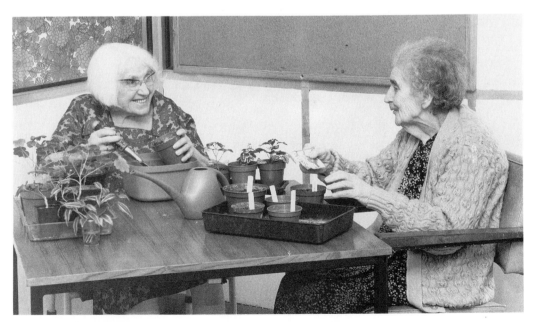

Fig. 7.3 Indoor gardening.

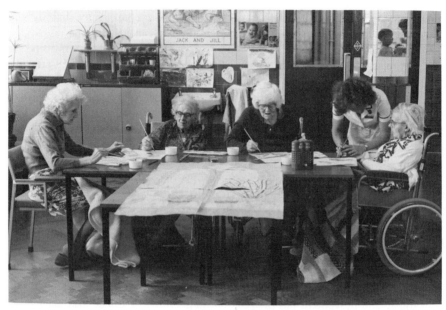

Fig. 7.4 Art group.

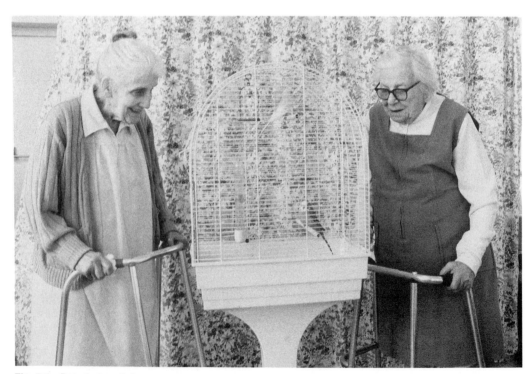

Fig. 7.5 Pets in hospital.

multidimensional effects is the use of pets or 'animal intervention'. Man's relationship with animals is long-standing, and for elderly people they may act as a familiar natural focus, evoking feelings of joy, comfort and security. Mugford and M'Comisky (1975) used the term 'social lubricant' to describe this aspect and demonstrated its impact in a study of birds as companions which found that they indeed helped pensioners to have a more positive attitude towards themselves (Fig. 7.5). There are however important factors to be aware of when introducing pets into an institutional environment, some of which are described by Cooper (1976).

Reality orientation

The majority of the activities already mentioned can, in one way or another, be employed as aids to orientation, but in recent years, the use of Reality Orientation (RO) has become an increasingly popular technique. An account of this method of treating confusion, disorientation and memory loss of elderly people, is provided in Chapter 19.

Reminiscence and life-review

RO may involve a comparison of life present with life past. The role of reminiscence as part of the life-review process is well recognized but not always viewed positively, the elderly being accused of preoccupation with the past. Butler (1974) felt the life-review process to be preventative and therapeutic for the mental, social and physical well-being of old people. It is a method of coming to a conclusion about the value of life and the balance of achievement within it. Reminiscence is a normal and valuable part of that process (Kastenbaum 1979) though it should be recognized that it will be of more value to some than others, and should therefore be used in a way that is sensitive to individual differences. Coleman (1986) investigated the function of reminiscence, exploring it in terms of life review, storytelling, the creation of a 'meaningful myth' (Lieberman & Tobin 1983) and the maintenance of self-esteem. Coleman's discussion highlights the point that whether a person will gain benefit will depend as much on her past history as on her present needs. For many people sharing reflections of the past can give a great deal of pleasure to both the listener and the teller (Fig. 7.6). It is an opportunity to look at the past objectively and thereby perhaps encourage a more positive assessment of one's past life. Preoccupation with the past is only detrimental if the past is denied, when it contributes to isolation.

Old people can be helped to reminisce simply by using tangible reminders of their past such as personal possessions; for example family albums, scrap-books and old letters (Holzapfel 1982). The use of more formal biographical studies have the potential to serve as a valuable focus for case study work, as well as an interesting experience for those participating in the project. Help the Aged (1981) have produced a tape/slide programme called 'Recall' which covers topics from childhood (pre–First World War) to the Space Age. Other organizations have developed ideas along similar lines which focus on their local area and community. The familiar pictures and sounds draw lively and informative discussions which are much enjoyed by all those involved. Sessions can be supplemented by items of everyday use or records of old-time music, which can be especially evocative. Family and friends, too, have an important role to play and this is frequently forgotten in the routine of institutional life. They hold many keys to the past and may be able to help reinforce the identity and individuality of the person in care. Their involvement may also help them to view their relationship more positively. Many carers feel very guilty when an old person is taken into an institution. They need support and reassurance in order to adjust to their new role and to be reconciled with their relative. Their participation in reminiscence and RO can be invaluable.

Much of what we do every day with our patients contains constituents of both RO and reminiscence, and arises from a philosophy of care that involves a belief in the potential worth and value of old people. Elderly people in institutions are, on the whole, dependent on other people in order to achieve life satisfaction. Unfortunately, interprofessional conflicts and inadequate organization of institutional routines often seem to work against

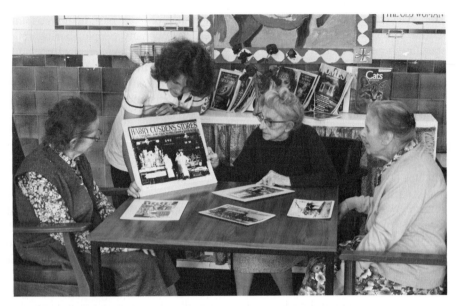

Fig. 7.6 Reminiscence.

the initiation of activity programmes (Davies 1982) even though their value is well recognized (Salter & Salter 1975). Change and overlap of roles are regrettably regarded has threatening instead of being viewed positively. Quality of life is a difficult concept to describe in concrete terms (Denham 1983) but its constituents are as applicable to us as to the old people we work with. We are the elderly of the future. If we recognize our own needs, likes and dislikes, we will see and understand many of theirs.

REFERENCES

Age Concern 1974 The attitudes of the retired and the elderly. Age Concern, London

Age Concern 1978 Profiles of the elderly, their mobility and use of transport. Age Concern, London

Age Concern 1988 Age well: planning and ideas pack. Health Education Authority, London

Bender M, Norris A, Bauckham P 1987 Group work with the elderly — principles and practice. Winslow Press, Oxford

Bromley D B 1974 Personality and adjustment in middle age and old age. In: Bromley D B (ed) The psychology of human ageing, 2nd edn. Penguin, London, p 235–240

Butler R 1974 Successful ageing and the role of life review. Journal of the American Geriatrics Society 12: 529–535

Cloke C 1983 Old age abuse in the domestic setting — a review. Age Concern, London

Coleman P 1986 Ageing and reminiscence processes: social and clinical implications. Wiley, Chichester

Comfort A 1974 Sexuality in old age. Journal of the American Geriatrics Society 12: 440–42

Comins J, Hurford F, Simms J 1983 Activities and ideas. Winslow Press, Buckingham

Cornish P 1983 Activities for the frail aged. Winslow Press, Buckingham

Cooper J E 1976 Pets in hospital. British Medical Journal 1: 698–700

Copple P 1983 The concept of exercise. Nursing Times 79(32): 66–69

Davies A 1982 Research with elderly people in long term care: some social and organisational factors affecting psychological interventions. Ageing and Society 2: 285–298

Department of Health and Social Security 1982 Handbook of wheelchairs and bicycles and tricycles. DHSS, Blackpool

Denham M J (ed) 1983 Care of the long-stay elderly patient. Croom Helm, London

Foott S, Lane M, Mara J 1975 Kitchen sense for disabled or elderly people. The Disabled Living Foundation. Heinemann, London

Glyn-Jones A 1975 Growing older in a south Devon town. University of Exeter

Goffman E 1961 Asylums: essays on the social situation of mental patients and other inmates. Doubleday, New York

Goldsmith S 1976 Designing for the disabled, 3rd edn. RIBA, London

Hamill C, Oliver R 1980 Therapeutic activities for the handicapped elderly. Aspen, London

Help the Aged 1981 Recall. Help the Aged Education Department, London

Hendricks J, Hendricks C D 1977 Ageing in mass society, myths and realities. Winthrop, Cambridge, Mass

Holzapfel S 1982 The importance of personal possessions in the lives of the institutionalised elderly. Journal of Gerontological Nursing 8(3): 156–158

Jones S 1983 Education and life in the continuing care ward. In: Denham M J (ed) Care of the long stay elderly patient. Croom Helm, London, p 122–148

Kastenbaum R 1979 Growing old — years of fulfilment. Harper and Row, London

Lieberman M A, Tobin S S 1983 The experience of old age. Stress: coping and survival. Basic Books, New York

Mace N L, Rabins P V 1985 The 36 hour day: caring at home for confused elderly people. Hodder and Stoughton in conjunction with Age Concern, London

McCormack D, Whitehead A 1981 The effects of providing recreational activities on the engagement level of long-stay geriatric patients. Age and Ageing 10: 287–291

Millard P, Smith C 1981 Personal belongings — a positive effect? Gerontologist 21: 85–90

Mugford and McComisky 1975 Some recent work on the psychotherapeutic value of caged birds with old people. In: Anderson (ed) Pets, animals and society. Ballière Tindall, London

Norman A 1985 Triple jeopardy: growing old in a second homeland. Policy Studies in Ageing No. 3. Centre for Policy on Ageing, London

Powell R R 1974 Psychological effects of exercise therapy upon institutionalised geriatric mental patients. Journal of Gerontology 29: 157–161

Reichard S, Livson F, Peterson P G 1972 Ageing and personality. Wiley, New York

Salter C de L, Salter C 1975 Effects of an individualised activity programme on elderly patients. Gerontologist 15: 404–6

Schulz R 1980 Ageing and control. In: Garber J, Seligman M E P (eds) Human helplessness: theory and applications. Academic Press, New York

Tunstall J 1966 Old and alone. Routledge and Kegan Paul, London

Turner A (ed) 1987 The principles of the activities of daily living in the practice of occupational therapy, 2nd edn. Churchill Livingstone, Edinburgh

Walker A 1986 Pensions and the production of poverty in old age. In: Phillipson C, Walker A (eds) Ageing and social policy. Gower Press, Aldershot

University of London Department of Extra Mural Studies 1986 Health and retirement — an ideas and resources pack for health educators with the Health Education Council. University of London

Wilshere E R 1985 Equipment for the disabled, 5th edn. Oxfordshire Area Health Authority, Oxford

Whilshere E R 1987 Equipment for the disabled, 6th edn. Oxfordshire Area Health Authority, Oxford

CHAPTER CONTENTS

The concept of mobility and prevalence of immobility 115
Prevalence of immobility 116
The role of physical fitness in maintaining mobility 116

Factors affecting mobility 117
Psychological and socioenvironmental factors 117
Physical factors 119

Gait and mobility problems related to pathological causes 120
Parkinson's disease 120
Hemiplegia 121
Arthritic conditions 121
Amputation 122
Falls 122

Assessing and managing immobility 124
Physical assessment and management 127
Lifting disabled old people 137

Stroke units 139
Stroke rehabilitation 140

Geriatric orthopaedic units 141

8

Mobility

Lynn Batehup, Amanda Squires

THE CONCEPT OF MOBILITY AND PREVALENCE OF IMMOBILITY

To be mobile implies having the ability to move around. It is a wide and diverse term which encompasses mobility required to care for one's self and the home environment, to move around outside the home in order to obtain the necessities for living, to take part in the social life of a community and recreation, and to be able to visit friends and relatives. The wide aspect of mobility is reflected in the way it is defined. According to Ebersole and Hess (1981) 'mobility is the pattern of how and where one moves about in personal and life space'. Barker and Bury (1978) stress the social aspect of mobility when they state that mobility is the key to active access to community, neighbourhood or friendship involvement, and that to be housebound tends to be a state of non-participant dependence, while mobility means self-sufficiency and engagement. Norman (1981) emphasizes the relative qualities of mobility: what may be relative immobility to one can be regarded as high-level mobility to another. In this era of 'constant movement' and ease of travel over long distances, those who cannot move so easily are increasingly at a disadvantage.

Loss of mobility is a common problem for ageing persons. A survey by Abrams (1978), which amongst other things enquired about the domestic mobility of two groups of elderly people, found that for the age group 65–74 years, 11% of the sample had a problem getting around the house, with this proportion rising to 25% for the 75+ years age group. For the 65–74 years age group

8% had difficulty getting out of bed, and this rose to 15% for the 75+ age group. Limitations of mobility affect all aspects of daily life including washing, dressing, eating and going to the toilet. An earlier survey by Harris (1971) found that of the total population over 65 years of age, 27% suffered some impairment which limited their daily activities of living, and this proportion rose to 37% for those aged 75 years and over.

PREVALENCE OF IMMOBILITY

The level of mobility an individual is able to achieve is usually classified into: (i) being able to move alone without difficulty; (ii) needing to have help going out; (iii) being housebound; (iv) being bedfast or chairfast. Within these levels there are wide variations and the person's own choice of level of independence should be considered. Those who are independent are usually able to negotiate pavements and roads and use public transport, while those who have difficulty are usually restricted to walking unless taken in a car. Those who are housebound or bedfast may be so temporarily because of ill health, but there still remains a group who are permanently either housebound or bedfast. The study by Hunt (1978) found that 1.9% of the over 85 years age group were permanently bedfast, and 18.7% were permanently housebound. In addition, 25% of the housebound lived alone and were therefore dependent on others to bring them the necessities for living. Furthermore, 42.5% of the bedfast and housebound had not been out of their houses for over a year, and 18.9% had not been out for three years. The conditions that are responsible for most mobility problems are of a chronic nature. These are arthritis and rheumatism, heart and lung conditions such as congestive cardiac failure and bronchitis, circulatory diseases, stroke illness, Parkinson's disease and problems with vision (Abrams 1978, Hunt 1978). There are, however, many people with mobility problems who report no illness or disability. Hunt (1978) reports that 44% of all men over 65 years, and 43.5% of all women 65 years and over with no illness or disability suffer from mobility problems.

THE ROLE OF PHYSICAL FITNESS IN MAINTAINING MOBILITY

Before discussing reasons for loss of mobility, the concepts of prolonging and maintaining functional capacity, especially of locomotor activity, into old age are briefly explored.

There is some agreement that in the absence of overt pathology there is often a slow decline in function with age, although individuals age at different rates. Also, different tissues and systems within a person demonstrate differences in rates of ageing (Weg 1975). One of the most critical age-related differences is the ability to respond to stress, both physical and emotional, and the rate of return to pre-stress levels of homeostasis (Selye 1970). This decrease in homeostatic capacity is most marked in neuroendocrine interaction. For the elderly person, stress reveals a declining capacity to achieve responses in, for example, heart rate and blood pressure, and whether it be physical stress, as in exercise, or emotional stress, as in fear and anxiety, the rate of recovery by the individual is slower with increasing age. Gerontologists agree that there is a decline of approximately 1% per year in functional capacity in most organ systems (Shock 1962), but it has been demonstrated that not all functional changes in older people are due to ageing. Some may be due to misuse or disease (de Vries 1970, 1974, and see Chapter 3).

Age-related changes in bone, muscle, and nervous tissue result in a decreased work capacity for the body. There is an overall decrease in bone mass which drops steadily from about the age of 45 years, and occurs more rapidly in women than in men (Exton-Smith 1978). This leads to a greater predisposition to fracture. There may be some thinning or even collapse of intervertebral discs. Muscle strength and size apparently diminish with age. There is prolongation of contraction time, latency period, and relaxation period by about 13%, and a decrease in the maximum rate of tension development (Goldman 1979). There are many changes with ageing in the nervous system, and also notable is the decrease in the overall co-ordinator–integrator role for the body's muscular, neuronal, glandular and circulatory systems (Shock 1962). Reduced efficiency of the heart muscle and contractile strength are reflected in a smaller cardiac output which is adequate for the average older person to function until additional and unaccustomed physical activity puts the individual under stress. When this happens, lower contractile strength, smaller cardiac output and reduced enzymatic performance cause the heart to respond to the work demand with less efficient performance and a greater energy expenditure than would be required by the same person years earlier (Ebersole & Hess 1981).

It is true in most Western societies that habitual activity of a person declines as she becomes older, and at retirement she is expected to slow down and 'take things easy'. The decline in physical activity with age is more evident in leisure occupations. A general finding is that the types of leisure activity change little with age, but as people grow older they spend less time in physical recreation and engage in them less energetically. A man in his twenties spends about five hours weekly in physical activities during his leisure time, but this is reduced to about three hours weekly when he is in his sixties (Lange et al 1978). A study by Wessel and Van Huss (1969) showed that age-related loss in physiological variables important to human performance were more highly related to the decreased habitual activity level than they were to age itself. The term 'hypokinetic disease' was first used by Kraus and Raab (1961) to describe the various bodily and mental derangements induced by inactivity, and may be one important factor involved in bringing about an age-related decrement in functional capacities (de Vries 1975). There is some support for this in a study by Saltin et al (1968), which describes changes similar to the age-related changes mentioned above in well-conditioned young men after three weeks of enforced bed-rest. It was found that maximal cardiac output decreased by 26%, maximal ventilatory capacity by 30%, oxygen consumption by 30% and the amount of active tissue decreased by 1.5%. Thus it seems that inactivity can produce losses in function entirely similar to those brought about more slowly in the average individual when he grows more sedentary as he grows older. This brings into question the losses of function attributed to ageing, and raises the question of how

much of the functional loss is due to long term deconditioning, and the sedentary life of the older individual.

There is some interest in the possibility of improving the physical capacity of older individuals by exercise training. A study by de Vries (1970) looked at 112 men aged 52–87 years. These men took part in a vigorous exercise programme and were tested at regular intervals on the following parameters: blood pressure, percentage of body fat, resting neuromuscular activation, arm muscle strength and girth, maximal oxygen consumption and oxygen pulse at heart rate of 145, pulmonary function, and physical work capacity on the bicycle ergonometer. A subgroup were also tested for cardiac output, stroke volume, total peripheral resistance, and the work of the heart at a workload of 75 watts on the bicycle. The most significant findings were related to oxygen transport capacity. Oxygen pulse and minute volume at a heart rate of 145 improved by 29.4% and 35.2% respectively, and vital capacity improved by 19.6%. A subsequent study looked at older women aged 52–79 years who participated in a vigorous three-month programme, and again physical fitness was improved (Adams & de Vries 1973). It seems that physical conditioning of the healthy older person can bring about significant improvements in the cardiovascular system, the respiratory system, the musculature and body composition. In general the result is a more vigorous individual who can also relax successfully. Other health benefits are likely to include a lower blood pressure and lower percentage of body fat, with concomitant lessening of the risk factors attributed to the development of coronary artery disease (de Vries 1975).

FACTORS AFFECTING MOBILITY

PSYCHOLOGICAL AND SOCIOENVIRONMENTAL FACTORS

For those individuals who are able to get out and about quite a high level of mobility is required. According to the Department of Transport (1975/6) 52% of journeys made by people over 65 years are made on foot, and it is the more frail elderly people who rely on walking as opposed to using public transport. Use of buses requires the mastery of considerable obstacles particularly associated with getting on and off and moving about within a travelling bus (Robson 1978). The elderly pedestrian is more likely to be involved in a road traffic accident than the younger adult pedestrian, with a casualty rate for those aged 70 years and over being five times that of the 25–39 age group (Goodwin and Hutchinson 1976). The difficulties encountered are those of coping with fast traffic when crossing roads even at pedestrian crossings and traffic lights, in negotiating hills, narrow uneven pavements, and steps and kerbs.

The internal environment of the home can harbour hazards to safe mobility, including poor lighting, narrow dark stairs, and slippery rugs. The danger of this type of hazard will be mentioned later in relation to falls. It is possible to prolong independent mobility for the elderly by simple adaptations such as handrails and correct seat heights. In a survey of mainly elderly and arthritic people living at home, it was found that ease in rising was rated as the most important factor in their choice of an easy chair (Munton et al 1981). Compared with young adults, older people are observed to take longer to rise from a chair and to rely on handgrip for balance, and to use thrust from arms and leg muscles (Shipley 1980). Loss of muscle strength, and the effects of illness on joint flexibility and muscle co-ordination may be part of the reason for difficulties in rising from a chair, but the problem may lie with the chair itself. Greater joint flexion and thrust will be needed if the seat platform and armrest are low, or the upholstery does not give firm support. A backward tilt in the angle of the seat or back support will require greater leverage (Finlay et al 1983). Though not in itself sufficient, ease in rising is clearly necessary for mobility.

The effects of an institutional environment such as a hospital ward or nursing Home can be detrimental to the elderly person. Lieberman et al (1971) found that patients placed in a cold dehumanized dependency-fostering environment show decline. Marlowe (1973) compared two groups of patients in two different institutions, and found

that those who became more active were in environments which encouraged autonomy and a personal approach, did not foster dependency by doing things for individuals that they could do for themselves, encouraged community integration and social interaction, and did not expect passivity and docility.

A home routine which includes walking to local shops, visiting friends or regularly walking a dog, may keep an elderly person fairly mobile. Admission to hospital for what ever reason will cut off these normal everyday reasons for getting out and about. Levels of mobility may rapidly deteriorate. It is probably true that many institutions, be they hospital wards or community Homes, foster dependency, unless it is a progressive atmosphere that encourages self-sufficiency. This may be related to the environment itself, or to the attitudes of the care staff or the residents' perceptions of how they are expected to behave. There is a tendency to overprotect elderly persons in institutions, to prevent them from moving around at will. This is a reflection of the fear for the person falling and sustaining an injury which will be blamed on inadequate supervision by nursing staff or relatives at home. If the mobile elderly person is not to deteriorate, and the rehabilitation of the person with impaired mobility is not to be impeded, then it is surely necessary to allow the individual more freedom of movement. Ensure that the environment is as safe and supportive as possible; by having beds, chairs and toilets at heights which make it easy to get in and out, on and off; by having non-slip floor surfaces, handrails, good lighting, identification of doorways; and by making sure that the person has her own glasses, hearing aid, and walking aid available if these are used. The choice to live dangerously is the prerogative of us all, and this should not be less so for elderly people.

Whether an individual retains a good functional level of mobility into old age is not totally reliant on physical ability or fitness, although it appears that medical problems are the major source of difficulties (Hunt 1978). Many people are mobile even though they suffer chronic conditions which cause much pain and discomfort, whilst others who are physically better may withdraw and become housebound. An individual's past experiences and others' perceptions and expectations of her and her abilities can together result in a reduction in mobility and activity. Loss of friends and relatives can reduce motivation required to make the effort to get out and about. Old people who on retirement move to a different geographical area can become isolated from their family and friends and become lonely, and this may be a cause of reduced mobility. Restriction or loss of mobility affects the ability of the individual to care for themselves adequately, and this may result in social isolation.

PHYSICAL FACTORS

An individual's mobility and independence are reliant to a great extent upon the normal functioning of the nervous, musculoskeletal, circulatory, and respiratory systems in a co-ordinated and integrated manner to produce a normal gait and posture. Injury or disease of one or more of these systems may lead to impairment of gait with subsequent reduction or difficulty with mobility (Imms & Edholm 1981). Disorders of gait, balance, and posture are common in the elderly, and they account for a large number of admissions to medical, geriatric, and orthopaedic wards (Nayak et al 1982). The term gait is defined by Galley and Forster (1982) as 'the manner of walking', and it includes locomotion or the act of moving from place to place. A 'gait cycle' consists of a step each by the right and left legs through the 'stance' and 'swing' phases. In normal walking, when approximately 50 to 60 steps/minute are taken, the stance phase comprises about 60% of the cycle and the swing phase 40%, with the two periods overlapping when the two feet are on the ground together for about 25% of the time (Galley & Forster 1982).

The gait of elderly people has been studied and compared with that of young normal subjects. Healthy old people showed on average a slower walking speed, shorter step length and lower frequency of stepping, with little difference in stride width (Guimaraes & Isaacs 1980). The slowing of the gait happened as a result of lengthening of the stance and double support phase, the period when both feet are on the ground simultaneously,

with little change in the length of the swing phase. According to Azar and Lawton (1964) this alteration in gait seems to be a physiological concomitant of ageing and it differs between the sexes. Women typically adopt a narrow walking and standing base and walk with a waddle, whilst men use a wide walking and standing base and a small stepped gait. On the other hand, results of a study of gait and mobility of elderly people (Imms & Edholm 1981) suggest that chronological age has only a minor effect on gait and mobility with pathological changes being more important. Findings by Visser (1983) show that patients with senile dementia of Alzheimer's type walked more slowly, took shorter steps, had a lower frequency of stepping, and a higher double support ratio when compared with matched normal controls. These gait characteristics closely match those described for normal healthy old people, and so it is probably the degree to which these changes have taken place in various groups that are the important factors. Support for this comes from Guimaraes and Isaacs (1980), who found that a group of patients who were hospitalized following falls had shorter steps, narrower stride lengths, slower speed, wider range of frequency of stepping, and a wider degree of variability of step length when compared with patients who either had not fallen or had fallen and were not admitted. All the groups showed some features of abnormal gait, with the highest level of abnormalities occurring in the oldest most disabled group. The commonest gait abnormalities have been listed by Caird and Judge (1976):

1. Abnormal elevation of the hip of the moving limb owing to a stiff hip.
2. Elevation of the moving limb due to a stiff knee.
3. The waddling gait of patients with bilateral hip disease or proximal muscle weakness.
4. The circumduction of a spastic hemiplegic leg in which the foot moves in an arc of a circle during forward movement.
5. The scissors gait, with crossing of the feet due to adductor spasm from bilateral pyramidal lesions, or more rarely, osteoarthrosis of the hips.
6. The apparent unequal length of steps in a

person with some degree of pyramidal tract disorder. The movements of the unaffected leg seem to carry the foot further than those of the affected leg.

7. The abnormal elevation of the limb, sometimes also with a little circumduction occuring in the presence of foot drop.

8. The shuffling gait with small hesitant steps, particularly when beginning to walk and turning, of the patient with Parkinsonism. She also tends not to swing the arms normally.

9. The wide-based staggering gait of the person with cerebellar disease.

10. The shuffling and tottery gait with small steps of the patient with severe brain disease whether vascular or non-vascular, and severe intellectual impairment. In general, those with vascular brain disease tend to have increased muscle tone and reflexes, and those with non-vascular disease mild rigidity and slowing of movement, with reduced reflexes. Both gaits may be difficult to distinguish from the gait of Parkinson's disease, although the patient with severe brain disease does not tend to have any greater difficulty in turning.

It is well to remember that old people are likely to have more than one abnormality, and previous traumas and congenital deformities should be noted.

Gait should be assessed with the patient wearing her normal footwear, and the shoes or slippers themselves should be examined for particular areas of wear. All parts of walking, including starting, turning, and stopping need assessment on different types of flooring, but essentially in conditions as similar to the patient's home as possible if assessment in the home is not feasible.

GAIT AND MOBILITY PROBLEMS RELATED TO PATHOLOGICAL CAUSES

PARKINSON'S DISEASE

Parkinsonism is a clinical syndrome characterized by a combination of rigidity and bradykinesia, and frequently including the following: resting tremor, a disorder of posture and balance, automonic dysfunction and dementia (Broe 1982). This syndrome produces a series of highly characteristic features which affect mobility. The standing posture is one of flexion of the knees, hips, trunk, neck, and elbows, with abducted shoulders. This posture has the tendency to push the centre of gravity too far forward resulting in a continuous acceleration of forward movement (festination) in order to prevent a forward fall. Or else the gait tends to be slow with small shuffling steps (Sabin 1982). Reduced ankle movements causes 'scuffing' of the toes, loss of heel strike, and the whole trunk and arms are moved as one unit with resultant loss of arm swing and shoulder rotation (Murray et al 1978).

This type of gait is highly unstable and falls are common. Individuals with this type of gait abnormality find it difficult or impossible to rise from a chair or bed. The sitting person fails to flex her legs close to her centre of gravity when trying to stand up, and so falls backwards. During walking, defective balance and righting mechanisms may cause the individual to lose balance when jostled, hurried, or when turning. The failure to lift the feet high enough off the ground means that tripping on such familiar and everyday things as the edge of a carpet or a small irregularity on the floor is likely. Difficulty in locomotion, i.e. inability to initiate or continue the forward shift of the body, can cause the person to remain rooted to the spot until given a small push which allows her to move her legs forward (Rosin 1982). Individuals may also have a tendency to run with small teetering steps — the 'festinating gait'.

It is obvious, therefore, that the range and speed of movements in Parkinsonian patients alter their ability to control locomotion, and it is thought that this gait pattern may be the result of adaptation to gain control of forward movement and balance with the actual power of motor control (Knutsson 1972). The effects of Parkinsonism vary in the degree to which they are seen in different individuals with only the severist sufferers displaying all these features. Patients with mobility problems related to Parkinson's disease require careful assessment in order to identify the abnormal patterns, and this should be followed by a programme of techniques and training to help alleviate the problem.

HEMIPLEGIA

The effects of a stroke on mobility are usually catastrophic, ranging from complete immobility, bedfast or chairfast, to a highly unstable staggering type of gait. From various studies it is understood that the inability of the hemiplegic patient to walk in a normal fashion appears to be related to:

1. Abnormal muscular activity resulting in loss of selective movement patterns.
2. A disorder of the normal postural mechanism — the righting and equilibrium reflexes.
3. A sensory deficit (Wall & Ashburn 1979).

The abnormal muscular patterns are usually characterized by increased flexion of the muscles of the upper limbs, trunk and neck, and increased extension of the muscles of the lower limbs. If the patient is able to walk, the hip is retracted with the leg hitched forward at the pelvis and with the toe or sole of the foot hitting the floor first rather than the heel. There may also be toe drag and inversion of the ankle. The affected leg is 'favoured' with the patient spending more time supported on the unaffected side. Disordered balance mechanisms result in an inability to sit without falling to the affected side, or to walk without leaning and perhaps falling to the affected side. These patients seem to be incapable of the integrated action necessary to align the body segments and bring their centre of gravity into balance with their feet below it (Adams 1974). The problems are further compounded by deficits in sensation and proprioception, so that signals from peripheral muscles and joints and from the environment are misinterpreted or not attended to at all. The combination of all these effects results in varying degrees of mobility restriction with loss of ability to attend to a wide range of activities of living. These patients require an intensive programme of retraining. Methods of therapeutic exercise described by Bobath (1978) aim to facilitate normal patterns of movement in response to tactile and proprioceptive stimuli, whilst inhibiting abnormal patterns of muscular activity. In addition, many

activities of living have to be relearnt and a safe and stimulating environment provided. There are several sources that describe rehabilitation methods for stroke patients (Johnstone 1977, Bobath 1978, Batehup 1983, Myco 1983, Hawker & Squires 1985) and further discussion can be found later in this chapter.

ARTHRITIC CONDITIONS

The commonest type of arthritic conditions which affect the elderly are osteoarthrosis and rheumatoid arthritis (Wright 1983), and it is generally acknowledged that these conditions are an important cause of mobility problems for the elderly.

Osteoarthrosis can be radiologically detected in almost all elderly people though it may be symptomless (Lawrence et al 1966). Generalized osteoarthrosis describes a widespread pattern of synovial joint involvement including, as well as hips and knees, terminal interphalangeal joints and thumb bases, with ankles and shoulders usually spared (Bird 1983).

Rheumatoid arthritis is a chronic systemic disorder affecting primarily the peripheral joints through inflammation and proliferation of the synovial membrane (Stevens 1983). The pattern of joint involvement is additive and symmetrical especially affecting proximal interphalangeal and metacarpophalangeal joints, wrists, knees, and small joints of the feet, but may also affect elbows, ankles, shoulders and hips (Stevens 1983). With some exceptions, the elderly person with inflammatory rheumatoid disease will have reached a 'burnt out' stage (Agate 1983), and, in common with osteoarthrosis, the most serious effects for an individual's mobility arises from problems in the main weight-bearing joints of the hips and knees. Pain and flexion contractures of hips with instability in the knee joints contributes particularly to immobility. To rise out of a chair or climb stairs, for example, requires a 90° range from almost full extension, and for ease in performing these activities a range of 110° flexion is necessary (Chamberlain 1983) in at least one leg.

Restoration of lost mobility can be especially difficult when the cause is arthritis of the rheumatoid type. Too often a permanent contracture in flexion of the knee for example has become established, and taking weight through such an abnormal joint is often very painful. It appears that attempts to correct flexion deformities with exercise or surgery for elderly patients is not wholly successful for a variety of reasons (Agate 1983), and prevention of this type of contracture in youth or middle age determines what capabilities exist when the patient reaches old age. This relies on enlightened care from doctors, nurses and physiotherapists. Much of what has been said also applies to osteoarthrosis, but it may be easier with the elderly osteoarthritic patient to reverse the immobility resulting from disuse. This can only be done by controlling pain, persuading the patient to stand and extend bent knees and hips, and straighten back and neck, and if necessary to walk with the help of some sort of aid. If in bed, patients should be encouraged to extend their knees and hips and to avoid pillows under the knees. When sitting in a chair a foot rest can be positioned to keep the knees straight. It is usually the case that the aim is not to return the person to work or some other form of outside activity, but rather to enable her to walk slowly and safely on one floor of a house, dress, and manage the toilet. Attention should also be paid to techniques of rising from and sitting down in chair, bed or toilet and to the height of these in order to promote independence. This limited range of mobility may be the difference between dependence and independence.

AMPUTATION

75% of new lower limb amputees are over the age of 60 years, and most have lost their limbs because of peripheral vascular disease or diabetic gangrene (Van de Ven 1984). These patients often have the associated problems of cardiac involvement, low exercise tolerance, arteriosclerosis with possible hemiplegia and diminished mental ability.

In the early stages after surgery it is important that attention be given to the position of the stump which should be extended at hip and knee and not raised on a pillow. A board under the mattress will help. According to Nichols (1976) the three main

factors contributing to the development of contractures after amputation are: pain, spasm, and immobility and bad posture either in bed or chair. Effective pain relief should help the muscle spasm. It is important that the stump should be positioned as stated, and lying prone with a pillow under the trunk for short periods throughout the day also helps to prevent contractures. Control of oedema in the stump by effective bandaging is essential to promote healing (Van de Ven 1984).

The team will decide on the most appropriate mobility regime and the condition of the remaining leg is an important factor. If an artificial limb is to be provided for mobility or aesthetic purposes, it should be worn as much as possible in order to maintain the shape of the stump. Protective footwear is advisable for the other leg. Wheelchair mobility may be more realistic for some elderly patients. A stump board on which the chair cushion is placed so that the stump can be extended, will prevent oedema and contractures. Boards can be provided for bilateral stumps, and can be folded down when the patient transfers or stands. The psychological benefits of being able to move around again should not be underestimated. Even though wheelchair mobility has to be accepted for some frail elderly persons, rehabilitation should never lack urgency, because in its own terms it can be highly successful in returning the person to an appropriate, largely domestic routine (Crowther 1982). Once mobility begins, it should continue as part of the day's routine. The patient should be encouraged to maintain an upright posture with weight bearing through the stump, so reducing the possibility of a circumduction gait. Some patients find the loss of one leg gives balance problems because of the altered weight distribution, and double amputees may find a similar problem in sitting because they feel unbalanced.

FALLS

Falls are a major problem for elderly people. It is not unusual to find that a person suffering from recurrent falls becomes housebound, even chair- or bedbound, immobile, demoralized and dependent upon the support of the social services (Exton-Smith & Overstall 1979). The majority of falls in old age result from a combination of factors. The ageing process, disease, drugs, and external hazards may all contribute (Campbell et al 1981). The rates of falls occurring in various settings have been reported in many studies. Exton-Smith (1977) found, in a survey of elderly people at home, that 31% of men and 47% of women over the age of 80 years reported falling. Brocklehurst et al (1978) found that in a group over the age of 85 years 46% had fallen during the previous year, and Overstall et al (1977) reported that 50% of his subjects aged 60 years and over had fallen for various reasons. This is obviously a problem of some magnitude. The outcome of falls is not always of a serious physical nature, but undoubtedly always causes some loss of confidence. The most common serious consequence of a fall for an older person is a fracture of the proximal femur (Fernie et al 1982).

Activity at the time of fall

Falling at home occurs most often in the bedroom or sitting-room, or when going to the toilet (Brocklehurst et al 1976, Wild et al 1981b). The study by Wild et al (1981b) shows that high numbers of falls occur on change of position such as getting up from bed, chair or toilet, going up stairs or walking on an irregular surface. There are also a large number of falls which happen unexpectedly with no accompanying symptoms or external hazards. In institutions most falls are associated with getting in or out of bed, on or off a chair, and when using the toilet or commode (Rodstein 1964, Ashley et al 1977).

Causes of falls

There is agreement that falls of the elderly can be attributed to extrinsic or intrinsic factors or a combination of both. Extrinsic factors include a wide range of environmental hazards such as loose carpets, trailing wires, dark stairs, uneven floors. Intrinsic factors include postural hypotension, cardiac dysrhythmias, muscle weakness, cervical spondylosis, and balance and righting problems. According to Wild et al (1981a) the concept that a fall in old age has 'a cause' is inadequate, and

they contend that the attribution of falls to perceived pathogenic mechanisms is often conjectural. Doctors rarely witness the fall, and so the 'cause' is often diagnosed from a combination of the patient's statement and the doctor's physical findings. Their evidence suggests that the patient's statements even when most carefully collected are not by themselves a very good guide to the possible cause. The elderly people in this study used the terms dizziness, giddiness, blackout, and lightheadedness when describing what happened, but all these terms lack a precise and unambiguous meaning. Falls result from uncorrected displacement of the body from its support base, which implies a difficulty with control of balance and posture.

Balance and falls

The term 'loss of balance' is frequently used in two different ways. It describes the single fall of a healthy person which is not otherwise explained by an accidental trip, and it describes those recurrent falls of a person who cannot maintain the upright posture unsupported (Isaacs 1982). It is also a term frequently heard in relation to elderly people, and implies usually that balance has been lost.

Balance is the set of functions which keeps the body upright during stance and locomotion by detecting and correcting displacements of the line of gravity beyond the support base (Isaacs 1982). The centre of gravity is the equivalent point within the body at which the whole body-weight may be considered to act, and in the upright position it lies within the pelvis at approximately the upper sacral region anterior to the second sacral vertebra (Galley & Forster 1982). It is beyond the scope of this chapter to describe the components of the balance mechanism in any great detail but, briefly, these include:

1 *Afferent mechanisms*, which detect displacements; these include vision, vestibular, and proprioceptive organs.

2. *Central mechanisms*, which receive and integrate information from the periphery and issue corrective instructions; these include stretch reflexes, righting reflexes, long loop reflexes which

help to control gait and posture, unexpected disturbances and voluntary movement, and tend to restore conditions to their previous state before displacement occurred (Grimm & Nashner 1978).

3. *Efferent mechanisms*, which transmit instructions to the muscles, including cells in the motor cortex and their connections with the spinal motor neurones, motor units, muscle fibres.

The rate of falls of the elderly has already been mentioned and it corresponds closely with failure of the balance mechanism in old age. The mechanisms involved in balance are particularly susceptible to age-related changes. According to Hasselkus (1974), although feedback is impaired by changes in joints, muscle spindles, and peripheral nerves, it is the slowing of central processes in the brain which perceive and integrate proprioceptive signals that is mainly responsible for increased reaction time. Therefore, the elderly person who stumbles finds that the speed of her postural reflexes is too slow to prevent a fall, and she has failed to correct the displacement of the body from its support base. Wild et al (1981a) have devised a classification of falls which is based on this idea. A fall or displacement can be of two types — initiated and imposed — and of two degrees — ordinary and extraordinary.

Initiated displacements

These are falls which the person herself induces in the course of her activities such as rising from a chair or bed, or during walking when the line of gravity is momentarily displaced beyond the support base. An 'ordinary initiated displacement' might result from an error on standing up, whilst an 'extraordinary initiated displacement' could be a fall from a chair or ladder or a sudden change of direction.

Imposed displacements

These are falls which occur from factors in the outside world such as irregular surfaces, and unexpected obstacles like pets and small grandchildren. There is normally sufficient capacity in the recovery mechanism for the detection and correction of the displacement, but as the balance mechanism becomes less efficient in later life the range and speed of recovery is reduced. An 'ordinary imposed displacement' might result from a trip on a loose carpet. An 'extraordinary imposed displacement' could occur when slipping on a patch of ice or a wet floor, or if a dog runs unexpectedly into one's path. Various medical factors such as reduced visual and vestibular function, reduction in proprioceptive mechanisms, pathology in the brain or spinal cord, and diseases of the peripheral nerves and muscles, may impair the balance mechanism. The advantage of this classification is that it becomes possible to categorize a fall on the basis of the information obtained from the patient or other onlookers, and may therefore be of some help in the prevention of falls (see Table 8.1).

Advanced old age is accompanied by an increased probability of falling even in quiet domestic surroundings. Elderly people adjust their gait to diminish the danger of falling by shortening and slowing the pace, broadening the base and lowering the height of their step (Murray et al 1978). Those at risk of falling are people aged 75 years and over who are housebound, who walk with shuffling irregular steps, and have a fear of falling whilst on their feet. Little evidence was found to support the statements frequently made that falls in old age are often caused by cervical spondylosis, vertebrobasilar ischaemia, etc. (Wild et al 1981b).

ASSESSING AND MANAGING IMMOBILITY

The multiple pathologies associated with ageing bring with them multiple problems, and for rehabilitation to be effective a thorough functional assessment of the patient's needs is essential to identify the real barriers to independence and to facilitate discharge. It is the patient's functional ability more than diagnosis, that will dictate future placement and so initially assessment is of the activities that the patient expects to undertake, followed by a physical assessment to identify the

Table 8.1 Prevention of falls

Displacement	Example	Causes	Prevention
Extraordinary imposed	Patch of ice Dog running into path	Environmental hazards	Avoid hazard Improve environment. Accidental falls due to an unsafe environment such as loose carpets, wet floors, dark stairs, account for a third to a half of all falls (Exton-Smith & Overstall 1979). Slippers and bare feet contribute to falls (Wild et al 1981a)
Ordinary imposed	Trips on rug or carpet	Trivial hazard Impaired perception of displacement	Correct hazard Patients with a history of falls place their feet unpredictably and may induce a displacement of which they are unaware (Guimaraes & Isaacs 1980). Perception of unsafe gait and retraining may be possible
Extraordinary initiated	Sudden movement of head	Hurried action	Teaching to help match activities to balance mechanisms, so that range and speed of activities is diminished to remain within the person's reduced competence
Ordinary initiated	Error on standing up	Disease Drugs	Identify cause The importance of psychotropic drugs in causing impaired balance of old people is increasingly recognized (Macdonald & Macdonald 1977). Wild et al (1981a) found that fallers were taking significantly more hypnotics, tranquillizers, and sedatives than were a matched control group

causes of any restriction to activity. It will be the diagnosis of these barriers to independence that subsequently dictate the type of treatment necessary.

When assessing any patient it is always essential to remember that improvement may not be possible, or desirable (Squires & Wardle 1988). Goals must be realistic and achievable, otherwise enthusiasm is lost by all involved. Accepting that a stage has been reached in life where deterioration or death are the most likely outcomes should not be seen as defeat, and goals must be set accordingly to ensure that dignity, relief from pain and other stresses are promoted.

The physiotherapist's assessment is aimed mainly at the components required for mobility, whilst the occupational therapist will focus attention on the daily living needs. Assessment is a continuing process and needs constant review. The initial assessment provides a baseline for the evaluation of subsequent treatments (Parry 1980). All professional staff have a legal and moral re-

sponsibility to do what is right for the patient, and failure to assess thoroughly may be viewed as negligence (Association of District and Superintendent Physiotherapists 1984). It is important to remember the atypical disease presentation, and biological factors which may affect rehabilitation, such as reduced exercise tolerance (Payton & Poland 1983). Also, an elderly person with a limited life expectancy may have priorities different from those of a younger person.

The rapport between patient and assessor is the key to the future relationship when treatment, often tiring and sometimes painful, with often slow progress, will stretch that relationship to the limit. Introductions, social skills and non-physical assessments can be used initially to pave the way. Some suggestions follow.

Communication

It is essential to check that the assessor and the patient can communicate with each other. This not only means checking speech, sight and hearing, but also language and dialect. The increasing number of people from ethnic minorities now reaching old age in this country is posing a challenge for health professionals. The old person may not have learnt English, or if a second language it may have been lost, which happens to people suffering with dementia or a stroke. An assessment of the patient's mental status should have been completed at the time of admission and this will be a useful indication of the level of mental ability that can be expected. Reassessment at intervals is essential and can reveal improvements in mental ability as the patient settles down to her new environment and becomes less confused. Denham and Jeffreys (1972) showed that a more realistic rehabilitation programme could be planned when the intellectual ability was known.

Occupation

The term 'old age pensioner' gives no insight into the life of the person being assessed. Time spent enquiring into the occupations held by the patient will give a fascinating view of a disappearing era, and may also indicate the physical tolerance likely to be available from either the work or recreational pursuits described. The last or current job held by an old person has been described as an 'end occupation' (such as caretaker or commissionaire) and previous occupations or hobbies should be investigated. There may have been contact with lead in metalwork or paint, leaving the patient with signs of neurological dysfunction; or with dust, resulting in chest diseases. Industrial accidents, war trauma and occupational hazards may have left the person with joint damage or limb deformity, and the neurological signs indicating the tertiary stages of syphilis, such as tremor and spastic paresis together with dementia, should not be overlooked.

Brief history

This can reveal the main problem if time is taken to investigate. In many cases breakdown in the person's ability to cope at home leads to hospital admission, and setting up domiciliary services may be more beneficial than rehabilitating someone who was managing quite well at home. On the other hand, the breakdown may reveal a situation that has been deteriorating for some time, and illness of the home help prevents the elderly person carrying on. Immediate intervention is necessary; waiting lists for a hospital bed or for outpatient treatment or community care are unacceptable.

Social circumstances

As the majority of elderly patients are referred from home, knowledge of the accommodation and available support is essential. Realistic rehabilitation cannot occur without information about door widths for walking aids, the number of stairs, the siting of the toilet, etc. Relatives, friends, community nurses and social services staff can often provide valuable information, and a visit to the home by a member of the team, preferably with the patient, early during her hospital stay is an advantage. The treatment of the patient within her own home has obvious advantages, but has yet to be fully developed in terms of community physiotherapy, and the social advantages of attending for outpatient treatment should not be overlooked.

Motivation

This is really the key to whether treatment is going to be effective or not, and motivation is just as necessary for the staff as for the patient. When one considers the incentives of the company, warmth, and interest provided in a hospital, it is not surprising that discharge home may sometimes be resisted. A similar situation may occur when a community nurse visits a lonely person at home and is her only visitor.

Diagnosis

Pathology increases with age, which means that a single symptom such as a stiff joint may have more than one cause and may have existed for some time. In addition, co-existing disorders may require treatments which are acceptable for one problem, but contraindicated for another. An example here is rheumatoid arthritis and spastic hemiplegia. Passive movements may be contraindicated in the former because of soft tissue involvement, but necessary in the latter to try to prevent contractures forming. The therapists must decide which problem poses the greater risk and select the appropriate treatment for each individual patient.

Functional assessment

The functions for assessment will vary with the individual team and assessment forms have been produced at some time by most units (Squires 1986). Ensuring that the patient's lifestyle is covered for the 24 hours of the day will mean that all the necessary activities for that individual are considered. It should be noted that a consistent finding is that ability to use the toilet is the most sensitive functional test.

Documentation is essential to ensure that team members neither omit nor duplicate an activity, and Rubenstein (1983) suggests that it should ensure an easy process, make a good teaching model, be reliable, allow transmission of information, facilitate smooth teamwork, provide valid data and measure progress. The method of documentation should be both succinct and sensitive to changes in ability; if it can also visually document change it will be easier for colleagues to appreciate and for patients to observe changes as well.

When skills are assessed they should be observed by the assessor, and statements by the patient and/or carers should not be accepted without proof (Coates & King 1982). Rubenstein et al (1984) found that the patient had the highest opinion of her abilities, and the relatives the lowest. Rubenstein and his colleagues felt that the patient's view may be due to optimism, shifted timeframe or concealment, and that the relatives' view may be influenced by fear of being overburdened.

The terminology used for the documentation is also important. All assessors must appreciate what terms such as 'independent' mean. For example, are walking aids and appliances allowed? Must appliances be put on independently as well? An idea of how the patient was functioning prior to the incident that brought her to our attention is vital. It is unlikely that any improvement on a pre-

viously comfortable lifestyle will be possible in many cases, and this level may become the aim of treatment. Rogers (1980) has pointed out that the trauma of admission causes confusion and anxiety to the patient and assessment should be delayed until later in the first week when the patient has settled. This can be a dangerous approach in cases in which dependence has been established within 24 hours. Payton et al (1983) point out that a loss of strength of 3% a day may occur during a period of immobility. A further assessment should be undertaken to record changes, and the progress that has been made a month after intervention commenced is a good indicator of eventual outcome (Stewart 1981). Following discharge, deterioration is most likely when equipment has not been provided (Sheikh et al 1979) or adaptations such as wider doorways have not materialized (Mahoney & Barthel 1965). Haworth and Hollings (1979) have suggested that social factors such as loss of confidence may also have an effect. As the goal of management of the patient is her relative independence at home, it is essential to ensure that the interventions are successful and follow-up assessment should be included immediately after discharge and also later when the patient and her carers have settled into their routine.

Following identification of the problems the patient is having during the 24 hours of the day, a physical examination will be necessary to identify the cause of the weakness, stiffness, loss of balance etc. so that appropriate intervention can be provided.

PHYSICAL ASSESSMENT AND MANAGEMENT
Neck

This can be a potent source of problems for old people. Intervertebral discs begin to degenerate from the second decade of life. The mechanics of the cervical spine are therefore altered and abnormal movement produces an increase in osteophyte activity and may subsequently cause cervical spondylosis. The increased bone formed can cause pressure on nerve roots, the vertebral artery or even the spinal cord, with the resultant problems of altered sensation, muscle weakness and reduced blood supply to the brain. The lower vertebrae tend to be more affected, and the first signs reported by the patient are usually weakness in the legs (Jeffreys 1980).

Unfortunately, little can be done except to advise less movement of the neck. Surgical collars have little to offer as they seldom fit and cannot be easily applied and removed. A cheaper, aesthetically more acceptable and probably more beneficial solution is to wear a thick scarf which will act as a warmer and will remind the patient not to turn her head too quickly. If the elderly person spends lengthy periods sitting in an armchair, this may increase the tendency to a flexion deformity of the neck, and a chair which allows relaxation in an upright posture may be more suitable.

Trunk

Thoracic deformities rarely start in old age and are usually congenital problems which were untreated owing to lack of facilities or finance. The main exceptions are deformities resulting from osteoporosis (Caird & Judge 1976). The consequences of thoracic deformity are that chest expansion will be reduced owing to calcification of the cartilages, and exercise tolerance and a powerful cough may also be reduced. Again, the condition cannot be reversed, but giving advice to the patient on posture in front of a mirror may prevent further deterioration, and diaphragmatic breathing can be taught so that as much of the lung capacity as possible is used. A wary eye should be kept on the deformity in case a pressure sore should develop on the apex of the curve, and attention to seating may be needed. Pain may be present from spinal deformity or joint degeneration, or wedge fracture of the vertebrae which occurs spontaneously in osteoporotic spines. One in 20 people over the age of 70 years experiences crush fractures of the spine (Nordin 1983). Surgical corsets may give some relief but are expensive, cumbersome and seldom worn correctly, and are often welcomed mainly for the warmth they offer, or worn out of habit. The elasticated abdominal support corsets can provide some support also to the lumbar and lower tho-

racic spine, and are easier to put on, washable, cheaper and warm, and can be supplied 'off the shelf'. Should a treasured corset be worn, it should be checked and renewed if necessary. Abdominal weakness is common in old age owing to poor posture and lack of exercise. Anyone undertaking a frantic keep-fit campaign after Christmas excesses will know the exceptional amount of effort required to strengthen these muscles, and although some strength can be regained by 'bridging exercises' on the bed and 'sit-forwards' on the chair, it may be that aids such as a bed ladder to get out of bed, and a wheeled frame to walk with will be needed as well.

Upper limbs

Assessment of the upper limbs will depend on the patient's requirements. A person living alone will need to be able to dress, cook and eat independently, whilst a patient living in sheltered accommodation may have help with some of these activities.

In old age the hands in particular can often provide a vivid picture of the life that has been led, showing callus formation, deformities and scars. In terms of function we must know what the patient needs to do and what is preventing her from doing it. An assessment of joint range and muscle power and sensation will show deficiencies, especially if compared with the opposite limb; and treatments to relieve pain, improve strength and range can be devised for the individual patient. Elevation of the arm will provide an indication of shoulder range and strength. Gripping the assessor's hand and trying to pull her or push her will assess grip strength and elbow mobility. The patient's hand should also be assessed for fine movements such as picking up a small object such as a pencil, or doing up a button. The ability to bring the hand to the mouth for eating will also assess range, strength, and co-ordination.

Muscle power is best assessed by comparing opposite limbs. The Medical Research Council gradings can be a useful baseline from which to work:

Grade 0   No contraction felt or seen

Grade 1   Flicker of activity felt or seen
Grade 2   Production of movement with gravity
          eliminated
Grade 3   Production of movement against
          gravity
Grade 4   Production of movements against
          gravity and an additional force
Grade 5   Normal power.

The hemiplegic patient who has had a severe stroke is likely to have a painful dislocated shoulder owing to the loss of muscle tone (Lind 1982), and so great care should be taken when handling and moving these patients. The patient may be unaware of the affected side and may even disown it, and she should be taught to attend to it by being encouraged to look for it, and handle and exercise it. Oedema is also a problem, and elevation throughout the day and night on a pillow will usually reduce it by means of gravity, but a lapse in surveillance allowing the patient's hand to be-

come dependent for even a short time will undo all the work the elevation achieved.

Massage may improve fluid absorption and venous return, and excellent results have been reported with pressure therapy units. The limb is elevated and placed within an air pressure sleeve, and air pumped into the sleeve provides gentle pressure on the limb so that effects similar to those of massage are achieved. The pressure can be individually selected for each patient, and can be constant, pulsed, or sequential in mode (Pflug 1975). Slings have gone out of favour in recent years because they reinforce the flexor spasticity of the hemiplegic arm, which may be in flexion, adduction, pronation, and internal rotation, and it is this spasticity which may contribute to subluxation (Bobath 1982). The arm is also prevented from functioning whilst encased in the sling. A more useful support is the 'figure of eight' bandage traditionally used for a fractured clavicle (Fig. 8.1), with the addition of a roll of foam placed in the

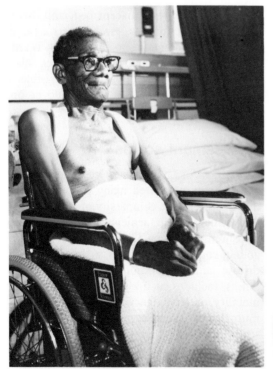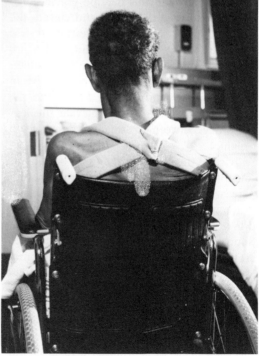

Fig. 8.1   Shoulder support for left hemiplegic patient: (a) front view; (b) rear view.

axilla of the affected side. This supports the shoulder and leaves the arm free for exercise (Bobath 1982).

Lower limbs

The lower limbs also require a functional assessment of joint range, strength and sensation. If the patient has to use the stairs, then hip, knee, and ankle mobility is necessary. The ability to rise from a chair and walk on the level must be assessed. There may be reduced range of movement of the ankles, and compensation for this may have to be taught, such as lifting the feet slightly higher to prevent tripping. Some deformities may be found, particularly of the knee, but perseverance by the patient and therapist, and application of innovative splints by the orthotist can overcome tremendous odds. In addition, the patient's feet must be examined, as painful feet will not welcome walking practice at any age, and may have been the cause of immobility in the first place.

Oedema of the lower limbs is a frequent problem for the elderly, and this may be gravitational owing to inability to get into bed and elevate the legs at night. This should be investigated, especially if the patient is attending hospital as an outpatient and practices at home are not known. Pressure therapy has been found to be effective in oedema of the lower limbs (Pflug 1975), and the patient should be encouraged to elevate the legs during the day between treatments and to go to bed at night.

The advice of the chiropodist should be sought. Shoes must be suitable; often attempts at rehabilitation are wasted when insufficient attention is paid to footwear. Suitable shoes that can be put on and taken off by the patient unaided are available. Slippers with adequate support and non-slip soles are also available for those with limited mobility, or for protection, and patients and relatives need advice before buying footwear. Shoes which will require any adaptation such as a raise or caliper must be well constructed, and advice should be sought. Unequal leg length should be checked and a decision made as to whether a raise should be applied or not. The patient may have adapted to long-standing shortening, but recent shortening, particularly from hip surgery, needs correction.

A caliper, if worn, should be examined and the repairs organized early. Fewer calipers are supplied these days as different treatment approaches have emerged, but some patients require supports, and the possibility should not be overlooked. The ability of the patient to get the caliper on and off and actually function with it must be assessed, and practice should be encouraged as with all daily living activities.

Skin condition

Although the nurse will be aware of any skin condition that the patient has, the other members of the team may not, and sharing this information is essential. For instance, one method of teaching transfers from a wheelchair to bed is to slide from one position adjacent to another. If a gluteal sore is present or likely, such friction will make it worse. Another method of transfer could be used, such as standing up from the chair, turning and sitting down on the adjacent bed, and this would prevent the friction risk. Any suspect areas should be discussed to ensure no further risk is entailed. For example, although bandaged leg ulcers of female patients wearing skirts are visible, those under trousers are hidden and should be brought to the therapist's attention.

Assessment scales

Assessment of physical activities and abilities after a stroke has presented many problems which are due mainly to the complexity of recovery patterns and difficulties in achieving objective and valid measurement tools. The assessment of other disabling conditions such as arthritis, Parkinson's disease, and amputation, in common with stroke illness, includes such aspects as activities of living, mobility, independence, motor deficit and neuromuscular performance. A discussion of assessment scales for stroke recovery therefore has relevance for the assessment of other chronic conditions.

Many scoring devices have been described to grade functional capacity and improvement during the rehabilitation process. Generally, these have been divided into organ system assessments, such as skeletal neuromuscular assessments (DeSouza & Langton Hewer 1980, Sheikh et al 1980, Ashburn 1982), and assessment of purposeful activities, such as eating, dressing, standing, walking, usually referred to as activities of living (ADL) (Katz et al 1963, Mahoney & Barthel 1965, Schoening & Iversen 1968, Sheikh et al 1979). For the purposes of research, it has been the practice for each study to develop its own assessment tools, and this tendency is criticized in a report by a group reviewing rehabilitation research and methods (Lancet 1982). This group identified 27 ADL scales, all of them representing minor variations on a common theme. Yet, if different therapeutic interventions in different settings are to be compared, a core of agreed measures has to be developed. In addition, many hospitals and rehabilitation centres have their own assessment tools which are used in physiotherapy and occupational therapy departments, and which are in the main untested.

Two assessment tools which may prove useful for widespread use are the motor assessment form for measuring physical disabilities following stroke (Ashburn 1982), and the ADL index devised for the Northwick Park stroke rehabilitation trial (Sheikh et al 1979), which has since been used for assessing disability across a wide range of conditions in a rehabilitation centre (Parish & James). A combination of these measures would provide a comprehensive picture of a patient's progress towards recovery, and in addition could be used for comparing different therapeutic techniques. Accurate measurement of disability is an essential component of rehabilitation; it provides a clear record of the patient's functional abilities, and should lead to the patient being discharged into a setting which is appropriate to her needs.

Problems associated with loss of balance, co-ordination and gait

The factors affecting balance have been described earlier. For treatment to be effective, a thorough clinical examination is necessary and it should be remembered that similar symptoms can be produced by several pathologies occurring together.

The problems related to loss of balance and co-ordination which can be treated by physiotherapy include the following conditions.

Pain

Pain can be reduced by heat or ice, both of which produce vasodilation which relieves vascular congestion and causes a reduction in the activity of the pain receptors (Lee & Warren 1978). Pain often causes muscle spasm and can therefore affect balance. Pain relief can also be achieved by transcutaneous nerve stimulation and by massage, which stimulate large diameter nerve fibres to close the 'gate' and reduce pain transmission (Melzack & Wall 1965).

Spasticity

This arises from hyperexcitability of the stretch reflex following an upper motor neurone lesion such as a cerebrovascular accident (Young & Delwaide 1981). The increase in skeletal muscle tone can produce patterns of abnormal flexion or extension. The posture and anxiety level of the patient at the time of assessment will affect the degree of spasticity. Spasticity is never confined to a single muscle but affects various muscle groups. Treatment by ice depresses the nerve conduction in the afferent nerves and reduces muscle tone (Lee & Warren 1978). Exercise of the muscle group antagonistic to those in spasm will reduce the spasticity (Knott & Voss 1968). Rhythmical passive movements through a normal pattern may also help. The most important component in promoting mobility of patients with spasticity is to start from a stable base, and patients should not be encouraged to mobilize until they have achieved a stable sitting and standing balance.

Reduced sensory input

A reduction in the activity of any of the senses which affect posture can occur in old age. Because of visual changes, older people may have trouble in adequately assessing environmental hazards. For example, there is a decline in visual acuity, with the pupil decreasing in size and becoming less responsive to changes in light (Riffle 1982). The older person requires more illumination in order to see well. With ageing, depth perception may become impaired (Riffle 1982), so the elderly person needs to be made aware of this change in relation to stepping off kerbs or stairs, and place her foot more consciously than before. Physical methods should be used to compensate wherever possible, for instance wearing spectacles and hearing aids. It is difficult, however, to compensate for lack of skin sensation and proprioception but knowledge that they exist is important.

Imbalance of muscle power

The treatment of muscle weakness is by repetitive exercise, preferably in the normal pattern for that part of the body, such as in proprioceptive neuromuscular facilitation techniques. Sensory stimulation over the working muscles increases input to the motor neurone pools, and techniques incorporating a stretch stimulation will also increase the input. Joint traction force assists flexion patterns, and joint compression facilitates extension patterns, as can be seen in normal weight bearing where the extensor patterns of the leg are brought into action. Stimulation can also be gained by using the body's natural righting reflexes (Atkinson 1977).

The Bobath method, which is suitable for a mixture of flaccid and spastic muscles as seen in hemiplegia, gives emphasis to re-educating movement in a bilateral way. The aim is to normalize tone and facilitate normal movement. The patient should be discouraged from using the unaffected arm and leg to compensate for the affected limb. Elderly patients with multiple pathology, which may include poor intellectual functioning, must be carefully assessed for a treatment regime which will be realistic for their needs. The whole team must be advised of the plan and must apply it continuously, from positioning of the unconscious patient through to mobilization.

Positioning the hemiplegic patient

Following a stroke the patient is left with a variety of sensory and motor deficits including loss of sen-

sation, visuospatial disturbances, disorders of body image, muscle paralysis, posture and balance disturbances, and abnormalities of muscle tone. By adequate positioning and handling of the patient, it is possible to prevent an undue increase in spasticity, contractures and shoulder pain (Parry & Eales 1976, Bobath 1982). The approach to positioning the stroke patient should be a co-operative effort with an informed patient and carer working with the nurses and physiotherapists to provide a consistent positioning routine.

It is helpful if the bed is firm and of variable height with locking wheels. This provides support for the whole body and aids the patient when transferring from bed to chair. If possible the bed should be placed to allow for an adequate amount of stimulation to the affected side.

Lying on the back (Fig. 8.2)

This position should be used as little as possible because it encourages extensor spasm (Johnstone 1977). The patient's head should be supported on one pillow and follow the straight line of the spine. The affected arm should be extended alongside the patient's body with the shoulder elevated. This can be achieved by placing a pillow lengthways under the shoulder and arm. The affected hip is supported on a pillow to prevent retraction and external rotation of the leg. Nothing should be placed in the patient's hand or against the sole of the foot as this encourages flexor spasticity. This applies to all positions.

Lying on the affected side (Fig. 8.3)

The patient's head should be supported on one pillow and follow the straight line of the spine. The affected arm should be eased forward with the palm of the hand uppermost. The affected leg is extended at the hip with the knee slightly flexed. The other leg is supported on a pillow. A pillow may be used to keep the trunk aligned.

Lying on the unaffected side (Fig. 8.4)

The patient's head should be supported on one pillow and follow the straight line of the spine.

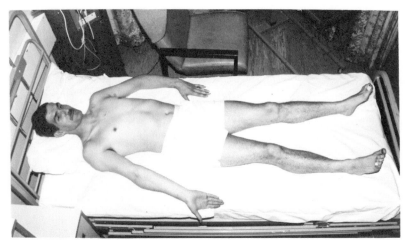

Fig. 8.2 Right hemiplegia: lying supine.

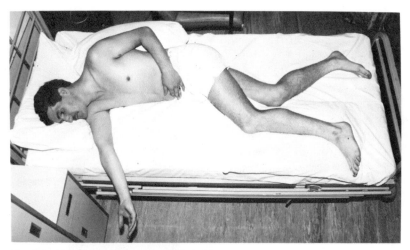

Fig. 8.3 Hemiplegia: lying on affected side.

The affected arm is brought forward with the palm facing down. The affected leg is brought forward, slightly flexed at the knee, and supported on a pillow. A pillow may be used to keep the trunk aligned and prevent the patient rolling backwards.

Sitting up in bed (Fig. 8.5)

The patient's head and trunk should follow a straight line well supported by sufficient pillows to prevent sagging. The posture should be as erect as possible. The affected shoulder should be brought forward, and this can be achieved by interlacing the fingers and extending the arms. The arms should be supported on one or two pillows. Both legs are extended.

Sitting in a chair (Fig. 8.6)

The chair should be of a height to allow the patient's feet to be placed flat on the floor with the knees at an angle of 90°. The back of the chair should be upright, and the armrests wide. The pa-

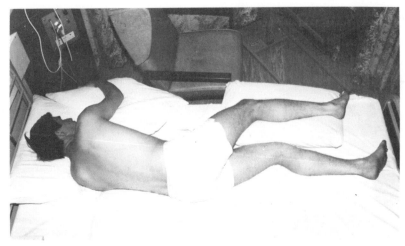

Fig. 8.4 Hemiplegia: lying on unaffected side.

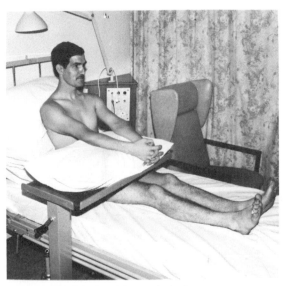

Fig. 8.5 Hemiplegia: sitting up in bed.

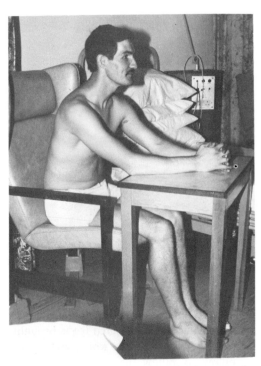

Fig. 8.6 Hemiplegia: sitting in chair raised to correct height for patient.

tient should sit upright in the chair, and, if the chair is suitable, supporting pillows should not be necessary. The shoulders should be placed forward, hands clasped and resting on a table.

Problems with shoes, feet and walking aids

All these need assessment and attention. Calluses and bunions can alter the body's balance, and the patient should be seen by the chiropodist. In a survey of walking-sticks used by elderly people, it was found that only 22% had been measured and of these only two thirds were the correct length, most of the others being too long (Sainsbury & Mulley 1982). Of the patients assessed in the survey who were fallers, 75% had sticks of an incorrect height. A survey by Kinsman (1983) showed that 75% of fallers wore slippers compared with 4% who wore lace-up shoes. Kinsman (1983) also found that 95% of the fallers were unsteady on their feet, but 48% improved after physiotherapy treatment.

Managing poor balance

When this is practised safely it ensures that someone can get up from a chair, or toilet, and can sit down on it safely. The prerequisites are a suitable chair (with appropriate height, arms, slant of back and seat), a non-slip floor, adequate strength and joint range and a reason to move. The chair most likely to be used at home can be adapted if necessary.

The usual method of chair drill is for the patient to position her feet parallel, slightly apart and slightly under the chair with her hands on the arms of the chair. She then wriggles towards the front of the chair, leans forward and pushes up from the chair and when upright places her hand on the aid if used. The reverse is performed when sitting down, in that the patient approaches the chair and turns around until the backs of the legs are touching the chair. She then feels for the arms of the chair with her hands, and gently lowers herself into the chair by bending in the middle. The same procedure should be followed when sitting or getting up from the toilet (Fig. 8.7).

Walking

The patient may walk incorrectly because an aid is used, particularly a frame. The patient should lift the frame (or push a wheeled frame), a pace in front of her and move first the weaker leg, and then the other leg up the frame but not inside it. She is then able to lift the frame again. Walking sticks are usually held in the hand opposite to the leg which is weaker or giving pain, but habits die hard and if an elderly person has always used a

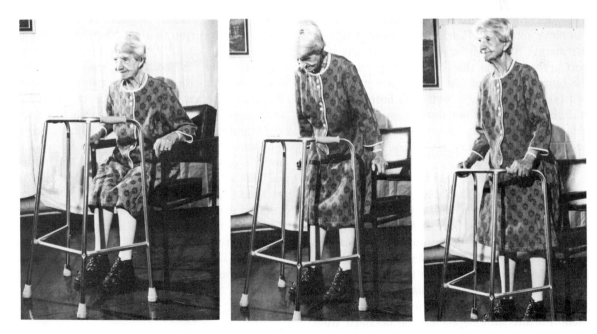

Fig. 8.7 Chair drill: (a) suitable chair, feet under and apart, hands on chair arms, lean forward; (b) push up from chair and lean forward; (c) hands on walking aid when upright.

stick in the right hand she will probably continue to do so.

The re-education of gait should relate to the patient's needs. Muscle strength, joint range, balance, correct walking aid, and footwear have all been discussed. The steps should be even in length, with even pace and even weight distribution, adequate abduction to prevent the legs crossing over and encouragement of a heel toe pattern (Lee 1978). The patient should practise going up and down steps and stairs if they are to be used at home. Provision of rails, or altering the house so that a one-level existence can be achieved may be wise since two thirds of the falls in the elderly occur on stairs (Caird & Judge 1976), and the majority of these occur when descending (Overstall 1978).

Patients should be encouraged to look ahead when walking and not at their feet, since this neck flexion results in a total body flexion pattern with bent knees and hips. A mirror or video system can be used so that the patient can see how she walks and can learn to control and improve it.

Mobility aids

These must be selected to ensure that the patient can move about safely; there is a variety of aids on the market. Gait will be abnormal with any support in the hands as this is not the natural gait for the human, but if an aid is necessary it must be suitable for the home as well as in hospital. Some wheeled varieties are not suitable on carpets. The aids must be carefully selected to meet individual needs, and those already in use should be checked for suitability and safety.

It has been suggested that the correct aid height is achieved when the handle is level with the distal crease of the wrist when the arm is down by the side of the body (Sainsbury & Mulley 1982). The patient's balance can be improved by raising or lowering the aid, and it is essential that only the aid that has been prescribed for the patient is used. The aid should be easily available to the patient on the ward if unaided mobility is to be encouraged. Further information can be obtained from the physiotherapy and occupational therapy departments.

Methods of getting up after falling

Isaacs (1979) estimated that three millon old people fall each year and yet little has been written about methods of getting up after falling. Priorities are warmth and calm, and a prearranged method of summoning help should be used. The elderly person living alone is the most vulnerable and should benefit from being taught different methods of getting up.

Roll and crawl. The faller must be able to roll onto her front, get on to all fours, and crawl to a chair which she then uses as a support to get up. The most frequent obstacle to this method is knee pain and weakness. The faller if hemiplegic should roll onto her front and push herself up into a side-sitting position using the unaffected side. She then shuffles on the floor in this position using the unaffected leg and arm until reaching a chair. Then using the unaffected arm and leg she can push herself up onto the chair (Robinson 1980).

Backwards shuffle. The faller gets into a sitting position on the floor and then, using her arms and legs, shuffles backwards to a low stool, ramp, or bottom stair and pushes herself up onto it until in a position to get up. This is particularly effective on the stairs as gradual progression up the stairs will bring the person to a good height to attempt to stand up.

Rescue chair. A mechanical device has been developed on the 'fork-lift truck' principle (Fig. 8.8). The seat of the chair can be lowered to the ground by the faller, who then shuffles back onto it and raises it electrically to a suitable height from which to stand up. It can also be used to lower a patient onto the floor from the sitting position so that conventional methods can be practised (Squires 1983). The faller should be encouraged to sit still for a while and recover before attempting to walk again. Remembering to pull the mobility aid along with her when moving across the floor after falling is wise so that it is ready by the chair when needed.

The long-stay patient

There will always be some patients who will have reached the limit of their physical capacity and for

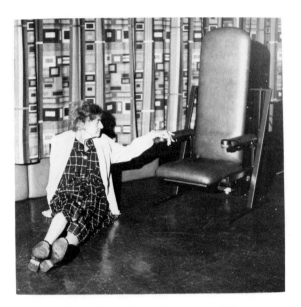

Fig. 8.8 Getting off the floor using rescue chair.

Patients being rehabilitated for discharge from hospital

These patients need constant advice, encouragement and supervision, which should be withdrawn gradually as the discharge date approaches. Communication between all the carers involved is necessary to ensure continuity of treatment and to prevent the problem of being too helpful. Activities achieved with the therapist should be continued by the nurses and other helpers every day. In a survey by Livesley and Graham (1983) it was found that of patients readmitted to hospital after discharge, the earliest admissions were due to insufficient notice being taken of the therapist's assessment and advice, whereas the later readmissions were generally for unavoidable clinical deterioration.

whom maintenance treatment is appropriate (Denham 1983). Passive movements to assist in nursing care may be undertaken by the therapist or taught to nursing staff where suitable. Hip abduction for hygiene, knee extension to prevent heel pressure, ankle movements to maintain circulation and upper limb movements to assist washing and dressing are fundamental. Full range passive movements to the joints of the limbs should be undertaken twice daily, taking care to support the limb throughout, to hold it and not pinch, and especially to be receptive to messages from the muscles or from the patient in terms of spasm or pain. A working knowledge of normal joint range is necessary and advice should be sought from the physiotherapist before undertaking passive movements if there is any doubt as to suitability or the range and pressure necessary (Martin-Jones 1962).

Where possible, standing will help by giving stimulation through the feet and initiating an extensor thrust movement which will prevent flexion patterns developing. Standing also aids bowel and bladder function and is particularly useful in preventing the accumulation of bladder calculi. Passive movements, handling and standing can be taught to interested relatives.

LIFTING DISABLED OLD PEOPLE

Research relating to nurses shows that low back pain is a major problem, accounting for between 35% and 47% of job-related injuries. The commonest alleged precipitating cause is lifting patients — this is implicated in 49–79% of all low back injuries (Stubbs & Osborne 1979). Although a variety of lifting methods is used, basic principles should be observed, as follows (Lloyd et al 1981):

- Assess the situation and see if the patient does need to be lifted, and if so how much she can do to help.
- Be aware of the medical condition present. Explain to the patient and any helper what you are going to do.
- Use mechanical aids if available and desirable.
- Ask for help if in any doubt of your physical limitations.
- Clear the area of hazards, wear safe shoes, prepare the destination.
- Position the feet correctly.
- Keep the patient as close to you as possible.
- Keep your back straight.
- Use your body as a counterbalance.
- Keep good time with your partner.

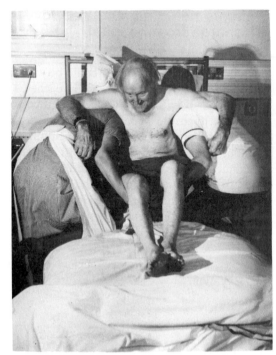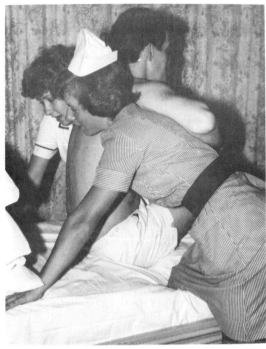

Fig. 8.9 Shoulder lift: (a) showing position of patient's arms and operators' arms; (b) method with leading hand on bed.

The shoulder lift (Fig. 8.9)

This has been shown to halve the back stress as compared with other methods (Stubbs & Osborne 1979), and can be used to move the patient up and down the bed, from chair to bed, and from floor to bed. Two lifters are needed. They face the patient, one on each side, place their shoulders nearest the patient under his axillae and their arms under his thighs, and clasp hands. The patient rests his arms along the backs of the lifters, or if this is not possible because of shoulder pathology the lifter on the affected side supports the patient's back with her other hand. The lifters point their leading feet in the direction they are moving and use their spare arms to press down on the bed, or hold the bed-head if going that way, which lessens the stress (Scholey 1982). The lifters lift and move the patient together, keeping their backs straight and bracing their free arms. It is essential to lift the patient and not drag him along the bed, so causing shearing forces on the skin. Lowering the

bed will make this lift easier as the lifter's back legs can kneel on the bed and give additional support.

The Bobath stand (Fig. 8.10)

This is an excellent method for standing and turning a patient, for example from bed to chair, when only one person is needed. It was developed for hemiplegic patients but can be successfully used for elderly people with other conditions. With the patient sitting on the edge of the bed either with bare feet or in non-slip footwear and feet slightly apart, the lifter places her feet outside those of the patient and her knees against his, slightly to the lateral side. The patient can either place his hands around the lifter's waist, or around her neck with the weaker hand being grasped by the stronger. When everything is ready, the patient is encouraged to lean forward whilst the lifter uses her body weight to counterbalance and help the patient to a standing position. When balance is gained, the

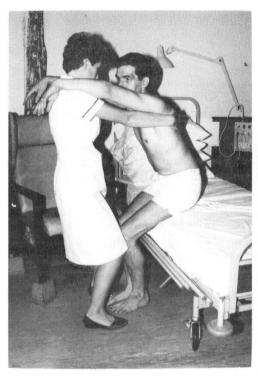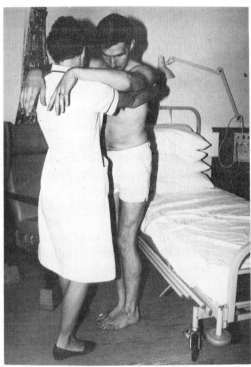

Fig. 8.10 Hemiplegia: (a) standing up; (b) stand and turn.

turn is controlled by the lifter and the patient is lowered by reversing the movements into the adjacent chair (Bobath 1982).

This method can be used to sit a patient back into a chair when she is slipping out, by helping her to stand and applying pressure to the knees which will push the hips back in the chair. When transferring patients from chair to bed and vice versa, both pieces of furniture must be stable and unable to move with the brakes on if available.

STROKE UNITS

Stroke patients account for 6% of all hospital running costs, 13% of all general medical bed-days, and 25% of geriatric bed-days (Carstairs 1976). The care of stroke patients in the United Kingdom, with some exceptions, is poor, and has failed to keep pace with developments in North America.

The question of stroke units is controversial, but there does seem to be agreement that changing the organization of stroke care to provide intensive care equipment, facilities and staffing, has no impact on overall mortality during the immediate period following the event (Akhtar & Garraway 1982). Therefore, interest has centred on the period following the acute phase, and the most effective means of organizing rehabilitation for the patients that have survived it. There is evidence that care in a specialized stroke unit is more effective for some patients than the care provided in a general medical unit. McCann and Culbertson (1976) found that those patients at 'level three' (those with severe impairment), attained significantly better results than similar patients on medical wards, although patients with moderate and profound impairment were no different.

Stroke severity ratings (McCann & Culbertson 1976) are as follows:

1. Mild   Patient has minor disabilities which slightly restrict ability to function at home and in community, can live independently.

2. Moderate   Patient has moderate disabilities, needs assistance of another person to help with some activities.

3. Severe   Patient has severe disabilities, needs supervision to function at home and in community.

4. Profound   Patient is completely dependent upon assistance of at least one person to carry out daily needs, not functionally competent in the home or community.

A study by Feigenson et al (1979) compared stroke unit patients with non–stroke unit patients, and found that more stroke unit patients were discharged home and that they walked better than non–stroke unit patients, but there was no difference between the two groups in ability to perform activities of daily living. There was also no difference between the two groups in length of stay in hospital. A British study supports these findings (Garraway et al 1980a). A higher proportion of patients discharged from the stroke unit, compared with those from the medical unit, were assessed as independent, although these findings were not supported at one year follow-up (Garraway et al 1980b). On the other hand, studies by Peacock and Lampteon (1972) and Waylonis et al (1973) did not support improved function of stroke unit patients. There are also advocates for stroke care at home (Smith 1981, Wade & Langton Hewer 1983) and as an outpatient (Smith et al 1981). Clearly then, the question of where stroke rehabilitation takes place remains unanswered, but there are some tentative conclusions that can be reached.

1. The group of patients in the middle range of impairment would probably do better in a disability-oriented stroke unit than in general medical or geriatric wards.

2. Those with minimal impairment will usually recover 'spontaneously' wherever they are, and those with very severe impairment will not recover more function if treated in a special unit.

3. Stroke units provide an environment in which communication between different members of the multidisciplinary team is extremely effective, providing a more consistent approach to stroke care than might be found in medical and geriatric wards.

4. Stroke units should improve patient interaction when participating in group activities with others suffering from similar disabilities.

5. Stroke units should improve carer knowledge and participation in the recovery process.

6. Stroke units have an important role in studying the value of different diagnostic and therapeutic interventions (von Arbin et al 1979)

A recent Consensus Statement produced by the Kings Fund Forum on the treatment of stroke suggested that no policy for stroke care exists at any level in the NHS for planning, organizing, implementing or evaluating care. A stroke policy should have standards, a comprehensive service and sufficient resources, including information for patients and carers. Assessment and rehabilitation should be a team effort with assessment, documentation, promotion of independence and a key worker (King Fund 1988).

The key to success is the ability to identify those patients who will benefit most from the facilities of a stroke unit. Some stroke patients will get better without any intervention. Some will never improve however much effort is put in by all members of the team.

STROKE REHABILITATION

There are conflicting views on the effectiveness of rehabilitation after stroke. Recent studies which attempt to evaluate rehabilitation methods for stroke patients are comparing mainly quantitative aspects of therapy such as the relative amounts of physical, occupational, and speech therapy received by patients in a controlled stroke unit/ward, with the amount received by patients in general medical wards (Garraway et al 1980, Smith et al 1981, Stevens et al 1984). An example of the amounts of physiotherapy, occupational therapy, and speech therapy received by patients in a stroke

Table 8.2 Therapy received by stroke patients.

	(SRW) Patients Patients Treated	Hours	General ward Patients Treated	Hours
Physiotherapy	112	4463	104	1486
mean		40		14
Occup. therapy	47	654	24	212
mean		14		8
Speech therapy	37	633	27	188
mean		17		7

Source: Stevens et al (1984).

rehabilitation ward as compared with therapy received by a group of patients in general wards is given by Stevens et al (1984) (Table 8.2).

A variety of remedial techniques may have been used in these studies but they have not been described. Modern exercise therapy for stroke patients takes into account the principles of neuromuscular facilitation. Various methods of facilitation have been developed (Brunstromm 1970, Kabat 1977, Bobath 1982), with each emphasizing a different aspect of the neurophysiological approach.

Neuromuscular facilitation

The neuromuscular mechanism, which includes the muscles, nerves, neural pathways and brain centres, initiates and achieves movement in response to a demand for activity (Gardiner 1981). To facilitate is to 'make easier', and neuromuscular facilitation is the process by which the response of the patient's neuromuscular mechanism is made easier. This is done by the therapist using specific techniques. The techniques developed by Bobath and Bobath (1950) and described by Bobath (1982) for the treatment of spastic hemiplegia, have received attention and recognition in the United Kingdom. This method is based on the concept that there exists a hierarchy of functions in the human nervous system, with a range from stereotyped and obligatory responses at the spinal cord level, to more variable selective ones integrated at subcortical and cortical levels. The influence of sensory stimuli and subsequent feedback, from the motor response produced, upon the integrative process is the basis of the treatment. Damage to the upper motor neurone, as in stroke, results in abnormal postural reflex activity with spasticity and disturbances in balance and righting mechanisms. The techniques are designed to increase, decrease or maintain muscle tone during a motor activity, and to facilitate active movements from a controlled posture (Flanagan 1967). Proprioceptive neuromuscular facilitation (PNF) (Kabat 1977) is another facilitation technique which relies mainly on stimulation of the proprioceptors for increasing the demand made on the neuromuscular mechanism to obtain and facilitate a response. Treatment by these techniques is very comprehensive and involves application of the principles of PNF to every aspect of the patient's handling.

There is doubt concerning the value of rehabilitative and physiotherapy procedures and the influence of therapy on recovery in the damaged central nervous system (Langton Hewer 1972). The major criticism is that the techniques of physical therapy for stroke patients, such as facilitation techniques, have not been evaluated in controlled trials. There are many factors which make research in the area of stroke recovery problematic, including cognitive and perceptual impairment, and spontaneous recovery (Lind 1982), but there still remains need for evaluation of specific methods of remedial therapy, especially in the light of doubts expressed by physicians and others.

GERIATRIC ORTHOPAEDIC UNITS

The increase in the incidence of fractured neck of femur especially in older women has led to planned co-operation between orthopaedic and geriatric specialties. This has either taken place on a specially planned joint ward, or has involved one team visiting the patient in the other team's ward. The Hastings approach is probably the best known. Success is attributed to high quality surgery, attention to medical and social needs, and the importance of the nursing role (Irvine 1984).

For maximum effect the selection of patients is crucial; Burley et al (1984) suggest that patients should be classified into three groups: members of group 1 are those who need little help; group 2 contains those who present with rehabilitation problems either physical, psychological or social and who might regain some independence with the team approach; group 3 consists of those who have no apparent prospect of returning to independence.

The studies that have been undertaken generally point to the key role played by the nursing staff in co-ordinating the efforts of the team round the clock, and the increased allocation of time from paramedical staff.

REFERENCES

Abrams M 1978 Beyond three score years and ten. Age Concern Publications, London
Adams G F 1974 Cerebrovascular disability and the ageing brain. Churchill Livingstone, Edinburgh
Adams G M, De Vries H A 1973 Physiological effects of an exercise programme upon women aged 52–79. Journal of Gerontology 28: 50–55
Association of District and Superintendent Physiotherapists 1984 Spring report. ADSP, London
Agate J N 1983 Physiotherapy problems and practice in the elderly: a critical evaluation. In: Wright V (ed) Bone and joint disease in the elderly. Churchill Livingstone, Edinburgh
Akhtar A J, Garraway W M 1982 Management of the elderly patient with stroke. In: Caird F I (ed) Neurological disorders in the elderly. Wright, Bristol
Ashburn A 1982 A physical assessment for stroke patients. Physiotherapy 68(4): 133–149
Ashley M J, Gryfe C I, Amies A 1977 A longitudinal study of falls in an elderly population II: Some circumstances of falling. Age and Ageing 6: 211–220
Atkinson H 1977 Principles of treatment. In: Cash J (ed) Neurology for physiotherapists. Faber, London
Azar G J, Lawton A H 1964 Gait and stepping as factors in the frequent falls of elderly women. Gerontologist 4: 83
Barker J, Bury M 1978 Mobility and the elderly: a community challenge. In: Carver V, Liddiard P L (eds) An ageing population. Hodder and Stoughton in Association with the Open University Press, Sevenoaks, Kent
Batehup L 1983 How teaching can help the stroke patient's recovery. In: Wilson Barnet J (ed) Patient teaching. Churchill Livingstone, Edinburgh
Bird H A 1983 Osteoarthrosis. In: Wright V (ed) Bone and joint disease in the elderly. Churchill Livingstone, Edinburgh
Bobath B 1978 Adult hemiplegia: evaluation and treatment, 2nd edn. Heinemann, London
Bobath B 1982 Adult hemiplegia: evaluation and treatment, 3rd edn. Heinemann, London
Bobath K, Bobath B 1950 Spastic paralysis: treatment of by the use of reflex inhibition. British Journal of Physical Medicine 13: 121–127
Brocklehurst J C, Exton-Smith A N, Lempert Barber S M, Hunt L, Palmer M K 1976 Fracture of the femoral neck. Report No 1 to the Department of Health and Social Security, London
Brocklehurst J C, Exton-Smith A N, Lempert Barber S M, Hunt I, Palmer M K 1978 Fracture of the femur in old age: a two centre study of associated clinical factors and the cause of the fall. Age and Ageing 7: 7–15
Broe G A 1982 Parkinsonism and related disorders. In: Caird F I (ed) Neurological disorders in the elderly. Wright, Bristol
Brunstromm S 1970 Movement therapy in hemiplegia: a neurophysiological approach, Harper and Row, New York
Burley L E, Scorgie R E, Currie C T, Smith R G, Williamson J 1984 The joint geriartic orthopaedic service in south Edinburgh. Health Bulletin 42(3): 133–140
Caird F, Judge T 1976 Assessment of the elderly patient. Pitman, London
Campbell A J, Reinken J, Allan B C, Martinez G S 1981 Falls in old age: a study of frequency and related clinical factors. Age and Ageing 10: 264–270
Carstairs V 1976 Stroke: resource consumption and cost to the community. In: Gillingham F J, Maudsley C, William A E (eds) Stroke. Churchill Livingstone, Edinburgh
Chamberlain M A 1983 Mobility of the elderly. In: Wright V (ed) Bone and joint disease in the elderly. Churchill Livingstone, Edinburgh
Coates H, King A 1982 The patient assessment. Churchill Livingstone, Edinburgh
Crowther H 1982 New perspectives on nursing lower limb amputees. Journal of Advanced Nursing 7: 453–460
Denham M 1983 Care of the long stay elderly patient. Croom Helm, London
Denham M, Jefferys P 1972 Routine mental testing in the elderly. Modern Geriatrics 2: 275
Department of Transport, National Travel Survey 1975/6. Department of Transport, Marsham Street London SW1P 3EB
De Souza L, Langton Hewer R 1980 Assessment of recovery of arm control in hemiplegic stroke patients. International Rehabilitation Medicine 2: 3–16
De Vries H A 1970 Physiological effects of an exercise training regime upon men aged 52–88. Journal of Gerontology 24: 325–336
De Vries H A 1974 Vigour regained. Prentice Hall, Englewood Cliffs, NJ

De Vries H A 1975 Physiology of exercise and ageing. In: Woodruff D S, Birren J E (eds) Ageing: scientific perspectives and social issues. Van Nostrand, New York

Ebersole P, Hess P 1981 Toward healthy ageing. Mosby, St Louis

Exton-Smith A N 1977 Functional consequences of ageing: clinical manifestations. In: Exton-Smith A N, Grimley Evans J (eds) Care of the elderly: meeting the challenge of dependency. Academic Press, London

Exton-Smith A N 1978 Bone ageing and metabolic bone disease. In: Brocklehurst J C (ed) Textbook of geriatric medicine and gerontology. Churchill Livingstone, Edinburgh

Exton-Smith A N, Overstall P W 1979 Geriatrics. MTP Press, Lancaster

Feigenson J S, Howard S, Gitlow S, Greenberg S D 1979 The disability oriented rehabilitation unit — a major factor influencing stroke outcome. Stroke 10: 5–8

Fernie G R, Gryfe C I, Holliday P J, Llewellyn A 1982 The relationship of postural sway in standing to the incidence of falls in geriatric subjects. Age and Ageing 11: 11–16

Finlay O E, Bayles T B, Rosen C, Millig J 1983 Effects of chair design, age and cognitive status on mobility. Age and Ageing 12: 329–335

Flanagan E M 1967 Methods for facilitation and inhibition of motor activity. American Journal of Physical Medicine 46: 1006–1011

Galley P M, Forster A L 1982 Human movement. Churchill Livingstone, Edinburgh

Gardiner M D 1981 The principles of exercise therapy. Bell and Hyman, London

Garraway W M, Akhtar A J, Prescott R J, Hockey L 1980a Management of acute stroke in the elderly: preliminary results of a controlled trial. British Medical Journal 281: 1040–1043

Garraway W M, Akhtar A J, Hockey L, Prescott R J 1980b Management of acute stroke in the elderly: follow-up of a controlled trial. British Medical Journal 281: 827–828

Goldman R 1979 Decline in organic function with age. In: Rossman I (ed) Clinical geriatrics, 2nd edn. Lippincott, Philadelphia

Goodwin P B, Hutchinson T P 1976 The risk of walking. In: Elkington P, McGlynn R, Roberts W (eds) The pedestrian: planning, and research. Transport and Environment Studies, Unpublished report by University College (London) Traffic Studies Group

Grimm R J, Nashner L M 1978 Progress in clinical neurophysiology 4: 70

Guimaraes R M, Isaacs B 1980 Characteristics of the gait in old people who fall. International Rehabilitation Medicine 2: 177–180

Harris A 1971 Handicapped and impaired in Great Britain, Part 1. Social Survey Division, Office of Population Censuses and Surveys, London

Hasselkus R 1974 Ageing and the human nervous system. American Journal of Occupational Therapy 28: 16

Hawker M, Squires A 1985 Return to mobility. The Chest Heart & Stroke Association, London

Haworth R J, Hollings E M 1979 Are hospital assessments of daily living activities valid? International Journal of Rehabilitation Medicine 1: 59–62

Hunt A 1978 The elderly at home – a study of people aged 65 and over living in the community in England in 1976. Social Survey Division, Office of Population Censuses and Surveys, HMSO, London

Imms F J, Edholm O G 1981 Studies of gait and mobility in the elderly. Age and Ageing 10: 147–156

Irvine R E 1984 The Hastings approach. The British Journal of Geriatric Nursing Jan/Feb, 12–14

Isaacs B 1979 Thoughts from a bathchair. Physiotherapy 65: 338–340

Isaacs B 1982 Disorders of balance. In: Caird F I (ed) Neurological disorders in the elderly. Wright, Bristol

Jeffreys E 1980 Disorders of the cervical spine. Butterworth, London

Johnstone M 1977 The stroke patient: principles of rehabilitation. Churchill Livingstone, Edinburgh

Kabat H 1977 Studies in neuromuscular dysfunction. In: Payton O D, Hirt S, New R A (eds) Neurophysiologic approaches to therapeutic exercise. Davies, Philadelphia

Katz S, Ford A B, Jackson B A, Jaffe M W 1963 Studies of illness in the aged: the Index of ADL, a standardized measure of biological and psychological function. Journal of the American Medical Association 184: 914–919

Kings Fund 1988 The treatment of stroke: Kings Fund consensus statement. Kings Fund Centre, London

Kinsman R 1983 Falls in the elderly. Unpublished audit, Barnet Health Authority

Knott M, Voss D 1968 Proprioceptive neuromuscular facilitation. Harper and Row, New York

Knutsson E 1972 An analysis of Parkinsonian gait. Brain 95: 475–486

Kraus H, Rabb W 1961 Hypokinetic disease. Thomas, Springfield, Illinois

Lancet 1982 Research aspects of rehabilitation after acute brain damage in adults. Lancet 2: 1034–1035

Lange K, Anderson R, Masironi R, Rutenfranz J, Seliger V 1978 Habitual physical activity and health. World Health Organization, Copenhagen

Langton Hewer R 1972 Stroke units. Lancet 1: 52

Lawrence J S, Bremner J M, Bier F 1966 Osteoarthrosis. Annals of the Rheumatic Diseases 25: 1–24

Lee J 1978 Aids to physiotherapy. Churchill Livingstone, Edinburgh

Lee J, Warren M 1978 Cold therapy. Bell and Hyman, London

Lieberman M A, Tobin S S, Slover D 1971 The effects of relocation on long term geriatric patients. Final report of Department of Mental Health, State of Illinois Project 17 328 (mimeo)

Lind K 1982 A synthesis of studies of stroke rehabilitation. Journal of Chronic Diseases 35: 133–149

Livesley B, Graham H 1983 Can readmissions to a geriatric medical unit be prevented? Lancet 1: 404–406

Lloyd P, Osborne C, Tarling C 1981 The handling of patients. Back Pain Association and Royal College of Nursing, Shears, Hants

Macdonald J B, Macdonald E T 1977 Nocturnal femoral fracture and continuing widespread use of barbiturate hypnotics. British Medical Journal 2: 483

McCann B C, Culbertson R A 1976 Comparison of two systems for stroke rehabilitation in a general hospital. Journal of the American Geriatrics Society 25: 211–216

Mahoney F I, Barthel D W 1965 Functional evaluation: the Barthel Index. Maryland State Medical Journal 14: 61–65

Marlowe R A 1973 Effects of the environment on elderly

state hospital relocatees. In: 44th Annual Meeting of the Pacific Sociological Association, Scotsfale, Arizona (mimeo)

Martin-Jones 1962 Passive movements: physiotherapy helps nursing. Nursing Times Publication, London

Melzack R, Wall P D 1965 Pain mechanisms: a new theory. Science 150: 971–978

Munton J S, Ellis M, Chamberlain A, Wright V 1981 An investigation into the problems of easy chairs used by the arthritic and the elderly. Rheumatology and Rehabilitation 20: 164–173

Murray M P, Sepic S B, Gardner G M, Downs W J 1978 Walking patterns of men with parkinsonism. American Journal of Physical Medicine 57: 278–295

Myco F 1983 Nursing care of the hemiplegic stroke patient. Harper and Row, London

Nayak U S L, Gabell A, Simons M A, Isaacs B 1982 Measurement of gait and balance in the elderly. Journal of the American Geriatrics Society 30: 516–520

Nichols P J R 1976 Rehabilitation medicine: the management of physical disabilities. Butterworth, London

Nordin B 1983 Preventing osteoporosis. Geriatric Medicine 13: 873–876

Norman A 1981 Barriers to mobility. In: Hobman D (ed) The impact of ageing. Croom Helm, London

Overstall P W 1978 Falls in the elderly: epidemiology, aetiology and management. In: Isaacs B (ed) Recent advances in geriatric medicine. Churchill Livingstone, Edinburgh

Overstall P W, Exton-Smith A N, Imms F J, Johnston A L 1977 Falls in the elderly related to postural imbalance. British Medical Journal 1: 261–264

Parish G, James D N 1982 A method for evaluating the level of independence during the rehabilitation of the disabled. Rheumatology and Rehabilitation 21: 107–114

Parry A 1980 Physiotherapy Assessment. Croom Helm, London

Parry A, Eales C 1976 Handling the early stroke patient at home and in the ward. Nursing Times 72: 1680–1688

Payton O, Poland J 1983 Ageing process — implications for clinical practice. Physical Therapy 63(1): 41–47

Peacock P B, Lampteon T D 1972 In: Stewart G J (ed) Trends in epidemiology. Thomas, Springfield, Illinois

Pflug J 1975 Intermittent compression in the management of swollen legs in general practice. Practitioner 215: 69–76

Riffle K L 1982 Promoting activity: an approach to facilitating adaptation to ageing changes. Journal of Gerontological Nursing 8: 455–459

Robinson G 1980 Multiple sclerosis — simple exercises. Multiple Sclerosis Society, London

Robson P 1978 Profiles of the elderly: their mobility and use of transport, vol 4, no 6, Age Concern Publications, London

Rodstein M 1964 Accidents among the aged — incidence, causes and prevention. Journal of Chronic Diseases 17: 515–526

Rogers J C 1980 Advocacy: the key to assessing the older client. Journal of Geriatric Nursing 6(1): 33–36

Rosin A J 1982 Parkinsonism. In: Isaacs B (ed) Recent advances in geriatric medicine. Churchill Livingstone, Edinburgh

Rubenstein L 1983 The clinical effectiveness of multidimensional geriatric assessment. Journal of the American Geriatrics Society 31(12): 758–762

Rubenstein L Schaver C, Weland G, Kane R 1984 Systematic bias in functional assessment of elderly adults: effects of different data sources. Journal of Gerontology 39(6): 686–91

Sabin T D 1982 Biologic aspects of falls and mobility limitations in the elderly. Journal of the American Geriatrics Society 30: 51–58

Sainsbury R, Mulley G P 1982 Walking sticks used by the elderly. British Medical Journal 284: 1751

Saltin B, Blomquist G, Mitchell J H, Johnston R L, Wildenthal K, Chapman C B 1968 Response to exercise after bedrest and after training. American Heart Association Monograph H23. The American Heart Association, New York

Schoening H A, Iversen I A 1968 Numerical scoring of self-care status: a study of the Kenny self-care evaluation. Archives of Physical Medicine and Rehabilitation 49: 221–229

Scholey M 1982 The shoulder lift. Nursing Times 78(12): 506–507

Selye H S 1970 Stress and ageing. Journal of the American Geriatrics Society 18: 669–690

Sheikh K, Smith D, Meade T, Goldenberg E et al 1979 Repeatability and validity of a modified ADL Index in studies of chronic disability. International Rehabilitation Medicine 1: 51–58

Sheikh K, Smith D, Meade T, Brennan P et al 1980 Assessment of motor function in studies of chronic disability. Rheumatology and Rehabilitation 2: 83–90

Shipley P 1980 Chair comfort for the elderly and infirm. Nursing 20: 858–860

Shock N W 1962 The physiology of ageing. Scientific American 206: 100

Smith A 1981 When home management of stroke was a success. Geriatric Medicine May: 65–70

Smith D S, Goldenberg E, Ashburn A, Kinsella G, Sheikh K, Brennan P J et al 1981 Remedial therapy after stroke: a randomized controlled trial. British Medical Journal 282: 517–520

Squires A 1983 Rescue chair. Multiple Sclerosis Society Bulletin 104: 1456

Squires A 1986 Physiotherapy assessment of the elderly patient. Physiotherapy 72(12): 617–620

Squires A, Wardle P 1988 To rehabilitate or not? In: Squires A (ed) Rehabilitation of the older patient. Croom Helm, London

Stevens M B 1983 Rheumatoid arthritis. In: Wright V (ed) Bone and joint disease in the elderly. Churchill Livingstone, Edinburgh

Stevens R S, Ambler N R, Warren M D 1984 A randomized controlled trial of a stroke rehabilitation ward. Age and Ageing 13: 65–75

Stewart C P U 1981 Mental status questionnaire, activities of daily living and discharge category in elderly patients undergoing rehabilitation. Journal of Clinical and Experimental Gerontology 3(4): 387–389

Stubbs D A, Osborne C M 1979 How to save your back. Nursing 3: 116–124

Van de Ven C M 1984 Amputations: Cash's textbook of general medical and surgical conditions for physiotherapists: Faber, London

Visser H 1983 Gait and balance in senile dementia of Alzheimer's type. Age and Ageing 12: 296–301

von Arbin M, Britton M, de Faire U, Helmers C, Miah K,

Murray V, Wester P O 1979 A stroke unit in a medical department. Acta Medica Scandinavica 205: 231–235

Wade D T, Langton Hewer R 1983 Why admit stroke patients to hospital? Lancet 1: April 9 807–809

Wall J C, Ashburn A 1979 Assessment of gait disability in hemiplegics. Scandinavian Journal of Rehabilitation Medicine 11: 95–103

Waylonis G M, Keith M W, Aseff J W 1973 Stroke rehabilitation in a mid-western county. Archives of Physical Medicine and Rehabilitation 54: 151–174

Weg R B 1975 Changing physiology of ageing: normal and pathological. In: Woodruff D S, Birren J E (eds) Ageing: scientific perspectives and social issues. Van Nostrand, New York

Wessel J A, Van Huss W D 1969 The influence of physical activity and age on exercise adaptation of women 20–69 years. Journal of Sport Medicine 9: 175–180

Wild D, Nayak U S L, Isaacs B 1981a Description, classification and prevention of falls in old people at home. Rheumatology and Rehabilitation 20: 153–159

Wild D, Nayak U S L, Isaacs B 1981b How dangerous are falls in old people at home? British Medical Journal 282: 266–268

Wright V 1983 Bone and joint disease in the elderly. Churchill Livingstone, Edinburgh

Young R R, Delwaide P J 1981 Spasticity. New England Journal of Medicine 304: 1 28–33

CHAPTER CONTENTS

The prevalence of foot problems 147
Ulceration, corn and callus   149
Superficial infections   150
Foot deformity   151
Soft tissue conditions   151
Toenails   152

Foot care advice   153
The chiropody service   154

9

Care of the foot

Mike C. Hobday

THE PREVALENCE OF FOOT PROBLEMS

Painful and deformed feet are very common problems for elderly people. Ebrahim et al (1981) surveyed 100 patients in an acute geriatic assessment and rehabilitation ward and found just one patient who presented no problem with her feet. Most of their sample had three or four specific foot problems which, apart from pitting oedema, excluded complications of systemic disease. Earlier, Hobson and Pemberton (1955) concluded that four out of five elderly people had foot disability on examination though not all complained of pain. More recent surveys of people aged over 65 years have shown that over half have difficulties with their feet and that, as would be expected, the incidence of problems increase with age (Kemp & Winkler 1983, Cartwright & Henderson 1987, Salvage et al 1988). Clark (1969) found that three quarters of people over 65 years reported trouble with their feet and the proportion recorded as having foot problems increased when they were professionally inspected. The attitudes of elderly people explain the well-documented discrepancy between their perceived need for chiropody treatment and their actual need for treatment (Townsend & Wedderburn 1965). Foot disability is frequently unreported by elderly people. It is seen as an inevitable accompaniment of ageing and many old people fail to seek help because of this (Williamson et al 1964, Kemp & Winkler 1983). The attitudes and expectations of patients have proved a difficult factor in many studies which seek to establish the incidence of foot problems in the population. Elderly people, particularly, seem to expect to have to endure painful feet with increasing years.

It is quite clear from surveys that a large majority of the elderly population do have problems associated with foot disorders. Kemp and Winkler (1983) found that some 88.7% of the elderly population was in need of foot care, if prophylactic advice and education were to be included in the concept of need.

Agate (1963) states that if a normal gait is to be preserved in the elderly then it is vital that the feet should not be painful or deformed. There is a clear relationship between foot problems and immobility of old people. Collyer (1981) concludes that an old person with painful feet may very easily become housebound and lose mobility, and this view is supported by Suvarna (1981). Mobility can be severely restricted by relatively simple foot problems. Most of these problems fall within the scope of practice of the state registered chiropodist, who can do much to alleviate these problems with palliative treatment and patient education. Loss of mobility will frequently exacerbate other problems from which a patient may be suffering, and general debility may be increased. Many common foot conditions which impair foot function can lead to, or contribute towards, falls (Helfand 1966).

There are many problems which can impair an elderly person's ability to cope with routine hygiene and care of the foot. Neglected feet are frequently an early sign of physical or mental deterioration. These problems include poor eyesight, rheumatic disease affecting the ability of patients to reach their feet or affecting the dexterity of the hands, obesity, neurological conditions and muscular weakness, hypertension, cardiac and pulmonary disorders which prevent old people from bending down to reach their feet.

Women over 65 years have a higher incidence of foot disorders than men over 65 (Clark 1969, Kemp 1988). The most prevalent problems which affect elderly people are corns and calluses, trouble with toenails, foot deformities resulting from badly fitting shoes in youth, and arthritis. Clark (1969)

found that 34% of the elderly people in her sample had difficulty in cutting toenails. Ebrahim et al (1981) found that of the 100 patients examined, 66 complained of difficulty in cutting toenails, 38 complained of onychogryphosis (thickening and deformity of the nail plate) and nine had ingrowing toenails. These are all high frequencies when compared to findings for the younger population. Clark (1969) found that 26% of elderly men and 49% of elderly women complained of corns, and that 25% of elderly men and 34% of elderly women complained of troublesome hard skin. Ebrahim et al found that 30 of the 100 patients exhibited corns and calluses and 15 complained of pain from corns and callosities. Heloma (corn) and hyperkeratotic lesions are caused by excessive pressure and are frequently secondary to badly fitting shoes, forefoot dysfunction and deformity of the toes. Hallux valgus has been found in 24% of people over 65 years old (6% in men, 35% in women), and lesser toe deformities in 70% of those over 65 years (Clark 1969). This figure for deformity of the lesser toes may well be low, as a hallux valgus angle of greater than 16° will in many cases impair the function of the adjacent toes. A compromised function of these toes, together with the deformity of the first metatarsal segment, will in most cases lead to pressure lesions under the central metatarsal area and give rise to metatarsalgia.

The expertise and scope of practice of the state registered chiropodist is today far wider than is generally understood. This presents real difficulties for other members of the health team concerned with foot care, who are uncertain whether or not to refer a problem to a chiropodist. As Kemp and Winkler (1983) state, 'The relationship of chiropody to the other foot care services remains ill-defined and hence the allocation of patients between them haphazard'. They tabulate a foot care spectrum (Fig. 9.1) which gives some indication of the scope of practice of chiropody.

The variable degree of debility of elderly people makes some surgical chiropodial procedures inappropriate. Chiropodists are trained to a high level of proficiency to recognize and evaluate the state of a patient's general health and the factors which would contraindicate the administration of local

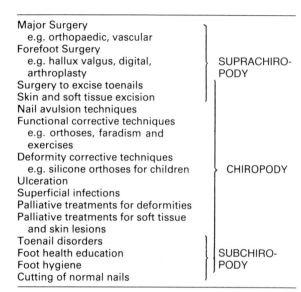

Major Surgery
  e.g. orthopaedic, vascular
Forefoot Surgery
  e.g. hallux valgus, digital,
    arthroplasty
Surgery to excise toenails
Skin and soft tissue excision
	SUPRACHIRO-
	PODY

Nail avulsion techniques
Functional corrective techniques
  e.g. orthoses, faradism and
    exercises
Deformity corrective techniques
  e.g. silicone orthoses for children
Ulceration
Superficial infections
Palliative treatments for deformities
Palliative treatments for soft tissue
  and skin lesions
	CHIROPODY

Toenail disorders Foot health education Foot hygiene Cutting of normal nails	SUBCHIRO- PODY

Fig. 9.1 The foot care spectrum. *Source: Kemp and Winkler (1983).*

analgesics and various topical drugs. Most elderly patients want to be free of discomfort and pain and are intolerant of radical therapies. As a result, much of the chiropodial treatment of the foot problems of elderly patients is of a palliative nature and is concerned with the lower half of the spectrum of treatments shown in Figure 9.1.

ULCERATION, CORN AND CALLUS

The aetiology of foot ulceration in elderly people is usually multi-factorial. Infection of skin abrasions frequently leads to intractable ulcerative lesions which require systemic antibiotic therapy because of compromised vasculature in the lower limb. A major factor, the importance of which is often underestimated, is trauma. Wall (1978) applies to the pathogenesis of foot ulceration the work of Barton (1977), which stresses the effects of pressure on the microcirculation. The pressure from ill-fitting shoes and from mattresses is an easily recognized problem. Less recognition has been given to skeletal deformity of the foot which can result in localized concentrations of pressure from footwear or from normal weight-bearing when standing or walking (Chodera & Cterceteko

1979, Snowden 1979), and ulceration associated with hyperkeratotic lesions results. Many of these ulcerations become secondarily infected (Hobday & Swallow 1973).

If an evaluation of the prognosis requires referral, then good teamwork is essential. A patient may well require systemic antibiotics, pathology and radiography examination or consultation with orthopaedic, diabetic or rheumatology specialists. Having made this assessment, the chiropodist will treat the ulceration by debridement of hyperkeratosis and necrotic tissue and with application of polyurethane sponge padding to dissipate high gradients of pressure which fall onto the lesion. Materials of higher density, or a combination of materials, may also be used.

Pressure ulcers on the foot differ from other pressure sores in several ways, the most important being their association with hyperkeratotic growth and their predilection to macerate because of the enclosed environment of hosiery and footwear. Because of these factors, together with the problems of reducing trauma to the ulcer, many of the topical drugs and applications used for gravitational ulcers and pressure sores prove disappointing. Most chiropodists will remove the overlying and surrounding hyperkeratotic tissue because it is a contaminant and so that evaluation of the state of the ulcer can be more accurately made. The calloused mass frequently becomes macerated with exudate and necrosis. The sedentary oedematous limb presents particular problems with maceration of such lesions.

Of particular importance in the treatment of plantar ulceration is the redistribution of pressure away from the ulcer site. Chodera and Cterceteko (1979), studying diabetic patients with and without peripheral nerve pathology, showed that an ulcer is always found at the site of localized maximum pressure with a steep pressure gradient. There is always a structural deformity and usually some loss of muscle function to the toes.

Padding such lesions, whether by application directly to the foot or in the form of an insole, is a major aspect of chiropodial treatment and is also used in the treatment of corn and callus. Figure 9.2 shows a foot with a moderately severe pressure lesion beneath the second metatarsophalangeal

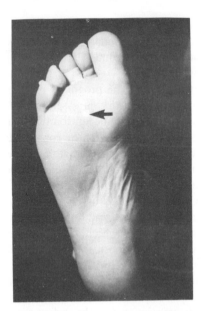

Fig. 9.2 Moderately severe heloma (arrowed) beneath the second metatarsal head.

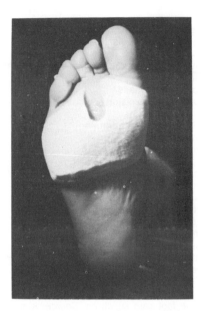

Fig. 9.4 The same foot with a felt protective pad.

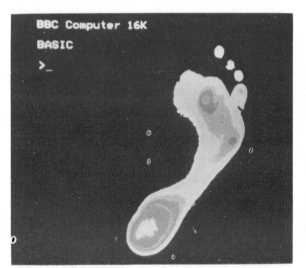

Fig. 9.3 Pedobarograph picture of the foot in Fig. 9.2.

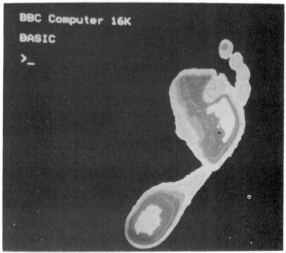

Fig. 9.5 Pedobarograph picture showing a reduction of pressure on the second metatarsal head area.

joint area. Figure 9.3 is a pedobarograph picture of the same foot in a static position showing that the calloused area has a high level of pressure and that there is a steep gradient of pressure. Figure 9.4 shows the foot after the hyperkeratotic mass has been removed and a felt pad has been applied to the forefoot to protect the area when weight bearing. Figure 9.5 is a pedobarograph picture which demonstrates the effectiveness of such a pad in deviating pressure away from the lesion.

SUPERFICIAL INFECTIONS

Plantar or digital warts are often asymptomatic on

the feet of elderly people and might be unnecessary to treat. They can be painful if periungual, and respond well over a period to applications of a mild caustic.

Pyogenic infections are usually associated with trauma which breaks the integument, so allowing opportunistic infection (Hobday & Swallow 1973). Serious infections with coagulase-positive staphylococci and haemolytic streptococci frequently develop cellulitis and lymphatic involvement and osteomyelitis of phalanges and metatarsals. The chiropodist visiting the elderly housebound patient is often the first to see such cases and will initiate medical supervision. Minor infections and septic paronychia are routinely treated topically and rarely give cause for concern, except for the severely debilitated and immunocompromised patient. The chiropodist frequently identifies maturity-onset diabetes or established diabetics who are not stabilized through treating such infections. Chiropody treatment is frequently incriminated in causing foot infections and subsequent gangrene (Gaunt et al 1984). State registered chiropodists who receive a three-year full-time course of training are very aware of these problems. Care must be taken to refer patients to practitioners who are state registered.

FOOT DEFORMITY

Pronation of the foot at the subtaloid joint complex resulting in a variable degree of valgus foot is most commonly the result of compensation for abnormality of the lower limbs or the result of rheumatic disease. In the young, biomechanical examination and treatment is of great benefit for this condition but, for elderly people, palliative relief of symptoms is often the most appropriate. There is a positive correlation between valgus foot and the incidence of hallux valgus with all the secondary forefoot problems associated with this. Soft protective insoles with adequate footwear, toes protected from trauma and debridement of corns and calluses give relief from pain and prevent ulceration of traumatized areas. Wright and Haslock (1977) found that 49% of their sample of rheumatic sufferers required chiropody. Many rheumatic diseases affect the feet in the early

stages. The elderly rheumatic patient is therefore likely to present with severe foot deformity and the above treatment regime is essential for the management of these cases. This treatment is particularly appropriate for people with rheumatoid arthritis but is also helpful for diabetics and other groups with microangiopathy and peripheral neuropathy.

Pes cavus, talipes conditions and other deformities of neurological origin will produce areas on the foot with very concentrated pressure lesions. Orthoses or pads designed to divert weight bearing or shoe pressure away from these lesions may be fitted for pain-free walking to take place.

Hallux valgus, hallux rigidus, dorsally dislocated lesser toes, hammer toes and clawed toes all present problems of disturbed forefoot function and adequate accommodation in footwear. Chiropodial orthoses for individual toes or multiple deformities prove useful for long-term management provided the patient can reach her feet. Otherwise protective dressings can be applied to the toes but these are of limited use. Digital or forefoot amputees may be fitted with either a prosthesis which fits to the foot or is incorporated into an insole to sit inside the shoe.

SOFT TISSUE CONDITIONS

The most prevalent soft tissue conditions encountered by elderly people are bursitis, chilblains and the degenerative effects of atrophic changes with vascular impairment.

An inflamed bursa may occur in the foot over any prominent bony deformity but is most frequently associated with the medial aspect of hallux valgus. Treatment is aimed at the alleviation of initiating mechanical stresses and the prevention of ulceration, sinus formation and sepsis. The danger is for penetration to occur into the joint space where the prognosis, with sepsis, almost always requires referral for orthopaedic procedures. Most uncomplicated cases of bursitis respond well to conservative measures.

The treatment of chilblains and the effects of cold and draughts on the feet of elderly people rely largely on prophylaxis. Thermo-insulating insoles issued in the autumn, together with advice on suitable hosiery and footwear are relatively simple preventive measures. However, patients who annually develop extensive or ulcerative chilblains should receive advice on diet and help with their living accommodation. Topical applications of rubefacients and other proprietory creams may give ephemeral relief of symptoms but are of unproven prophylactic use.

Most elderly chiropody patients exhibit degenerative changes of the soft tissues of the foot and lower limb. The ageing process and atrophic changes lead to fragility and loss of elastic properties of the skin and diminished adiposity of the superficial fascia. This loss and modification of the soft tissue under the principal weight-bearing areas of the foot, the heel and metatarsal heads, may lead to inflammatory conditions or pressure lesions. It is often important to compensate for this thinness of the feet by recommending microcellular rubber-soled footwear and/or soft cushioning insoles.

Plantar fasciitis, tenosynovitis, strains and sprains are less frequent local conditions seen by chiropodists working with the elderly. Interdigital maceration of the toe webs is more common, especially in neglected cases, and also poor hygiene and leg oedema.

TOENAILS

The management of normal nails of old people should present no problem for friends, relatives, health care personnel, or the patients themselves to cope with, provided the general state of the patient's feet is considered and simple guidelines are followed. Normal nails will not be painful to touch, will not be excessively brittle, thickened, friable, discoloured or dystrophic (structurally affected by changes to digital blood supply). The lateral margins of the nail plate will be free of each sulcus and the transverse and longitudinal curvature will not be exaggerated.

After cleansing, three or four separate cuts using toenail nippers should be used rather than attempting to cut in one. A cut from each corner towards the middle should be made first and then the residue trimmed straight across the free edge of the nail plate. Nails should not be cut too short.

A common fault in nail cutting is to cut towards the sulci, leaving a rough spike within the sulcus. This penetrates the skin causing onychocryptosis, that is, an ingrown toenail where the nail has penetrated the soft tissue of the nail sulcus. In the debilitated person this can lead to a serious infection. After cutting, any roughness at the free edge should be filed smooth using a nail-file or emery board to prevent inadvertent excoriation of the skin of the leg or adjacent foot whilst the patient is in bed.

Pathological nails require the attention of a chiropodist. Onychogryphosis and onychomycosis (fungal infection of the nail plate) are probably the most frequent local conditions which cause difficulty with cutting nails. A chiropodist will reduce the thickness of these nails by using a nail drill, which is a skilled exercise (Figs. 9.6 and 9.7). In

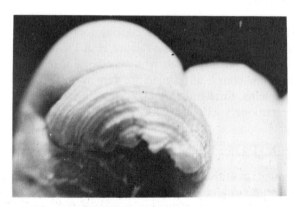

Fig. 9.6 Onychogryphosis before chiropody treatment.

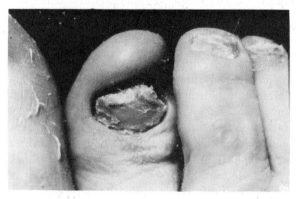

Fig. 9.7 Onychogryphosis after treatment.

cases of neglect, gryphotic nails may attain such length as to curve under or over the toes preventing walking and frequently leading to ulceration. If traumatized, subungual ulceration or paronychia may result if onychogryphosis is not treated.

Partial or total nail avulsion techniques (sterilization of the nail matrix) for onychocryptosis have a high success rate with the younger patient but are not often appropriate for elderly people, and conservative management is most often employed. The excision of the penetrating nail spike must be achieved before resolution occurs.

Arterial impairment and vasospastic disorders cause dystrophic thinning and sometimes absence of the nail plate. Residual slow nail growth and periungual roughness should be reduced with an emery board rather than nippers or scissors and an emollient cream applied.

FOOT CARE ADVICE

Much of the foot care advice needed by elderly people is fundamental and commonsensical but enquiry by patients is rarely made until signs and symptoms are present. This can be well into adult life, if not old age. Swallow (1976), writing about the problems that diabetics have with their feet, gives extremely good advice, much of which is relevant to old people in general. They should be encouraged to wash their feet daily, or on alternate days, in warm water (40–45°C), but not to soak them, which causes excessive dryness. The feet should be dried using a soft towel with particular attention given to the interdigital spaces but without forcing the toes apart. If feet are moist or hyperhidrotic (affected by excessive sweating) then a spirit-based swab followed by a light dusting of talc should be recommended. If the feet are dry, the patient should use a hand cream or emulsifying ointment, but not between the toes if moist.

This routine hygiene can present a problem for many elderly housebound patients because of disability. The help of members of the household or friends and relatives should be sought to carry this out. Certainly, debilitated patients should

inspect their feet or have them checked weekly for abrasions, blisters, colour changes, swelling or any suppurative lesion, especially if they have loss of sensation in the feet or lower limb.

Any open wound should be covered with a sterile dressing, and if healing is delayed or infection ensues then it must be brought to the attention of the health care team. Housebound patients should have a telephone number or address readily available and the reticent person should be actively encouraged to seek medical help.

Burns on the feet of elderly people with sensation loss are common and often lead to intractible ulceration. Hot-water bottles should be discouraged unless used only to warm the bed before retiring and bath water should not be too hot. Accidental scalding of the feet is not uncommon. A relatively large number of old people have erythema ab igne of the legs and feet. This is a brown-red reticular patterned discolouration owing to exposure to heat. These patients should be advised to use a rug or blanket over their legs to prevent burning when sitting by a fire.

Socks and stockings should be loose-fitting to avoid restriction to the superficial circulation, particularly over the toes and heels. Garters should never be used. Patients should not walk about the house barefooted in case of injury, and many styles of bedroom slippers are unsuitable to wear for long periods of time or for anything but short walks around the house. Slippers are usually a poor fit to the foot and constrict the toes if too short and narrow or traumatize the toes when walking if too large. If carpet slippers are the footwear of choice they should be of a style which extends high up the dorsum of the foot with some form of fastening.

Patients will often purchase or be given proprietary products to ease painful feet. It is important to advise patients not to use corn plasters containing caustic medicaments, some solutions advertized to cure ingrown toenails and devices for cutting corns and callosities. Some of these products may be harmless but others contain strong keratolytics which may cause ulceration and lead to infection. Corn planes and other sharp instruments should not be used because of the danger of injury.

THE CHIROPODY SERVICE

The aims of the community and hospital chiropody service are to promote pain-free healthy feet and maintain the mobility of the disabled and elderly population; to evaluate the effects of local and systemic disorders; to educate the patient in foot health, and to liaise with members of the health care team for overall patient management.

An efficient and successful foot care service for elderly people relies on a multidisciplinary approach involving surgeons, doctors, nurses, physiotherapists, chiropodists, other paramedicals, voluntary bodies, friends and relatives. Co-ordination of personnel to respond to the needs of elderly people usually operates through the patient's general medical practitioner. State registered chiropodists employed within the National Health Service are in extremely short supply. The number of state registered chiropodists in the UK is only about 6000, and only about half this number work for the NHS (Kemp 1988). The chiropody service is inadequate to meet the demand for treatment of the priority groups (Department of Health and Social Security 1979). The *Survey of Manpower Resources in the NHS Chiropody Service* (Association of Chief Chiropody Officers 1980) revealed that in order to give an adequate service more than double the number of practitioners is needed. The ACCO calculation is an underestimate of manpower shortage since it did not take account of the true prevalence of foot problems of the elderly. The adequacy of the chiropody service for old people varies according to residence. Wade et al (1983) reported that 75% of residents in private nursing Homes found the service adequate, compared with 63% of old people living at home, 38% in hospital and 36% in local authority residential Homes.

It is impossible for the chiropody service to achieve its aims and potential and play a full part in the foot care team. Nurses are in a particularly good position to help old people with general foot care, whether they are in hospitals, residential Homes or at home. Whilst it is recognized that hospital and community based nurses have a heavy workload, it would be an easy, efficient and inexpensive exercise to organize training programmes for nurses. Nurses have good opportunities to gain insight into the elderly patient's circumstances and problems and could deal with hygiene and the cutting of normal nails, footwear advice and the recognition of serious lower limb conditions which require medical attention. This would free the chiropodist to utilize his or her time more effectively and ensure that more elderly people receive chiropodial foot care. It would also keep more old people mobile, independent and at home.

Information sources

The following organizations are useful sources of information and educational leaflets and materials.

- Association of Chief Chiropody Officers, 3 New Road, Aston Clinton, Aylesbury, Bucks HP22 5JD.
- Chiropodists Board, The Registrar, Council for Professions Supplementary to Medicine, 184 Kennington Park Road, London SE11.
- Disabled Living Foundation, 380 Harrow Road, London W9
- Health Education Authority, Mabledon Place, London WC1
- Shoe and Allied Trades Research Association, Rockingham Road, Kettering, Northants NN16 9JH.
- Society of Chiropodists, 53 Welbeck Street, London W1M 7HE.
- Society of Shoe Fitters, 19 Woodgreen, Calmore, Southampton S04.

REFERENCES

Agate J 1963 The practice of geriatrics. Heinemann, London
Association of Chief Chiropody Officers 1980 Survey of manpower resources in the NHS chiropody service. ACCO, Aylesbury, Bucks
Barton A A 1977 Prevention of pressure sores. Nursing Times 41: 1593–95
Cartwright A, Henderson G 1987 More trouble with feet. HMSO, London
Chodera J D, Cterceteko G 1979 The application of the Pedobarogram in patients with diabetic neuropathic ulcers. A preliminary report, Biomedical Research and

Development Unit, Bioengineering Centre, Roehampton, London

Clark M 1969 Trouble with feet. Occasional Papers on Social Administration, no 29 G Bell, London

Collyer M I 1981 Maintaining the elderly patient's mobility. Geriatric Medicine 11(12): 27–30

Department of Health and Social Security 1979 staffing of the National Health Service (England): an analysis of the demand and supply position in the major staff groups. DHSS, London

Ebrahim S B J, Sainsbury R, Watson S 1981 Foot problems of the elderly: a hospital survey. British Medical Journal 283: 949–950

Gaunt N, Rogers K, Seal D, Denham M, Lewis J 1984 Necrotising fasciitis due to group C and G haemolytic streptococcus after chiropody. Lancet 1: 516

Helfand A E 1966 Foot impairment — an etiologic factor in falls in the aged. Journal of the American Podiatry Association 56: 326–330

Hobday M C, Swallow A W 1973 A pilot survey to investigate the incidence of bacterial types isolated from ulcerative lesions found on the feet of chiropody patients. Chiropodist 28: 260–266

Hobson W, Pemberton J 1955 The health of the elderly at home. Butterworth, London

Kemp J 1988 Feet and footwear of older people. In: Squires A J (ed) Rehabilitation of the older patient. Croom Helm, London

Kemp J, Winkler J T 1983 Problems afoot: need and efficiency in footcare. Disabled Living Foundation, London

Salvage A V, Vetter N J, Jones D A 1988 Attitudes of the over 75s to NHS chiropody services. The Chiropodist 43: 103–105

Snowdon C 1979 Pressure sores and patient support systems. Biomedical Research and Development Unit, Bioengineering Centre, Rochampton, London

Suvarna R R 1981 In: Neale D (ed) Common foot disorders: diagnosis and management. Churchill Livingstone, Edinburgh

Swallow A W 1976 Chiropody for the diabetic foot. British Journal of Hospital Medicine 23: 235–238

Townsend P, Wedderburn D 1965 The aged in the welfare state. G Bell, London

Wade B, Sawyer L, Bell J 1983 Dependency with dignity: different care provision for the elderly. Occasional Papers on Social Administration no 68. Bedford Square Press, London

Wall B 1978 The pathology of pressure sores and factors which influence their healing. Chiropodist 33: 442–445

Williamson J, Stokoe I H, Gray S et al 1964 Old people at home: their unreported needs. Lancet i: 1120–70

Wright V, Haslock I 1977 Rheumatism for nurses and remedial therapists. Heinemann, London

CHAPTER CONTENTS

Normal ageing of the respiratory system 158
Implications of physiological changes 158

Pathological, environmental and lifestyle factors 158
Protection of vulnerable individuals 159
Acute and chronic respiratory problems 159

Nursing implications 159
Maintaining sufficient intake of air 164
Maintaining sufficient intakes of food and water 167
Provision of care associated with elimination processes 167
Maintaining a balance between rest and activity 168
Maintaining a balance between solitude and social interaction 168
The promotion of normalcy 168

Conclusion 169

10

Breathing

Christine M. Hanks

Oxygen is required at a cellular level to produce sufficient energy for an organism to function. Carbon dioxide is produced as a by-product. Oxygen is made available to all the cells of the body and carbon dioxide is removed by an elegant transport system, which begins when atmospheric oxygen is drawn into the lungs via the respiratory tract and brought into contact with the alveolar membrane. The surface area of this membrane (which allows exchange of gases) has been estimated to be roughly the size of a badminton court, but is folded in such a way that it fits neatly into the thoracic cavity. The air on the pulmonary side of the membrane is separated from the capillary blood by only 0.2 mm. It is across this tiny divide that oxygen diffuses into the blood and carbon dioxide diffuses into the alveolar air.

Just as the pulmonary capillary network ensures swift and efficient gas exchange, a similar network exists in all body tissues to bring about the whole function of the respiratory system: that is, to provide oxygen for, and to remove carbon dioxide from, the cells of the body.

The mechanism by which atmospheric gases are delivered to the alveolar membrane and alveolar gases are expelled is termed ventilation. Ventilation is effected by the action of the muscles of the thorax, and controlled by the respiratory centre in the brain stem via the phrenic and intercostal nerves. The respiratory centre is, in turn, stimulated mainly by raised levels of arterial carbon dioxide and also by lowered levels of arterial oxygen (see Guyton 1986, or any general physiology text, for a more detailed discussion). Breathing is not normally under conscious control, although it can be stopped for a few seconds at will; breathing is modified unconsciously during eating, drinking, talking and exercise.

NORMAL AGEING OF THE RESPIRATORY SYSTEM

It has been difficult to assess physiological ageing processes of the respiratory system, since few aged lungs will be free of some pathological or environmental insult. Changes found in the 'normal' lung have, however, been described (e.g. by Brandstetter & Kazemi 1983).

In old age, there is a loss of the protein elastin and therefore of the elasticity which maintains the patency of the small airways. The loss results in the underventilation of many alveoli, except during deep breathing, with a resultant mismatch between the parts of the lung that are ventilated and the parts of the lung that are well perfused with blood, particularly at the bases of the lungs. Brandstetter and Kazemi (1983) note that the loss in elasticity is demonstrated by the fact that the prompt collapse of the lung at autopsy may no longer be exhibited, retractibility is sluggish and deflation is incomplete; alveolar dilation, which also occurs, is a common finding in senescence: the so-called 'senile emphysema' (Cander & Moyer 1964).

Changes also occur in the composition of the protein collagen. Crosslinks form between the subunits of the collagen resulting in increased rigidity, which is thought to be at least partly responsible for the alterations of mechanical properties of the lung, as described in Table 10.1.

There is a loss of muscle tone and strength in the diaphragm, intercostal muscles and accessory muscles; together with a decrease in sensitivity of the upper respiratory tract, this leads to a less responsive and effective cough reflex. Some cilia are lost and those which remain have a reduced efficiency; epithelial mucus production is increased and macrophages become less efficient. The above changes, then, conspire to impair the protective mechanisms of the respiratory system.

Table 10.1 Alteration of pulmonary function with age. *Source: Brandstetter and Kazemi (1983).*

Vital capacity	Decreases
Forced expiratory volume in 1 second	Decreases
Lung recoil pressure	Decreases
Closing volume	Increases
Functional residual capacity	Increases
Residual volume	Increases
Total lung capacity	Remains same
Diffusing capacity	Decreases
Arterial oxygen tension	Decreases
Arterial carbon dioxide tension	Remains same

General musculoskeletal changes of ageing also affect the respiratory system, so that osteoporosis of the ribcage and vertebrae can result in kyphosis, which can be observed in the generally stooped posture of some elderly individuals. Kyphosis will compromise respiratory movements and thus reduce the extent of lung inflation.

IMPLICATIONS OF PHYSIOLOGICAL CHANGES

The respiratory system of the young adult can respond to a challenge (for example, heavy exercise or an infection) by using compensatory mechanisms (e.g. increasing respiratory depth and rate; strong cough reflex), but where changes due to age have occurred that option is reduced. It is for this reason that elderly people are more susceptible to the adverse effects of pathological processes and adverse environmental conditions.

PATHOLOGICAL, ENVIRONMENTAL AND LIFESTYLE FACTORS

Environmental conditions, both at home and at work, past and present, will affect the respiratory status of the individual. The elderly person has had a longer period of time in which to succumb to unfavourable environmental conditions; in addition, some may have been exposed, without protection, to conditions which are not tolerated today, such as asbestos dust or mustard gas. A cold, damp home environment will reduce resistance to infection, thus predisposing the occupant to bronchitis and tuberculosis. A diet deficient in nutrients will have a similar effect; iron-deficiency anaemia will result in a reduction of the oxygen-carrying capacity of the blood, which, if severe, will cause further embarrassment of the respiratory system.

Although a life of healthy practices gives the best chance of healthy later years, the majority who reach old age do so without this ideal situation. It is never too late, even for elderly people, to benefit from non-smoking and regular exercise. Cigarette smoke is the chief initiating and potentiating agent in the development of chronic obstructive airways disease (Caird & Akhtar 1972). It stimulates mucous glands to hypertrophy, and predisposes the smoker to infection by reducing the number and efficiency of the epithelial cilia. Tobacco smoke has recently been shown to play a major role in the development of emphysema, which is now considered to be due to an imbalance between protease and antiprotease mechanisms in the lung. Excess protease activity damages and dissolves alveolar walls and small airways. Cigarette smoke induces the proliferation of alveolar macrophages, which contain proteases. On the death of the macrophages, the proteases are released exceed the neutralizing capacity of the antiprotease system (Howard 1987). Cigarette smoke is also carcinogenic.

Regardless of the now incontrovertible evidence for the adverse effects of smoking cigarettes, consideration should be given to the individual who cannot or does not wish to stop smoking. The habit was begun when it was not only acceptable to smoke, but considered chic and sophisticated.

Weak ventilatory muscles are thought to contribute to lowered maximal ventilatory volumes, and, since it appears to be inactivity which plays a major part in causing the muscle weakness and lack of stamina commonly found among the old, then a programme to improve the mobility and activity of elderly people would be beneficial to this group.

PROTECTION OF VULNERABLE INDIVIDUALS

Old people can be protected from influenza by vaccination, which confers a substantial degree of protection when the vaccine used corresponds with the antigenic structure of the virus (Barker & Mullooly 1980). Frail elderly people may be protected from cross-infection by restricting contact with infected individuals, be they carers or friends. A balance must be made, however, between protection and isolation. If the patient/client is made aware of the dangers of cross-infection, and yet chooses to continue the contact, her point of view should be respected. With clear explanation to both the patient and the visitor, however, separation for a period may be tolerated more easily.

Nurses in the community are ideally placed to note poor environmental conditions and to assist the client in obtaining the help and advice needed to improve their circumstances.

ACUTE AND CHRONIC RESPIRATORY PROBLEMS

Chronic respiratory problems develop throughout life and are often associated with smoking and/or environmental factors. The disabling effects tend to increase with age, leaving some individuals housebound. Chronic obstructive airways disease (COAD) is the term used to encompass conditions such as chronic bronchitis, emphysema and asthma. Chronic bronchitis is defined clinically as the presence of a cough and sputum produced most days of the week for a minimum of three months of the year and for at least two successive years. Patients with chronic asthma have the major symptom of breathlessness, rather than cough or sputum. Patients with emphysema have abnormal enlargement of the air-spaces distal to the terminal bronchioles, accompanied by destruction of the alveolar walls. Acute respiratory problems such as influenza are seen at any age; however, in elderly people, this may be complicated by COAD, or simply by the changes we have identified as being associated with ageing.

NURSING IMPLICATIONS

The aim of all care is to preserve independence for as

Table 10.2 A care plan for a widowed 75-year-old woman with an acute chest infection and chronic obstructive airways disease.

Assessment of the patient may be initially somewhat cursory, prior to initiating urgent medical therapy. It will, however, include the monitoring of vital signs:

Colour and state of skin
Quality and rate of respirations
Pulse rate
Blood pressure.

Vital social information can be obtained from the patient or significant others.

		Agency		
Requisite	Demand	Knowledge	Motivation	Skill
Universal Maintenance of oxygenation	Increase level of oxygenation	Knows which positions allow easiest breathing Knows that oxygen will help her feel better	Desperately wants to be able to breathe more easily Wants to use oxygen	Weak and unable to position herself well. Can use equipment when in reach
	Reduce amounts of mucus present	Knows the importance of expectoration	Feels a little embarrassed to expectorate in the ward	Presently finds expectoration tiring
	Reduce the viscosity of mucus	Does not know that keeping well hydrated will help expectoration	Finds water distasteful	Can drink without help provided that she is well positioned, and the drink is within reach
Therapeutic Administration of medication	Administer antibiotics prescribed by the physician	Patient knows why the antibiotics have been prescribed; how and when they should be taken	Patient wants to comply with the physician's instructions	Has ability to self-administer but too weary to remember at present
	Increase bronchodilation	Does not know how to use the nebuliser	Patient wants to comply with the physician's instructions	Can use mask when it is prepared
Maintenance of oxygenation	Reduce oxygen demand	The patient knows that increased activity increases breathlessness	Wants to reduce her breathlessness	She is able to modify her activities
		She has noticed that anxiety also increases her breathlessness		She finds relaxation difficult

Table 10.2 (continued)

Early in the admission, further relevant information can be obtained and at this time an effective relationship can be entered into with the patient and her family (or significant others). The nurse can take this opportunity to 'determine the existing and projected self-care requisites, their particular values, and expected changes in their values' (Orem 1985, p 227)

Self-care deficit	Nursing system	Methods of assistance
Needs help with positioning and maintaining optimum position. Needs oxygen and humidification unit to be provided and regulated	Partially compensatory	The nurse will assist in positioning to provide optimum chest expansion using pillows Nurse will provide and regulate humidified oxygen, and remind patient of dangers of occluding vent holes in the mask. Nurse will monitor the patient's use of oxygen mask
Requires reassurance that it is OK to expectorate	Educative/supportive Partially compensatory Requires sputum pot and tissues	Discuss, encourage and teach deep breathing exercises and effective expectoration Provide sputum pot and tissues Enlist help of physiotherapist
Patient needs provision of fluids, to know why this is important, and motivation to drink	Partially compensatory Educative/supportive	Explain to the patient why hydration is important: agree type and amount of fluids to be taken in 24 hours. Discuss with patient and carers the variety of drinks she can provide
Needs presentation of medication in correct dose, at correct time	Partially compensatory	The nurse will administer the medication as appropriate and monitor its effect and any side-effects. She will complete the appropriate records
As above, but to be administered by nebuliser		As above. The nurse will also explain the functioning of the nebuliser to the patient
Requires recognition of decrease in mobility and help with activities aimed at reducing the effects of immobility	Supportive Partially compensatory	The nurse will assist the patient in all physical activities in order to reduce her energy expenditure
Patient requires information on relaxation techniques She needs protection from situations which provoke unnecessary anxiety	Educative/Supportive	Discuss ways of enabling relaxation. Identify situations which the patient finds stressful and explore ways of minimising these Ensure effectiveness of above measures by: Monitoring- Patient's arousal level and ability to attend Patient's skin colour (pallor or cyanosis), skin temperature, presence of perspiration. Patient's respiratory rate, depth and quality Presence of breathlessness, cough, wheeze or pain on breathing Temperature, pulse rate and blood pressure

Table 10.2 (continued)

	Agency	Agency		
Requisite	Demand	Knowledge	Motivation	Skill
Universal Maintenance of sufficient intake of food and water		Patient is aware of need for good nutrition	Eating causes breathlessness and nausea	Activity of eating causes weariness
The provision of care associated with elimination processes and excrements	Provision of facilities in view of immobility	Patient is aware of needs for regular elimination	Patient is motivated to ensure regular bowel movements	Patient is able to sit on commode. No ill effects without oxygen for trip to toilet. Tired after act
	Provision to prevent possible constipation	Knowledge needs updating	As above	Sometimes so weary that cannot make an effort to defaecate
Therapeutic requisite Risk of heart failure and/or renal hypoxia	Monitor urinary output in view of risk	No knowledge of these risks		
Universal Maintenance of balance between rest and activity	Reduction of anxiety/relief of boredom	Patient knows she feels anxious at times	Wants to reduce her	Not skilled in relaxation techniques
	Gradual increase in activity	Knows she must increase mobility eventually	Does not feel much like activity at present and does not want to think about it	Presently, any movement tiring
Maintenance of balance between solitude and social interaction		Has knowledge of her own feelings	Motivated to optimize balance	Has ability to express feelings when allowed so
Universal/ developmental Promotion of normalcy	Increase self-esteem	Has little insight	Not convinced she can improve the way she feels	Limited at present due to immobility

Table 10.2 (continued)

Self-care deficit	Nursing system	Methods of assistance
Requires help in planning strategies aimed at reducing breathlessness nausea and tiredness	Educative/supportive Partially compensatory	1. Activities in preceding section should begin to improve the situation 2. Allow a period of rest before meals 3. Offer a mouth-wash before meals 4. Present small meals and do not rush the patient 5. Discuss with patient and carer the provision of preferred snacks 6. Monitor amounts and types of food eaten
1. Requires provision of commode 2. Help with transferring to commode 3. Move to toilet	Partially compensatory	1. Provide buzzer within easy reach 2. Answer buzzer quickly 3. Ensure warmth and modesty on transfer to commode 4. Ensure buzzer within reach in toilet 5. Help with cleaning after evacuation 6. Monitor bowel movements and record if patient has difficulty in remembering
		1. Rest before usual time for defaecation 2. Prevent dehydration 3. Encourage high fibre diet 4. Adminster aperients if required 5. Help with mobilization when possible
Nurse required to measure and record urine output	Wholly compensatory	1. Measure and record urine output 2. Evaluate 8-hourly 3. Inform physician of oliguria or gradual positive fluid balance
Requires enablement to discuss anxieties	Educative/supportive	Identify with patient anxieties; explore ways of alleviating or coping with them. Suggest use of relaxation techniques and teach if patient is interested
Help required in planning gradually increasing activity	Educative/supportive	Draw plan of gradually increasing activity with help of patient and significant others. Monitor activity levels and record. Re-evaluate plan regularly to ensure realistic goals and compensate for relapse in expected progress
Needs to be enabled to express herself	Educative/supportive	Nurse will allow time for the patient to feel comfortable and allow her to discuss her fears and explore possible ways of dealing with these
Requires encouragement and support for her self-care	Educative/supportive	The nurse will foster a positive but realistic attitude in the patient, focusing on what she can do and on expected improvements.

long as possible and to this end nurses must learn the most basic skill of all, that of knowing when to do, and when to forbear. (Brysson Whyte 1988, p. 7)

It is with these thoughts in mind that aspects of Orem's (1985) self-care model of nursing will be used to outline the management of an elderly person with breathing difficulties. According to Orem, a person is a 'functional, integrated whole with an overall motivation to achieve self-care'. Orem sees nursing intervention as necessary when the individual (or his/her significant others) is unable to achieve and maintain a balance between self-care abilities and the current demands of self-care. These current demands are made up of three aspects:

1 Universal self-care requisites, i.e. the needs of any healthy individual, identified by Orem as

   a) The maintenance of a sufficient intake of air

   b) The maintenance of a sufficient intake of water

   c) The maintenance of a sufficient intake of food

   d) The provision of care associated with elimination processes and excrements

   e) The maintenance of a balance between activity and rest

   f) The maintenance of a balance between solitude and social interaction

   g) The prevention of hazards to human life, human functioning, and human well-being

   h) The promotion of human functioning and development within social groups in accord with human potential, known human limitations, and the human desire to be normal.

2 Developmental self-care requisites, i.e. those associated with human developmental processes; conditions occurring during the life cycle; and events adversely affecting development.

3 Health deviation self-care demands. These are those demands made by virtue of the disease or illness of the patient. This may be a need for a wound to be dressed, or medication to be taken.

When there is a mis-match or 'deficit relationship' between the client's capabilities and requirements, then it is the role of the nurse to help the client make up the 'deficit'. In order to do this both parties (nurse and patient/significant others) must identify the same problems and agree on the action required. The relationship between the two, therefore, is contractual in nature, and implies an equality in the relationship. This focus may, to some extent, combat the ageist attitudes held by many people, including health care professionals, that can cause them to fail to promote a positive outlook in old age (see Ch. 31 for further discussion on ageism).

In the following consideration of the health-care needs of an elderly patient with breathing problems, the first six of the self-care requisites will be used; prevention of hazards and promotion of normalcy will be related to each in turn. Developmental self-care requisites and health deviation self-care requisites will be considered at the same time where appropriate.

A care plan has been devised in the form of a table (Table 10.2).

MAINTAINING SUFFICIENT INTAKE OF AIR

The patient may have a problem taking in that quantity of air required for normal functioning. This fact may be determined by observation of, and communication with, the patient. Nursing assessment will make use of the observations made on the patient, and communications with the patient (or significant others). Information about previous episodes of respiratory difficulty, history of smoking (observation of nicotine staining will also give an indication), cough or chest pain, and what has been found to relieve it will help in planning care. An account of normal exercise tolerance should also be sought.

Observations which will be useful are identified in Table 10.2. One particular observation — that of consciousness — will be dealt with in more detail.

If an individual is unable to maintain appropriate arterial oxygen and carbon dioxide levels, she is said to be in respiratory failure. An elderly person with a compromised respiratory system as a baseline, who then undergoes a further assault, such as an acute respiratory tract infection, is at risk of moving into respiratory failure. It is important that the early manifestations of restlessness, dizziness and disorientation are recognized as symptoms of impending respiratory failure, and not accepted as 'senility'.

The problem of clouding of consciousness may be as distressing to family and friends as to the patient herself. The nurse, may be alerted to alteration in conscious level by the patient's relatives, who may notice the subtle changes more quickly than the nurse. In situations where the nurse has worked closely with the patient, the nurse may be first to notice the difference and be able to support the relatives, explaining the changes they see.

Once the assessment has been made, the self-care deficit (termed 'nursing diagnosis' by some authors) can be identified, and nursing action planned. The nursing actions identified in Table 10.2 are discussed here in more detail.

Removal of secretions

The nurse should work with the physiotherapist in teaching the patient how to cough effectively: the patient will be shown how to inspire deeply, pause, and then cough forcibly to expel secretions. If this activity is too exhausting for the patient, then the nurse may suggest deep breathing, with particular attention on long exhalation. This may move secretions sufficiently to stimulate the cough reflex. The patient may also be taught how to breathe through pursed lips, which increases pressure in the respiratory tree during expiration, thus increasing the period during which gas exchange is possible in the alveoli.

Expectoration is seen by most adults (particularly women) as an anti-social activity. The nurse can help by providing disposable sputum pots and tissues, and by encouraging the patient to recognize its necessity.

The patient may be helped to maintain a position conducive to maximum lung expansion. An upright posture, either in bed or in a chair can be maintained by careful positioning of pillows to give support to the back and will allow the thorax, and so the lungs, to fully expand, thereby permitting maximum ventilation. Positioning may be particularly difficult where osteoporosis has

resulted in kyphosis. The patient may find she is best able to manage lung expansion by leaning forward over a cushioned table (the orthopnoeic position).

If this patient has a pyrexia, then she may become dehydrated; this, in turn, will result in making the sputum she produces even more sticky and tenacious. It is important, therefore, that this patient understand the need to maintain her hydration.

Another way to help with the removal of secretions may be by the use of mucolytic drugs which reduce the stickiness of secretions and make them more easily expectorated; however, some authorities suggest that plain water inhalation may be just as effective.

Bronchoconstriction

Bronchoconstriction may be present along with increased secretions, and so, in addition, bronchodilating drugs are administered. These may be given by the oral route, and/or by inhalation. The drug given by inhalation quickly reaches the site of action in the bronchioles, and so because of this useful and direct route, less of the drug is needed for effective action. A common example of this type of drug is salbutamol (Ventolin®) which is a B_2 adrenergic receptor stimulant. Corticosteroids (e.g. prednisolone) are also administered to patients with airways obstruction, for their anti-inflammatory action on the bronchial mucosa. The alleviation of inflammation reduces oedematous swelling, making air entry and exit easier and less noisy. The smallest possible effective dose must be given because elderly people are most susceptible to the distressing side effects such as sodium and water retention, osteoporosis, impaired glucose tolerance and hypokalaemia.

The inhaled drug is often given in hospital via a nebulizer, which is connected in line between an oxygen or air supply and the patient's oxygen mask; or, alternatively, the drug may be presented as a fine dry powder and given via an inhaler. The bronchodilator is taken first, and time is given for it to be effective (about ten minutes), so that when the corticosteroid is inhaled, it is delivered far down into the respiratory tree to the tiny bronchioles, where the anti-inflammatory effect is required.

The nebulizer requires a minimum of co-operation by the patient, but the metered dose inhaler (MDI) needs a degree of co-ordination for effective use. Various studies have shown that up to 89% of patients of all ages are unable to use MDIs correctly, and even after tuition 30% are still unable to co-ordinate their use (Jarrett 1988). The elderly patient with chronic respiratory weakness and poor co-ordination may find them difficult to use. To make this as easy as possible for the patient, time should be taken to teach her exactly how to use the inhaler. The information is best presented in small amounts and repeated; if possible the information should be written down, too, and the nurse should ask the patient to relate the information back to her (in a non-condescending manner) to check that she has understood and remembered. Although this procedure is necessary when giving information to all patients, the elderly individual may have some loss of hearing or sight, or may be reluctant to admit that she did not grasp the information the first time.

Reduction of anxiety

The elderly patient with breathing problems who has been admitted to a busy medical ward will be the focus of social interaction. The activity around her — bustling nurses, porters, doctors, radiographers, phlebotomists — may make her feel anxious and flustered; she may feel powerless and dependent, aware of things being done to her, but almost uninvolved. The anxiety stimulates her sympathetic nervous system and further increases her respiratory rate (tachypnoea) and her heart rate (tachycardia). These, and other manifestations, make the patient more aware of her emotional state and begin a vicious circle. The situation can be made much less stressful if the carers have a calm and restful approach, allowing time for interaction. Breathlessness makes talking difficult, and an oxygen mask may muffle the patient's words. Even listening may be a chore when breathing requires all one's attention. Reassurance that there is plenty of time, and that she is not inconveniencing the carer will help the patient to relax.

The relief afforded by these means may be the nearest that the patient comes to enjoying breathing as a pleasurable experience.

Hazards associated with maintaining sufficient intake of air: oxygen administration

A patient with COAD whose condition is deteriorating may suffer from additional complications as a result of chronic hypoxaemia, which can be alleviated by administering oxygen (Ziment 1982). Normal values for partial pressure of arterial oxygen (PaO_2) and partial pressure of arterial carbon dioxide ($PaCO_2$) are 11.3–13.3 kPa (85–100 mmHg) and 4.8–5.9 kPa (36–44 mmHg) respectively (Oh 1985). However, Wheeler (1980) gives the normal values for a 70-year-old man as PaO_2 80 mmHg and $PaCO_2$ less than 50 mmHg.

A patient with COAD will have developed a tolerance to higher $PaCO_2$ levels, and will have adapted to being stimulated to breathe by low PaO_2 levels. The major hazard for patients with COAD on oxygen therapy, is that an increased PaO_2 may diminish the individual's hypoxic ventilatory drive, thus exacerbating respiratory failure with accompanying increases in $PaCO_2$.

In view of this danger only just enough oxygen should be given to reduce hypoxia without reducing the ventilatory drive. An inspired oxygen percentage (FIO_2) of between 24%–28% is usually the optimum level. This percentage of oxygen can be delivered most accurately to the patient who is spontaneously ventilating through a specially designed face mask (e.g. System 22 with blue (24%) or white (28%) Venturis®).

In addition to ensuring that the correct mask and correct flow rate are set, the nurse should be vigilant in her observations that the patient has not either:

(a) reduced her intake of oxygen by removing her mask, or by wearing it over her mouth only, or

(b) increased her intake of oxygen by occluding the ventilation holes with her hands or bedclothes.

By explaining to the patient why she has been prescribed oxygen and how the mask works, the nurse should aim to achieve maximum patient co-operation.

Oxygen therapy can be made available in the home, and the preferred method is to utilize an oxygen concentrator, which relieves the need for oxygen cylinders.

MAINTAINING SUFFICIENT INTAKES OF FOOD AND WATER

In the acute situation the most pressing problem for the patient will be that she has no time or energy to eat or drink, because all her time and energy is concerned with breathing. In addition to this, hypoxia makes her feel anorexic; and tenacious, foul-tasting sputum will remove any remaining inclination to eat or drink.

In order to help the patient maintain sufficient intake of food and water, the nurse should help her to keep her mouth fresh; this can be achieved by using a soft-bristled toothbrush after meals and encouraging frequent small drinks. The amount of fluids to be taken by the patient should be identified and discussed with her. If fluid intake is to be encouraged, then appropriate fluids should be available, that is, fluids that the patient likes, in a container that she can lift, and in a place that she can reach.

To encourage the patient to attempt eating, the nurse can help by ensuring that the patient is presented with a small amount of preferred food. A large amount of hot food will quickly cool, while the patient slowly chews. Even when the patient improves sufficiently to be able to consume large amounts of food, this is not to be recommended, because abdominal distension will interfere with lung expansion and therefore ventilation; small frequent meals are preferable.

Older people have an increased requirement for protein, some vitamins and calcium (Hanks 1986) and those with infections also have an increased demand for carbohydrates (to meet increased metabolic demands) and protein (to support the immune system).

In some conditions the patient suffers from a non-productive cough, which has not only no protective function, but which exhausts the patient and traumatizes the oropharynx. The patient may find that sipping warm drinks or sucking sweets or lozenges may be soothing.

It is important to emphasize the pleasurable experience of eating and drinking, when difficulty in breathing can make them seem a chore. Eating may be preferred in a social context by some individuals, whereas others may feel constrained by their own physical limitations (or, in some situations, by the socially unacceptable behaviour of their fellow diners). At home, or in homelike accommodation, a glass of wine or sherry before meals may enliven the appetite.

PROVISION OF CARE ASSOCIATED WITH ELIMINATION PROCESSES

Constipation may be a problem for the patient with COAD for a number of reasons:

a) general lack of mobility and activity reduces the motility of the bowel following meals (Holdstock et al 1970)

b) it has previously been established that this patient may be dehydrated

c) the energy required for defaecation may be more than the dyspnoeic patient can manage

d) in a hospital ward, the lack of opportunity for privacy may discourage the individual from making the effort.

Clearly, each of these points can be taken up by the nurse. In addition to improving hydration, the nurse could arrange where possible for the patient to use the toilet, and to minimize the activity of the patient prior to the visit, so that the effort of defaecation is not too much for her.

As her condition improves, the nurse can guide the patient in her choice of high-fibre foods, and improving mobility will also ease the situation.

Some degree of heart failure may be an additional problem for the elderly patient with COAD, and therefore fluid retention will be a problem, with resulting oliguria; oliguria is also a result of severe hypoxia, because there is insufficient oxygen supply to the kidneys. Urinary output, therefore, should be monitored in those who are at risk.

MAINTAINING A BALANCE BETWEEN REST AND ACTIVITY

First, to consider rest and activity for the patient with COAD, it may be found that far from being in balance, this elderly person with acute breathing difficulties is desperately in need of rest, and cannot find the energy for even the simplest activity. Her rest is disturbed by dyspnoea, which is aggravated if she falls into an unsuitable position. She may have a cough which also disturbs her. She will be disturbed by the nurse as she helps her to change position in order to prevent pressure sores and consolidation in the dependent parts of her lung.

There can be little in life as frightening as not being able to breathe, or fighting for each breath; the fear of sliding into sleep and not waking is very real. This anxiety can turn a restful night into a time of terror.

Hypnotics cannot be used to help this patient because of the depressive effect they have on respiration. Ways must be found, therefore, of easing the mind and the body of this patient. She may find comfort in being in a bed near the nurse's station, so that she can see the nurses. Alternatively, a quieter place in the ward may allow her to sleep without disturbance. The patient may be helped if she is allowed time to express her feelings, and to explore with the nurse the ways she might find most useful to deal with them.

If sleep during the night is limited, and the effort of breathing is exhausting the patient, then periods of rest during the day should be encouraged; this is often difficult on the busy medical ward, and it requires organization on the part of the nurse to arrange the patient's activity in bursts, so that time can be made for rest (and protection from unnecessary disturbance).

In addition to ensuring sufficient rest, it is also vital to consider the importance of activity for this patient. During the period when the patient's breathing problems are at their worst, movement is probably restricted to helping her change her position, in order to prevent areas of collapse in dependent portions of the lung, and also to prevent pressure sores. As we have seen, the position of the patient is important; a recumbent position will reduce the capacity for gas exchange, exacerbate any hypoxia, and could result in the patient becoming confused, thus increasing the risks to this patient.

It is important, therefore, that early mobilization is achieved. This should not be a haphazard process, but should be planned with the patient. Movement and exercise should be increased each day, with short sessions scheduled for morning and afternoon (Guthrie & Petty 1970).

MAINTAINING A BALANCE BETWEEN SOLITUDE AND SOCIAL INTERACTION

Solitude and social interaction can have both positive and negative connotations for anyone. It has been established that bustling staff may increase the anxiety of the patient, but once the activity has passed the patient may find that she has some solitude. She may enjoy the peace of not having to interact with any other person, although solitude may also be a frightening experience. She may worry that if she stopped breathing no-one would know. She feels confined, since she has no strength to seek others; she may feel abandoned. If the nurse explains what is happening, when she will next come to see her, and that she need only press the call button for a swift response, she can do much to make the situation for the patient more tolerable.

THE PROMOTION OF NORMALCY

The patient suffering from a chronic disability is likely to have lowered self-esteem and loss of motivation to enjoy life; the potential for depression and social isolation in elderly people compound the problem. The nurse can give the patient the opportunity to learn how to increase her own self-care, in order to increase her morale. She may also be able to facilitate improved communication between the patient and her relatives and friends.

CONCLUSION

The aspects considered here of nursing an elderly patient with breathing difficulties are not based on an individual but on many assumptions about elderly people and how they may react to a situation. 'The elderly', however, are not an homogeneous group; every year of our existence gives us more experiences, more reasons to differ from our fellows, more time to develop our idiosyncrasies.

Only by working with our clients/patients as partners can we effectively use our knowledge and their knowledge, experience and perspectives, to devise a plan of care that can be effective for the individual, and not just fit for a book.

REFERENCES

Allen S C 1988 How respiration and cardiac reserves decline in old age. Geriatric Medicine 18(4): 23

Barker W H, Mullooly J P 1980 Influenza vaccination of elderly persons. Journal of the American Medical Association 244: 2547–2549

Brandstetter R D, Kazemi H 1983 Aging and the respiratory system. Medical Clinics of North America 67:(2) 419–431

Caird F I, Akhtar A J 1972 Chronic respiratory disease in the elderly. Thorax 27: 764–768

Cander L, Moyer J H 1964 Aging of the lung. Grune Stratton, New York

Guthrie A, Petty T 1970 Improved exercise tolerance in patients with chronic airways obstruction. Physical Therapy 50: 1333

Guyton A C 1986 Textbook of medical physiology. Saunders, Philadelphia

Hanks C M 1986 Digestion and nutrition in the elderly. Geriatric Nursing and Home Care 6(5): 12–15

Howard P 1987 Chronic chest disorder: positive approach pays off. Geriatric medicine 17(10): 49–59

Holdstock D J, Misciewicz J J, Smith T, Rowlands E N 1970 Propulsion (mass movements) in the human colon and its relationship to meals and somatic activity. Gut 11: 91–99

Jarrett D R J 1988 Differential diagnosis: asthma and its mimics. Geriatric Medicine 18(7)

Oh T E 1985 The manual of intensive care. Butterworths, Sydney

Orem D E 1985 Nursing concepts of practice. McGraw-Hill, New York

Wheeler H H 1980 A patient with chronic bronchitis, emphysema, cor pulmonale and pulmonary embolism. Nursing Times 76: 1339–1345

Whyte B 1988 On growing old: a personal view. In: Wright S G (ed) Nursing the older patient. Harper and Row, London

Ziment I 1982 Management of respiratory problems in the aged. Journal of the American Geriatrics Society, Supplement, 30(11): S36–S45

CHAPTER CONTENTS

Risk factors affecting the nutritional status of elderly people 173

Specific nutritional problems 175
Anorexia 175
Dehydration 175
Anaemias 175
Vitamin C deficiency 176
Vitamin D deficiency 177
Diet-related bowel disorders 177
Swallowing problems 178

Assessment of nutritional status 179

Helping the elderly patient to eat 179

Nutritional services in the community 181

Dental services for elderly people 182

11

Eating and drinking

Susan Thomas

Until recent times knowledge of the dietary needs of elderly people was based largely on folklore and tradition. It was assumed that old people needed less to eat and that they enjoyed the mythical 'geriatric' diet. However, current thought suggests that old people may need less energy (kilocalories) than younger people, but their requirements for all nutrients is similar and, in some instances, actually increased (see Table 11.1). Yet, for a variety of medical and social reasons, many old people reduce not only their energy intake, but also their intake of many vital nutrients, resulting in malnutrition. What is the extent of malnutrition amongst elderly people in the United Kingdom? Prior to 1967, two major nutritional surveys had been carried out: Bransby and Osborne (1953) completed a survey of old people living alone or with their spouses in Sheffield, and Exton-Smith and Stanton (1965) carried out a smaller survey of elderly women living alone in two London boroughs. These surveys dispelled some of the rumours that old people exist mainly on a diet of bread, butter, jam, biscuits and cups of sweetened tea. However, more detailed research was needed in order to ascertain the actual extent of malnutrition which existed amongst the elderly.

In 1967 the Department of Health and Social Security undertook a nationwide nutrition survey of elderly people living in the community (DHSS 1972) in which they found that 3.2% of the subjects were suffering from clinical malnutrition. Five years later they repeated the study on those of the original sample still alive and willing to co-operate (DHSS 1979b). Seven per cent of the subjects had clinical malnutrition at the time of this survey. For the majority of these the malnutrition was found to be secondary to a medical

Table 11.1 Comparison between recommended daily amounts of food energy and nutrients for the elderly and younger age groups in the UK.
Source: Department of Health and Social Security (1979a).

Age range years	Occupational Category	Energy MJ	Energy kcal	Protein g	Thiamin mg	Riboflavin mg	Nicotinic acid equivalents mg	Total folate µg	Ascorbic acid mg	Vitamin A retinol equivalents µg	Vitamin D cholecalciferol µg	Calcium mg
Men												
18–34	Sedentary	10.5	2510	63	1.0	1.6	18	300	30	750	(i)	500
35–64	Sedentary	10.0	2400	60	1.0	1.6	18	300	30	750	(i)	500
65–74	Assuming a sedentary life	10.0	2400	60	1.0	1.6	18	300	30	750	(i)	500
75+		9.0	2150	54	0.9	1.6	18	300	30	750	(i)	500
Women												
18–54	Most occupations	9.0	2150	54	0.9	1.3	15	300	30	750	(i)	500
55–74	Assuming a sedentary life	8.0	1900	47	0.8	1.3	15	300	30	750	(i)	500
75+		7.0	1680	42	0.7	1.3	15	300	30	750	(i)	500

(i) No dietary sources may be necessary for children and adults who are sufficiently exposed to sunlight, but during the winter children and adolescents should receive 10 µg (400 i.u.) daily by supplementation. Adults with inadequate exposure to sunlight, for example those who are housebound, may also need a supplement of 10 µg daily or psychological condition, which could lead one to conclude that a decline in physical or psychological well-being leads to a decline in nutritional status.

For every diagnosis of clinical malnutrition, there must be many more old people suffering from subclinical malnutrition. Overt clinical malnutrition only appears after a long latent period of inadequate food intake. During this time the body's nutrient stores are gradually depleted, but there are no outward signs of deficiency. However, during a crisis causing physiological stress such an individual has few nutritional reserves to draw on and thus slides into a state of malnutrition.

RISK FACTORS AFFECTING THE NUTRITIONAL STATUS OF ELDERLY PEOPLE

Based on a list drawn up by Exton-Smith (1978), the following risk factors may all predispose elderly people to malnutrition.

Loneliness

For some old people, dining alone heightens their feelings of solitude. Many women, used to a lifetime of cooking for their husbands and families, lose the incentive to cook for one.

Ignorance

The generation reaching old age today were brought up in times of great hardship, when financial limitations governed food choice. Housewives relied heavily on both sugar and fats in order to satisfy their family's appetites. This paved the way for a lifetime of poor eating habits. One of the groups of old people most at risk are widowers who, on the death of their wives, may be forced to fend for themselves with neither culinary skills nor nutrition knowledge.

Budget

Eating well on a pension demands that the individual be skilled at budgeting and motivated to shop wisely, taking advantage of special offers. Brockington and Lempert (1967) found that those old people with a supplementary income had a better diet than those who relied on their pension alone. Each person's priorities differ; to some, food may be less important than heating, bingo, alcohol or cigarettes.

Physical disability

Any disability, however great or small, can hinder the shopping, cooking or even eating of food. For example, one old lady who suffered from severe arthritis had her store cupboard well stocked with tinned food but ate none of it because she was unable to manipulate a can-opener.

Mental confusion and depression

Dementia affects 5% of the population aged 65 and over in this country. It brings with it a lack of awareness of the basic human needs — a confused old person may simply forget to eat, unless someone is there to remind her. Demented patients may demonstrate bizarre eating patterns, which, due to their poor nutritional balance, could lead to malnutrition. For example one patient was found drinking pickle and HP sauce, and another ate soap. Depression is also an important cause of anorexia in the elderly.

Iatrogenic factors

The continuation of special diets long after they are needed can cause malnutrition. For example, adherence to low fat diets 10 or 15 years after cholecystectomy can cause chronic weight loss and deficiency of the fat-soluble vitamins. The old 'gastric regime' for ulcers, which excluded some fruit and vegetables could, in the long term, precipitate scurvy. The indiscriminate use of 'special' diets could also damage a patient with a precarious nutritional state. For example, overweight patients subjected to rigorous reducing regimes on admission to geriatric wards may well have an underlying subclinical malnutrition, which would be compounded by the diet. Many elderly people have a patchy knowledge of nutrition. This can lead to abstention from certain nourishing foods for no logical reason and a heavy reliance on other foods or vitamin pills, believing them to be the panacea of all ills. Both situations can lead to disaster.

Alcoholism

Alcohol may be drunk in excess quantity by an old person for pain relief, to dull loneliness, for warmth or, as one old man told me, for the maintenance of a last surviving vice. The elderly alcoholic may be difficult to detect because, like younger alcoholics, they tend to be secretive about their drinking habits. However, it is imperative that those with an excessive alcohol intake be identified in order to give appropriate nutritional supplements and advice, thus preventing the more harmful nutritional consequences of alcohol abuse. On investigating a patient suspected of drinking, a history from relatives, friends or the social services might be invaluable. One cachexic old man admitted to a geriatric unit in an acute confusional state was unable to give any sort of diet history. The doctors had rejected any thought that the patient was an alcoholic, but a routine call to the home help organizer revealed that the only way the old man would eat his meals-on-wheels was if the meal was delivered to the local public house, where he spent most of his day.

Deficiencies of the vitamin B complex, particularly thiamine and folic acid are commonly seen in the alcoholic.

Drugs

There are many harmful interactions between drugs and nutrition. Certain medications (e.g. digoxin, phenformin and chemotherapy agents) can cause nausea and loss of appetite. Others may induce depletion of the body's mineral stores; thus penicillamine depletes zinc; purgatives deplete phosphate; diuretics deplete potassium; and zinc depletes magnesium (Roe 1977). Aspirins and salicylates may cause internal bleeding, leading to an iron deficiency anaemia. Certain other drugs can interfere with vitamin metabolism, but conversely the same vitamin, when given in therapeutic doses, can interrupt the drug metabolism, as in the long-term use of anti-convulsants with folic acid and vitamin D (Dent et al 1970, Labadarios et al 1978).

Taste and smell perception

Whilst it is accepted that both sight and hearing might decline with ageing, the impairment in the senses of taste and smell is seldom considered. Other factors which contribute to a decline in taste and smell perception include disease state, drugs, poor oral hygiene and smoking. Food choice and appetite may be seriously affected by disorders of taste and smell, resulting in malnutrition.

Dentition

Lack of dentition or ill-fitting dentures may influence food choice, causing the elderly individual to select a diet high in soft starchy foods, at the expense of meat, fresh fruit and vegetables. Poor oral hygiene may mask taste perception.

Malabsorption

Malabsorption is a potent cause of malnutrition in elderly people. Conditions such as ischaemic bowel, post-gastrectomy syndromes and gluten sensitivity can all cause malabsorption, resulting in weight loss, with deficiency of folic acid, vitamin B12 and the fat-soluble vitamins.

Increased nutritional requirements

Elderly patients recovering from surgery, those on prolonged bed-rest and those with pressure sores may all have an increased nutritional requirement. However, it is just these patients who lose their appetite and eat less rather than more food.

Cultural and religious factors

Many of the Asian immigrants to Britain, particularly elderly Asians, have not adopted Western eating habits, preferring to purchase their own familiar foods. Items such as imported leafy green vegetables are both costly and low in vitamin content owing to transportation problems. Many

Hindu Asians are strict vegetarians, and a deficiency of iron and vitamin B12 may occur in those who take no animal products. Osteomalacia is also seen among the Asian community. Hindus fast on special festivals in their calendar and, in addition, many fast on one or two days each week. Muslims fast during Ramadan, and although they are exempt if ill many will insist on fasting, regardless of their condition. Such practices could compound an underlying malnutrition.

SPECIFIC NUTRITIONAL PROBLEMS

ANOREXIA

Loss of appetite, or anorexia, in elderly people is an important sign of loss of physical or emotional well-being, which needs thorough investigation. Whatever the cause, a sudden onset of anorexia, sometimes with total refusal of food, will result in a state of acute starvation within days of onset. A chronic loss of appetite can often go unnoticed, unless nursing staff are vigilant at mealtimes. Patients who survive on 500–600 kilocalories (kcal) daily or less can slowly slip into a state of semi-starvation. In addition to the physical signs of starvation, with weight loss, poor wound healing and physical debility, the starved individual experiences mental changes. A starved patient may be withdrawn, depressed, emotionally labile and might express a death-wish. Treating this type of patient can be difficult and will be discussed further on.

DEHYDRATION

A person can survive for some weeks without food, but without fluids she will die within a matter of days. Provided there is free access to water, the fluid balance is carefully regulated by the body and a balance between input and output maintained. The optimum fluid intake is 1.0–1.5 litres (6–9 cups) daily, yet many old people drink far less, some believing that they need less fluid as they grow older. Davies (1981) noted that certain old people limited the time of their last drink in the day, usually because they preferred not to get up in the night. Dehydration involves more than a change in water balance — there are also accompanying changes in electrolyte balance. When water supply is restricted, or losses excessive, owing to fever, vomiting, burns or haemorrhage, the rate of water loss exceeds the rate of electrolyte loss. The extracellular fluid becomes concentrated and osmotic pressure draws water from the cells into the extracellular fluid in compensation.

In mild cases of dehydration, the encouragement of oral fluids may be all that is required. Offering tea, coffee, milk, fruit juice and carbonated drinks rather than water alone will encourage the patient to take fluids. In severe cases of dehydration, however, the patient may be unable to tolerate a sufficient quantity of oral fluids and intravenous infusion will be necessary.

ANAEMIAS

Anaemia is the term used to describe any condition where the oxygen-carrying capacity of the blood falls below normal. Symptoms vary with the type and severity of the anaemia, but can include tiredness, breathlessness on exertion, dizziness, pallor of the mucous membranes, palpitations, ankle oedema and, occasionally, angina in elderly people.

Iron-deficiency anaemia

Iron deficiency causes a microcytic, hypochromic anaemia. In addition to the usual symptoms of anaemia described above, iron-deficient patients may have brittle, spoon-shaped nails (koilonychia) and a sore, red, smooth tongue. Iron-deficiency anaemia in elderly people is usually associated with chronic internal bleeding or acute haemorrhage. Poor diet is rarely the sole cause of microcytic anaemia in this age group, but may be a contributory factor. Iron deficiency is usually treated with oral iron tablets, such as ferrous sulphate or ferrous gluconate. In severe cases blood transfusions are given. Advice on increasing the iron content of the diet is also important. Rich sources are liver and liver products such as liver paté and liver sausage, corned beef, kidney, red meats and eggs. Other good sources include wholemeal bread, fortified breakfast cereals, lentils and green vegetables.

Vitamin B12 deficiency anaemia

Vitamin B12 deficiency anaemia causes a megaloblastic anaemia. Other symptoms may include a red raw tongue, and, if advanced, there may be a subacute combined degeneration of the cord, peripheral neuropathy and mental changes. The deficiency can be caused by malabsorption owing to lack of intrinsic factor (pernicious anaemia) or chronic atrophic gastritis. It is also a long-term complication of partial or total gastrectomy. In rare cases, vitamin B12 deficiency has been diagnosed in people following Vegan diets, which exclude all animal products, including milk. Treatment is with monthly injections of vitamin B12 for life.

Anaemia due to folic acid deficiency

Folic acid deficiency also causes a megaloblastic anaemia, and in addition to the symptoms common to all anaemias, the patient may have a red, raw tongue. Unlike iron and B12 deficiency, this type of anaemia is often associated with poor diet, particularly in elderly people. In the DHSS survey of the elderly in 1972 (DHSS 1979b), approximately one fifth of the men and one quarter of the women had evidence of long-term folate deficiency. There has been interest in the significance between dementia and poor folate status in elderly people (Sneath et al 1973). It is most probable that the dementia leads to inadequate dietary intake and, in turn, folate deficiency, although the likelihood that the folate deficiency itself leads to impaired mental function cannot be excluded. Rich sources of folic acid include liver and dark-green leafy vegetables. This vitamin is easily destroyed by prolonged cooking, and therefore those old people who rely upon institutional catering such as meals-on-wheels or hospital food, may have a low intake of folate. Treatment of this anaemia is with folic acid tablets and dietary advice.

VITAMIN C DEFICIENCY

Scurvy, caused by severe vitamin C deficiency, is seldom seen today. However, occasional cases are still diagnosed amongst the elderly people, particularly old men living alone — hence the term 'widower's scurvy'. Symptoms include swelling and bleeding of gums (except in edentulous individuals), 'sheet' haemorrhages in the skin of the arms and legs, anaemia and mental changes. One such case of scurvy was diagnosed in an old lady who was admitted to hospital from her own home. On admission she was emaciated, dehydrated and unable to respond to even the simplest command. 'Sheet' haemorrhages on both arms were noted and these spontaneously opened and bled within 24 hours of admission. Urinary saturation tests (Harris & Ray 1935) substantiated the provisional diagnosis of scurvy, which was confirmed by the diet history obtained from relatives: three weeks' supply of meals-on-wheels were found, unopened, in the old lady's kitchen and the only other food in the house was half a packet of biscuits. There was also evidence that she had been drinking her own urine. With rehydration, feeding and vitamin C this old lady made a remarkable improvement and soon became an alert, although slightly confused, member of the ward. She chose not to return to her own home, but moved into a private nursing Home.

Subclinical vitamin C deficiency is a more common finding in elderly people. Davies (1981) carried out research into the nutritional intake of elderly recipients of two meals-on-wheels per week in Portsmouth. It was reported that 40% of the subjects were taking less than the recommended daily amount (RDA) of vitamin C (DHSS 1979b), and that the vitamin C intake on the 'meals' days was less than on other days. The risks of rapid vitamin C destruction in institutional catering have long been recognized (Platt et al 1963) and yet vitamin C deficiency still occurs in institution-bound old people. Thomas et al (1982) reported that, of a group of elderly long-stay psychiatric patients, those who were not drinking a regular glass of orange juice had serum ascorbic acid levels suggestive of scurvy. Signs and symptoms of subclinical vitamin C deficiency are difficult to detect, but may include an increased tendency to bruising, poor wound healing, listlessness and depression. Schorah et al (1979) reported that there was a slight but significant improvement in appetite, daily living activities and interest when a group of elderly long-stay patients, known to have low vitamin C levels, were given a one month course of this vitamin.

A quick way to assess whether there is enough vitamin C in the diet is to find out whether the old person takes one of the following daily: citrus fruit, e.g. orange or grapefruit; fresh orange juice; freshly cooked greens; raw tomato. If none of these is included, a deficiency should be suspected. Useful suggestions of vitamin C foods for the housebound elderly person and those not receiving regular supplies of fresh fruit and vegetables, include (fortified) blackcurrant juice, (fortified) dried instant fruit drinks and (fortified) instant mashed potato powder, which all have added vitamin C.

VITAMIN D DEFICIENCY

From the age of 40 our bones begin to atrophy, although the speed with which this happens is subject to individual variation. This is a commonly occurring concomitant of ageing, known as osteoporosis, for which there is little remedy except to take regular exercise and to ensure an adequate calcium intake, unless hormone replacement therapy is prescribed. A more treatable condition, osteomalacia or adult rickets is also prevalent amongst elderly people, particularly those who are housebound. Anderson et al (1966) diagnosed oesteomalacia in 4% of female admissions to a geriatric unit. Aaron et al (1974) reported that 20–30% of women and 40% of men presenting with fractured proximal femur had osteomalacia. Thomas et al (1982) found that 43% of elderly psychiatric patients in long-stay care were at risk of osteomalacia.

Osteomalacia is caused by lack of vitamin D, which is needed to transport calcium from the diet to the bones. Symptoms of this deficiency disease include bone pain, muscle weakness and an increased susceptibility to falls and fractures. In Britain most of our vitamin D is derived from the action of sunlight on the skin, with a small contribution from diet. Osteomalacia can easily be prevented by adequate exposure to sunlight. Regular walks or rests in the sunshine should be encouraged. No stripping off is needed — open shirt collars and rolled-up sleeves are sufficient. Direct sunlight is not necessary — a seat in the shade will be adequate. For those who are completely housebound, a seat on a balcony or beside an open window would be beneficial. Serving afternoon tea in the grounds might encourage elderly residents of Homes and hospitals to take a little sunshine. Regular use of the foods containing vitamin D will help to boost the body's stores, particularly in the winter months when none can be derived from sunlight. Good sources of vitamin D include oily fish, margarine, Ovaltine, liver, eggs, evaporated milk.

It should be remembered that diet alone will not prevent osteomalacia. If an old person is completely housebound, with no access to sunlight, then he or she should be referred to a doctor for vitamin D tablets. Finally, a word of warning, vitamin D can be extremely toxic and so self-medication should be discouraged.

DIET-RELATED BOWEL DISORDERS

Constipation

Causes of constipation in elderly people include lack of dietary fibre, lack of fluids, insufficient exercise, loss of muscle tone and the effects of drugs. Many patients during the first few days of hospital admission experience constipation. This is due to a change of environment, change of diet and emotional disturbance, but the constipation will usually settle within a few days.

The use of purgatives, although helpful in certain cases, should not become a ward routine. There are four different types of purgatives:

- Bulk-forming drugs, e.g. methylcellulose, Fybogel® and Isogel®.
- Stimulant laxatives which increase intestinal activity, e.g. bisacodyl, danthron, senna, castor oil.
- Faecal softeners which either soften the

whole stool, e.g. docusate sodium, or add lubrication, e.g. liquid paraffin.
- Osmotic laxatives maintain the volume of fluid in the bowel by osmosis, but do not act directly on the faeces, e.g. magnesium sulphate, lactulose.

An adequate intake of fibre will help to prevent constipation. The diet should include wholemeal bread, high fibre breakfast cereals such as Weetabix, Shredded Wheat, Branflakes, Puffed Wheat, muesli and porridge, and plenty of fruit and vegetables. Whenever possible, encourage your patients to eat the skin of potatoes, tomatoes and apples since this will also supply valuable fibre. Avoid the liberal use of bran in your patients' diets because, as well as being unpalatable, bran chelates certain trace elements, notably calcium and zinc, making them less available to the body. Old people should be encouraged to take plenty of fluids (1.0–1.5 litres daily). Physical activity will help to stimulate the tone of the bowel muscle. Exercise classes for elderly people, whether in day centres, Homes or hospitals, can be very beneficial. Even the effect of laughter will stimulate the body. Constipation is discussed in more detail in Chapter 12, Eliminating.

Diverticular disease

Diverticular disease becomes more prevalent with increasing age and is common in old people. It is the presence of small pouches in the large intestine which are harmless in themselves, unless they become inflamed or, as occasionally happens, perforated. Evidence suggests that deficiency of fibre in the Western diet is responsible for this disease. Treatment is based on increasing the fibre content of the diet, using high fibre foods first and added bran only if necessary. Some patients may experience abdominal discomfort after starting a high fibre diet. It is important to reassure them that this is only transient and should resolve once the body has adapted to the change in diet.

SWALLOWING PROBLEMS

Management of the patient with swallowing diffi-culties requires the joint skills of the nurse, speech therapist, occupational therapist and the dietitian. Patients most likely to have swallowing problems include those with head injuries, strokes, multiple sclerosis, motor neurone disease and Parkinson's disease. When nursing staff first notice that a patient has difficulties, a prompt referral to the therapists is necessary to prevent the patient suffering from starvation.

The physiotherapist will advise on the correct posture to facilitate easy feeding. Wherever possible the patient should sit in a chair, rather than in bed. Feet should be flat on the floor, ensuring good flexion of the hips. In the case of the stroke patient, the affected side of the body should be brought forward, by lifting the weaker arm onto the table. Non-stick mats will prevent the patient's plate from moving. Feeding cups should be used with caution, since certain conditions such as Parkinson's disease actually prevent the patient from being able to tip the head back sufficiently to drink from the feeding cup. A glass or cup and saucer with a straw may be more appropriate and less demoralizing than a feeding cup. If a nasogastric tube is in place the patient may be unable to swallow normally (Waterhouse 1983). Nasogastric feeding can be an essential nutritional support during the acute phase of illness, but should be discontinued as soon as the patient is taking sufficient oral nutrition. During the period of total dependence on tube feeding it is important regularly to moisten the tongue with drops of strong flavours, e.g. lemon juice, peppermint oil, in order to stimulate the taste buds. When patients are learning to bite (an essential pre-swallowing activity) allow them to practise on French toast or cream crackers wrapped in gauze. On the introduction of food, thought must be given to the correct texture required. A monotonous diet of sloppy foods such as mince will not help the patient's progress to normal eating. A variety of textures are preferable, but not mixed together as in stew, where solid lumps in a fluid sauce would create problems. Suitable main courses include boneless fish, chopped meat such as chicken, skinless sausages, corned beef and savoury egg custards. Root vegetables, cauliflower and tinned tomatoes are good accompaniments, but peas, cabbage and 'stringy' vegetables should be avoided. Desserts present fewer problems; tinned pears, custards, icecream and yoghurts are all easily managed.

ASSESSMENT OF NUTRITIONAL STATUS

The primary cause of hospital admission is seldom identified as malnutrition, yet many old people are admitted with a subclinical malnutrition which may be overlooked. This can lead to poor wound healing, delayed recovery and inability to cope at home after discharge. A simple routine of screening all new admissions to the geriatric ward would identify those most likely to be malnourished and steps can then be taken to improve their nutrition and with it, their speed of recovery. Factors to be considered are listed below.

Diagnosis

The patient's diagnosed condition may hold a clue to malnutrition. For example, motor neurone disease or severe Parkinson's disease might cause physical difficulties in either eating or swallowing. A patient with bad pressure sores or leg ulcers may need extra nutrients for wound healing. A previous medical history of partial or total gastrectomy is worth noting, particularly if the patient is losing weight, as this might be due to the nutritional problems associated with gastric surgery.

Medication

In addition to recording the list of medications currently taken by the patient, ascertain whether purgatives are taken on a regular basis. An enquiry about any vitamin tablets or 'tonics' is also useful.

Weight

A record of each patient's weight on admission is essential and should be compared with the patient's normal 'healthy' weight, in order to assess whether there is any weight loss. Past medical notes may provide details of old weights. Each patient should be questioned about their normal healthy weight; many old people have little idea about recent weight, but may well remember their weight on entering the army, getting married or before having children. This is important information because, although the proportion of lean body mass to fat decreases with ageing, total weight should remain unaltered throughout adult life (Forbes and Reina 1970).

Social history

Routine questions about each patient's social status, home situation and social services are all relevant to the assessment of nutritional well-being.

Diet history

If the patient is a good historian, a simple diet history would be valuable. This should include the following points:

Number of meals consumed daily.
A brief account of the content of the meals.
Does the patient take meals-on-wheels?
• What time does she receive them?
• What time does she actually eat them?
Is fresh fruit or fresh fruit juice taken regularly?
Does the patient drink alcohol? (specify type and amount)
How much fluid is consumed daily (in cupfuls)?
How many meals are eaten out each week?

If the patient is an unreliable historian, confirmation of the diet history could be obtained from relatives, neighbours or home help.

HELPING THE ELDERLY PATIENT TO EAT

Menu planning

Meals are the focal point of the day for many patients, punctuating an often monotonous daily ward routine. It is of vital importance, therefore, that the menu is the best that funds will allow.

The menu cycle should be at least 3–4 weeks long to avoid becoming repetitive. The use of different menus for summer and winter, which incorporate seasonal foods, will add interest to the meals. All hospitals should be able to offer patients a choice of food, which should include a soft alternative to the main course for those with chewing or swallowing problems. However the use of purée, sometimes known as 'geriatric' food, should be strongly discouraged because it is usually unnecessary and always unappetizing.

However rushed you are on your ward, make time to help patients fill in their menu cards. Encourage the more able patients to help the others with their menus. If patients are given the chance to choose their own meals they may become more interested in eating. Some success has been achieved in using a visual menu made up of food photographs for confused patients.

Elderly patients tend to prefer the meal patterns they enjoyed when they were younger: a cooked breakfast for those who want it and a light breakfast for others; a cooked main meal at lunch and a high tea rather than a large evening meal. This might not match the catering manager's ideas, but perhaps there is room for compromise. In one hospital the catering manager wrote a separate supper menu for the childrens' and elderly wards together — including items such as scrambled eggs on toast, jacket potatoes and cheese, sausages and baked beans and homemade soups. It met with great approval from young and old alike.

The current nutrition guidelines recommended by the National Advisory Committee on Nutrition Education (NACNE, 1983) have initiated changes in hospital catering. However, the dietary guidelines recommended for the rest of the population must be interpreted with care for the over-75s.

A fat restriction in old age is unlikely to confer benefits to health and it may even have a harmful effect on intake of the fat soluble vitamins. The restriction of salt is not particularly beneficial to elderly people and may reduce enjoyment of food for those who suffer from loss of taste acuity, and those accustomed to adding salt. Similarly, a reduction in the sugar content of meals might detract

from the taste of the food. However, it would be wise to discourage sugar and sugary foods between meals because they dull the appetite. A high fibre diet is important in old age but the fibre should come from food rather than bran supplements; plenty of fluids should be encouraged to accompany a high fibre diet.

When writing a menu try to include dishes with names which describe the basic ingredients; for example, rather than dazzling the patients with 'chilli con carne' call the dish 'spicy mince'. Avoid the use of bland foods because the frequently voiced complaint that 'food does not taste like it used to' is more likely to be a reflection of loss of taste and smell acuity than a complaint about hospital food. Celebrations and festivities should be the ideal time for special meals; reminiscence could be stimulated by the occasional use of traditional foods such as jellied eels or 'bubble and squeak'. All of this will help to make the ward less frightening and more of a home to the patients.

The dining environment

Communal dining can encourage sociability amongst the patients and help to increase the appetite. Round tables break down barriers between the diners. Tableclothes and flowers add style to even the plainest hospital fare.

If the hospital uses bulk food trolleys, why not acquire some serving dishes and allow the patients to serve themselves and each other with vegetables and gravy? The tactful segregation of the messy eater might save embarrassment. Serving the slowest eaters first will enable them to enjoy their meal, without feeling hurried. Feeding the dependent patients is a time-consuming task, but one which, if carried out with kindness and understanding, will strengthen the bond between patient and nurse.

The management of loss of appetite

Accurate nursing observation at mealtimes will provide essential information on the patient's progress. If a patient appears to be taking insufficient food and/or drink, it is useful to keep a food chart. This should record the amount of food/drink served to the patient and the quantity left on the plate, together with any special observations. This information, once analyzed by the dietitian, will form the basis of dietetic treatment.

The first step to take when loss of appetite has been observed, is to discuss it with the doctor, since this may be an important symptom of illness. Dietary supplements should be offered to the patient between meals. This could be a high protein milk drink such as Build-Up® (Nestlé) or Complan® (Crookes Healthcare Ltd), fruit juice and caloreen or a snack of daintily served sandwiches. A small amount of alcohol, such as a glass of sherry, 20 minutes before a meal, may help to whet the appetite. In certain cases where the loss of appetite is due to acute illness or following surgery, a short course of appetite stimulants may be appropriate.

Tube feeding

The decision to tube feed a patient may present a moral dilemma for staff. It should only be considered as an interim means of nutritional support for the patient temporarily unable to sustain his or her own nutritional intake, for example, after major surgery or during the initial recovery period after a stroke. Tube feeding may also be beneficial to supplement oral intake for the undernourished patient. Bastow et al (1983) reported improvements in the clinical outcome of very thin patients with fractured neck of femur, when they were given supplementary overnight tube feeding. One severely undernourished lady with advanced Parkinson's disease was built up with supplementary overnight tube feeding sufficiently to be allowed home for some precious extra months before she required long-term care.

The usual method of tube feeding is via a fine-bore nasogastric tube. In recent years a range of commercially prepared sterile tube feeds, such as Clinifeed® (Roussel Laboratories) have replaced the need for homemade hospital tube feeds. A range of soya-based feeds are available for lactose intolerant patients or those temporarily unable to tolerate milk. The preferred method of administering the feed is by continuous drip because this minimizes the problems of diarrhoea associated with bolus feeding. A balance can be struck between the two methods by giving mobile patients a few hours' break from continuous tube feeding each day, allowing them the freedom to walk around unencumbered by drip stands and bottles.

Try to recommend that a time limit is set on the duration of the tube feeding and make sure that the relatives understand that it is temporary. The feeding regime can then be reviewed at the end of the allotted time and either continued or discontinued with the minimum of emotional upset. The idea of fixing review dates may prevent a situation of 'open-ended' tube feeding, when it is clearly inappropriate to continue to tube feed a patient, but morally difficult to call a halt to it.

The role of special diets

Special diets have a limited role to play in the nutritional care of old people. Reducing diets should be limited to cases where obesity hinders the patient's mobility and rehabilitation. Initially the diet should exclude sugar and sugar-containing foods, such as sweets, chocolate, squashes, Lucozade® and other carbonated drinks, because these supply 'empty' calories with little nutritive value. If a stricter diet is necessary, the dietitian should be asked to draw up a regime which will restrict kcals whilst providing balanced nutrition. Elderly diabetics who are treated either by diet and tablets or by diet alone can usually be controlled by simple advice on eating regular meals and excluding sugar and sugar-containing foods. However, those diabetics taking insulin injections may need more extensive advice. Other special diets are seldom necessary for elderly people, but if they are needed, diet sheets should be simple and concise.

NUTRITIONAL SERVICES IN THE COMMUNITY

The meals-on-wheels service which first began during the Second World War and was run by the Women's Voluntary Service (WVS, now Women's Royal Voluntary Service), is now organized jointly by local authorities and the WRVS. It supplies a hot midday meal to 2.5–3.0% of the elderly population in Britain. The cost and quality of the meal varies between areas, as does its nutritional content. Hitherto the service also provided a valuable daily social contact with housebound old people, but as greater demands are put on the service that social contact has become minimal in some areas. Local authorities strive to provide between five and seven meals per week for many recipients but Davies (1981) suggests that it might be more beneficial to spread the net wider and offer two to three meals per week for a greater number of old people, and perhaps spur them on to cook for themselves on the other days. Davies also suggests that there should be more reassessment of the clients because some old people only need meals-on-wheels as a temporary measure, to help them over a period of illness or bereavement, but the meals may be continued longer than necessary. Home helps are invaluable in the maintenance of many old people's nutrition. In the limited time allocated to each client the home help might be asked to do both the shopping and cooking of food. Luncheon clubs and day centres can provide both company and a good meal for many mobile old people. A few centres provide wheels-to-meals, thus enabling the housebound elderly to enjoy the benefits of these facilities, rather than dining alone. Several adult education centres run 'cook and eat' classes, which have the dual purpose of teaching culinary skills whilst offering the students a well-balanced meal.

There is much to be done in the field of nutrition education for elderly people. Pre-retirement classes are an excellent forum for nutrition teaching, because the individual is on the threshold of a major change in lifestyle and is often receptive to advice. Nutrition education is also disseminated via organizations such as Age Concern, by broadcasting and in the press. Education of all people involved in the caring network available for dependent elderly people is essential if our aged population is to be well nourished.

DENTAL SERVICES FOR ELDERLY PEOPLE

Research into the dental requirements of elderly people suggests that they feel the need for dental care less and less with advancing age although evidence suggests that advanced periodontal disease in old people is a serious problem (British Dental Journal 1983). By the age of 65 years over 79% of the population are edentulous (Todd et al 1978). A large proportion of this age group wear dentures. These should be replaced every 5–10 years. However, in a survey carried out by Osbourne et al (1979) 16% of the respondents had been wearing their present dentures for 30 years or more. Neill (1972) concluded that masticatory performance was no better in subjects who wore dentures of indifferent quality than in edentulous individuals. The dental service makes no special financial concessions for old people who normally have to pay the full dental fees unless they are exempt from prescription charges. However, dentists do run a domiciliary service for the housebound elderly for no extra charge. Osbourne et al (1979) noted that many elderly people were reluctant to visit the dentist. Of the subjects who complained of dental problems, 32% never attended a dentist. Reasons cited included prohibitive cost of treatment, waste of time, difficulty in travelling and fear of the dentist. If the nurse could take time to ask about her patients' state of dentition and encourage them to seek expert help from the dentist, this may add to the pleasure of eating.

REFERENCES

Aaron J E, Gallagher J C, Anderson J, Stasiak L, Longton E B, Nordin B E C, Nicholson M 1974 Frequency of osteomalacia and osteoporosis in fractures of the proximal femur. Lancet 1: 229–233

Anderson I, Campbell A E R, Dunn A, Runciman J B M 1966 Osteomalacia in elderly women. Scottish Medical Journal 11: 429–435

Anonymous 1983 Do we fail our elderly? British Dental Journal 155: 6–179

Bastow M D, Rawlings J, Allison S P 1983 Benefits of supplementary tube-feeding after fractured neck of femur: a randomised controlled trial. British Medical Journal 287: 1589–1592

Bransby E R, Osborne B 1953 A social and food survey of the elderly living alone or as married couples. British Journal Nutrition 7: 160–180

Brockington F, Lempert S M 1967 The Stockport study: the social needs of the over 80's. University Press, Manchester

Davies L 1981 Three score years . . . and then? Heinemann, London

Dent E C, Richens A, Rowe D J F, Stamp T C B 1970 Osteomalacia with long-term anticonvulsant therapy in epilepsy. British Medical Journal 4: 69

Department of Health and Social Security 1972 A nutrition survey of the elderly. Report by the Panel on Nutrition of the Elderly. HMSO, London

Department of Health and Social Security 1979a Recommended daily amounts of food energy and nutrients for groups of people in the United Kingdom. HMSO, London

Department of Health and Social Security 1979b Nutrition and health in old age. HMSO, London

Exton-Smith A N 1978 Nutrition in the elderly. In: Dickerson J W T, Lee H A (eds) Nutrition in the clinical management of disease. Edward Arnold, London

Exton-Smith A N, Stanton B R 1965 Report of an investigation into the dietary of elderly women living alone. King Edward's Hospital Fund, London

Forbes G B, Reina J C 1970 Adult lean body mass declines with age: some longitudinal observations. Metabolism 19: 653–663

Harris L J, Ray S N 1935 Diagnosis of vitamin C subnutrition by urine analysis. Lancet 1: 71–77

Labadarios D, Dickerson J W T, Parke D V, Lucas E G, Obuwa G H 1978 The effects of chronic drug administration on hepatic enzyme induction and folate metabolism. British Journal Clinical Pharmacology 5: 167–173

NACNE 1983 A discussion paper on proposals for nutritional guidelines for health education in Britain. The Health Education Council, London

Neill D J 1972 Masticatory studies. In: A nutritional survey of the elderly. DHSS. HMSO, London

Osbourne J, Maddick I, Gould A, Ward D 1979 Dental demands of old people in Hampshire. British Dental Journal 146: 351–355

Platt B S, Eddy T P, Pellett P L 1963 Food in hospitals. Nuffield Foundation, Oxford University Press

Roe D A 1977 Drug induced malnutrition in geriatric patients. Comprehensive Therapy 3(10): 24–28

Schorah C J, Scott D L, Newill A, Morgan D B 1979 Clinical effects of vitamin C in elderly patients with low blood vitamin C levels. Lancet 1: 403–405

Sneath P, Chanarin I, Hodkinson H M, McPherson C K, Reynolds E H 1973 Folate status in the geriatric population and its relationship to dementia. Age and Ageing 2: 177–182

Thomas S J, Millard P H, Storey P B 1982 Risk of scurvy and osteomalacia in elderly long-stay psychiatric patients. Journal of Plant Foods 4: 191–197

Todd J E, Walker A M, Dodd P 1978 Adult dental health survey UK. OPCS Volume 11. HMSO, London

Waterhouse C 1983 Feeding and swallowing problems after stroke. Geriatric Medicine 13: 433–435

CHAPTER CONTENTS

Introduction 185

Elimination needs 186
Identifying an acceptable place 186
Ability to get there 187
Ability to hold excreta 187
Ability to empty 188
Toilet-related skills 188

Defaecation 188
Assessing defaecation 188
Recording defaecation 188
Planning care 189
Constipation 189
Faecal incontinence 191

Micturition 191
Bladder dysfunction in old age 191
Incontinence in institutional care 193
Bladder training 194

Management of intractable incontinence 194
Incontinence aids 194
Indwelling catheters and elderly people 195
Community services for the incontinent person 196

The continence advisor 196

12

Eliminating

Christine Norton

INTRODUCTION

The passage of urine and faeces is, for most people in Western society, a very personal and private function, which many are able to take for granted. Considerable control over micturition and defaecation is necessary for the commonly accepted criteria of continence to be met. This involves a complex neuromuscular co-ordination, in conjunction with an awareness of societal norms. This control may become vulnerable for many older people, most especially at times of illness or disease, amongst disabled elderly people and those in residential or hospital care. The nurse has a key role, in both hospital and community settings, in identifying those elderly people at risk of elimination problems. By a thorough assessment of each individual's needs, appropriate care can be planned to maintain normal function and prevent problems, or to remedy those problems already apparent.

Traditionally, nurses approached elimination care in a routinized manner — most nurses were familiar with bedpan rounds, bottle rounds, bowel books and four-hourly toileting regimes. Care of bowel and bladder tended to be seen as a low-status task which required little knowledge or expertise, and was often left to the most junior or untrained staff. Working with elderly people was often identified as synonymous with an endless routine of changing incontinent patients and wet beds. Indeed, this may be partly responsible for the unfavourable image of 'geriatric nursing' held by some nurses. Yet the majority of old people manage to maintain normal elimination function to the end of their days. Problems are not a necessary or inevitable concomitant of ageing and should never be passively accepted. Problems do not 'just happen'; there must always be a cause or reason for them. If this can be discovered it can often be remedied, or at least the effects upon the individual minimized.

Elimination is a difficult subject for most older people to talk about. Many were brought up with Victorian attitudes towards bodily functions — that these are somehow shameful and should never be mentioned in public. Commonly, failure to maintain normal function was thought to reflect adversely on the character of the sufferer. Elimination difficulties were a cause for shame, embarrassment and guilt and were typically kept hidden. Consequently, many people who have problems do not seek help. For example, only a tiny proportion of incontinent people reveal the fact to health or social service agencies (Thomas et al 1980). Simons (1985) found that most older women felt that incontinence was normal and inevitable. A nurse must approach the subject with the utmost sensitivity and tact if a good rapport and trust are to be established. She must also be alert to the possibility of problems with every patient, not just those with overt difficulties. Nurses may be reluctant to bring the subject into the open, either accepting problems as irremediable or pretending nothing is wrong in order to spare the patient's embarrassment. Schwartz (1977) has described this as an attitude of 'mutual pretence' between nurses and patients, leading to problems being coped with rather than constructively confronted. Nurses are notoriously good at 'coping' in unsatisfactory circumstances. This is not always in the patient's long-term interests. Elimination problems cause misery, discomfort, can be a burden to carers, and may even rob an individual of the ability to live independently. They merit a serious nursing effort to provide optimum care.

Elimination has repeatedly been identified as a major problem for geriatric nursing. From the time of Norton's study onwards (Norton et al 1962), it has been known that problems such as incontinence occupy a high proportion of nursing time and energy. Wells (1980) compared several studies which found between 4% and 8% of nursing activity related to elimination. Maybe not surprisingly, she found that the amount of time spent 'promoting continence' was inversely related to the amount of incontinence on a ward. Trained nurses were found to have 'confused, inaccurate' knowledge about the causes of bladder or bowel problems. Negative attitudes and inadequate knowledge do seem to be becoming less common, however. There is a rapidly growing literature on promoting continence and today the motivated nurse has considerable scope for positive management of elimination.

Although bowel and bladder care is primarily seen as a nursing concern, the importance of other professions should not be forgotten. Ideally, the multidisciplinary team will work together to maximize function. This chapter will highlight the nursing component in the team's approach to care.

ELIMINATION NEEDS

Certain basic needs are common to both micturition and defaecation. Millard (1979) has argued that the individual must be able to identify an acceptable place for elimination; to be able to get to that place; and be able to hold excreta until that place is reached. The ability to empty the bowel or bladder easily, completely and in private once there, and to perform a number of toilet-related skills, could be added to this. This may sound obvious, but failure in these abilities is so common that each will be considered in turn, along with possible measures to solve problems.

IDENTIFYING AN ACCEPTABLE PLACE

An older person's ability to identify correctly an acceptable place for elimination may be impaired in several ways. Most people expect to use a lavatory, behind a locked door. In unfamiliar surroundings, this presumes an ability to follow signposts and read and correctly interpret labels on doors. Impaired vision, dim lighting or unclear (or absent) signs will create difficulties. Sometimes male and female symbols can be difficult to distinguish. The problem is often compounded by a reluctance to ask for help. In some instances of cerebrovascular disease, the individual loses the ability to recognize the function of common objects (e.g. a lavatory). The confused or demented person may likewise experience difficulty correctly identifying right and wrong receptacles and may, for instance, use a sink or wash-basin in error. In hospital, expectations are different from those in general society, and people are asked to void into bedpans, bottles, commodes, behind curtains or doors without locks (or even without a door or any privacy). It is easy to see how a disoriented person may not be able to identify which is the 'acceptable' place. The very confused person may lose all 'socially acceptable' behaviour, and the concept of continence or incontinence becomes irrelevant to the individual.

Correct identification can be aided by clear explanations of what is expected, ensuring good lighting, signposting and labelling of facilities and, if necessary, improving vision by provision of spectacles. Gilleard et al (1981) have demonstrated how training can improve ward orientation with psychogeriatric patients.

ABILITY TO GET THERE

It is no good knowing that there is a correct place for elimination unless that place can be reached. The problem may be an unsuitable environment or an individual's physical disabilities. At home, many elderly people have a lavatory which involves climbing stairs or is outside. If shared with others it may be occupied when needed. Public lavatories are often difficult for anyone with even a slight disability to use and are usually in sparse supply. With council cutbacks they may be closed, or vandalized and not repaired. Many older women have a horror of public lavatories (believing that they risk catching diseases) and would rather avoid their use. It has been estimated (Scottish Home and Health Department 1970) that elderly people in hospital should be a maximum of 12 metres from the lavatory. Yet many of our geriatric wards were built in the days when all pa-

tients were nursed in bed — lavatories have been built on as an after thought, often at the opposite end of the ward to the dayroom and down a corridor or around a corner. The British Standards Institution (1979) has drawn up guidelines for recommended lavatory design for disabled people, but these seem seldom to be adhered to, even in new buildings or upgradings.

Mobility is essential in getting to the lavatory. This may be helped by ensuring that beds and chairs are of the correct height and design to aid rising; that routes are uncluttered with obstacles (e.g. loose mats in the house); and that the individual has the optimum mobility aid for her needs. Good footcare and well-fitting shoes can make a great difference. Opening the lavatory door and getting into the compartment may present problems if design is poor. The height of the lavatory and availability of grab-rails will often determine whether sitting and rising are possible. Manual dexterity is crucial in removal of clothing, positioning and cleansing. Appropriate clothing, a raised seat or a dressing aid can facilitate independent toileting.

Sometimes depression or apathy may result in lack of motivation to attempt to reach the lavatory. The individual with an impoverished social environment may simply cease to try. This is particularly a problem in long-stay care if incontinence has become the norm and no expectation is put upon the individual to attempt to be continent. Occasionally, incontinence seems to be a protest or sign of despair from an individual in an unacceptable personal situation. A positive atmosphere should be the aim.

Where physical disabilities are severe, an alternative such as a hand-held urinal (male or female) or a commode may be more appropriate, if privacy in their use can be ensured.

ABILITY TO HOLD EXCRETA

The individual needs to be able to control bladder and bowel contents reliably while getting to the lavatory. This requires competent urethral and anal sphincters and the ability to inhibit detrusor (bladder muscle) and rectal contractions. Any of these may be impaired by disease or ageing (see below). With increasing age, sensation tends to diminish and the individual gets less warning and often experiences increased urgency of micturition or defaecation. It is a cruel fact that this urgency may coincide with decreased ability to hurry.

ABILITY TO EMPTY

Constipation and bladder voiding difficulties are common in old age and have many possible causes (see below). Privacy is an important component in enabling complete evacuation.

TOILET-RELATED SKILLS

Sitting or standing in the correct position for long enough, using lavatory paper, flushing the lavatory, handwashing and many other incidental skills are all part of independence in toileting. The nurse's assessment will determine which, if any, of these prerequisites for successful elimination are lacking for each individual. Care should be planned which aims to maximize each individual's potential for independent continence. The physiotherapist, occupational therapist, chiropodist, optician and planner may each have a contribution. Wells (1980) has described how many nurses often accept an unsuitable environment without considering how it might be improved.

DEFAECATION

Many older people seem obsessed by their bowels. Having lived through an era when the medical profession extolled the virtue of at least one bowel motion per day and weekly purgation, many become distressed if they do not achieve this. In fact, the range of 'normality' is wide and lies between three motions per day and one every three days (Connell et al 1965).

ASSESSING DEFAECATION

Nurses often assess bowel function very superficially, simply determining whether the bowels have been opened or not. Wright (1974), in a study of bowel function of hospital inpatients, found that no ward routinely asked about a patient's usual pattern on admission, and that bowel problems caused considerable worry amongst the patients studied. Problems were most likely amongst bedpan or commode users and for old people, with one in three patients experiencing decreased bowel frequency in hospital.

Figure 12.1 gives a checklist which may be used to guide assessment of bowel function. Privacy is essential during this assessment. A common vocabulary must be established — most patients understand 'opening bowels', but this can never be presumed. By finding out the patient's usual bowel pattern the nurse will avoid imposing her own, possibly arbitrary, criteria for evaluating the success of bowel care. As far as possible care should conform to the individual's usual habit, providing this was problem-free. The term 'constipation' may be used by the patient if an expected daily motion is missed, but more properly describes motions which are hard and difficult to pass as well as infrequent. Consistency of motions is difficult to assess accurately but, generally, distinction can be made between hard pellets (scybala), soft motions and unformed diarrhoea.

If the patient has urgency, this must be considered in relation to mobility and the environment. Mobility itself is a major stimulant of colonic mass movements. Poor diet or low food intake may underlie problems. If dietary regulation is planned, the patient's preferences must be respected — spooning bran onto porridge uninvited may cause food to be left, rather than the intended benefit to bowel function. Many (possibly most) old people use laxatives (Brocklehurst 1978). Often this is for no good reason and can be stopped, especially if diet is improved (Bass 1977, Battle & Hanna 1980). A long history of laxative abuse may lead to colonic damage. Any alteration of an established regime should be carefully monitored.

RECORDING DEFAECATION

Accurate records are vital in assessing the success of bowel care. If the patient cannot communicate,

Name: Assessment
                               date:

Patient's usual term for
defaecation:
Usual frequency of bowel action: Range:
Usual time of day:
Any associated habits/events:

Does patient complain of
constipation?
If so, what is understood by this?

Does patient get sensation of the
need to defaecate?
Average time taken for bowel
action:
Does patient have to strain?
Is defaecation associated with
pain?
Any bleeding: Fresh or altered
                   blood:
Mucus:
Problematic flatus: Continent
                       of flatus:
Scybala: Ribbon
                       stools:
Usual consistency of faeces:
Usual amount of faeces:
Does patient experience urgency?   Time of warning:

Diet: Any food taken for bowels:
       Any food avoided for
       bowels:
       Average daily fluid intake:

Laxative use: Present:
                Past history of use:
Any constipating drugs taken:
History of perianal problems:

Faecal incontinence?
If yes: Nature of soiling:
         Sensation of incontinence:
         Frequency of incontinence:

Result of rectal examination if
done:
Any recent change in bowel
habits?

Toilet facilities
       Problems with using
       lavatory:
       If bedpan/commode used,
       reaction to this:

Ability to cleanse after
defaecation:
Mobility impaired?

Are any bowel problems
anticipated with current
illness/condition?

Fig. 12.1 Assessment of defaecation.

or is thought to be an unreliable witness, the nurse must inspect excreta. A simple Yes/No response is inadequate; note should also be made of amount, consistency, ease or difficulty of passage, whether laxatives were used, and if the patient feels the rectum has been cleared. If constipation or impaction is suspected, a digital rectal examination will confirm this. Immobile, confused patients with a tendency to impaction should be examined regularly to check that the rectum is not becoming loaded with faeces.

PLANNING CARE

Bowel care should involve active nursing policies, not an assumption that all is well until problems arise. A routine which is sensitive to each person's needs should be planned, and changed over time if those needs change. Table 12.1 gives a sample care plan which illustrates that comprehensive care often involves many different aspects.

CONSTIPATION

There is little evidence that constipation is an inevitable accompaniment to old age (Brocklehurst 1978). Many of the reasons older people experience infrequent, hard, difficult motions are reversible. A variety of physiological causes may underlie constipation; for example, a bowel lesion, neurological or metabolic disease, or psychological illness (e.g. depression). These will be aggravated by immobility, poor diet or fluid intake, inappropriate environment, drug side-effects, and ignoring the call to stool (Exton-Smith, 1972). Constipation should be investigated and appropriate treatment instigated for any of these problems.

The virtues of a high-fibre diet have been extolled in the prevention and management of constipation. The evidence for the efficacy of this diet is far from unassailable (Pollman et al 1978). For elderly people, caution should be taken against intestinal obstruction, metabolic effects and lowered food intake due to satiety. Most studies have measured success of fibre by a decrease in laxative use, but often without evidence that laxatives were necessary in the first place.

Where constipation is known to be a problem,

Table 12.1 Sample care plan — Mrs S W.

Date	Problem	Goal	Planned action	Review date	Outcome
17.1	Admitted incontinent of fluid stool many times each day. Found to be faecally impacted	Faecal continence within one week	Administer one micro-enema each morning until no further return	24.1	No further return from enemas. Faecal continence now restored
17.1	Embarrassment at communicating need to defaecate	Able to ask for lavatory facilities	Explain hospital terms. Frequent, discreet enquiries of needs. Ensure privacy	21.1	Seems less shy but still will not ask for lavatory. Continue to ensure she is asked if she needs to go
19.1	Worried other patients will be offended by smell when uses commode	Patient is less worried about other patients	Avoid use of bedpan or commode. Take to lavatory at quiet times. Reassure	22.1	Patient happier using lavatory, but feet do not reach the floor
19.1	Inability to reach lavatory independently	Independence in reaching lavatory within one week	Refer to physiotherapist for advice on mobilization. Ensure correct height bed and chair	23.1	Can walk slowly with walking frame. Requires encouragement and sometimes becomes disoriented
19.1	Difficulty removing clothes and wiping bottom because of arthritic hands	Independence at toilet within 2 days	Refer to occupational therapist. Allow time and give encouragement for independence	21.1	Patient provided with more suitable pants and a wrap over skirt, which she finds easier to remove. Uses bottom-wiper
20.1	Need to prevent future constipation and recurrence of impaction	Frequent (every 1 or 2 days), soft, easy motions	Encourage fluid intake (at least 1500 ml/24 h) and high fibre diet	25.1	Motion achieved on alternate days but still hard and difficult to pass. Dislikes high fibre diet and fluids
22.1	Feet do not reach floor when on lavatory	Patient reaches optimal position for easy defaecation	Provide foot block	24.1	Foot block aids bowel evacuation — continue use
26.1	Dislikes high fibre diet and high fluid intake	Takes acceptable alternative to prevent constipation	Obtain prescription for laxative. Provide preferred drinks (Bovril® or lemonade)	30.1	Motions now softer and more regular. Patient understands importance of this continuing after discharge from hospital

prophylactic laxatives may be of benefit. Godding (1972) reviewed the mode of action of the commonest laxative agents, which are essentially bulking, lubricant or stimulant in function (see Ch. 11 for further discussion). Evidence on the criteria for selection is sparse and seems to rest largely on the physician's preference. It is now well established that liquid paraffin should not be used because of the risk of inhalational pneumonia and paraffinomas.

FAECAL INCONTINENCE

Faecal incontinence may be a symptom of a number of different disorders, e.g. severe diarrhoea, neurogenic bowel, muscular damage or, most commonly in elderly people, faecal impaction with overflow incontinence or spurious diarrhoea (Parks 1980). Impacted faeces, resulting from chronic constipation, can usually be presumed to be the cause of faecal incontinence in elderly people, especially those in long-term care. Action of mucus and bacteria cause diarrhoea-like discharge which seeps around the faecal mass. If the rectum is chronically distended the anus becomes patulous and allows free passage of this and small pieces of formed stool. Hard (or occasionally soft, putty-like) faeces can be felt digitally in the rectum in 98% of instances. Treatment involves relief of the impaction, usually with a course of enemas (e.g. 7–10 days of a daily micro-enema) until the colon is cleared (this may be checked by plain abdominal radiography) and then care provided to prevent future constipation.

If the faecal incontinence is neurogenic in origin (i.e. a failure to inhibit rectal emptying), then management by induced constipation with planned evacuation (e.g. alternating a constipating agent with suppositories) may help keep incontinence under control. This, of course, requires meticulous

---

CASE REPORT

Mr F C was an 82-year-old resident in a Part III residential Home. A chronic schizophrenic, his usual behaviour pattern had been inactive and co-operative according to the staff. When this changed and Mr F C became noisy, restless, aggressive and doubly incontinent, he was referred for geriatric care, since the Home felt they could no longer cope with him. On examination he was found to be faecally impacted. The district nurse visited the Home daily and eight consecutive enemas were given before the bowel was cleared. Thereafter Mr F C became his old self again. Future problems were avoided by increasing his fluid intake and mobility, adding more fruit, vegetables and high-fibre bread to his diet and administering a dose of senna at night if no good bowel action had occurred in the previous 36 hours.

---

monitoring if problems are to be avoided, and a regime must be evolved to suit each individual.

MICTURITION

Disorders of micturition become increasingly common with age. Nocturia (rising at night to pass urine) affects most old people. Many also experience diurnal frequency, urgency and, between 10–20%, some degree of urinary incontinence (Thomas et al 1980, Vetter et al 1981). Between 16% and 19% of people in residential care are regularly incontinent (Masterton et al 1980), and in geriatric wards 30–60% of patients, with an average of 44%, are reported to be incontinent (Gilleard 1981). In psychogeriatric wards, complete continence has been found to be rare (McLaren et al 1981). Urinary tract infection is present in 17% of older people (Brocklehurst et al 1968) and up to 50% of those in institutional care. One in 10 men are likely to experience symptoms attributable to prostatic hypertrophy.

As with bowel problems, causation is often complex and multifactorial. Each patient requires a detailed assessment of his individual needs and problems prior to planning of care. Figure 12.2 shows a checklist which covers the different aspects of this assessment. An accurate chart will supplement and clarify this assessment and reveal any pattern to problems.

BLADDER DYSFUNCTION IN OLD AGE

Most people with urinary symptoms have an underlying bladder dysfunction. Indeed, in old age two or even three separate problems may be present in combination. It is important to obtain an accurate diagnosis, since the treatments are different. Usually a careful history and examination will indicate the cause, but if in doubt urodynamic studies are necessary to distinguish the bladder dysfunctions.

Detrusor instability

Detrusor instability, or the 'unstable bladder', is

Name:	Assessment date:
Patient's usual term for micturition:	
Daytime frequency:	Range:
Nocturia:	
Urgency:	Time of warning:
Urge incontinence:	
Stress incontinence:	
Passive incontinence (just wet):	
Nocturnal enuresis:	

If patient is incontinent:
  When did this start?
  How much is leaked?
  How often?
  What events cause
  incontinence?

Symptoms of voiding difficulty:
  Does patient experience bladder
  sensation?
  Hesitancy?
  Is stream good?
  Straining to void?
  Post-micturition dribbling?

Dysuria:
Haematuria:
Medical conditions which might
affect bladder:
Drugs:
Parity:

Any mobility/dexterity problems?
Observe toileting and comment on
problems:

Examinations:
  MSSU result:
  Skin condition:
  Rectal examination:
  Atrophic vagina or prolapse:
  Post-micturition residual urine
  volume:

Fig. 12.2 Assessment of micturition.

the commonest bladder dysfunction in old age, and may, indeed, be the norm for elderly people (Brocklehurst & Dillane 1966). The patient, usually because of neurological impairment (e.g. cerebrovascular disease), loses the ability to reliably inhibit detrusor (bladder muscle) contractions and so experiences urgency and frequency. If this is severe, or the sufferer is immobile, asleep or no lavatory is at hand, incontinence may result. This is treated most successfully by a combination of anticholinergic medication (e.g. imipramine 10–25 mg at night) and bladder training (see below).

Incompetent sphincter

This complaint is commonest for post-menopausal, parous women and may be associated with atrophic changes in the vagina and urethra or prolapse. It causes symptoms of stress incontinence (leakage upon physical exertion such as cough). If incontinence is slight, relief can be gained from pelvic floor exercises, with hormone replacement therapy if indicated. The patient is taught to interrupt micturition midstream to identify the sensation of a pelvic floor contraction, and then to practise this contraction on a very regular basis. More severe stress incontinence usually requires surgical correction, for which advanced age is no contraindication (Stanton & Cardozo 1980). Sometimes a vaginal ring pessary will produce symptomatic relief.

Outflow obstruction

Prostatic enlargement in men is the commonest cause of outflow obstruction. It may occur also in either sex because of faecal impaction or a pelvic mass. The patient usually experiences frequency and difficulty voiding. Residual urine may accumulate in the bladder and overflow incontinence usually presents as a continuous non-specific dribbling. Treatment involves relief of the obstruction.

Atonic bladder

If the detrusor muscle fails to contract for micturition, or if the contraction is not sustained until the bladder is empty, a chronic residual collection of urine may be present. This may become infected and lead to overflow incontinence. Common in both diabetics and demented people, this may be a feature of any neurological disease. The use of intermittent (in–out) catheterization to drain off this residual urine is widespread for younger patients with a hypotonic bladder. Its use for elderly people has not yet been widely reported, but initial results are promising. Some patients can be taught to self-catheterize in which case a clean, non-sterile, technique is taught; for others, a relative or nurse must do the catheterization. Some patients seem to regain detrusor tone with this management and resume normal voiding; for others, the intermittent catheterization must become long-term management.

Urinary tract infection (UTI)

The presence of 'significant' bacteriuria (commonly accepted as 100 000 organisms per ml of urine) is so high (Brocklehurst et al 1968, Milne et al 1972) that it must call into question the criteria of significance adopted for the younger people. Milne et al could find no symptoms clearly associated with infection, and Brocklehurst et al found that infection correlated with frequency and difficulty in passing urine. Neither study demonstrated a relationship between incontinence and urinary tract infection (UTI).

Probably the most useful way to treat UTI is to distinguish between acute and chronic infection. The patient with a sudden onset of the symptoms of cystitis — dysuria, pain, frequency, pyrexia and possibly confusion — should receive the appropriate antibiotic therapy. A chronic infection is often asymptomatic, will not respond to antibiotics, or will soon return, and should seldom be treated (Brocklehurst 1977). Routine treatment of UTI, regardless of symptoms or needs, risks the emergence of resistant organisms and should be avoided.

It is wise to remember that for older women, symptoms of atrophic urethritis may mimic cystitis. Inspection of the vulva will reveal if atrophic changes such as dry, inflamed mucosa are present.

INCONTINENCE IN INSTITUTIONAL CARE

Incontinence in residents in Homes or hospitals is often associated with multiple, undiagnosed and untreated problems (King 1979, 1980, Lepine et al 1979) which, if remedied, lead to restoration of continence for a proportion of residents. It cannot be overemphasized that an individual assessment is the crucial first step in any nursing intervention. If the resident is confused, a behavioural assessment is indicated (Maney 1976, McCormick & Burgio 1984). A behaviour modification programme, which rewards the desired behaviour

(continence) and gradually extinguishes the unwanted behaviour (incontinence) may be devised and is often successful if implemented consistently. (See Smith and Smith (1987) for a review of behavioural approaches to training.)

Promotion of continence

Where incontinence levels are high, there is much evidence that the situation can be improved considerably by the introduction of a more reality-oriented, therapeutic environment (Volpe & Kastenbaum 1967, Storrs 1982). Even without any specific elimination management, continence can be promoted, it seems, by motivating patients and stimulating an interest in life and activities. However, the difficulties of introducing innovative programmes to treat incontinence and motivating staff to comply should not be underestimated (Igou 1986). Much depends on the attitude and ethos of care and it should be remembered that elimination care will not be beneficial unless general care is individualized in intent and content.

Toileting and changing

Both Reid (1974) and Ramsbottom (1980) have studied toileting and changing routines in hospital, and describe the sacrifice of privacy and dignity to speed, with care delivered in a purely routine fashion. Ramsbottom concludes that 'care is not focused on patients' needs but on routines which might or might not be appropriate for each patient'. Nursing auxiliaries were observed to give most care. It is still common for a ward or Home to have toileting times (e.g. before or after meals) when everyone is toileted, regardless of needs. For some people whose elimination exhibits no pattern, this might be the best policy, but it is hardly likely to suit a whole group of people who are likely to have a variety of requirements.

Reid (1974) identified the ward environment as a major obstacle to better care once incontinence has occurred. The problem is particularly acute where an increasing number of patients are ambulant and spend a proportion of each day in a communal day area with no facilities for changing wet pads or clothes. This problem needs further attention and the development of nursing practices to cope with it.

BLADDER TRAINING

Bladder training is a very misused term in nursing. Many nurses claim to be implementing 'bladder training' when really all that is happening is that the patient is toileted at pre-set intervals, usually at times which fit the ward routine. This might train staff not to forget toileting, but does little to 'train' a bladder. Routine toileting at rigid intervals has a place for patients who have not responded to bladder training, and may decrease incontinence. Bladder training refers to a more specific management. The individual's own pattern of micturition and incontinence is carefully charted on a baseline chart and then individualized toileting times are devised to anticipate these needs. This may need to be frequent initially, and the interval may vary (e.g. more often in the morning after a dose of diuretic, less often in the evening). Gradually the intervals between toilet visits should be extended until a more normal and convenient pattern is restored. This training is most suitable for patients with detrusor instability and may be used in hospital and community settings. Careful selection of suitable patients is the key to success. A variety of other scheduling regimens have been reported (Hadley 1986).

MANAGEMENT OF INTRACTABLE INCONTINENCE

Even with the best available management and care, some patients remain incontinent. It is important that this is recognized as inevitable and that nurses do not feel guilty about it. The individual can usually be helped to maintain dignity and comfort in some way. The nurse should teach the patient, or her family, the most suitable management techniques, and she has an important supportive role in care.

INCONTINENCE AIDS

A good incontinence aid will enable the incontinent person to be socially accepted and to lead a relatively normal life. Despite the huge range and variety of aids now available (Association of Continence Advisors 1988), some function poorly. An aid must be carefully selected with regard to the individual's degree, type and pattern of incontinence, local anatomy, physical and mental abilities, personal preference, washing or disposal facilities, and cost. No one aid will suit everyone and a range should be provided (Fader et al 1986). The nurse must be the patient's advocate in this and be prepared to make a case for the supply of the most appropriate items. Ryan-Woolley (1987) gives a critical review of the major categories of aids and the literature relating to their selection.

Body-worn pads and pants

Most incontinent women, and some men, use a disposable, absorbent pad held in place by pants to collect urine or faeces. Sanitary towels are the most commonly used, but will not cope with any but minimal leakage. Plastic pants are undignified, uncomfortable and can cause considerable skin problems and should not be in routine use. The first alternative to plastic pants were 'marsupial' pants, with 'one-way' material and a waterproof pocket for the pad. These remain popular, especially in male and female styles. They are unsuitable for faecal incontinence, can be difficult for the manually disabled to use and many people do not like the idea of wetting their pants directly. Other pads are plastic-backed and held in place with stretch pants. All pads are only as good as the quality of their constituents and design. Gaining in popularity are the all-night body pads and all-in-one diaper systems for people with heavy incontinence. Some pads now have 'super-absorbent' gel to augment capacity. Most recently washable, re-usable pads and pants with absorbent gussets are available.

Male appliances

Some men are able to use a penile sheath or an

appliance in preference to a pad. A retracted penis or poor manual dexterity make their use difficult. A penile sheath should be carefully selected for appropriate size and is most satisfactory if a self-adhesive variety is used, or if held in position with a double-sided adhesive strip. It should be connected to a leg-bag. Appliances (e.g. pubic pressure urinals) should always be fitted by an experienced appliance fitter.

Bed and chair protection

Bedpads or underpads are the most commonly used incontinence aid in the Health Service. Ramsbottom (1980) has reviewed the literature and found no clear criteria or body of nursing knowledge regarding their uses. In clinical observation she found that many disintegrated, adhered to the skin or leaked, and in 54% of instances more than one was used, thereby cancelling any cost advantages. Nurses were found to put up with poor performance of aids and 'make do' with poor quality and quantity of supplies, having no channel of communication to express dissatisfaction. Bedpads do have their uses but are often expected, quite unrealistically, to cope with all incontinence needs. Washable bedsheets with a stay-dry surface have proved to be comfortable, popular and cost-effective, but in some instances laundry provision is inadequate to cope with them.

Nurses must consider more carefully the use of bed and chair protection, possibly refocusing care from protection of the environment to protection of the patient.

INDWELLING CATHETERS AND ELDERLY PEOPLE

Generally, the use of an indwelling catheter should be seen very much as a 'last resort' when all other methods of managing micturition have been tried and have failed. Widespread, indiscriminate use of catheters has fallen into disrepute, as has their use solely for nursing convenience (Crow et al 1988). A move away from catheters can be shown to benefit even severely incontinent patients in many instances (e.g. Brandberg et al 1980).

The decision to use a catheter should only be made for clear and valid reasons, with a definite goal which can be evaluated, and in full consultation with all concerned, especially the patient. The individual's quality of life should be the prime consideration — will the use of a catheter significantly improve independence, comfort and dignity? For some patients (e.g. someone with severe incontinence which is poorly controlled by an aid) a catheter can be a great benefit, even enabling community rather than hospital care. Each decision should be made on an individual basis and re-evaluated at intervals.

Managing a catheter

Many long-term catheters are poorly managed (Kennedy et al 1982, 1983). Confused, ignorant management and a lack of knowledge of the principles of catheter drainage were found to be widespread. For example, 30% of nurses said that they would increase catheter size if leaking occurred — the exact opposite of optimal practice. The majority of catheters (57%) were changed before their expected lifespan was reached, usually because of blocking or leakage. Only 10% of catheters were not problematic. It was found that smaller catheters were associated with fewer problems and this accords with advice from urologists that small catheters allow drainage of the paraurethral glands and there is therefore less risk of stricture or abscess formation (Blandy 1981). Small (5–10 ml) balloons are also recommended for routine use.

If a patient has to live with a catheter, drainage must be made convenient. For day use, a leg-bag or a bag attached to a waist-belt, garment holder or in a pocket inside trousers or a skirt will hide the urine from public view. Some systems allow direct connection of night bags to the bottom of day bags without breaking the closed system (Kennedy 1984b), which is a benefit in hospital although less vital in the community. The outlet tap should be simple to use and to understand, but many fail to meet these criteria (Kennedy 1983).

Patient teaching and individualized care will overcome many problems. The importance of diet, exercise, fluid intake, personal hygiene and avoiding constipation should be emphasized (Blannin

1982). Sexual function should be discussed, and if the patient is sexually active an alternative to an urethral catheter considered. Sometimes the patient or a partner may be taught to remove and replace the catheter, thus increasing independence. Individual solutions can often be reached for problems (Kennedy 1984a). Leaking may be caused by too large a catheter or balloon, or by an unstable bladder (which may respond to anticholinergic therapy). Routine washouts should be used only when a catheter is found to block persistently. Infections are almost inevitable with long-term catheter drainage (Hart 1985) and should only be treated if the patient is symptomatic (Brocklehurst 1977). If a catheter causes repeated problems, its use should be questioned since the patient may be better off without it.

COMMUNITY SERVICES FOR THE INCONTINENT PERSON

A variety of services are available for the incontinent person who lives at home. Male sheaths and appliances, catheters, bags and some deodorants and skin-care products are available on prescription from the chemist. District nursing services usually provide a range of absorbent products and waterproof sheeting (e.g. mattress covers), but the quality and quantity of such provisions varies greatly between health authorities. Most also provide loan of commodes and hand-held urinals, although this is sometimes left to voluntary organizations such as the Red Cross. District nurses may give help with personal hygiene, bathing and management of catheters and appliances.

Social service departments are usually responsible for aids to daily living, such as walking aids, grab-rails and modifications to the home (e.g. provision of a downstairs lavatory). Some departments employ community physiotherapists and occupational therapists who can suggest a range of aids to independence and teach relatives the easiest way of lifting and transferring if this is necessary. A home help may be able to assist with laundry. Some local authorities also provide a laundry service for incontinent people which collects soiled

items and delivers them back clean, and a soiled pad collection service.

Various financial benefits may be obtained by disabled incontinent people. Attendance allowances are available to those who need frequent attention from a carer in connection with bodily functions (the claimant must have been in need of care for six months). Social security offices can give advice on this, and on the Social Fund (loans for special needs) and the Independent Living Fund (help with employing carers).

THE CONTINENCE ADVISOR

With the recognition of the very positive role of the nurse in managing incontinence, the concept of the nurse specialist has grown. By 1987 approximately half of all Health Authorities in the United Kingdom had at least one continence advisor in post (Association of Continence Advisors 1987). These nurses have a very diverse role — from clinical casework and running incontinence and urodynamics clinics to teaching, research, acting as a resource and information centre, product development and appraisal, and supplies liaison (Norton 1986).

This role has not yet received comprehensive evaluation. The only study which has examined the role of the continence advisor did not demonstrate clear clinical or cost advantages (Ramsbottom 1982), but researchers admit considerable methodological problems, and 'improvement' in incontinence is difficult to document (Badger et al 1983). Certainly costs were increased as more people received services. A nursing clinic which offers advice to patients considered 'hopeless' by medical staff achieved continence for 10% of patients (Shepherd et al 1982). A similar clinic has been reported in the United States (Brink et al 1983), and it was found that teaching constituted a major demand on time.

Some nurses fear that a nurse specialist will fragment care. Continence is surely the responsibility of every nurse? In an ideal world this would be true, but it does seem at present that many nurses and patients can benefit from the expertise and teaching of a continence advisor. Nursing care can move towards its prime goal in this area — problem-free elimination for the patient.

REFERENCES

Association of Continence Advisors 1987 Index of continence advisory services. ACA, London

Association of Continence Advisors 1988 Directory of continence and toileting aids. ACA, London

Badger F J, Drummond M F, Isaacs B 1983 Some issues in the clinical, social and economic evaluation of new nursing services. Journal of Advanced Nursing 8: 487–494

Bass L 1977 More fiber–less constipation. American Journal of Nursing 77(2): 254–255

Battle E H, Hanna C E 1980 Evaluation of a dietary regimen for chronic constipation. Journal of Gerontological Nursing 6: 527–532

Blandy J P 1981 How to catheterise the bladder. British Journal of Hospital Medicine 25(7): 58–60

Blannin J P 1982 Catheter management. Nursing Times 78: 438–440

Brandberg A, Seeberg S, Bergstrom G, Nordqvist P 1980 Reducing the number of nosocomial Gram-negative strains by using high absorbing pads as an alternative to indwelling catheters in long-term care. Journal of Hospital Infection 1: 245–250

Brink C, Wells T, Diokno A 1983 A continence clinic for the aged. Journal of Gerontological Nursing 9: 651–655

British Standards Institution 1979 Access for the disabled to buildings. BS 5810

Brocklehurst J C 1977 Urinary infections: not all patients need treatment. Modern Geriatrics 7(3): 33–36

Brocklehurst J C 1978 The large bowel. In: Brocklehurst J C (ed) Textbook of geriatric medicine and gerontology, 2nd edn. Churchill Livingstone, Edinburgh

Brocklehurst J C, Dillane J B 1966 Studies of the female bladder in old age. Gerontologica Clinica 8: 285–319

Brocklehurst J C, Dillane J B, Griffiths L, Fry J 1968 The prevalence and symptomatology of urinary tract infection in an aged population. Gerontologica Clinica 10: 242–253

Connell A M, Hilton C, Irvine G, Lennard-Jones J E, Misiewicz J J 1965 Variations of bowel habit in two population samples. British Medical Journal 2: 1095–1099

Crow R, Mulhall A, Chapman R 1988 Indwelling Catheterization and related nursing practice. Journal of Advanced Nursing 13(4): 489–495

Exton-Smith A N 1972 Constipation in geriatrics. In: Avery Jones F, Godding E W (eds) Management of constipation. Blackwell, Oxford

Fader M J, Barnes K E, Malone-Lee J, Cottenden A 1986 Incontinence garments: results of a DHSS study. Health Equipment Information, No 159, DHSS, London

Gilleard C J 1981 Incontinence in the hospitalised elderly. Health Bulletin 39: 58–61

Gilleard C, Mitchell R G, Riordan J 1981 Ward orientation training with psychogeriatric patients. Journal of Advanced Nursing 6: 95–98

Godding E W 1972 Therapeutic agents. In: Avery Jones F, Godding E W (eds) Management of constipation. Blackwell, Oxford

Hadley E C 1986 Bladder training and related therapies for urinary incontinence in older people. JAMA 256(3): 372–379

Hart J A 1985 The urethral catheter — a review of its implication in urinary tract infection. International Journal of Nursing Studies 22(1): 57–70

Igou J 1986 Incontinence in nursing homes. Clinics in Geriatric Medicine 2(4): 873–885

Kennedy A 1983 Long-term catheterisation. Nursing Times 79(17): 41–43

Kennedy A 1984a Catheters in the community. Nursing Times Community Outlook 80(6): 51–55

Kennedy A 1984b Drainage system on trial. Nursing Mirror 158: 19–20

Kennedy A, Brocklehurst J C 1982 The nursing management of patients with long-term indwelling catheters. Journal of Advanced Nursing 7: 411–417

Kennedy A, Brocklehurst J C, Lye M D W 1983 Factors related to the problems of long-term catheterisation. Journal of Advanced Nursing 8: 207–212

King M R 1979 A study of incontinence in a psychiatric hospital. Nursing Times 75: 1133–1135

King M R 1980 Treatment of incontinence. Nursing Times 76: 1006–1010

King's Fund Project Paper 1983 Action on incontinence. King's Fund Centre, London

Lepine A, Renaut R K, Stewart I D 1979 The incidence and management of incontinence in a home for the elderly. Health and Social Service Journal 89: E9–12

McLaren S M, McPherson F M, Sinclair F, Ballinger B R 1981 Prevalence and severity of incontinence among hospitalised, female psychogeriatric patients. Health Bulletin 39: 157–161

McCormick K A, Burgio K L 1984 Incontinence: an update on nursing care measures. Journal of Gerontological Nursing 10: 16–23

Maney J Y 1976 A behavioural approach to bladder retraining. Nursing Clinics of North America 11: 179–188

Masterton G, Holloway E M, Timbury G C 1980 The prevalence of incontinence in local authority homes for the elderly. Health Bulletin 38: 62–64

Millard P H 1979 The promotion of continence. Health Trends 11: 27–28

Milne J S, Williamson J, Maule M M, Wallace E T 1972 Urinary symptoms in older people. Modern Geriatrics May: 198–212

Norton C 1986 Nursing for continence. Beaconsfield Publishers, Beaconsfield

Norton D, McLaren R, Exton-Smith A N 1962 An investigation of geriatric nursing problems in hospital. National Corporation for the Care of Old People, London

Parks A G 1980 Faecal incontinence. In: Mandelstam D (ed) Incontinence and its management. Croom Helm, London

Pollman J W, Morris J J, Rose P N 1978 Is fiber the answer to constipation problems in elderly people? A review of the literature. International Journal of Nursing Studies 15: 107–114

Ramsbottom F J 1980 Toileting and changing elderly patients in hospital. Unpublished Report Department of Geriatric Medicine, University of Birmingham

Ramsbottom F J 1982 Is advice really cheap? Journal of Community Nursing 5(11): 9–16

Reid E A 1974 Incontinence and nursing practice. M. Phil Thesis, University of Edinburgh

Ryan-Woolley B 1987 Aids for the management of incontinence. Kings Fund Centre, London

Schwartz D R 1977 Personal point of view. Health Bulletin 35: 197–204

Scottish Home and Health Department 1970 Geriatric accommodation report. SHHD, Edinburgh (Mimeographed)

Shepherd A M, Blannin J P, Feneley R C L 1982 Changing attitudes in the management of urinary incontinence — the need for specialist nursing. British Medical Journal 284: 645–646

Simons J 1985 Does incontinence affect you? — incontinence and self-concept. Journal of Gerontological Nursing 11(6): 37–42

Smith P S, Smith L J 1987 Continence and incontinence: psychological approaches to development and training. Croom Helm, London

Stanton S L, Cardozo L D 1980 Surgical treatment of incontinence in elderly women. Surgery 150: 555–557

Storrs A 1982 What is care? British Journal of Geriatric Nursing 1(4): 12–14

Thomas T M, Plymat K R, Blannin J, Meade T W 1980 Prevalence of urinary incontinence. British Medical Journal 281: 1243–1245

Turner R K 1980 A behavioural approach to the management of incontinence in the elderly. In: Mandelstam D (ed) Incontinence and its management. Croom Helm, London

Vetter N J, Jones D A, Victor C R 1981 Urinary incontinence in the elderly at home. Lancet 4: 1275–1277

Volpe A, Kastenbaum R 1967 Beer and TLC. American Journal of Nursing 67: 100–103

Wells T J 1980 Problems in geriatric nursing care. Churchill Livingstone, Edinburgh

Wright L 1974 Bowel function in hospital patients. Royal College of Nursing, London

CHAPTER CONTENTS

Physiological aspects of thermoregulation 201
Normal body temperature 201
Normal thermoregulation 202

Changes with ageing 205

Other effects of the cold on elderly people 206

Raised body temperature 207

**Measurement of body temperature in elderly
people** 208

Low body temperature 209
Social factors 210
Behavioural factors 211

Prevention 211
Money 212
Heating 212
Keeping warm 213

Early detection 213

**Care of an elderly person with a low body
temperature** 214

**Care of an elderly person with a raised body
temperature** 217

Conclusion 218

13

Maintaining body temperature

*Rosamund A. Herbert,
Miriam Rowswell*

The ability of elderly people to maintain a normal body temperature is one aspect of homeostasis that has been widely discussed over the past few years not only within the caring professions but also by the general public. It became popularized by reports of hypothermia and the effects of the cold on the old. We hear much less about the effects of the heat and hot temperatures on elderly people. Without a doubt, this over-emphasis on the problem of hypothermia has obscured the fact that by far the majority of older people maintain a normal body temperature throughout their lives. This is an example, perhaps, of how it is possible to get a misrepresentative — and an unduly pessimistic — view of biological changes with ageing (see Ch. 3). As always, we must consider the enormous variability of age-related changes from one individual to another. Most older people are able to maintain a normal body temperature under usual conditions; nevertheless, both severe cold weather and heat waves do lead to a considerable increase in mortality and morbidity among elderly people. This increased mortality is not due to a failure in thermoregulation, i.e. the body's ability to maintain a normal body temperature, but rather to other consequences of the heat or cold on the body's physiology. It is now generally accepted that the number of deaths from all causes provides a more valid measure of the effects of extremes of temperature on the elderly than simply the number of deaths (as revealed by death certification) due to hypothermia or heat illness.

More attention in the UK has been given to the effects of the cold on elderly people than to the effects of heat. There is an overall excess winter mortality of about 40 000 every year in England and Wales (Keatinge 1987). This increased mortality is particularly noticeable in people over 60 years of age. In the past these excess deaths have been associated with hypothermia, i.e. simple cooling of the body core until death occurs, but in reality the actual recorded deaths from hypothermia account for fewer than 1% of these excess deaths; deaths where there is any mention of hypothermia on the death certificate average between 500–600 per year (OPCS 1987). Epidemiological work shows that the excess cold-related mortality is due predominately to myocardial infarctions, cerebrovascular accidents (strokes) and respiratory tract infections (Bull & Morton 1978). Certainly, hypothermia is a relatively infrequent cause of death in elderly people.

Although hypothermia is an infrequent cause of death it has received much publicity and attention because it is in most circumstances considered to be preventable and, when it does actually occur, has a potentially poor prognosis. Brocklehurst (1973) reported up to a 50% mortality with hypothermia in the elderly, although the death rate can be higher if there is concurrent illness. Hypothermia is said to exist when the deep body temperature (for example, rectal temperature) falls below an arbitrarily defined limit of 35°C (Royal College of Physicians 1966). However, 35°C is not a physiologically defined lower limit of normality and problems can ensue from body temperatures that are low but do not reach that of the RCP's definition.

The prevalence of low body temperatures in elderly people is difficult to establish with any accuracy. Estimates of the extent of hypothermia have been made from surveys of the temperature of individuals being admitted to hospital, from surveys of body temperature in elderly people living at home and from mortality statistics. Each of these approaches has given different estimates, and values often differ widely as to the prevalence of hypothermia.

Initial estimates of mortality from hypothermia were high. Taylor (1964) estimated that the deaths from hypothermia each winter numbered between 20 000 and 100 000 among elderly people. This es-

timate was based on oral temperature measurements, which have since been shown to be unreliable indicators in cold conditions (Fox et al 1973a). Examination of death certificates from before 1979 is unhelpful, since hypothermia was not recorded as a separate category in the mortality statistics until 1979.

One study of old people admitted to the University College Hospital group in London found that 3.6% of elderly patients admitted were hypothermic; this survey assessed the deep body temperature of patients admitted during three winter months in selected hospitals (Goldman et al 1977). In contrast to this, a study undertaken at The London Hospital during January and February in which the body temperature of all patients entering the hospital as emergencies was measured, found that only three patients (all ages) had body temperatures below 35°C, representing 0.04% of a total 7579 admissions to the Emergency Department (Coleshaw et al 1986). This study supports other literature that says that the number of hypothermic patients admitted to hospital is small and those patients who are hypothermic are usually cold only because drink or drugs or serious illness caused them to collapse in cold surroundings (Keatinge 1987).

In the winter of 1972, two large-scale surveys of body temperature in elderly people living at home were performed (Fox et al 1973b). This involved a national random sample of 1000 elderly people aged over 65 living at home. Simultaneously, 1000 elderly people in the London borough of Camden were assessed and an intensive domiciliary and hospital investigation was performed on a subgroup of the Camden residents. Only 0.58% of the national sample (0.32% in Camden) was found to have a deep body temperature of 35°C or below. However, a significant number (9.5% of the national sample and 10% in Camden) were found to have a deep body temperature below 35.5°C. So these surveys did not find a high incidence of hypothermia in the elderly at home, but a large 'at risk' group with low body temperatures between 35°C and 35.5°C.

Findings such as these partly account for the large amount of attention that hypothermia received in the 1970s and early 1980s. However, further work has clarified the relationship between the excess winter mortality and elderly people: first, there have been refinements in the methods used to study hypothermia (some of the earlier methods almost certainly overestimated the occurrence of a low body temperature); secondly, it is now recognized that it is not hypothermia per se that is responsible for the majority of the excess winter deaths. Part of the complexity of investigating and studying the area is that many different factors are involved, including physiological changes with increasing age, superimposed disease conditions, and important socioeconomic factors.

An analysis of recorded monthly deaths in England and Wales for the years 1962–67 first showed the fundamental relationship between environmental temperature and death rates (Bull & Morton 1978), although the phenomenon was known about in the 19th century. The effect is most clearly seen in the population group older than 60 years. When comparisons are made between various countries with respect to cold-related deaths the UK fares particularly badly. Cold-related deaths amount to 12% of total deaths in England and Wales, 11% in Scotland, but only 4–6% in other countries investigated, e.g. France, Sweden, USSR, USA, Canada (Grut 1987). These figures demonstrate clearly the importance of factors other than biological ones in excess winter mortality. Standards of housing, the type and cost of heating, poverty and cultural factors have all been implicated. The 'Old and the Cold' has become something of a political issue.

Having put the subject of the effect of environmental temperature in perspective it is now appropriate to consider the factors that influence the ability of elderly people to maintain a normal body temperature under various conditions. Temperature regulation is an excellent example of homeostasis and, as discussed in Chapter 3, most homeostatic mechanisms function quite adequately in older people. This chapter will first consider the factors normally involved in thermoregulation and then consider the aspects that change with ageing. Physiological, behavioural and social issues will be examined. The last part of the chapter considers the appropriate nursing care and interventions for older people with abnormal body temperatures.

PHYSIOLOGICAL ASPECTS OF THERMOREGULATION

There are many factors to take into account when considering the possible susceptibility of older people to extremes of environmental temperature. Again, to emphasize a key point, many elderly people will never have problems with maintaining a normal body temperature. As discussed in Chapter 3, there are many variables that affect an individual's homeostatic capabilities; physiological fitness and training, diet, lifestyle and concurrent illness will all have a direct influence on an individual's thermoregulatory capacity.

NORMAL BODY TEMPERATURE

As discussed above, many factors are involved in allowing an individual to maintain a normal body temperature. It is essential to maintain a 'normal' deep body or core temperature for optimum function of the metabolic processes in the cells of the so-called vital organs — brain, heart, lungs, liver, etc. For instance, enzymes in the cells of these organs are very temperature-dependent; in contrast, the cells of the peripheral tissues can function at and withstand lower temperatures. So, regardless of the environmental temperature, homeotherms (warm-blooded animals) maintain a constant deep body temperature. This is achieved at the expense of quite wide variations in the temperatures of the peripheral tissues (sometimes referred to as the shell of the body) e.g. hands and feet. Deep body temperature varies with the site of measurement (e.g. rectal, oral) and is different from the skin temperatures recorded at the surface of the body. Thus each part of the body has its own temperature. Core temperature is normally in the range of 36–37°C, whilst the temperature of the skin and extremities is lower. For instance, oral temperature might be 36.8°C, skin temperature of the back might be 33°C and the feet 27°C.

There has been some debate as to whether the normal core temperature is the same in older people as in, say, younger adults; some initially suggested that core temperature was lower in the elderly, but the evidence is far from conclusive. So many factors influence the level of body temperature that it is difficult to attribute any temperature change to ageing per se. So, to all intents and purposes the normal range for core temperature of 36–37°C should still be used for older people, although you might expect an older person to have a temperature nearer the lower limits of normal. Getting a low temperature measurement should not be automatically explained by saying the patient is old.

NORMAL THERMOREGULATION

In order for the deep body temperature to remain constant in an individual, heat gain must equal heat loss. This is expressed in the first Law of Thermodynamics:

$$M = E \pm C \pm K \pm R \pm S$$

where

M = heat produced by metabolism
E = heat lost by evaporation
C = heat lost/gained by convection from the air
K = heat lost/gained by conduction from solids/liquids
R = heat lost/gained by radiation
S = term for heat storage in the body.

The ideal ambient (surrounding) temperature for comfort and thermal equilibrium for a person sitting down wearing normal indoor clothes is approximately 21°C; the temperature gradients, namely from core to skin and skin to air under these conditions are just adequate to transfer excess heat from the metabolically active tissues to the surroundings. Heat always flows down temperature gradients. If the ambient temperature is decreased and the temperature difference between the skin and environment increases, heat loss through convection and radiation increase. Thus the body ceases to be in thermal equilibrium. The opposite occurs if the individual is in a hot environment; then the body gains heat from the atmosphere by convection and radiation (and also by conduction if in direct contact with something hot, e.g. a hot water bottle).

Factors such as clothing and the amount of body fat will also affect heat loss from the body. It is generally believed that fatter individuals are better insulated than their thinner counterparts, but the importance of fat is unclear. It is probably of greater significance in water (e.g. the blubber of marine animals), since water is a better conductor of heat than air. Clothing is the most appropriate insulation for humans.

In order to maintain a constant and normal body temperature, a balance must be maintained between the heat lost and heat gained by the body. The main features of temperature regulation are shown in Figure 13.1. The major source of heat production is the body's metabolic processes: the chemical processes that provide energy for all the metabolic reactions in the body also produce heat. The blood circulating around the body then distributes the heat generated as a by-product of metabolism around all the tissues. If the metabolic rate increases, for example with exercise or diseases like thyrotoxicosis (the thyroid hormones directly influence the rate of metabolism), more heat will be produced in the body. In order to maintain a normal core temperature under these circumstances heat loss from the body must be increased — otherwise the body temperature will rise. It is simpler for the body to regulate the amount of heat lost rather than to alter the metabolic rate.

Thus there is a constant balancing act going on in the body: if the core temperature is elevated, heat loss mechanisms are necessary to restore the equilibrium; whereas if the core temperature falls, a combination of heat conservation and heat gain mechanisms are necessary.

One of the main ways that we regulate heat loss from the body is by varying the blood flow to the surface of the body. If we need to lose heat vasodilatation occurs, which has the effect of increasing blood flow to the periphery (the skin becomes red and warm) and heat is lost by convection and radiation because the temperature of the surface is higher than the temperature of the surrounding air and objects. If an individual needs to conserve heat within the body, a widespread peripheral vasoconstriction occurs, reducing blood (and hence heat) flow to the limbs especially (the skin appears pale and feels cold to touch); this has

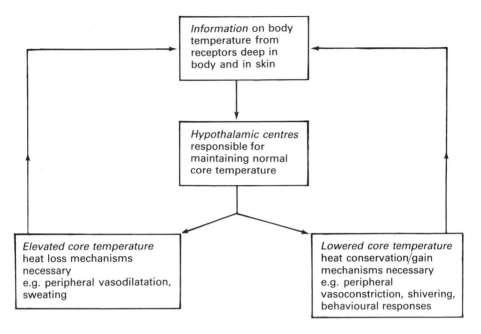

Fig. 13.1 Simplified diagram showing the main features of temperature regulation. Constant feedback is an essential part of maintaining homeostasis.

the effect of retaining heat in the core of the body as the temperature differential between the surface of the skin and the atmosphere is reduced. So less heat is lost. This vasoconstrictor/vasodilator response is described as the vasomotor tone and is controlled by the sympathetic nervous system (see Fig. 13.2).

The extent of the vasoconstrictor response varies from one region of the skin to another. For example, little change occurs in the cutaneous vessels in the head, whereas in the hands and feet there is considerable nervous control over the calibre of blood vessels. Appreciable quantities of heat can be lost through the head, especially in people who are bald or have thinning hair; hence the reason for wearing a hat in cold environments.

In colder conditions people will need to increase heat production as well as to reduce heat loss by vasoconstriction and this is achieved by increasing metabolic heat production. The simple response of clapping hands together or moving generates more heat as a by-product of muscle metabolism. Shivering is also a way of increasing heat production. Shivering consists of synchronous contractions of small groups of voluntary muscles which contract out of phase with other groups, so that no useful movements of the joints are produced — it simply generates heat. The shivering metabolic response to cold exposure is not great; for short periods a four-fold increase in metabolic rate can be produced and a two-fold increase can be maintained over a period of several hours. Ordinary dynamic muscular work is a much more efficient way of increasing metabolic rate, since the rate may increase tenfold or more.

Babies are unable to shiver (the nerve pathways that control the shivering response have not developed fully) and they depend on a process known as non-shivering thermogenesis (NST). NST relies on the high metabolic activity of brown adipose tissue or brown fat. The occurrence of NST due to brown fat in adults remains a contentious issue, although there is some evidence for brown fat in cold-adapted adults (Lean & James 1986), but under usual conditions brown fat is not thought to play a significant role in adult thermoregulation in the cold.

Sweating is an important mechanism in aiding

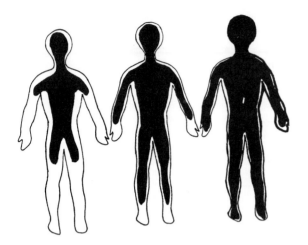

(a) cold environment   (b) neutral environment   (c) hot environment

Fig. 13.2 Diagram showing the relationship between vasomotor tone and environmental temperature. The core temperature of the body must be maintained between 36–37°C whatever the external environmental temperature. In cold environments the peripheral vasoconstriction 'reduces' the size of the core of the body (shown in black) and the size of the 'shell' increases (a); in hot environments the peripheral vasodilatation 'expands' the core of deep body temperature and the shell size is reduced (c).

heat loss from the body. The sweat produced in the sweat glands is passed by ducts to the skin surface and then evaporates from the surface of the body. In order to evaporate the fluid uses heat from the body (the latent heat of vaporization); thus heat is removed and the skin cooled. It is the evaporation of sweat that cools an individual — it is pointless to wipe off any sweat from the skin, say after exercise, since this will eliminate any cooling effects.

Of course under normal circumstances we do not rely only on physiological mechanisms to maintain a normal body temperature; behavioural and social aspects are important too. If we are cold we put on additional clothing (which is a good insulator) and this reduces heat loss from the surface of the body. We might also move around more, increase the heat supply to the environment (e.g. put on the fire) and have a hot drink. Eating in-

creases the metabolic heat production because the specific dynamic action of food (especially proteins) causes heat to be generated during the absorption and metabolism of the nutrients.

Conversely, if we are too hot we remove items of clothing and manipulate our environment appropriately; we also tend to move around less or move more slowly to minimize heat production, and to have an ice-cold drink.

The environment that we are in as well as our general fitness level affect our ability to thermoregulate. In a very hot environment an individual might gain heat through convection from the air and radiation from the sun. The presence of any air movement and the level of humidity affect our ability to lose or gain heat. If we are in an area with a breeze or draught, convective air loss from the surface of the body will increase as air warmed by heat from the body is constantly replaced by cooler air. If we are in a humid environment, the sweating response is less effective as the air is already partly saturated with water vapour and so less able to accept more water vapour from sweating; an extreme example of this would be in a sauna. Sweat gland activity is more efficient in fit people who take regular exercise since physical activity demands efficient disposal of heat; thus a fit person has in effect 'trained up' many of his or her heat loss mechanisms, e.g. sweating. In general the human body's physiological mechanisms are more efficient at coping with hot environments than cold ones; this is because man has, as it is believed, evolved in tropical climates. Water is a better conductor of heat than air is, and so exposure to hot or cold water in a bath or swimming pool will alter conductive heat loss or gain.

An inherent part of any homeostatic mechanism is the central monitoring and control of the system; receptors to detect the variable being controlled are essential in passing sensory information to the control centre. The hypothalamus is the 'control centre' for thermoregulation and sensory information is passed to the hypothalamus from the temperature sensors in the skin and deeper structures in the body. It is generally accepted that thermal information from the skin surface summates in some manner with that from the body core to stimulate integrated thermoregulatory activity. Information is also fed to the cerebral cortex to give the awareness and perception of body temperature. Temperature perception is important if an individual is to bring into operation the appropriate behavioural responses to aid temperature regulation.

Individual variability

Even in young subjects there is considerable inter-subject variation in response to heat or cold stress. For example, in the cold some people exhibit very good vasomotor control and others seem to rely on increased heat production to maintain body temperature. It has also been suggested that females have a greater reliance on vasomotor control and this is certainly observed in hot environments (Fox 1974). Differences between males and females may also be explained by variations in body fat and in the differences in quantity of metabolically active mass of the body.

CHANGES WITH AGEING

The factors that determine thermoregulation have been discussed in some detail so that the reasons why some elderly people may be more at risk than younger individuals can be clearly understood. Thermoregulation does not actually fail in elderly people but the potential for coping with extreme temperatures is diminished. This is in line with the general decline in homeostatic efficiency in the elderly when the body is stressed. With alterations in environmental temperatures the physiological responses of the elderly are more variable and body temperature oscillates between wider limits of internal temperature.

There are some physiological changes with ageing that may affect thermoregulation. For instance, vasomotor responses to the cold have been shown to be less efficient in minimizing heat loss in some elderly people, i.e. there is a reduction in the efficiency of the vasoconstrictor response. It has been suggested that some 20% of a normal

healthy elderly group do not constrict significantly on cooling (Collins 1987a). This reduced vasoconstrictor effect does seem to be an age-related phenomenon and may be due to autonomic dysfunction developing. This effect might be further exacerbated in people with arteriosclerosis (Collins 1987b).

Some elderly people also show a reduced metabolic response to cold stress when compared with younger subjects. Many factors interact. There is a smaller proportion of actively functioning cells in the elderly and so the basal metabolic rate (BMR) is slightly decreased; the BMR decreases significantly until the age of approximately 30 and then there is only a gradual decline into old age. Metabolic heat production in older people is generally lower because of reduced activity and a smaller energy intake (people may consume less protein or eat less in general). A few older people also suffer a degree of hypothyroidism, which will reduce metabolic heat production.

In some elderly people the shivering response is altered. Earlier work suggested that shivering was reduced or absent in the elderly; however, more recent work (Collins et al 1981a) has shown that shivering ability is not lost with ageing, even in those 80 years of age, but changes in the character of shivering do occur. The shivering is often less vigorous and a longer latent period is required to initiate maximum shivering. Detraining is probably a major contributory factor, as well as ageing changes in muscle cell function. Some work has shown that the older people who exhibited the 'best' shivering response were those who showed marked loss of efficiency in their vasomotor response to the cold; this demonstrates the adaptability of human physiology even in old people.

There is no evidence at present to show changes in the central nervous control of thermoregulation in elderly people. Some older people may be more susceptible due to the prescription of drugs that interfere with thermoregulation, e.g. phenothiazines, hypnotics, and some antidepressants. Alcohol has a marked peripheral vasodilator effect which tends to increase heat loss. Alcohol should never be given to anyone whom you suspect may have a low body temperature; although alcohol gives a general feeling of warmth it will tend to increase heat loss.

Sensory systems do become less sensitive with age (see Ch. 3) and a reduced ability to sense cold or changes in temperature may clearly put some old people at risk. Some elderly people do appear to have a blunted perception of temperature changes and thus do not experience 'coldness' until environmental temperatures have lowered below those that make younger people feel cold (Watts 1972, Collins et al 1981b). Collins et al found a deterioration with age in the ability to discriminate between environmental temperatures and this could contribute to the vulnerability of the old. Investigations of behavioural thermoregulation indicate that elderly people often lack the precision of environmental temperature control shown by younger people (Collins et al 1981b). If an individual lacks the awareness of 'being cold', he or she might not make use of the important behavioural adaptations to the cold and, for example, may not put on additional clothing or turn up the heating.

However, cultural or economic factors (such as the cost of heating) rather than a blunted temperature sense may cause some elderly people not to increase the heat supply to the environment. Similarly, it may be more difficult for some old people to increase metabolic heat production by moving around, due perhaps to arthritis or some other health problem. Financial or social factors, e.g. cost and living alone, may also limit the food intake and this in turn will reduce the diet-induced thermogenesis. Several studies have shown a link between undernutrition and poor thermoregulation in the elderly; thus undernutrition may predispose to hypothermia. It has also been suggested that there might be a link between undernutrition, hypothermia and fracture of the femoral neck in the winter months (Bastow et al 1983, Fellows et al 1985).

Added to these problems is the fact that many elderly people in the UK live in a poor standard of housing which stretches physiological responses even further. There is evidence of very low temperatures in the homes of the elderly and this will particularly stress an ageing thermoregulatory system.

In addition to the above factors, clinical or subclinical diseases present in the elderly, e.g. hypothyroidism and cardiovascular or neurological disorders, may interfere with normal thermoregulation if they decrease an individual's ability to respond to the cold. Prolonged immobility due to conditions such as arthritis, unsteadiness and postural hypotension will reduce heat production. If a person is less active this may lead to a reduced food intake and less diet-induced thermogenesis. Reduced physical fitness will also contribute to this vicious cycle. People with confusional states or dementia are also likely to be at risk.

The importance of these endogenous and exogenous factors is indisputable, but sometimes spontaneous hypothermia occurs that cannot be accounted for by these factors; in such cases, failure of the thermoregulatory processes themselves should be considered.

OTHER EFFECTS OF THE COLD ON ELDERLY PEOPLE

There are other genuine effects of exposure to the cold that can give rise to concern for elderly people and also help to explain the increased mortality and morbidity in cold weather. Being in a cold environment has other effects on the body besides challenging temperature homeostasis. For instance, it has a negative effect on dexterity; a low peripheral temperature leads to a loss of sensation which is especially noticeable in the hands and feet. There is a loss of manipulative ability, probably due to an increased viscosity of the synovial fluid in the joints (joints often feel stiffer in the cold) and increased muscle viscosity (Ramsey 1983). So the cold affects neuromuscular and sensory function and this would lead to an increased likelihood of accidents occuring, e.g. while getting up at night. It has been suggested that these changes contribute to the dramatic increase in incidence of fractured neck of femur that occurs indoors in winter (Lloyd 1987).

A seasonal pattern of blood pressure variation has been recognized for some time, with blood pressure being higher in the winter months (in the order of 5 mmHg for both systolic and diastolic pressures) (Rose 1961). However, experimental work with old people exposed to cold environments for a short period of time has shown that some elderly people have a greater increase in blood pressure than younger people (Collins et al 1985); there was also a strong association between the fall in deep body temperature and increase in systolic blood pressure. Raised blood pressure in the cold may have a long-term effect in the aetiology of arterial thrombosis and this may help to explain winter mortality from coronary and cerebral thrombosis. Keatinge et al (1984) have demonstrated other changes in the blood; they have shown that there is an increase in size and number of platelets in the blood, an increase in the number of red blood cells and a 20% increase in the viscosity of the blood during mild cooling. These factors together may contribute to the increase in arterial thrombosis in cold conditions, especially in people with atheromatous vessels.

It is known that exposure to cold has other effects on the body's physiology. Cardiovascular reflexes are initiated by cold air on the face and can result in a slowing of the heart rate and changes in blood pressure; these reflexes affect people of all ages but might precipitate illness in the elderly. Cold also places an additional strain on the heart and circulation by increasing the volume of blood circulating in the core of the body; this may in turn take a significant toll on unfit elderly people during the winter. Certainly, exercise combined with exposure of the face and extremities to the cold produces a number of cardiovascular responses that increase the strain on the heart and circulation.

As already mentioned at the beginning of this chapter, the high winter mortality is due to deaths from myocardial infarctions, strokes and respiratory disorders. The 'typical' pattern of illness is an increased incidence of myocardial infarctions occurring two to three days after a cold spell; strokes occurring after about a week and an increase in respiratory infections at about 10 days. The changes described above in the blood and the cardiovascular system are thought to account for the raised incidence of cerebral and coronary thrombosis. Exposure to cold air is also known to induce

bronchoconstriction and wheezing and it may also alter mucin production and depress ciliary activity. Immunological impairment in the elderly and the greater risk of exposure to bacterial and viral agents during the winter months together with these physiological responses might combine to render some elderly people more susceptible to respiratory tract infection and explain the trends that are observed in respiratory disease.

Thus the cold does have a potentially damaging effect on old people, even if not by hypothermia. It was initially thought that exposure to cold indoor conditions was the major problem. However, a study by Keatinge (1986) looked at the seasonal mortality in people who lived in homes with unrestricted heating (housing association homes where the heating bills were paid by the authorities). The continuous high daytime temperatures did not prevent the mortality among the residents from rising in winter by a percentage similar to that among the general population. Extensive outdoor excursions by able-bodied residents and the preference for open windows and no heating at night, provided their only substantial exposure to cold. The simplest explanation is that though the quality of life was higher with heated housing, the beneficial effects on mortality of the high indoor temperatures were balanced by the adverse effects of increased exposure to cold outdoors. The results of this study therefore suggest that the traditional tendency of the British to expose themselves to fresh air may be as important as poor heating in causing excess mortality during the winter.

RAISED BODY TEMPERATURE

Less work has been conducted on the effect of heat and hot environments on elderly people; the adverse effects of high environmental temperatures are not usually a problem in the UK, but have been observed in Australia and the USA. The excess mortality of elderly people during heatwaves is attributed mainly to an increased number of deaths from ischaemic heart disease and, to a lesser extent, CVAs (Foster et al 1976). While the high incidence of cardiovascular and cerebrovascular disease in the elderly is probably the primary cause of their enhanced vulnerability, impairment of thermoregulatory function may also be partly responsible. Foster and colleagues have shown a reduced sweating response in some of the elderly people tested which was especially pronounced in women. Other work has also shown this diminished sweat response, as well as a delayed development of vasodilatation on warming their elderly subjects. These changes reflect a deterioration in sweat gland or blood vessel function, possibly as a consequence of structural changes in the skin and/or changes in autonomic function. Impairment of the skin circulation is a considerable disadvantage since the physical routes of heat loss call for an increased surface temperature. Diminished thermal perception may also contribute to impairment of homeostasis.

An older person who develops hyperthermia or heat illness is at a disadvantage: the frequency of death from hyperthermia increases rapidly after the age of 60 years (Kenney 1989). The effect of high heat loads is cumulative, and the incidence of hyperthermia increases steadily as a hot spell continues. This progressive morbidity is probably due to failure to maintain water and salt balance. The increased demand on the circulation in heat calls for good vascular filling, and sweating requires the availability of large volumes of fluid. The older person may be unaware of the need or be incapable of acquiring the necessary fluid. The course of hyperthermia once initiated can be rapid. When the body temperature reaches 41°C, the central control mechanisms become depressed, and at this point the chemical reactions of metabolism take place at an increasing rate so that a positive feedback situation develops. In this phase the body temperature rises rapidly and death, usually from respiratory depression, ensues when it reaches around 44°C.

Perhaps more frequent is high body temperature occurring during a fever. Infection is a common problem in the elderly and it is often said that old people do not manifest a raised body temperature with an infection. It has been known for many years that the febrile response is diminished in elderly people and this may in part be due to ageing changes in the immune system itself. Part of the

problem also stems from the difficulty in defining the upper limit of normal body temperature in the elderly and also from difficulties in getting an accurate measurement of core temperature in older people. McAlpine et al (1986), however, maintain that with careful and effective monitoring pyrexia is detectable in the majority of infected elderly patients. It is obviously important to use, wherever possible, each individual as her own control, i.e. 37°C might indicate pyrexia in an individual whose normal temperature was in the range of 36–36.5°C. Certainly the extent of temperature increase may be less marked in older people, but older people do react like younger ones by developing fever in response to acute and chronic infections, neoplastic growths, deep vein thromboses, myocardial infarctions and other inflammatory conditions.

MEASUREMENT OF BODY TEMPERATURE IN ELDERLY PEOPLE

It is obviously important if we are concerned with temperature homeostasis to be able to measure core or deep body temperature accurately; measuring body temperature in the elderly needs careful attention. The most commonly used route is oral or sublingual measurement. Several studies have shown that this method can be unreliable in elderly people, especially if used to assess low body temperatures or in cold environments (Fox et al 1973a). A study by Sloan and Keatinge (1975) compared sublingual and oesophageal temperatures in subjects in various air temperatures (oesophageal temperature is often used for research purposes since it gives an excellent measurement of core body temperature). In warm air (25–44°C) Sloan and Keatinge found that sublingual temperature stabilized within 0.45°C of oesophageal temperature, but in air at room temperature 18–24°C they were sometimes as much as 1.1°C below, and in cold air (5–10°C) the oral temperatures were as much as 4.4°C below oesophageal readings. Thus caution should be exercised in the use of oral temperatures in cold environments. Indeed it is thought that some of the high incidences of hypothermia reported in early work was due to oral temperatures being taken. Another potential problem for some older people is keeping a thermometer in the correct place under the tongue for 5 minutes and keeping the mouth firmly closed.

A study by Nayagam et al (1986) looked at the best route for recording temperatures in older people. Nayagam et al compared oral, axillary and rectal temperatures. Oral measurements were taken in two ways: once by the nurses using their normal ad hoc timing method and once by the researchers with the thermometer left in situ for 5 minutes. The results showed that oral temperature was unreliable and would miss over 30% of fevers. Axillary temperature in the study was found to be higher and more consistent than ad hoc oral temperature recordings, but still error prone. The authors recommended that rectal temperature was the best method; they also said that the lack of fever with infection in the elderly is commonly due to faulty technique rather than the true absence of fever, though the temperature is often only modestly elevated.

So rectal temperature is still the method of choice if there is particular concern about the level of an individual's temperature and should certainly be the method used if considering low body temperature. Of course a low reading thermometer (range 25–40°C) should be used since the scale of the usual clinical thermometers starts only at 35°C.

One method that gives reliable measurements of core temperature and has been shown to be acceptable to older people is the use of urine temperature measurements with a Uritemp® bottle (see Fig. 13.3). This was used by Fox et al (1973c) and is simply a plastic container with a funnel in the top and a low reading thermometer placed inside. The funnel has some small holes in it to allow excess urine to flow through. Providing at least 100 ml of urine is passed the urine drains slowly through the funnel and the urine temperature is recorded on the thermometer. Since clinical thermometers have a 'kink' in the column of mercury, the maximum temperature is recorded permanently on the thermometer. So, for example, a district nurse could come and read the value at some convenient point later. The early morning temperatures are likely to be the lowest, since tem-

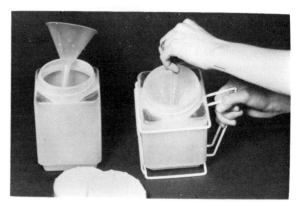

Fig. 13.3 The Uritemp® apparatus.

perature drops during the night due to the circadian rhythm, inactivity and possibly also unheated or cold bedrooms.

There is no easy answer as to the best route of temperature monitoring for older people and so a nurse should use a combination of methods (perhaps also monitoring room temperature) and other clinical skills to assess whether a patient has a normal, high or low body temperature.

LOW BODY TEMPERATURE

As has been suggested above, the development of a low body temperature in an elderly person results from a complex interaction of physiological, social and behavioural factors. Hypothermia as defined by the Royal College of Physicians (deep body temperature below 35°C) can be divided into primary and secondary hypothermia. Primary hypothermia occurs because of dysfunction of the thermoregulatory system itself. It is most frequently seen during the cold winter months but can happen at any time of the year. Accidental exposure to severe cold alone may also lead to primary hypothermia. Secondary hypothermia occurs as the result of concomitant illness or disability that renders the elderly person more susceptible to the cold. A survey of 100 consecutive cases of hypothermia conducted by Maclean and Emslie-Smith (1977) found that 85% were over the age of 60 years. Almost half the cases had been found lying on the floor after falling accidentally or as the result of an illness and few of the elderly cases had no predisposing illness. The authors concluded that hypothermia is uncommon in elderly people in the absence of any underlying disease or incapacity. The following section examines in greater detail how social and behavioural factors contribute to the problem of low body temperatures in elderly people.

SOCIAL FACTORS

There are currently about 10 million people over retirement age in the United Kingdom and the proportion of elderly people in the population is predicted to rise well into the next century, with the greatest increase being in the number of people over 85 years of age. A large number of elderly people live alone (currently about three million), often in large houses which were once family homes. Older people tend to live in older properties which are less thermally efficient and less well maintained. Scandinavian countries and regions of North America where extreme winter conditions are the rule have built housing that incorporates thick walls, window shutters, triple glazing, well insulated roofs and efficient heating systems. Insulation standards in many of these countries are much higher than our own, although housing built in the UK since 1970 has been found on average to be about 3°C warmer than properties built before 1914. Unfortunately, this has not benefited many elderly people and in 1986 it was reported by Age Concern that 60% of pensioners still occupied properties that had no loft insulation and that even more had inadequate draught-proofing. Many pensioners occupy privately rented accommodation and may have landlords who have not bothered to undertake renovations and repairs. Others, who are owner-occupiers, may have lost the inclination or physical ability to maintain the property themselves, or have lost their partner who may have been the one responsible for upkeep of their home. Many simply cannot afford the services of builders, plumbers, carpenters and the like.

Housing, fuel and food are the major expenses for elderly people and the cost of these may account for three quarters or more of their income. Pensioners spend a larger proportion of their income on fuel relative to the national average but this represents less in absolute terms because of their small pension relative to average earnings. Despite the fact that more time is spent at home and that heat is needed throughout the day it has been estimated that many old people spend less on heating in winter than families do in summer and live in cold environments. A national survey conducted in 1972 and reported by Wicks (1978) discovered that 90% of pensioners in the study had morning living room temperatures below the 21°C minimum proposed for old people by the then Ministry of Housing for periods when the outside temperature was −1°C. 75% of pensioners had morning living room temperatures of less than the 18.3°C minimum recommended by the Parker Morris Report on council housing, and 54% had room temperatures below 16°C, the legal minimum established by the Offices, Shops and Railways Act. These findings were confirmed by a later and smaller survey of pensioners living in the Glasgow area.

Many pensioners' homes are equipped with obsolete and ineffective heating appliances that are expensive to use. Most fuel costs rose steeply in the late 1970s and early 1980s; this has forced pensioners to economize further on heating in order to make ends meet, at the same time as they have grown older and become more incapacitated. Bedrooms, bathrooms, lavatories and passages are often left unheated and living rooms may be heated only intermittently. This situation may be very hazardous. Lloyd (1986) suggests that the warmth of the air in a room that is only intermittently heated may be sufficient to abolish vasoconstrictor activity in the skin whilst radiant heat loss to the cold walls may continue without the individual feeling cold. Falls in unheated parts of the home are then potentially disastrous.

In addition to shelter and heating in winter, to keep warm people need to eat well, have warm clothing and keep active. The intake of food at regular intervals during the day makes an important contribution to thermogenesis. A diet that is restricted by financial limitations, by the individual's physical difficulties in obtaining supplies, manipulating cooking and eating utensils or by disorders of the digestive tract, are all factors that will render the vulnerable elderly person more susceptible to the cold. Weight loss results in a reduction in lean body mass and loss of insulating fat and a relative increase in heat loss from the body surface due to a high surface-area : body-mass ratio.

Clothing worn by elderly people may deteriorate or be neglected for various reasons. There may be a reluctance to spend money on clothes if the budget is tight, and warm winter wear is relatively expensive. There may be a loss of pride in personal appearance, especially after the death of a spouse, and if the spouse was the partner responsible for maintaining and replacing clothing this aspect of self-care may lapse. In addition, it can be hard for older people to obtain items of warm clothing appropriate to their generation. Many have to rely on distant specialist stockists or mail order because multiple high street stores concentrate on the young fashion market.

Regular exercise is also an important way of keeping warm. To save on their fuel bills many elderly people spend longer in bed. This has the unfortunate effect of creating a vicious cycle of muscle weakness, reduced capacity for exercise and immobility.

Social isolation and distance from family aggravate the risk of hypothermia. With rising age, many elderly people become increasingly isolated. This may be due partly to physical deterioration but factors such as poor public transport, cost of travel on public transport, fear of being a victim of street crime and death of members of their peer group all contribute to an increasingly isolated existence. Neighbouring families may all be out during the day and social contacts may be few and far between. This can easily lead to situations where the early warning signs of potential hypothermia may be missed or overlooked.

BEHAVIOURAL FACTORS

Many elderly people have certain attitudes and beliefs which cause them to be reluctant to spend money on heating even when they can afford it. Such attitudes are notoriously difficult to change

and may be hard for carers of a different generation to understand or respect. The fear of debt is particularly prevalent and the concept of respectable debt relatively new. Many professionals caring for the elderly will themselves have mortgages, overdrafts and credit cards, but most elderly people have never owed money, and do not intend to start doing so.

Quarterly bills for gas and electricity may present difficulty to those on a weekly budget and fears about inflation and rising costs may increase levels of anxiety. It was much easier to see how quickly a pile of coal was diminishing than it is to work out how much gas or electricity is being used. In addition, coal was bought and used, whereas modern fuels are used and then bought.

Older people are proud of their independence and were brought up in an era before the welfare state. Many are reluctant to claim state benefits, preferring to live in impoverished situations relying solely on their state pension rather than engage with the bureaucracy of the social security system, which for these people still means the indignity of the means test and the stigma of charity.

Also prevalent amongst the older population are attitudes concerning the healthy qualities of fresh air. In the past, tuberculous patients were nursed in open wards and many people believe it is healthy to sleep in cold bedrooms and to keep windows open at night whatever the temperature outside. Electric blankets and duvets may be perceived as modern and new-fangled and offers to purchase these by family members may be resisted unreasonably. Such attitudes and beliefs should be addressed with sensitivity and tact; a sustained and strenuous public education programme targeted at older people is needed in this regard.

PREVENTION

The most effective solution to the hypothermia problem is to prevent it, and to relieve the worry and discomfort experienced by many elderly people each winter. It has been encouraging that since 1979 the number of hypothermia-associated deaths has declined.

It is important not to become complacent about the problem, especially when the winters are mild. Oliver (1983) reported the findings of a study by the Institute of Consumer Affairs that indicated that 87% of elderly people had never seen any of the numerous leaflets or pamphlets available which give advice about keeping warm or about heating problems. There have been subsequent campaigns by government agencies and voluntary bodies such as Age Concern and Help the Aged to rectify this at both the national and local level, through use of the mass media and through targeting groups working with and for elderly people.

There are three main ways of preventing hypothermia:

1. by obtaining as much money as possible for elderly people
2. by 'burning' that money as efficiently as possible to produce heat
3. by keeping as much as possible of the warmth produced in and around the old person.

MONEY

It is important that older people are kept aware of all the benefits and grants they may be entitled to and encouraged to apply for these (e.g. new arrangements related to introduction of the Community Charge). Age Concern produces an annual publication, 'Your Rights', and a Freephone helpline exists to give information and advice (0800 289 404). Income Support replaced the Supplementary Benefit in April 1988 for those with limited savings and a low income, and a Social Fund is operated by the Department of Social Security from which loans and grants may be made to meet special needs. In very cold weather pensioners on Income Support may be entitled to Cold Weather Payments to help with the cost of extra heating, although qualification for this varies according to local average temperatures.

Various budget schemes are operated by the gas regions and electricity boards to assist people paying for fuel. These include coin and token meters; stamps; weekly, fortnightly, monthly or flexible payment schemes; or, in the case of those on Income Support, direct deductions from benefits to clear a debt. All pensioner households are pro-

tected from disconnection between October and March by a Code of Practice operated by the fuel industry. In case of difficulty in meeting payment, it is important that the Gas or Electricity Board is notified as soon as possible.

Grants are also available to assist pensioners with loft insulation, the lagging of water pipes and tanks, and towards the cost of draught-proofing. For those who receive Income Support or Housing Benefit, this can amount to 90% of the cost.

HEATING

Insulation and draught-proofing are important ways of preventing generated heat from escaping. In addition to the grant aid provided for materials, a number of local community projects provide help with installation. Simple measures such as letterbox covers, heavy curtains over the front door, fabric 'sausage' draught excluders and blocking unused fireplaces can be both cheap and effective. Double glazing is very expensive, but curtains with thermal linings or temporary double glazing with plastic film, combined with aluminium foil behind radiators on outside walls will all help to conserve heat. However, it is important to remind pensioners that some ventilation is essential when using paraffin, gas, Calor® gas or solid fuel heaters. Economies on water heating can be made by ensuring there is an insulating jacket on the hot water tank and checking that the thermostat of the immersion heater is not set too high. Dual immersion heaters are useful, but expensive. Dripping taps should be repaired as soon as possible, and the use of a bowl for washing hands and dishes rather than a running hot tap may produce savings.

It is important that elderly people are familiar and confident with their heating appliances and the controls. Heating systems or appliances with thermostats are a great advantage provided the thermostat is allowed to control the temperature rather than being used as a switch. Equipment should be checked regularly for safety, preferably before the cold weather begins, and all open fires should be guarded. It can be very tempting to sit too close to a source of heat and old people should be warned about the dangers of this, especially if they were to fall asleep. Bedrooms should be heated in cold weather and for at least one hour before going to bed. Electric blankets or hot water bottles filled with warm rather than scalding water provide useful supplementary heat when going to bed. There are various types of electric blanket commercially available. Certain overblankets can be kept on all night and there is at least one very low voltage underblanket that can be kept on and which has the added advantage of being waterproof if occasional incontinence is a problem.

Thermometers can be helpful in monitoring room temperatures in rooms that are regularly used. In very cold weather, some elderly people choose to live and sleep in the same room to economize on heat. If this is done the bed should be kept away from the outside walls to prevent conductive heat loss. As suggested earlier, leaving parts of the home without heat is not the best solution because the possibility exists of a fall in some unheated area of the home.

KEEPING WARM

Hot drinks and meals have been identified as important for keeping warm and healthy in winter and for providing comfort. Meals on Wheels is an invaluable service and complete meals and convenience foods, though expensive, are nutritious and useful for those who cannot be bothered, or for those unaccustomed to cooking, provided they are dextrous enough to open tins and packaging. Pressure cookers, slow cookers and divided saucepans enable small amounts of food to be heated more efficiently. A balanced diet with protein, carbohydrate and fibre will help to prevent undernourishment and weight loss but food supplements and soups or frequent light snacks can be very helpful for those with small appetites. A hot drink left in a vacuum flask by the bed is often advisable to provide a warm drink in the night or early in the morning.

Any form of exercise, however leisurely, will generate heat and promote warmth. It is important to encourage elderly people to keep as mobile as possible and to avoid sitting for long periods. Even gentle exercises will help and jobs should be spaced out to alternate resting times with periods of activity.

Warm thermal underwear and several layers of thin clothes are more effective insulation against the cold than one thick layer. Natural fibres tend to be warmer than synthetics and an extra loose wool jumper may be as effective as a two degree rise in room temperature. It is particularly important for old people that they keep all exposed areas, feet, hands and head covered, especially if going outside. Even inside, bed socks and a night cap will help to reduce heat loss in a cold bedroom.

EARLY DETECTION

Vigilance on the part of formal and informal carers, friends, neighbours and anyone who even occasionally visits old people is an important part of protecting our elderly population from the effects of the cold. Hypothermia is notoriously difficult to identify because its symptoms are non-specific and its onset can be insidious and may mimic those of other conditions. It is essential that all who come into contact with elderly people in the community know what to look out for and are alert to cold room temperatures, lack of food in cupboards, heating appliances turned off, inappropriate dress for the ambient temperature, apathy and drowsiness, as well as hazards such as trailing flexes and poor lighting that might precipitate an accident in a cold house.

Ideally, it should be possible to construct 'At Risk' registers of the elderly. These would identify the very aged with multiple pathology, those receiving polypharmacy and those whose social history suggests they are at risk. This might enable better targeting of scarce community resources and enable community nurses, social services staff and workers in the voluntary sector to co-ordinate their work more effectively. For example, some local authorities, charities and housing associations provide alarm systems for elderly people, but the criteria for qualifying for these vary from area to area. Some of these emergency alarm systems can be extended to work automatically if sensors detect a low room temperature or if there has been an extended period of inactivity. These systems might be a valuable asset to an old person known to be at high risk.

Certain warning signs should alert carers to the possibility of hypothermia. These include:

- no complaints of feeling the cold even in a very cold room
- drowsiness and apathy
- slurred speech and a husky voice
- skin that is cold to the touch. This applies not just to the extremities but to areas that would normally be warm such as the abdomen, between the thighs and under the arms
- a puffy face that may appear pale or grey in colour
- apparent confusion and slow responses
- slow and shallow breathing.

Figure 13.4 illustrates the typical facial appearance of a hypothermic patient. This can readily be mistaken for myxoedema.

After summoning help, steps should be taken to warm up the room whilst avoiding subjecting the

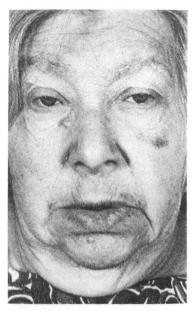

Fig. 13.4 Facial oedema of an elderly hypothermic woman.

elderly person to any direct source of heat such as a hot water bottle, a hot bath or a heater. Further heat loss should be prevented by wrapping her up well, including her head, in light coats, blankets or a duvet. If the victim is conscious and alert, then warm, nourishing drinks can be given but alcohol, which causes vasodilation, should not be given since this would increase heat loss.

As the core temperature drops, the vital organs become progressively functionally defective. Respiration becomes more difficult and is often wheezy, and gaseous exchange becomes increasingly ineffective. Eventually, respiratory arrest develops. The victim becomes confused and unable to respond sensibly, then lapses into coma, and may have convulsions and die. There may be tachycardia initially but, with increasingly poor cardiac output, bradycardia develops. Arrhythmias develop, the most serious being asystole or ventricular fibrillation, which cause immediate cardiac arrest. In the presence of other diseases such as chronic bronchitis, dementia, or ischaemic heart disease, the clinical effects may develop earlier, i.e. with relatively mild hypothermia, and cardio-respiratory arrest may be precipitated by cooling in susceptible people even before severe core hypothermia is established. Table 13.1 illustrates the effects of dropping core temperature even in the absence of other pathologies.

Hypothermia can only be diagnosed accurately by the use of a low reading thermometer; an elderly person with an oral temperature of 35°C or less should always have her rectal temperature recorded. Patients whose hypothermia is secondary to underlying disease may present with a mixture of signs and symptoms and it is essential to obtain an accurate core temperature in these individuals. Full diagnosis of their condition may be possible only after rewarming has taken place.

CARE OF AN ELDERLY PERSON WITH A LOW BODY TEMPERATURE

There is no standard treatment for hypothermia in the elderly person and careful consideration of each individual case is required, taking into ac-

Table 13.1 Signs and symptoms of hypothermia

RECTAL TEMPERATURE	SIGNS AND SYMPTOMS
37–35°C	Cold, pale skin Poor muscle co-ordination Shivering Hyperpnoea Piloerection Tachycardia
35–32°C	No shivering Cold skin Waxy appearance Puffy face Confusion Bradypnoea
32–30°C	Rigid muscles Dilated pupils Poor reflexes Low blood pressure Bradycardia Coma Convulsions
30–28°C	Flaccid muscles Bradycardia or tachycardia Fixed dilated pupils Atrial fibrillation Risk of cardiac arrest
28°C and below	Cyanosis Barely detectable vital signs Cardiac arrest

Table 13.2 Common investigations in hypothermia

INVESTIGATION	RATIONALE
Chest X-ray	To detect bronchopneumonia or pulmonary oedema
Abdominal X-ray	To detect severe gastric dilation and risk of aspiration pneumonia
ECG monitoring	To detect sinus bradycardia and atrial fibrillation. Often shows characteristic J wave
Arterial blood gases	To indicate degree of hypoxaemia
Blood cultures	To detect underlying septicaemia
Blood biochemistry	To assess fluid and electrolyte requirements, detect blood sugar abnormalities, renal impairment, etc.
Haematology	May detect haemoconcentration, raised white cell count, thrombocytopenia, etc.

count any known current disease and the degree of hypothermia. Although severely hypothermic patients may be mistakenly considered dead it may be ethically inappropriate to initiate intensive treatment in a patient who, for example, has obviously suffered a catastrophic stroke.

Previously healthy people with a mild degree of hypothermia (core temperature 32–35°C) may not need admission to hospital and may be gently and passively rewarmed at home under careful supervision (Collins 1988). A potential risk of circulatory collapse during rewarming exists and for this reason hospitalization should always be considered. Opinions differ as to whether hypothermic patients can be managed satisfactorily in general wards or whether they should be cared for in intensive care units. Wherever they are, it is important that they can be monitored closely with facilities to hand to institute rapid intervention should complications arise. Initial investigations that are required are shown in Table. 13.2.

To end this section, four problems associated with hypothermia are identified, together with their nursing goals and the actions designed to alleviate or prevent them.

Problem

Manifestations of hypothermia caused by low body core temperature (see Table 13.1).

Goal

The patient will suffer no further heat loss and rewarming will occur at a rate of approximately 0.5°C per hour.

Nursing actions

The patient is normally nursed in a room or cubicle where the room temperature can be kept between 25–30°C. Insulation from further heat loss is achieved by the use of light blankets or a duvet or a space blanket. If using a space blanket the patient should be placed on the silver side and swaddled. Lloyd (1986) suggests that space blankets may be disadvantageous because they are noisy and that this may increase confusion and restlessness in an elderly hypothermic patient. The efficacy of space blankets appears to be unproven and if the patient does not start to generate heat then the blanket is only insulating a cold body and should be removed. Whatever insulating covering is used, the patient's head must also be included, since this is a major source of heat loss.

Conservative rewarming methods with elderly patients appear to be more generally favoured than the aggressive active rewarming used with younger victims of accidental hypothermia. In some centres, rapid central rewarming techniques such as warm gastric or colonic lavage, warm mediastinal irrigation and peritoneal dialysis with warmed solutions have been used in intensive care settings. Miles and Thompson (1987) claim successful use of the Clinitron® bed for rewarming in two case reports and this may offer useful advantages.

Problem

Potential complications of rewarming, e.g. hypotension, hypoxia, pulmonary oedema, etc.

Goal

No complications will occur whilst maintaining spontaneous rewarming.

Nursing actions

Continuous rectal monitoring of core body temperature is recommended using an electronic probe. Respirations, blood pressure and pulse should be recorded half-hourly to hourly. If the pulse becomes irregular, if blood pressure falls or if the temperature rises too rapidly then the rate of warming should be slowed and the patient re-cooled until the vital signs stabilize. This situation occurs when cutaneous vasodilatation reduces the peripheral resistance, blood flows away from the vital organs, and cardiac output is unable to compensate. An alternative to re-cooling is to maintain the blood pressure with administration of dopamine. In addition, cold blood returning to the core from the extremities may produce an 'after drop' in core temperature and induce cardiac dysrhythmias.

Warmed oxygen at an appropriate concentration via a mask is frequently administered to correct hypoxaemia. A substantial number of patients require positive pressure ventilation because lung function deteriorates as a result of pulmonary oedema or because of the development of atelectasis, and it is therefore of importance to observe respiratory function closely.

The patient's level of consciousness should be assessed regularly and should steadily improve as she rewarms. Hypoglycaemia may also correct itself during rewarming, although in the case of hypoglycaemic diabetics or the severely malnourished, intravenous glucose may be administered.

Problem

Risk of pressure sores as indicated by assessment using Norton or Waterlow scale (see Ch. 14).

Goal

No pressure sores will develop.

Nursing actions

Hypothermic patients may have been immobile and lain or sat in one position for many hours with poor skin perfusion as a result of cutaneous vasoconstriction. Immediate action should be taken to protect their pressure areas. Use of a pressure support system such as a low air loss bed, Pegasus® bed, ripple bed or Clinitron® bed is advocated since any unnecessary movement of the patient can precipitate ventricular fibrillation (see Ch. 14 for further information on pressure sore prevention).

Problem

Potential fluid imbalance due to cold induced fluid shifts.

Goal

Arterial and venous pressures will remain within normal limits and urine output will be adequate.

Nursing actions

Since blood pressure falls when the body temperature is very low, water moves from the plasma to the intestinal compartments giving rise to oedema and to the characteristic bloated appearance (Fig. 13.4). These cold-induced fluid shifts often reverse spontaneously on rewarming and intravenous fluids are given based on individual requirements. If given, they should be prewarmed. Oliguria is not uncommon but diuresis should improve as the temperature of hypothermic patients rises. Passage of catheters to monitor urine output and nasogastric tubes to relieve gastric dilation and avoid aspiration of gastric contents has to be balanced against the risk of inducing ventricular fibrillation, and is best avoided whilst core temperature remains below 30°C.

Current practice suggests there are no indications for routine use of thyroxine or steroids although coexisting disease may need drug therapy (Maclean 1987). A broad spectrum antibiotic is usually administered prophylactically to treat overt or suspected bronchopneumonia.

If the clinical course of rewarming progresses favourably then recovery is likely. One or more complications indicate a poorer prognosis. Once the patient has been rewarmed, attention must be directed at discharge planning and establishing the home circumstances. Returning an individual who has been hypothermic to the same environment without adequate support or change in her situation will predispose to further attacks.

CARE OF AN ELDERLY PERSON WITH A RAISED BODY TEMPERATURE

When an elderly person develops a fever in response to some infectious agent or inflammatory process, then treatment involves management of the underlying cause as it would in a younger person, bearing in mind that the febrile response may be less marked. The principles of treating hyperthermia or heat illness are also the same for both older and younger patients.

Problem

Dehydration due to water and sodium depletion.

Goal

Rehydration and correction of fluid and electrolyte balance.

Nursing action

Whenever the patient's condition permits, oral rehydration with cold drinks is the preferred method since this is a more 'physiologically' normal route. When the patient is confused or unable to tolerate frequent drinks, intravenous rehydration will be required. This involves carefully controlled administration to ensure that the cardiovascular system is not further stressed by the rapid infusion of large volumes of fluid. Vital signs should be carefully monitored and the infusion rate varied accordingly. Urine output also should be observed as rehydration progresses to establish whether or not renal function has been impaired.

Problem

Impaired/ineffective heat loss mechanisms.

Goal

Heat loss will increase and body temperature will drop.

Nursing actions

The patient should be nursed in a cool room with the minimum of light coverings. Air movement can be created by use of an electric fan, air conditioning or other ventilation systems and this will increase heat loss by convection from the surface of the body. Further heat loss can be promoted by careful use of tepid sponging which will enhance evaporation of moisture from the skin. Body temperature should be monitored before and after this procedure and the patient observed closely to ensure that the shivering mechanism is not activated as this would be counter-productive.

CONCLUSION

This chapter has considered some of the important issues concerning temperature homeostasis in the elderly. Most elderly people are more than able to maintain a normal body temperature under most circumstances. Our emphasis has been on low body temperatures since this is a particular concern in the UK. However, health professionals should not forget other situations where the thermoregulatory systems can be stressed. For example, low body temperatures are a problem during and after surgery due to the mode of action of anaesthetic drugs and physical exposure. Even hot or cold baths could be stressors in some vulnerable individuals.

REFERENCES

Bastow M, Rawlings J, Allison S 1983 Undernutrition, hypothermia and injury in elderly women with fractured femur. Lancet Jan 22: 143–146

Brocklehurst J C 1973 Hypothermia in old age. Update Oct: 1019–1025

Bull G M, Morton J 1978 Environment, temperature and death rates. Age and Ageing 7: 210–224

Collins K J 1987a Physiological changes in the elderly predisposing to hypothermia. In: Maudgal D P (ed) Hypothermia: medical and social aspects. Pergamon Press, Oxford

Collins K J 1987b Effects of cold on old people. British Journal of Hospital Medicine Dec: 506–514

Collins K J 1988 Hypothermia in the elderly. Health Visitor 61(2) Feb: 50–51

Collins K J, Easton J C, Exton-Smith A N 1981a Shivering thermogenesis and vasomotor responses with convective cooling in the elderly. Journal of Physiology 320: 76P

Collins K J, Exton-Smith A N, Dore C 1981b Urban hypothermia: preferred temperature and thermal perception in old age. British Medical Journal 282: 175–177

Collins K J, Easton J C, Belfield-Smith H, Exton-Smith A N, Pluck R A 1985 Effects of age on body temperature and blood pressure in cold environments. Clinical Science 69(4): 465–470

Coleshaw S R, Easton J C, Keatinge W R, Floyer M A, Garrard J 1986 Hypothermia in emergency admissions in cold weather. Clinical Science 70: 93–94P

Fellows I W, MacDonald I A, Bennett T, Allison S P 1985 The effect of undernutrition on thermoregulation in the elderly. Clinical Science 69: 525–532

Foster K G, Ellis F P, Dore C, Exton-Smith A N, Weiner J S 1976 Sweat responses in the aged. Age and Ageing 5: 91–101

Fox R H 1974 Temperature regulation with special reference to man. In: Linden R J (ed) Recent advances in physiology No 9. Churchill Livingstone, Edinburgh

Fox R H, MacGibbon R, Davies L, Woodward P M 1973a Problem of the old and the cold. British Medical Journal 1: 21

Fox R H, Woodward P M, Exton-Smith A N, Green M F, Donnison D V, Wicks M H 1973b Body temperatures in the elderly: a national study of physiological, social and environmental conditions. British Medical Journal 1: 200–206

Fox R H, Macdonald I C, Woodward P M 1973c A hypothermia survey kit. Journal of Physiology Jan: 4–6P

Goldman A, Exton-Smith A N, Francis G, O'Brien A 1977 A pilot study of low body temperatures in old people admitted to hospital. Journal of Royal College of Physicians 11(3) 291–306

Grut M 1987 Cold-related deaths in some developed countries (Letter). Lancet Jan 24: 212

Keatinge W R 1986 Seasonal mortality among elderly people with unrestricted home heating. British Medical Journal 293: 732–733

Keatinge W R 1987 Hazards of cold weather. In: Maudgal D P (ed) Hypothermia: medical and social aspects. Pergamon Press, Oxford

Keatinge W R, Coleshaw S R, Cotter F, Mattock M, Murphy M, Chelliah R 1984 Increases in platelet and red cell counts, blood viscosity and mean arterial pressure during mild surface cooling: factors in mortality from coronary and cerebral thrombosis in winter. British Medical Journal 289: 1405–1408

Kenney R A 1989 Physiology of ageing: a synopsis, 2nd edn. Year Book Publishers, Chicago

Lean M, James P 1986 Brown adipose tissue in man. In: Trayhun P, Nicholls D (eds) Brown adipose tissue. Edward Arnold, London

Lloyd E L 1986 Hypothermia and cold stress. Croom Helm, London

Lloyd E L 1987 Cold-related deaths in Britain (Letter). Lancet Feb 14

McAlpine C H, Martin B J, Lennox I M, Roberts M A 1986 Pyrexia in infection in the elderly. Age and Ageing 15: 230–234

Maclean D 1987 Emergency management of hypothermia: a review. Journal of the Royal Society of Medicine 79: 528–531

Maclean D, Emslie-Smith D 1977 Accidental hypothermia. Blackwell Scientific Publications, Oxford

Miles J M, Thompson G R 1987 Treatment of severe accidental hypothermia Using the Clinitron bed. Anaesthesia, April 42(4): 415–418

Nayagam D, Shah S, Fairweather D S 1986 Which route for recording temperature in the old. Clinical Science 71 (suppl 15) 16P

Oliver C 1983 Old and cold. Nursing Times 79(43) Oct 26: 8–9

Office of Population Censuses and Surveys 1987 1985 mortality statistics — Cause. HMSO, London

Ramsey J 1983 Heat and cold. In: Hockey R (ed) Stress and
Fatigue in Human Performance. Wiley, Chichester
Rose G 1961 Seasonal variation in blood pressure in man.
Nature 189: 235
Royal College of Physicians 1966 Report of the Committee
on Accidental Hypothermia. Royal College of Physicians,
London
Sloan R E, Keatinge W R 1975 Depression of sublingual
temperature by cold saliva. British Medical Journal
1: 718–720

Taylor G 1964 The problem of hypothermia in the elderly.
The Practitioner 193: 761–767
Watts A J 1972 Hypothermia in the aged: a study of the
role of cold sensitivity. Environmental Research
5(1): 119–126
Wicks M 1978 Old and Cold. Hypothermia and Social
Policy. Heineman, London

CHAPTER CONTENTS

The skin 221
Assessment of the skin 221
Nursing management 222

The mouth 223
Care of the mouth 223

Pressure sores 224
The extent of the problem:
  pressure sore prevalence 225
Location and classification of pressure sores 225
Causes and predisposing factors in pressure
  sore development 226
Assessment of the patient at risk 228
Preventing pressure sores 231
The management of pressure sores 234
Evaluation 239

14

Maintaining healthy skin

Sally J. Redfern

THE SKIN

The skin, that most sensitive of organs, is the part of ourselves which is visible to others and which can reflect our emotions, well-being and state of health. The effects of ageing on the skin are regarded, particularly in Western societies, as negative, unwanted and to be avoided as far as possible. A tremendous amount of time and money is spent on skin and hair in an attempt to retain one's youthful appearance for as long as possible.

Normal ageing results in changes to the significant functions of the skin: protection, heat regulation, conveying sensation and body image, storage of water and fat, and absorption and excretion (see Chapter 3 for further discussion of physiological changes with age). All of these changes may affect an elderly person's comfort and the extent to which she interacts with the environment. If she also suffers from a skin disorder, then the effects of that, together with the perceived negative consequences of an ageing skin, may cause the old person to withdraw from public view completely.

ASSESSMENT OF THE SKIN

A careful assessment of the skin can give the nurse clues about a patient's emotional state and lifestyle as well as about her state of health. Physical assessment should include observation of:

● Moisture — dry, oily, sweaty, discharge (e.g. vaginal)

- Texture — smooth, rough
- Temperature — difference between trunk and extremities
- Colour and areas of discolouration (e.g. bruising, pigmentation)
- Thickness and turgor, wrinkles
- Oedema
- Blemishes — scars, rashes, soreness
- Infestation — head lice, body lice, scabies
- Areas of discontinuity — blisters, cuts, ulcers, pressure sores.

Skin lesions are common in elderly people and observation should be made of their location, their structural characteristics, their size, colour and grouping (e.g. in tissue folds, following nerve pathways). Skin lesions can be classified into primary and secondary categories (Carnevali & Patrick 1979). Primary skin lesions include non-elevated macules (such as drug rashes, petechiae, senile purpura, freckles), elevated papules, nodules and tumours (such as senile warts, neurofibromas, psoriasis, insect bites, basal cell carcinomas), and elevated fluid-filled vesicles (such as blisters, second degree burns, infected pimples and boils).

Secondary skin lesions can be crusts from serum, blood or pus (such as in impetigo), scales (as in psoriasis, exfoliative dermatitis), lichenification from excessive scratching (as in atopic dermatitis), erosion (as in syphilitic chancre), ulcers (stasis or varicose ulcers, pressure sores), scars (keloid or hypertrophied scarring), and atrophy.

NURSING MANAGEMENT

Nursing management of the elderly person's skin should be based on the nursing history and assessment. The aims of nursing care are to help the patient prevent skin problems, to maintain a maximum level of skin function and structure and to promote return to a healthy skin state. The common problems of elderly people with skin disorders are:

1. Discomfort from pruritis, pain, dryness, extremes in temperature, trauma.

2. A low self-concept of body image related to perceived or actual disfigurement.

3. Disruption of lifestyle as a result of the need for treatment, and dependency on others for assistance with treatment and coping with activities of living.

4. Systemic disturbance, such as fatigue, sleep loss, fluid loss.

5. Potential for developing complications such as infection, skin breakdown, depression. The likelihood of multiple pathology of the frail elderly, coupled with their slower recovery rates in comparison to younger people, means that their tolerance for additional stress will be low and they may be unable to resist further complications.

Skin discomfort

Generalized pruritis can result from oozing, weeping lesions such as eczema, pemphigus and localized excoriations (e.g. pruritis vulvae, pruritis ani), or it may indicate systemic disorders such as kidney disturbance, diabetes, anaemia, polycythaemia or barbiturate withdrawal. Such conditions require specific medical treatment, but if the main problem is pruritis resulting from dry skin, the nurse can do much to help the patient minimize discomfort. For example, soap removes protective oils and increases skin dryness (see Torrance 1983) and so should be used on axillary and genital areas only. A daily tub bath is unnecessary and water for washing should not be too hot. A non-perfumed emollient containing lanolin applied after washing prevents loss of moisture from the skin. Cotton underclothes are more comfortable to the skin than synthetics. The ambient humidity of living rooms can be increased with humidifiers to prevent skin dryness.

Discomfort also results from the relative inability of elderly people to cope with extremes in temperature (see Chapter 13, Maintaining Body Temperature). Action can be taken to promote optimum blood flow to the skin to maintain body temperature by attending to clothing, bedclothes and electric blankets, ambient temperature, avoiding the 'wind/chill factor' or excessive heat, adequate nourishment, fluids and exercise, and avoiding certain sedatives and tranquillizers (e.g.

phenothiazine derivatives) that depress cerebral function and circulation and increase the sensation of cold.

The elderly person has thin, fragile, inelastic skin which is susceptible to trauma and bacterial invasion. The nurse can raise the person's awareness of potential problems and can encourage actions to prevent trauma, for example:

1. Wearing protective clothing such as gloves for dishwashing and gardening.
2. Padding exposed body surfaces such as knees when gardening, using thimbles when sewing.
3. Avoiding direct contact with extreme heat or cold, such as hot water bottles, fires, radiators, frozen foods.
4. Avoiding tight clothing which can restrict circulation, such as tight waistbands, tight stockings or socks.
5. Keeping skin abrasions clean and exposed to air to allow drying, unless a dressing of some kind is necessary.

Low self-concept

Skin disorders can be unsightly and from ancient times have carried the stigma of physical and moral uncleanliness with subsequent self-rejection, feelings of guilt and unworthiness. Responses like these can increase the stress which underlies the condition and its severity might increase, and response to treatment decrease. Possible outcomes to such responses are raised anxiety and depression and insomnia.

Sensitive nursing care can be instrumental in enhancing a patient's self-esteem by, for example, touching the affected skin without wearing gloves (unless contraindicated), by looking at the patient without distaste or disgust, by talking with and listening to the patient and her family and friends, and by explaining to the patient and family the nature of the disorder, clarifying misconceptions, and encouraging them to help with the care required.

Disruption of lifestyle

Skin disorders can be extremely long lasting, debilitating and the focus of a patient's life if the treatments are time-consuming. The manifestations of the disease (e.g. pruritis, oozing, pain, depression, withdrawal), the treatments required (baths, lotions, creams, dressings), the systemic responses which may occur as a result of the disease or the treatment, and the effects of other disabilities of the old person (such as arthritis, immobility, loss of sight), all add to the likelihood of a way of life which is disrupted and which focuses on the skin complaint. The nurse can do much to encourage the old person to continue as far as possible with previous activities and social contacts, and to avoid isolation.

THE MOUTH

Oral problems commonly experienced by elderly people are edentulousness, dental caries, stomatitis and peridontal disease. These problems can lead to discomfort, a decrease in taste sensation, an increase in infection, and a reduction in nutritional and fluid intake. Saliva is necessary for oral health and factors which interfere with its production include mouth breathing, anticholinergic drugs and radiotherapy (McConnell 1988). Broad-spectrum antibiotics can lead to fungal infections such as Candida albicans, and trauma to the oral mucosa may result from badly fitting dentures. Peridontal disease such as gingivitis can result from vitamin deficiency and other aspects of malnutrition (see Chapter 11).

CARE OF THE MOUTH

It is not uncommon for old people to neglect their oral hygiene. Dental care is expensive and they may not have participated in preventive dental health care throughout their lives. The reduced manual dexterity caused by arthritis, stroke and other neuromuscular disorders make oral hygiene procedures difficult to perform. Depression, confusion and brain failure may impair judgement or reduce the motivation necessary for adequate self-care. Also, some old people may not appreciate the importance of proper oral hygiene, and may continue to believe that loss of one's teeth is an inevitable consequence of ageing.

A nursing assessment of the mouth should include careful inspection of the mucous membranes, the tongue, the teeth and any dentures, together with determining any dehydration, malnutrition or drug effects. Jenkins (1989) has developed an oral risk assessment scale similar to the Norton pressure sore risk scale (Fig. 14.1). Jenkins' scale considers the patient's age, oral condition, mastication ability, nutritional state and airway.

A considerable amount of nursing research has been carried out on the effectiveness of mouth care procedures, including the use of specific mouthwashes, toothbrushes and foam applicators, and the frequency of mouth care. No firm conclusions have been reached about the best mouthwash although lemon-glycerine has been criticized for its drying effect on oral mucosa, its lack of cleansing properties, and its tendency to decalcify the teeth (McConnell 1988). Similarly, lemon-glycerine swabs have been criticized. A toothbrush or a foam applicator seem to be equally effective but the swabbing procedure using forceps is ineffective and uncomfortable (Howarth 1977, Harris 1980). Harris concluded that a child's small-headed toothbrush is the best implement to use.

Adequate nutrition and hydration are the most effective means of keeping the mouth clean, moist and healthy. It is the person who is reluctant to eat and drink who becomes dehydrated and develops a dry, encrusted and dirty mouth rather than the unconscious patient. Such reluctant patients are likely to be found in elderly care wards and old people's Homes.

Sodium bicarbonate is an effective cleaning agent for encrusted mouths, but Howarth (1977) reported that patients find it unpleasant and so it should be used sparingly. Bocasan® and hydrogen peroxide are both mucosolvents, but Bocasan® can burn oral mucosa if inadequately diluted and hydrogen peroxide can break down normal tissues if used frequently (Jenkins 1989). Glycothymoline gives temporary refreshment only. Howarth found that glycerine, or glycerol, was used regularly for lubricating the lips, but although early nursing textbooks gave warning of its astringent proper-

ties, no mention of dilution appeared in any procedure sheet or later textbook that she consulted. As she pointed out, since cosmetics firms use 20% glycerol for moisturising creams and 40% for astringent lotions, it would be wise for nurses to do the same or to abandon glycerol for something less damaging, such as lanolin.

The available evidence suggests that the following regime is effective for patients requiring mouth care:

1. A child's small-headed toothbrush with either fluoride toothpaste or chlorhexidine gel, which is effective in inhibiting the development of dental plaque and gingivitis (Gibbons 1983). Harris (1980) recommended an electric toothbrush, each patient being provided with a personal brush head. Interdental gum massagers and dental floss should be much more in evidence (Speedie 1983, Jenkins 1989).
2. Tap water or sodium chloride solution at 0.9% (Jenkins 1989).
3. Vaseline® or lanolin for the lips, which are soothing and last longer than other materials.
4. Whole mouth brushing which should include the teeth, gums, palate and tongue and so is suitable for edentulous patients. Since over 80% of the population over 75 years do not have their own teeth (Sofaer 1979), nurses should encourage patients to brush their gums as much as they do their dentures.

This regime is more effective than traditional mouth care using swabbing techniques, and, as Gibbons (1983) observed, is cheaper than the packs issued by the hospital sterile supply departments.

PRESSURE SORES

Although pressure sores (decubitus ulcers) have been a constant plague for the debilitated and chronically ill since the beginning of recorded history (Bennett 1983a), the problem we now face is a relatively new one. With increasing numbers surviving into extreme old age, and with improvements in medical care which enable people to survive the multiple pathology and serious illnesses of old age, the number of those at risk of pressure sores has increased. The costs of a pressure sore to the patient are incalculable and the cost to the National Health Service is staggering. Fernie (1973) estimated this is to be £60 million per year, Scales et al (1982) put the figure at more than £150 million, and Exton-Smith (1987) estimates the hospital cost to be at least £420 million per year today.

More recently, Hibbs (1988) has calculated the additional cost of treating a patient with a fractured hip and a deep, gangrenous pressure sore. This patient spent 180 days in hospital at a total cost of £25 905.58, or £143.92 per day. The cost per day for the 'standard' orthopaedic patient at this hospital was calculated at £112.06, and the average length of stay was 10.9 days. The conclusion reached was that 51 additional days in hospital were required to restore the patient to health which could have been used by other patients if the pressure sore had been prevented.

THE EXTENT OF THE PROBLEM: PRESSURE SORE PREVALENCE

Comparisons among the prevalence studies which have been published are difficult because of the different populations sampled and methods used. A Danish study (Peterson & Bittmann 1971) showed a prevalence rate of 43 people with sores per 100 000 of the general population, and rates for patient samples ranged from 1.5% to 94% depending on type and location of patient (Torrance 1983) and definition of sore. In a one-day survey of two Scottish Health Board areas (Jordan & Barbenel 1983), the prevalence rates in the hospital and community patient population were 8.8% and 9.4% respectively. More recently, a survey in 132 hospitals in four health regions in England reported 961 patients with pressure sores, a prevalence rate of 6.7% (David et al 1983). This compares with a prevalence rate of 5.8% in hospitals within the Nottingham Health Authority (Nyquist & Hawthorn 1987). In a Swedish hospital study, Ek and Bowman (1982) found a rate of 4% but this was based on the total number of beds,

some of which may have been unoccupied, rather than on the total number of patients, and so the rates are not comparable. A recent review of the literature has suggested that between 3% and 10% of patients develop pressure sores during their hospital stay (Maklebust 1987).

What is clear is the association of pressure sores with age, with two thirds or more of patients with sores being over 70 years. Other related factors are level of consciousness, immobility, incontinence and medical condition. Cerebrovascular, cardiovascular and arthritic diseases as well as neoplasms are commonly related to higher pressure sore incidence. It is in the elderly care and orthopaedic wards that the vulnerable patient, presenting with a number of these interrelated contributing factors, is likely to be found.

LOCATION AND CLASSIFICATION OF PRESSURE SORES

22 unique types of sore were located on 17 body sites by David et al (1983), but over half the sores were found in the pelvic region and over a quarter on the lower extremities, notably the heels (David et al 1983, Torrance 1983, Maklebust 1987). These findings are confirmed by Nyquist and Hawthorn (1987) who found that 65% of the sores were on the sacrum, buttocks, hip or trochanter.

Various classifications of pressure sore type have been suggested (Berecek 1975, Torrance 1983), but the Type 1 and Type 2 distinction described by Barton and Barton (1981) is widely used. A Type 1 sore occurs when sustained pressure causes superficial blistering, and if pressure is unrelieved, it spreads into the deeper tissues to form a deep ulcer. The local blood vessels become occluded with erythrocytes and the endothelial cells of the vessels swell but remain intact. In the case of the Type 2 sore, damage starts in the deeper tissues and spreads up to the skin surface. The blood vessels are occluded with platelets and the vessels' endothelial cells become separated and damaged (Bennett 1983a). When skin breakdown is first seen, deep tissue damage has occurred for some time and a deep ulcer is inevitable. Either type of sore usually occurs over bony prominences where there is little opportunity for pressure to be dissipated through fatty tissues. The Bartons have also described a third type of sore, the inactive or indolent sore, which is unlikely to heal and normally occurs in dying patients.

The Type 1 sore shows a temperature difference of more than 2.5°C between the ulcer margin and adjacent healthy tissue, whereas the Type 2 sore shows a smaller temperature difference (about 1°C) and is much slower to heal. The totally inactive sore is cold and there is no or very little temperature difference between the sore margin and surrounding skin.

Many systems for classifying pressure sores are available (Maklebust 1987), one of which is the five grades or stages described by Bennett (1983a):

Grade 1a   Blanching erythema. Reactive
           hyperaemia causes a distinct
           erythema after pressure is
           released. Light finger pressure will
           cause blanching of this erythema,
           indicating that the
           microcirculation is intact.
      1b   Non-blanching erythema. The
           erythema remains when light
           pressure is applied, indicating a
           degree of microcirculatory
           disruption and inflammation.
Grade 2   Superficial damage — epidermal
           blister.
Grade 3   Dermal ulcer — whole skin
           thickness including necrosis and
           eschar.
Grade 4   The lesion extends into the
           subcutaneous fat.
Grade 5a   Involvement of deeper soft tissues.
      5b   Involvement of bone and/or joints.

This classification cannot indicate whether the sore is deteriorating or showing signs of healing. David et al (1983) attempted to overcome this problem by recording the presence of granulation tissue, scar tissue, scab formation, necrotic material and purulent smell. The more knowledgeable nurses are about the underlying pathology and predisposing factors contributing to pressure sores, the more

likely will they plan effective preventive and treatment regimes.

CAUSES AND PREDISPOSING FACTORS IN PRESSURE SORE DEVELOPMENT

The factors which contribute to the development of pressure sores are numerous and interactive, and although direct pressure is one of the most important, not every patient exposed to pressure will develop a sore. The healthy person can lie immobile for several hours without injury, yet a susceptible patient can develop a sore within an hour. This is because the susceptible patient is victim to several predisposing factors which together render him or her extremely vulnerable.

Direct pressure compresses tissues and if it is greater than the average arterial capillary pressure (32 mmHg), then the capillaries in this region are occluded and the tissues they supply are deprived of blood and the oxygen and nutrients it carries (see Maklebust's review, 1987). If the pressure is prolonged for more than about two hours, then a pressure sore will develop in the susceptible patient, although some patients, notably paraplegics, can develop sores in less than two hours. There is universal agreement that the principal cause of pressure sores is constant pressure sustained for prolonged periods (Maklebust 1987). Complications of pressure are shear and friction forces which can occur when the patient slides down the bed or is dragged up it. Shearing forces cause local vessels to be obliterated, kinked and ruptured, so forming thromboses and destroying the microcirculation, as occurs in the Type 2 sore.

The predisposing factors which increase a patient's vulnerability to pressure sores are often divided into intrinsic and extrinsic factors.

Intrinsic factors

Body type

The bonier body is more susceptible to pressure sores, but the obese, immobile patient who is difficult to lift is vulnerable to shearing forces and friction.

Immobility

Normally, excessive pressure causes discomfort and a spontaneous change of posture even during sleep. A healthy person changes position once every 15 minutes or so during sleep, and a reduction in the number of spontaneous body movements during sleep is directly related to an increase in the incidence of pressure sores (Exton-Smith & Sherwin 1961). Therefore, any condition which reduces mobility or the sensation of pain, such as paralysis, anaesthesia, clouding of consciousness, sedation, mental apathy or very poor physical condition, can contribute to sores (Berecek 1975).

Nutritional state

Malnutrition may be more common in institutionalized patients than is realized and increases susceptibility to pressure sores through devitalization of tissues. The nutrients particularly important for the prevention of pressure sores are proteins, carbohydrates, vitamins and minerals, especially zinc (Torrance 1983, Bobel 1987, Maklebust 1987). A negative nitrogen balance is associated with oedema and this renders the patient extremely susceptible to pressure sores.

Incontinence and excessive moisture

Norton et al (1962) found that 38% of incontinent patients developed pressure sores compared with 7% who were continent. The exact nature of the relationship between pressure sores and incontinence is not clear (Gosnell 1987), but wet skin or clothing and bedding can cause maceration of the skin and damage from friction on movement, and can reduce the resistance of the skin to ulceration (Maklebust 1987). It is likely that the incontinent patient is susceptible to pressure sores because of other factors such as immobility and neurological disease.

Increased temperature and infection

Pyrexia produces an increase in metabolic rate and demand for oxygen which will endanger existing ischaemic areas and areas at risk (Maklebust 1987). Bacteria further increase the demand on local metabolism for their own requirements and those of the body's defence mechanisms. And severe infection weakens the body's reserves by causing nutritional disturbance (Torrance 1983).

Anaemia and vascular disease

A reduction in the threshold level of pressure which tissues can withstand will occur with any condition which decreases the quality or quantity of blood reaching those tissues, and pressure injury is more likely. Thus cardiac disorders, anaemia, peripheral vascular disease and arteriosclerotic disease are important predisposing factors in pressure sore development (Berecek 1975, Crow 1988).

Neurological disease

Whether it is the disease itself or the consequent lack of sensation and mobility of patients with such conditions as paraplegia, multiple sclerosis, Parkinsons disease and cerebrovascular accidents, their susceptibility to pressure sores is well known (Maklebust 1987, Crow 1988). Other intrinsic factors are age and illness of any kind. Ageing skin loses its elasticity and subcutaneous fat and some muscle atrophy occurs. Furthermore, because of the likelihood of multiple pathology, elderly people are particularly at risk, for example, those with diabetes mellitus, rheumatic disease, orthopaedic conditions, muscle–wasting diseases, burns and renal disease (Torrance 1983).

Psychological factors

The emotional stress of illness and disability stimulates the adrenal glands to increase production of glucocorticoids. This leads to an inhibition of collagen formation and an increase in risk of tissue breakdown (Maklebust 1987).

Extrinsic factors
Skin hygiene

The traditional practice of washing patients' pressure areas every two hours as a matter of course is, fortunately, out of favour. Although frequent washing of the incontinent patient is necessary, overzealous use of soap and water can be harmful because protective oils are lost, the skin pH is altered, and dehydration occurs (Lowthian 1982, Torrance 1983).

Massage

Vigorous skin massage is another traditional practice which can be dangerous to vulnerable tissues, particularly where non-blanching erythema suggests existing early damage (Barbenel et al 1983, Torrance 1983). Dyson (1978) reported a reduction of 38% in the incidence of pressure sores in a group of elderly patients whose skin was not rubbed, compared with a group who received the usual pressure area massage. Post-mortem examination of tissues from the massaged group showed extensive damage compared with virtually none in the non-rubbed group.

Patient positioning, lifting and bedmaking

Patient positioning, lifting and bedmaking can contribute to pressure sore development if done incorrectly so that damage from pressure, friction and shear forces occur. These forces are particularly hazardous for the patient sitting up in bed, and tight bedding can completely restrict the movement of the debilitated patient.

Drugs

Any drug which decreases sensation or mobility can increase the likelihood of pressure sores. Thus, sedatives, tranquillizers, opiates and alcohol should be used with care. David et al (1983) reported that 41% of patients with pressure sores were receiving sedatives or narcotics. Prolonged use of oral steroids and anti-inflammatory drugs should be avoided because they delay the healing process.

The patient support system

The support system, be it a bed, chair, operating table or theatre or casualty trolley, can contribute to pressure sore development in two ways: its inability to distribute or relieve pressure on the body and its effect on the interface between skin and support surface. A hard surface increases areas of high pressure such as on the sacrum and heels, and the mattress or cushion cover can be so tight as to cause a hammock effect which increases the load on the tissues. This can be reduced by ensuring that the mattress or cushion moulds round the body yet is sufficiently thick to avoid 'grounding', where the body is not kept clear of the bed or chair base.

A soft surface is more likely than a hard one to distribute pressure evenly and reduce pressure sufficiently to avoid tissue distortion, but if the support is one of uniaxial rather than triaxial or hydrostatic loading, then tissue distortion can occur (Torrance 1983). Uniaxial, or one-directional pressure on the tissues causes stretching and compression of the blood vessels, whereas triaxial loading directs pressure on the tissues in three directions simultaneously, so avoiding damage to vessels.

The ordinary foam mattress of the hospital bed does not provide triaxial support; it is often too thin to prevent grounding, and the mattress cover may be too tight to avoid pressure from hammocking. In addition, the waterproof material of the cover and of pillows and drawsheets may have adverse effects on the skin, causing heat retention, high skin humidity and sweating. Thus the patient will be both uncomfortable and at risk of developing a pressure sore.

ASSESSMENT OF THE PATIENT AT RISK

The nursing assessment of any elderly patient should include a pressure sore risk assessment. The continuing dwindling of resources in the National Health Service makes it increasingly important for nurses to know with confidence which patients are at risk and where the resources should be focused. Assessment of risk can be done very

Table 14.1 The pressure sore risk rating scale (Norton scale). *Source: Norton D, McLaren R, Exton-Smith A N 1962. Reproduced by permission of NCCOP.*

A		B		C		D		E	
Physical condition		Mental condition		Activity		Mobility		Incontinent	
Good	4	Alert	4	Ambulant	4	Full	4	Not	4
Fair	3	Apathetic	3	Walk/help	3	Slightly limited	3	Occasionally	3
Poor	2	Confused	2	Chairbound	2	Very limited	2	Usually/urine	2
Very bad	1	Stuporous	1	Bedfast	1	Immobile	1	Doubly	1

Instructions for use
1. Score patient (1–4) under each heading (A–E), and total the scores.
2. A score of 14 or less indicates the patient is at risk and preventive care is necessary.
3. When sacral oedema is present the patient might be at risk even with a high score.
4. Assess the patient regularly.

Table 14.2 The Knoll scale for liability to pressure sores. *Reproduced by permission of Knoll Pharmaceutical Co., New Jersey.*

PARAMETERS	0	1	2	3	Score
General state of health	Good	Fair	Poor	Moribund	————
Mental Status	Alert	Lethargic	Semi-comatose	Comatose	————
			Count these conditions as double		
Activity	Ambulatory	Needs help	Chairfast	Bedfast	————
Mobility	Full	Limited	Very limited	Immobile	————
Incontinence	None	Occasional	Usually of urine	Total of urine and faeces	————
Oral nutrition intake	Good	Fair	Poor	None	————
Oral fluid intake	Good	Fair	Poor	None	————
Predisposing diseases (Diabetes, neuropathies, vascular disease, anaemias)	Absent	Slight	Moderate	Severe	

The higher the score the greater is the potential to develop decubitus ulcers.
Patients with scores above (12) should be considered at risk.

easily by nurses using one of the rating scales available, although the nurse should also use her clinical judgement in assessing risk since none of the scales have been shown to be completely reliable in identifying the susceptible patient (Barratt 1987, Crow 1988). The most well-known scale, the pressure sore risk rating scale (Norton scale) (Table 14.1), was developed by Norton and her colleagues (1962) over 25 years ago, and has only recently begun to be used by practising nurses. Girvin and Griffiths-Jones (1989) found that only 23% of 57 wards in their survey were using a risk assessment scale.

Although simple to use and becoming increasingly popular among nurses, the predictive validity of the Norton scale has been called into question by several researchers, particularly with regard to its tendency to over-predict (for a review see Taylor 1988).

Many of the more recently developed risk assessment scales are based on the Norton scale but include additional factors in an attempt to improve their applicability and predictive ability (Gosnell 1973, 1987, Pritchard 1986, Knoll 1982, Waterlow 1985). Poor nutritional status is an important factor in skin breakdown and its ommission in the Norton scale is a serious limitation (Barratt 1987).

The Knoll scale (Table 14.2) developed by Abruzzesse (1985) is more detailed than Norton's but also simple to use. It takes into account oral

Table 14.3 The Waterlow pressure sore risk assessment. *Reproduced by kind permission of Nursing Times, where this Scale first appeared in an article on February 18, 1987.*

Build/weight for height		Visual skin type		Continence		Mobility		Sex Age		Appetite	
Average	0	Healthy	0	Complete	0	Fully mobile	0	Male	1	Average	0
Above average	2	Tissue paper	1	Occasionally	1	Restricted/	1	Female	2	Poor	1
Below average	3	Dry	1	incontinent		difficult		14–49	1	Anorectic	2
		Oedematous	1	Catheter/	2	Restless/	2	50–64	2		
		Clammy	1	incontinent		fidgety		65–75	3		
		Discolour	2	of faeces		Apathetic	3	75–80	4		
		Broken/spot	3	Doubly	3	Inert/	4	81+	5		
				incontinent		traction					

Special risk factors:
(1)	Poor nutrition e.g. terminal cachexia	8		
(2)	Sensory deprivation e.g. diabetes, paraplegia, cerebrovascular accident	5	Assessment value	
(3)	High dose anti-inflammatory or steroids in use	3	At-risk —	10
(4)	Smoking 10+ per day	1	High risk —	15
(5)	Orthopaedic surgery/fracture below waist	3	Very high risk —	20

nutritional and fluid intake and predisposing diseases (diabetes, neuropathies, vascular diseases, anaemias) as well as general state of health, mental status, activity, mobility and incontinence. It also weights certain factors by doubling the score of patients with high (i.e. at risk) scores on certain factors. The scoring system is the reverse of that for the Norton scale, so that high scores (above 12) indicate that the patient is at risk. Some evidence has been found for the predictive ability of the Knoll scale, although its reliability increased when nutritional intake, fluid intake and predisposing diseases were removed as risk factors (Towey & Erland 1988). This is not to suggest, however, that these three are unimportant as risk factors. Rather, it seems more likely that their assessment is more complex than the simple ticking of a category required by the scale, which resulted in rater disagreement.

The Waterlow scale (Table 14.3) has been developed more recently, and is claimed to be able to identify a wider range of patients at risk than the Norton scale (Waterlow 1987). It takes into account the patient's build, skin type, age and appetite as well as mobility and continence. Special risks, such as factors contributing to tissue malnutrition, neurological deficits, drugs, smoking and major surgery or trauma are also included. Like the Knoll scale, the higher the score the higher the risk, and minimum scores for 'at

risk', 'high risk' and 'very high risk' have been identified.

The Braden scale assesses mobility, activity, sensory perception, skin moisture, friction and shear, and nutritional status (Bergstrom et al 1987a, 1987b). Each dimension is rated from 1 (least favourable) to 3 or 4 (most favourable) and the score range of the total scale is from 6 to 23. A score of 16 or less indicates pressure sore risk, although the authors recommend that each clinical area should determine its own cut-off point. The scale has been validated with elderly, medical-surgical and intensive care patients. Its reliability and validity are high and this scale is favoured over the Norton and Gosnell scales (Taylor 1988).

A more sophisticated technique for pressure sore risk assessment is thermography or radiometry which can detect temperature differences in the tissues and can identify damaged (i.e. relatively avascular) tissue before anything is noticeable clinically. A portable instrument was developed and tested by Newman and Davis (1981) and shown to give a precise and reliable indication of early tissue damage. Its use could be justified in clinical areas containing a high proportion of vulnerable patients.

Ultrasound has also been used to detect early tissue damage, for example at the Stoke Mandeville spinal injuries unit, and transcutaneous oxygen tension is a valuable technique for measuring skin hypoxia (Jakobsen & Christensen 1987). No doubt more sophisticated techniques will continue to appear, but nurses should use one of the existing rating scales which are simple and relatively unambiguous.

PREVENTING PRESSURE SORES

Preventing pressure sores for the patient at risk is a responsibility for all members of the care team and particularly the nursing staff who have the most contact with the patient. Relieving pressure on the patient is one of the fundamental aims of prevention and this applies as much to chairbound as to bedbound patients. In fact, the totally helpless chairbound patient might be at greater risk than the same patient in bed because body weight is not distributed over such a large area, and preventive measures are not applied so rigorously. Jordan and Barbenel (1983) found that 29% of totally helpless chairbound patients had pressure sores, compared with 9% of totally helpless bedbound patients.

Pressure-relieving or automatic turning beds remove the need for manual turning, but if these are not available or not indicated then the patient or nurse must take on the responsibility. Two-hourly pressure relief is the usual practice for patients at risk but individual needs vary. Lowthian's (1979) 24-hour turning clock is a simple aid which can be adjusted to the patient's needs and reduces the possibility of the care being forgotten (Fig. 14.1). It is also suitable for the chairbound patient who can be taught to shift position and do regular push-ups in the chair every 15 minutes or so. The obese hemiplegic patient may not, however, be able to do push-ups, and should regularly be helped to stand and gain balance, or be taken for frequent walks to relieve pressure areas.

Careful positioning of the body and limbs is important to prevent contractures and pressure sores where bony prominences touch each other. Judicious use of pillows and back supports can help and bed cradles can relieve the weight of bedclothes. Patients should be taught the dangers of pressure and to manage their own pressure relief regime as far as possible.

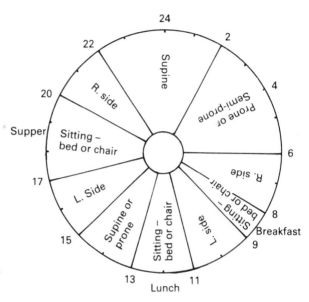

Fig. 14.1 Twenty-four hour 'turning clock' for a mainly bedfast patient at risk of pressure sores. *After Lowthian 1979.*

Nurses should be taught correct lifting techniques which ensure patients are lifted clear of the support surface. The shoulder lift is advocated for heavy patients (Scholey 1982) and is less back-breaking for the nurse than the standard lift, yet, in our experience, it is used less frequently.

A healthy nutritional state is essential for pressure sore prevention, and old people are more at risk from malnutrition than many other patient groups. There is evidence that a diet adequate in fluid, protein, iron, vitamin C and zinc sulphate is necessary to prevent tissue damage and promote healing (Abbott et al 1968, Moolton 1972, Taylor et al 1974, Guttman 1976, Bobel 1987).

Bearing in mind the dangers mentioned earlier of excessive washing of skin and vigorous massage of pressure areas, skin should be kept clean and dry, and massage avoided. The value of most of the topical applications used in the prevention of pressure sores is doubtful and astringents such as surgical spirit, alcohol and witch hazel can be harmful (Torrance 1983). Dry skins which have lost their natural oils will benefit from the application of oil-based creams, and barrier creams containing silicone or zinc can help prevent skin maceration of incontinent patients.

Preventing pressure sores involves attending to all those risk factors mentioned earlier which may be present. Without appropriate medical treatment of anaemia, cardiovascular, peripheral vascular and neurological conditions, and without recognition of the contribution of certain drugs to the development of pressure sores, the preventive nursing care outlined here will achieve little success.

Patient support systems in preventing pressure sores

The ideal support system for the susceptible patient should fulfil the following requirements (Torrance 1983, p. 29–30) and be comfortable for the patient:

1. Distribute pressure evenly to avoid tissue distortion and disruption of the microcirculation, or
2. Provide frequent relief of pressure by varying the areas under pressure
3. Minimize friction and shearing forces
4. Provide a comfortable ventilated interface environment
5. Be acceptable to the patient and not restrict movement
6. Not impede nursing procedures
7. Be easy to lift patients on and off
8. Be readily adaptable for external cardiac massage
9. Easily maintained and cleaned
10. Realistically priced

No support system available fulfils all the requirements. The effective ones are complicated to use and extremely expensive. Torrance (1983) has classified the numerous support systems available into four types: those which alternate the area of the body under pressure; those which reduce and distribute pressure evenly (moulding devices); those which assist or simulate normal movement and turning; those which protect specific body areas.

Devices which alternate the area of the body under pressure

The alternate pressure mattress (APM), or ripple mattress, is one with which all nurses are familiar and which operates by exerting intermittent high pressure on the body so that no part of the body is continuously under high pressure. The original small-cell APM has been shown to be ineffective in preventing pressure sores, but the large-cell APM is effective if it is working properly and used in conjunction with a regular turning regime (Bliss et al 1967, Jakobsen & Christensen 1987). It is often the case that APMs are incorrectly installed or are faulty, and even though the red warning light is on, no action is taken by the nurses. This can be extremely dangerous for the patient.

Other types of APM are available, some with longitudinal cells or 'bubble' pads, but the only one which will be mentioned here is the Pegasus® air wave system. This is similar in principle to the ripple mattress except that there are two layers of air cells and every third cell is deflated in turn. The mattress is ventilated by pinholes through which air passes and is dispersed around the patient. The air wave system (AWS) has been shown to be more effective than the large-cell ripple mattress in preventing pressure sores and reducing the severity of existing sores (Exton-Smith et al 1982). The AWS did not break down during the trial, whereas the ripple mattresses did on several occasions.

Pillows or foam blocks can be placed strategically on an ordinary mattress so that there are gaps at pressure points. This can be effective if used with regular turning, but pressure and shear stresses are relatively high on either side of each gap.

Devices which reduce and distribute pressure evenly

These surfaces mould themselves to the body contours, so reducing any points of high pressure. They tend to be fairly sophisticated devices which must have sufficient volume to displace the patient's weight without 'grounding', and have an enveloping membrane which is not so tight that it causes 'hammocking'. They also aim to provide triaxial rather than uniaxial loading so avoiding tissue distortion.

Examples of these systems are cut foam mattresses, water beds which achieve true flotation, the Clinitron® air-fluidized bed (SSI) and the low air loss bed system (Mediscus, SSI). Many of these beds have been subjected to fairly rigorous research trials and found to be effective in preventing and treating pressure sores (Kenedi et al 1976), but the most efficient systems tend to be complicated, cumbersome and expensive. The cost, however, pales to insignificance if it is compared with the cost to the patient and to the National Health Service of treating pressure sores.

The Slumberland Vaperm® patient support system has been developed at the Royal National Orthopaedic Hospital, Stanmore (Lowthian 1983, Scales et al 1982). It consists of five densities of fatigue-resistant polyurethane foam and has pressure-relieving channels inside the foam at vulnerable body sites such as the sacrum and heels. It is claimed to be effective in preventing pressure sores and in providing a compatible dry micro-climate between the skin and mattress because the covering material is waterproof but permeable to water vapour.

Measuring the interface pressure between the skin and the support surface using pressure transducers is recommended before a new and often expensive patient support system is introduced (Exton-Smith 1987, Clark 1988). Interface pressures have been compared between different support systems using healthy volunteers as subjects. The Mediscus® low air loss bed and feather pillows on a foam mattress produced significantly lower surface pressures than the interior sprung hospital mattress, the foam mattress on a linked spring base, a water bed, operating tables and the floor (Redfern et al 1973). Marshall and Overstall (1983) recommended the Nuclea® foam mattress over the standard foam mattress, the Talley® ripple mattress, two water beds, the Mecabed® net suspension bed and the Spenco Silicore® bed-pad. The Nuclea® foam mattress is a relatively cheap system which combines the properties of water and foam. Maklebust and her colleagues reported interface pressures below 32 mmHg for an air-fluidized bed, a low air loss bed and a three-layered air cushion (Maklebust 1987).

Jakobsen and Christensen (1987) compared transcutaneous oxygen tension ($tcPO_2$) over the sacrum of volunteers lying on different support systems. They found the $tcPO_2$ was significantly lower for the standard sprung mattress compared with all the others, and resulted in total anoxia for most of the subjects. The best mattresses were the Talley® ripple mattress (when cell deflated) and the Spenco Silicore® bed-pad, both of which gave significantly higher $tcPO_2$ readings (greater oxygenation) than a water mattress, an artificial sheepskin and the sprung mattress.

The research outlined here is limited in its applicability because not all support surfaces have been tested in comparative studies, nor have patients at risk from pressure sores been included as subjects.

Devices which assist or simulate normal movement and turning

The main feature of these systems is that they help the nurse or patient to relieve pressure by assisted turning. Simple devices are the overhead hand-grip, handblocks for the patient to lift herself clear of the bed, and the rope ladder fixed to the end of the bed with which the patient can pull herself forward. Other systems assist turning with manual, electric or automatic controls. The Co-Ro® constant turning bed automatically turns the patient from side to side 15 times an hour. The Egerton® tilting and turning bed and the Stryker Circo-electric® bed have attendant-controlled electric motors which assist in turning. Net suspension beds (Mecabed®, Egerton®) are open-mesh nylon hammocks in which the patient can be turned very easily by one nurse operating two handles.

Devices which protect specific body areas

These devices include pads, fleeces, cushions and heel, elbow and sacral protectors. Natural and artificial fleeces are extremely popular; they are soft and comfortable and keep the skin dry. They are not, however, very effective in relieving pressure and avoiding tissue distortion and they can have very high friction values (Lowthian 1983). Laundering was a problem with early products but modern fleeces wash well as long as the manufacturers' instructions are followed. In a comparison of 11 natural and synthetic fleeces, Denne (1983) found the synthetic fleece Mullipel® to be the best in terms of accommodation depth, laundering and degree of matting. However, in an earlier study, Denne (1979) concluded that natural fleeces were more effective than synthetics in reducing friction and in keeping the skin dry; and so the decision on what to buy is not easy.

Numerous pads and cushions are on the market, such as foam, siliconized hollow fibres, bead, gel, water, air alternating pressure cushions and mixtures (e.g. gel or water and foam). It is important that the cushion is fitted to the patient and chair or wheelchair in which it will be used. The occupational therapy department in hospitals can give nurses and patients advice on wheelchair adaptation and maintenance, and a comprehensive book has been published by the Royal Association for Disability and Rehabilitation (RADAR) on choosing the best wheelchair cushion to suit individual needs (Jay 1983). Most cushions are unable to relieve pressure to such an extent that manual pressure relief is unnecessary, and the cushion cover may reduce the efficiency of the cushion's pressure distribution properties. Thus pressure relief is still necessary by patients doing regular push-ups or being helped to stand and walk where possible.

There are a number of sacral, elbow and heel protectors available made of foam, gel, siliconized hollow fibres, air padding and bandages. It is unlikely that these make a great contribution to the prevention of pressure sores, and some may be harmful by restricting the blood supply, such as the heel 'doughnut' made from bandages (Lowthian 1983). There is no doubt that with high quality nursing care more pressure sores can be prevented. The bewildering array of aids on the market for preventing and treating pressure sores makes choosing what is best in terms of cost and effectiveness very difficult. More valid evaluative research is required and should be used by the

health team to make an informed choice on what to buy. So often a bulk order for a piece of equipment is continued unquestioningly without thought for new developments which may be cheaper and more effective. The ubiquitous ripple mattress is a case in point.

Very few of the aids available remove totally the need for continued preventive care by nurses. Most, at best, reduce the frequency with which pressure relief is required, and if nurses do not appreciate the principles on which the device works and its limitations, then the patient is in considerable danger.

THE MANAGEMENT OF PRESSURE SORES

Meticulous attention to preventive care, both systemic and local, can avoid the development of pressure sores for most patients. However, in the case of inactive sores, which almost always occur in the terminally ill, nothing is likely to be effective, and nursing care should focus on the promotion of comfort even if this means that the patient lies or sits directly on the sore.

Management of the patient with pressure sores must focus on pressure relief, removing and avoiding predisposing factors, and wound care. Relief of pressure has been discussed in some detail already, and general management should focus on the predisposing factors mentioned earlier. For example, the medical condition of the patient should be stabilized, anaemia treated with blood transfusion if severe, oedema removed with diuretics, systemic infection treated with antibiotics, and incontinence investigated and treated. A balanced fluid and nutritional intake is essential, with supplements of protein, vitamin C, iron and zinc where necessary. Drugs should be prescribed cautiously and if possible, those known to delay healing, such as corticosteroids and anti-inflammatory drugs avoided.

Assessment of pressure sores

It is impossible to judge the rate of healing or deterioration of a wound or the effectiveness of local treatments without an assessment of the size and severity of the sore. The difficulty in finding a valid method of measuring sore size and healing rate has dogged many researchers who have attempted to evaluate local treatments. Techniques used include measurement of wound diameters, tracing the sore outline on transparent film, photographing the sore against a centimetre measure, using a computer-aided photographic method (Anthony & Barnes 1984), or using thermography. These measures cannot document changes in wound volume or in the general state of the wound (degree of smell, pus, inflammation, necrosis, etc.). Some researchers have attempted to solve this by developing complex rating scales or calculating 'healing indices', which, for example, measure wound size in relation to days of healing. Others have measured wound volume with dental impression-making material; the Silastic Foam Dressing® (Dow Corning) used to dress deep, granulating wounds; a 'profilometer'; tomography; or stereophotogrammetry (Anthony 1987). These are sophisticated techniques more suitable for research in which accurate measurement is important. The nurse needs a simple, easy-to-use assessment technique which is reasonably valid. The sore outline traced on transparent film provides a useful guide to healing if done regularly (say, weekly) and filed in sequence in the patient's notes.

Wound healing

Intense cellular and biochemical activity occur during the process of wound healing in which there are four stages of repair (Westaby 1981a): traumatic inflammation (0–3 days), destructive phase (1–6 days), proliferative phase (3–24 days), maturation phase (24 days–1 year). Two mechanisms which are extremely important to the process of healing are contraction and epithelialization (Westaby 1981b). Large sores can be closed by contraction and, since skin elasticity is retained, the result functionally and cosmetically is good. Epithelialization occurs in conjunction with contraction. Hair follicles and the wound margins provide the main sources of epidermal regeneration, and in shallow wounds which contain viable hair follicles, migration of epidermal

cells across the wound surface can occur fairly rapidly. Winter (1976) demonstrated that it takes seven days to bridge the gap between two hair follicles. For deeper wounds, healing is much slower because the sources of epidermal regeneration, other than the wound margins, are lost.

Epithelialization occurs over living tissue and travels under any scab that has formed. It has been established (Winter 1976) that epithelialization is much faster if it occurs in a moist environment compared with the dehydration which accompanies scab formation. This has important implications for choice of wound dressing materials. Winter found that 100% epidermal regeneration occurred two to three times faster with wounds covered with an occlusive, oxygen-permeable dressing, such as Op-Site® (Smith & Nephew), compared with wounds covered with a conventional dry dressing.

More recent research has called into question the existence and the need for an oxygenated local environment in the promotion of wound healing (Varghese et al 1986). Varghese and his colleagues compared the local environment of chronic full-thickness ulcers (some of which were pressure sores) treated with either an oxygen-permeable polyurethane film (Op-Site®) or an oxygen-impermeable hydrocolloid dressing (Duoderm®/Granuflex®). They found that the oxygen tension in the fluid under the polyurethane film was very low even though it was oxygen permeable; and the fluid under the hydrocolloid dressing was totally hypoxic. Both dressings promoted healing by providing a moist wound environment, impeding eschar formation and so stimulating epithelial migration. The authors support recent evidence that oxygen-impermeable dressings are more effective than oxygen-permeable ones and the oxygen required for wound healing is provided through the blood supply.

Debriding and cleaning wounds

There is a bewildering number of substances available to put on pressure sores, yet very few have been tested systematically for their contribution to wound healing. Debriding a pressure sore of all necrotic tissue is necessary before healing can begin, and surgical, chemical or enzymatic debriding is used. The quickest method is to debride and clean the wound surgically under a general anaesthetic which often precedes wound closure by skin or muscle flap graft. This technique tends to be used only for large pressure sores which have not responded to other treatments, but a certain amount of debriding of necrotic tissue can be done by the nurse with scissors or scalpel.

The chemical debriding agents in frequent use in the United Kingdom are the hypochlorite solutions (Eusol®, Milton®), hydrogen peroxide and creams such as Aserbine® (Beecham) and Malatex® (Norton). Hypochlorite solutions are still used extensively in the National Health Service although there is a growing body of research evidence recommending that they should be withdrawn from use (Thomas 1988, Spanswick et al 1990). It was known as long ago as 1919 that the bacteriocidal effects of hypochlorites is minimal (Fleming 1919) yet their use has continued. Now it has been confirmed that the antimicrobial activity becomes ineffective when the hypochlorite solution reacts with proteins and cellular debris in the wound (Cotter et al 1985, Leaper et al 1987). More seriously, hypochlorites are toxic to cells and delay wound healing by increasing the inflammatory response, by interfering with collagen synthesis and by damaging epithelial cells (Brennan et al 1986, Deas et al 1986, Johnson 1986, 1987, Tatnall et al 1987, Kozol et al 1988). Even though this research has been done on animals, it seems that the hypochlorites are, at best, ineffective and, at worst, extremely damaging.

Proteolytic enzymes which liquify and debride necrotic wounds have apparently been more extensively used in the United States than in Britain. Varidase® (Lederle) is now popular in this country and it desloughs the wound without damaging healthy tissue (Torrance 1983). Varidase® can be applied either directly to the wound or as a soaked gauze pack. It can also be injected under a scab or the scab can be scored with a scalpel until oozing occurs and a Varidase®-soaked gauze dressing applied.

There is evidence for the effectiveness of Varidase®, and nurses should persist with its use,

because the sore may initially appear to enlarge due to the removal of slough. Signs of healing will not be apparent for several days.

Dextranomer beads (Debrisan®, Pharmacia) are porous and hydrophilic and absorb fluid from the surface of moist, suppurating wounds, so acting as an effective cleansing and debriding agent. They absorb any bacteria in the wound exudate and allow tissue granulation to occur in a moist environment. Debrisan® dressings should be changed at the point of bead saturation, and care should be taken to remove all used beads before applying more. There is evidence for the effectiveness of Debrisan®, particularly in comparison with hypochlorites (Goode et al 1979, Nasar & Morley 1982). The seaweed dressings (calcium alginates) are also polysaccharide 'xerogel' dressings like Debrisan®, and are effective in their ability to absorb exudate, bacteria and odour (Thomas 1985, Turner et al 1986). These dressings should be used on moist, exuding, sloughy wounds to promote granulation.

The more usual methods of removing bacteria from pressure sores are by mechanical cleaning and application of a topical antiseptic. Mechanical cleaning is usually done by swab and forceps or gloves, or by irrigating the wound. Antiseptic lotions such as cetrimide, chlorhexidine, povidone-iodine and hydrogen peroxide are frequently used on infected pressure sores. Their value is now considered to be dubious since they have been found in culture to be toxic to fibroblasts even at high dilutions and are rapidly inactivated (Deas et al 1986, Leaper et al 1987, Cameron & Leaper 1988). Further research is necessary for conclusive results, but since there is no evidence that bacterial contamination delays healing (Deas et al 1986, Leaper 1986, Gilchrist & Reed 1988), it would be wise for wounds to be cleaned with normal saline alone.

Wound dressings

Turner (1982) lists the criteria necessary for the optimum dressing:

1. To maintain high humidity between the wound and the dressing
2. To remove excess exudate and toxic compounds

3. To allow gaseous exchange (although oxygen permeability is now considered unnecessary, Varghese et al 1986)
4. To provide thermal insulation to the wound surface
5. To be impermeable to bacteria
6. To be free from particles and toxic wound contaminants
7. To allow removal without causing trauma during dressing change (p. 43)

No dressing as yet achieves all these requirements, but some fairly recent products do help in the healing process (Turner et al 1986). Different pressure sores of course require different dressings, but in order to aid healing the dressing should prevent dehydration and contamination. The conventional dry gauze dressing achieves neither; it exposes the wound surface to dehydration so allowing scab formation, and the dressing fibres often become entangled in the scab, resulting in fresh trauma when the dressing is removed. For a healthy person, allowing a fairly superficial wound to become dehydrated presents few problems because healing will occur, but if a dressing is needed at all, a non-adhesive one would be wise.

With a debilitated elderly person, healing may be prolonged and nurses should take action to reduce discomfort to a minimum. In this case, a fairly shallow wound should be covered with a polymeric film dressing which prevents dehydration, such as Op-Site® (Smith & Nephew), Tegaderm® (3M) or Bioclusive® (Johnson & Johnson). These occlusive oxygen-permeable adhesive dressings create a moist wound environment. No dehydration occurs and so no scab is formed, which enables rapid migration of epidermal cells across the wound surface. After cleaning and any necessary debriding, the shallow wound should be covered by the film dressing, and left undisturbed until healing is complete, unless clinical signs of infection occur. Eventually, the dressing will slough off during washing. Nurses often find it difficult to leave it alone because wound exudate collects under the membrane and may look contaminated. This collection of fluid is beneficial because it helps to loosen necrotic debris by autolysis, and may promote healing (Leaper 1986). If the membrane bulges excessively with exudate this can be aspirated through the dressing

with a needle and syringe, and the puncture site covered with another piece of film. There is increasing evidence for the effectiveness of these film dressings on shallow wounds (Lawrence 1986).

The film dressings now available are replacing the non-adhesive paraffin-impregnated dressings (Tulle Gras®, Jelonet®, Sofratulle®, Unitulle®). These do retain a moist environment until they dry out, and they are usually covered with gauze which can become incorporated into the wound. They have the same disadvantages as dry gauze dressings unless they are changed frequently before they dry out.

The deeper pressure sore presents a different problem because it will almost certainly be infected (unless it has been surgically debrided) and will require regular cleaning and debriding. Dehydration of a deep wound which has dermal as well as epidermal damage is a much more serious problem than for shallow wounds because an already impoverished environment for healing is damaged further. Dehydration destroys the remnants of any hair follicles left, so removing all sources of epidermal regeneration except the wound edges. Furthermore, if a deep sore has been surgically or chemically debrided and then left with a dry dressing or one which dries out rapidly, then newly exposed healthy tissue and its vasculature die, and granulation cannot occur.

There does not seem to be a single best dressing material for the deeper sore, except of course, skin in the form of grafts or flaps. These are usually applied after surgical debridement, which is an effective but relatively rare choice of treatment for elderly patients with deep pressure sores. The polymeric sheet *foam* dressings which have a hyrophilic film wound-contact surface and foam backing which absorbs exudate are considered to be effective (see Turner et al 1986). Examples of these dressings are Release® (Johnson & Johnson), Coraderm® (Armour Pharmaceuticals), Allevyn Burn Dressing® (Smith & Nephew) and Lyofoam® (Ultra Laboratories). These dressings provide a moist wound environment, and require changing frequently when wound exudate is profuse and contaminated. If exudate is excessive, highly absorbent pads could be placed over the polymeric foam dressing so that a moist environment retained. As with films, nurses should persist with these hydrophilic foam dressings, even if the wound looks messy and macerated. This is normal and it is only after about six days that a dramatic improvement will be seen.

The Silastic Foam Dressing® (Dow Corning/Wellcome) has advantages over the now-discredited ribbon gauze packing which has been the standard treatment for cavity wounds for so long. Silastic Foam® is non-adherent, highly absorbent and more comfortable for the patient than the gauze pack, and can be replaced by many patients themselves (Harding 1986). Silastic Foam® is made up from two liquids, a base and a catalyst, which are mixed together and poured into the wound. After two to three minutes the mixture expands to four times its original volume and sets to a solid spongy consistency. It therefore conforms accurately to the contours of the wound and should be removed, rinsed clean, soaked in antiseptic, squeezed dry and replaced once or twice daily. This dressing is not appropriate for deep wounds with irregular contours, cavities and sinuses because pieces of the foam may break off and get left behind in the wound when the dressing is changed.

Over the last decade hydrogels and hydrocoloids have been developed as advances in dressing materials. The *hydrogels* are hydrophilic, semipermeable water polymer gels which are highly absorbent, conformable, non-adherent, they promote granulation and provide pain relief (Turner et al 1986). They come in sheets or sachets and are useful for irregularly shaped cavity wounds and leg ulcers. Examples of hydrogels are Vigilon® (Bard), Geliperm® (Geistlich) and Scherisorb® (Schering Chemicals).

Hydrocolloid dressings have similar properties to hydrogels except that they are impermeable to moisture and gases. The impermeable outer layer of the dressing adheres strongly to the skin surrounding the wound. The inner hydrocolloid layer of the dressing absorbs the wound exudate to form a gel which swells as it absorbs the exudate and retains a moist environment whilst it conforms to the wound contours (Turner et al 1986). Examples of hydrocolloid dressings are Granuflex® (also

known as Duoderm®, Squibb Surgicare), and Comfeel® (Coloplast). The dressing should be left in place for about five days, or until the absorption of the hydrocolloid with the wound exudate reaches the edge of the dressing, as indicated by a change in the colour of the dressing. When the dressing is removed, the gel remains in the wound cavity and should be washed away with saline before a new dressing is applied. The effectiveness of hydrocolloid dressings for leg ulcers and pressure sores has been established (Harkiss 1985, Deas et al 1986, Turner et al 1986, Gorse & Messner 1987).

A completely different group of dressings, not based on plastic films, foams, gels and colloids, are *biodressings*. The most well-known natural biodressing is, of course, human skin, but research is progressing on other natural biodressings such as foetal sac membranes (amnion and chorion), the dura mater and animal skin, particularly from the pig. These dressings provide optimal healing, adherence, sterility, hypoallergenicity, non-toxicity, non-pyrogenicity and permeability (Lofts 1987). Attempts are being made by cell biologists to 'culture' the patient's own cells into dressing sheets. These dressings would produce no immunological problems of rejection and would be particularly appropriate for dressing burns.

Work is also being carried out to develop biosynthetic dressings which have the advantages of the natural biodressings but are made from a combination of a silicone elastomer and animal or human collagen. The theory is that endothelial cells and fibroblasts migrate from the wound into the dressing material and the associated collagenases degrade the dressing material, so providing nutrients for the production of more endothelial cells and fibroblasts (Lofts 1987).

The search for increasingly effective dressing materials for the chronic wound is continuing to move ahead at a tremendous rate. Dressings have evolved from the traditional 'passive' absorbent plugs and dry covers, to the 'interactive' dressing with its controlled environment, and on to the 'active' dressings which deliver or stimulate delivery of substances active in the healing process (Fairbrother 1988).

EVALUATION

The bewildering variety of products available which purport to assist in the prevention or healing of pressure sores means that evaluating the treatment and care given to each patient as well as systematic product evaluation with valid research studies is essential. Evaluating the effects of nursing care and treatment is not something which comes naturally to many nurses. But evaluation need not be difficult as long as an effective assessment of the patient's problems is made before treatment begins, using measurement where possible. Assessment of the extent to which the patient is at risk of developing pressure sores should include use of one of the rating scales mentioned earlier and knowledge of the intrinsic and extrinsic factors known to contribute. The effects of treatment should be evaluated at regular intervals by repeated assessments which are compared with the initial baseline assessment. A similar assessment is required for the patient who has a pressure sore, together with some kind of measurement of the sore size before treatment and at regular intervals during treatment.

Pressure sores are wounds which have a complex aetiology and pathology. It follows that their prevention and treatment are also complex and cannot be the sole responsibility of any one health professional. Adequate assessment, care and evaluation requires a team effort which includes the patient.

Improving the basic education of nurses, doctors and paramedical staff would expand their knowledge of preventive and treatment practices, but knowledge continues to increase with new research and development, and it is difficult for practising nurses and doctors to keep up to date. A pressure sore team, consisting of doctors, nurses, physiotherapists, etc. with particular interest and knowledge could provide assistance and a monitoring role. A clinical nurse specialist in pressure sore care is another solution (Dowding 1983, Waterlow 1987, Simpson 1988). Specialists like these could be instrumental in promoting sound practice and disseminating new information to nurses and others, and in redrafting and up-dating procedure manuals.

The increase of very old, frail people is continuing and therefore the number of patients at risk from pressure sores is rising. In these days of dwindling resources, prevention is much cheaper than cure, as well as being more effective and acceptable to patients. In order for patients to receive high quality care, nurses and their colleagues must expand their knowledge and incorporate the results of valid research into their planned individualized patient care.

REFERENCES

Abbott D F, Exton-Smith A N, Millard P H, Temperly T M 1968 Zinc sulphate and bedsores. (Letter) British Medical Journal 2: 763

Abruzzesse R 1985 Early assessment and prevention of pressure sores. In: Bok Y L (ed) Chronic Ulcers of The Skin. McGraw-Hill, New York

Anthony D 1987 The accurate measurement of pressure sores. In: Fielding P (ed) Research in the Nursing Care of Elderly People. Wiley, Chichester

Anthony D, Barnes E 1984 Measuring pressure sores accurately. Nursing Times 80(36): 33–35

Barbenel J C, Forbes C D, Lowe G D O (eds) 1983 Pressure sores. Macmillan, London

Barratt E 1987 Pressure sores: putting risk calculators in their place. Nursing Times Feb 18, 65–70

Barton A, Barton M 1981 The management and prevention of pressure sores. Faber, London

Bennett G C J 1983a Pressure sores revisited. Geriatric Medicine 13(5): 415–418

Bennett G C J 1983b Treating pressure sores. Geriatric Medicine 13(6): 493–494

Berecek K H 1975 Etiology of decubitus ulcers. Nursing Clinics of North America 10(1): 157–170

Bergstrom N, Braden B J, Laguzza A, Holman V l987a The Braden scale for predicting pressure sore risk. Nursing Research 36(4): 205–210

Bergstrom N, Demuth P J, Braden P J 1987b A clinical trial of the Braden scale for predicting pressure sore risk. Nursing Clinics of North America 22(2): 417–428

Bliss M, McLaren R, Exton-Smith A N 1967 Preventing pressure sores in hospital: controlled trial of a large-celled ripple mattress. British Medical Journal 1: 394–397

Bobel L M 1987 Nutritional implications in the patient with pressure sores. Nursing Clinics of North America 22(2): 379–390

Brennan S S, Foster M E, Leaper D J 1986 Antiseptic toxicity in wounds healing by secondary intention. Journal of Hospital Infection 8: 263–267

Cameron S, Leaper D J 1988 Antiseptic toxicity in open wounds. Nursing Times 84(25): 77

Carnevali D, Patrick M L 1979 Nursing management for the elderly. Lippincott, Philadelphia

Clark M 1988 Measuring the pressure. Nursing Times 84(25): 70–72

Cotter J L, Fader R C, Lilley C, Herndon D N l985 Chemical parameters, antimicrobiol activities and tissue toxicity of 0.1 and 0.5% sodium hypochlorite solutions. Antimicrobiol Agents and Chemotherapy 28: 118

Crow R 1988 The challenge of pressure sores. Nursing Times 84(38): 68–73

David J A, Chapman R G, Chapman E J, Lockett B 1983 An investigation of the current methods used in nursing for the care of patients with established pressure sores. Nursing Practice Research Unit, Northwick Park Hospital and Clinical Research Centre, Harrow, Middlesex

Deas J, Billings P, Brennan S, Silver I, Leaper D 1986 The toxicity of commonly used antiseptics on fibroblasts in tissue culture. Phlebology 1: 205–209

Denne W A 1979 An objective assessment of the sheepskins used for decubitus sore prophylaxis. Rheumatology and Rehabilitation 18: 23–29

Denne W A 1983 Prevention of pressure sores: a study of the mechanical properties of fleeces. Nursing Focus May/June: 8–9

Dowding C 1983 Tissue viability nurse — a new post. Nursing Times 79(24): 61–64

Dyson R 1978 Bedsores — the injuries hospital staff inflict on patients. Nursing Mirror 146(24): 30–32

Ek A-C, Bowman G 1982 A descriptive study of pressure sores: the prevalence of pressure sores and the characteristics of patients. Journal of Advanced Nursing 7(1): 51–57

Exton-Smith A N 1987 The patient's not for turning. Nursing Times 83(42): 42–44

Exton-Smith A N, Sherwin R W 1961 Prevention of pressure sores: significance of spontaneous bodily movements. Lancet 2: 1124–1126

Exton-Smith A N, Wedgwood J, Overstall P W, Wallace G 1982 Use of the 'air wave system' to prevent pressure sores in hospital. Lancet 1: 1288–1290

Fairbrother J E 1988 Beyond occlusion and back again. In: Ryan T J (ed) Beyond Occlusion: wound care proceedings. London, Royal Society of Medicine

Fernie G R 1973 Biochemical aspects of the aetiology of decubitus ulcers on human patients. Unpublished PhD Thesis, University of Strathclyde, Glasgow

Fleming A 1919 The action of chemical and physiological antiseptics in a septic wound. British Journal of Surgery 7: 99–129

Gibbons D E 1983 Mouth care procedures. Nursing Times 79(7): 30

Gilchrist B, Reed C 1988 The bacteriology of leg ulcers under hydrocolloid dressings. In: Ryan T J (ed) Beyond occlusion: wound care proceedings. London, Royal Society of Medicine

Girvin J, Griffiths-Jones A 1989 Towards prevention. Journal of the Wound Care Society. Nursing Times 85(12): 64–66

Goldstone L A, Goldstone J 1982 The Norton score: an early warning of pressure sores? Journal of Advanced Nursing 7(5): 419–426

Goode A W et al 1979 The cost effectiveness of dextranomer and eusol in the treatment of infected surgical wounds. British Journal of Clinical Practice 33(11/12): 325, 328

Gorse G J, Messner R L 1987 Improved pressure sore healing with hydrocolloid dressings. Archives of Dermatology 123: 766–771

Gosnell D J 1973 An assessment tool to identify pressure sores. Nursing Research 22(1): 55–59

Gosnell D J 1987 Assessment and evaluation of pressure sores. Nursing Clinics of North America 22(2): 399–416

Guttman L 1976 The prevention and treatment of pressure sores. In: Kenedi R M, Cowden J M, Scales J T (eds) Bedsore biomechanics. Macmillan, London p 153–160

Harding K G 1986 Clinical experience of silastic foam dressing. In: Turner T D, Schmidt R J, Harding K G (eds) Advances in wound management. Wiley, Chichester

Harkiss K J 1985 Cost analysis of dressing materials used in venous leg ulcers. Pharmacy Journal 253: 268–269

Harris M D 1980 Tools for mouth care. Nursing Times 76(305): 340–342

Hibbs P 1988 Pressure area care for the City and Hackney health authority. Unpublished Report, City and Hackney Health Authority

Howarth H 1977 Mouth care procedures for the very ill. Nursing Times 73(10): 354

Jakobsen J, Christensen K S 1987 Transcutaneous oxygen tension measurement over the sacrum on various anti-decubitus mattresses. Danish Medical Bulletin 34(6): 330–331

Jay P 1983 Choosing the best wheelchair cushion: for your needs, your chair and your life style. Royal Association for Disability and Rehabilitation, London

Jenkins D 1989 Oral care in the ICU: an important nursing role. Nursing Stardard 4(7): 24–28

Johnson A 1986 Cleansing infected wounds. Nursing Times 82(37): 30–34

Johnson A 1987 Wound care — packing wound cavities. Nursing Times 83(36): 59–62

Jordan M M and Barbenel J C 1983 Pressure sore prevalence. In: Barbenel J C, Forbes C D, Lowe G D O (eds) Pressure sores. Macmillan, London

Kenedi R M, Cowden J M, Scales J T (eds) 1976 Bedsore biomechanics. Macmillan, London

Knoll Pharmaceutical Co 1982 The Knoll scale of liability to pressure sores. In: McFarlane J, Castledine G A guide to the practice of nursing. Mosby, St Louis

Kozol R A, Gillies C, Elgebaly S A 1988 Effects of sodium hypochlorite (Dakin's Solution) on cells of the wound module. Archives of Surgery 123(4): 420–423

Lawrence J C 1986 Film dressings. In: Turner T D, Schmidt R J, Harding K G (eds) Advances in wound management. Wiley, Chichester

Leaper D J 1986 Antiseptics and their effect on healing tissue. Nursing Times 82(23): 45–47

Leaper D, Cameron S, Lancaster J 1987 Antiseptic solutions. Nursing Times Community Outlook, April, 30–34

Lofts P F 1987 Biodressings. In: Turner T D et al (eds) Advances in wound management. Wiley, Chichester

Lowthian P T 1979 Turning clocks system to prevent pressure sores. Nursing Mirror 148(21): 30–31

Lowthian P T 1982 A review of pressure sore pathogenesis. Nursing Times 78(3): 117–121

Lowthian P T 1983 Nursing aspects to pressure sore prevention. In: Barbenel J C, Forbes C D, Lowe G D O (eds) Pressure sores. Macmillan, London

McConnell E S 1988 Nursing diagnoses related to physiological alterations. In: Matteson M A, McConnell E S (eds) Gerontological nursing: concepts and practice. Philadelphia, W B Saunders

Maklebust J 1987 Pressure ulcers: etiology and prevention. Nursing Clinics of North America 22(2): 359–377

Marshall M, Overstall P 1983 Mattresses to prevent pressure sores. Nursing Times 79(24): 54–59

Moolton S E 1972 Bedsores in the chronically ill patient. Archives of Physical Medicine and Rehabilitation 53: 430–438

Nasar M A, Morley R 1982 Cost effectiveness in treating deep pressure sores and ulcers. Practitioner 226: 307–310

Newman P, Davis N H 1981 Thermography as a predictor of sacral pressure sores. Age and Ageing 10: 14–18

Norton D, McLaren R, Exton-Smith A N 1962 An investigation of geriatric nursing problems in hospital. Re-issued 1975. Churchill Livingstone, Edinburgh

Nyquist R, Hawthorn P J 1987 The prevalence of pressure sores within an area health authority. Journal of Advanced Nursing 12: 183–187

Peterson N C, Bittmann J 1971 The epidemiology of pressure sores. Scandinavian Journal of Plastic and Reconstructive Surgery 5: 62–66

Pritchard V 1986 Calculating the risk. Nursing Times 82(8): 59–61

Redfern S J, Jeneid P A, Gillingham M E, Lunn H F 1973 Local pressure with ten types of patient-support system. Lancet ii: 277–280

Roberts B V, Goldstone L A 1979 A survey of pressure sores in the over sixties on two orthopaedic wards. International Journal of Nursing Studies 16(4): 355–364

Scales J T, Lowthian P T, Poole A G, Ludman W R 1982 'Vaperm' patient-support system: a new general purpose hospital mattress. Lancet 2: 1150–1152

Scholey M 1982 The shoulder lift. Nursing Times 78(11): 506–507

Simpson G 1988 Time to specialise. Nursing Times, Community Outlook, June, 22–24.

Sofaer B 1979 The loss of dentures in hospital. Nursing Times Occasional Paper 75(21): 85–88

Spanswick A, Gibbs S, Ekelund P 1990 Eusol — the final word! The Professional Nurse, January, 211–212

Speedie G 1983 Nursology of mouth care: preventing,

comforting and seeking activities related to mouth care. Journal of Advanced Nursing 8(1): 33–40

Tatnall E M, Leigh I M, Gibson J R 1987 Comparative toxicity of antimicrobiol agents on transformed human keratinocytes. British Journal of Dermatology. 117 Supplement 32: 31–32

Taylor K J 1988 Assessment tools for the identification of patients at risk for the development of pressure sores: a review. Journal of Enterostomal Therapy 15(5): 201–205

Taylor T V, Rimmer S, Day B, Butcher J, Dymock I W 1974 Ascorbic acid supplementation in the treatment of pressure sores. Lancet 2: 544–546

Thomas S 1985 Use of calcium alginate dressing. The Pharmaceutical Journal 235(634): 188–190

Thomas S 1988 Pressure points. Nursing Times, Community Outlook, October, 20–22

Torrance C 1983 Pressure sores: aetiology, treatment and prevention. Croom-Helm, London

Towey A P, Erland S M 1988 Validity and reliability of an assessment tool for pressure ulcer risk. Decubitus 1(2): 40–48

Turner T 1982 Which dressing and why — 1. Wound care series no. 11 Nursing Times 78(29): 41–44

Turner T D, Schmidt R J, Harding K G (eds) 1986 Advances in wound management. Wiley, Chichester

Varghese M C, Balin A K, Carter M, Caldwell D l986 Local environment of chronic wounds under synthetic dressings. Archives of Dermatology. 112: 52–57

Waterlow J 1985 A risk assessment card. Nursing Times 81(48): 49–55

Waterlow J 1987 Calculating the risk. Nursing Times 83(39): 58–60

Westaby S 1981a Healing: the normal mechanism—1. Wound care series no. 3 Nursing Times 77(47): 9–12

Westaby S 1981b Healing: the normal mechanism—2. Wound care series no. 4 Nursing Times 77(51): 13–16

Winter G 1976 Some factors affecting skin and wound healing. In: Kenedi R M, Cowden J M, Scales J T (eds) Bed-sore biomechanics. Macmillan, London, p 47–54

CHAPTER CONTENTS

Introduction 243

Normal adult sleep 244
Sleep stages 244

Sleep of elderly people 246
Sleep length and sleep cycles 246
The relationship between night-time and daytime
behaviours 247

Causes of sleep problems in elderly people 247
Biological rhythms, ageing and sleep 248
Sleep deprivation 249
Environmental causes of sleep disturbance 250
Drugs associated with sleep disorders 252
Illness and sleep disturbance 253
Conclusions 256

Assessment of sleep 256
Sleep assessment format 257
Patient goals/objectives regarding sleep 259
Nursing intervention to promote sleep 259
Reassessment or continuing assessment of
sleep 260
Finally, a word on loneliness 260

15

Sleep and rest

Morva Fordham

Fond words have oft been spoken of thee, sleep!
And thou hast had thy store of tenderest names;
The very sweetest words that fancy frames
When thankfulness of heart is strong and deep!
Dear bosom child we call thee, that dost steep
In rich reward all suffering, balm that tames
All anguish, saint that evil thoughts and aims
Takest away, and into souls dost creep
Like a breeze from heaven. Shall I alone,
I surely not a man ungently made,
Call thee worst tyrant by which flesh is crost?
Perverse, self-willed to own and to disown,
Mere slave of them who never for thee prayed,
Still last to come where thou are wanted most!

William Wordsworth

INTRODUCTION

Sleep is a state of reduced responsiveness (or increased threshold) to external stimuli. In other words it is an altered state of consciousness from which a person can be aroused if the stimulus is sufficient. It is the inactive part of the circadian sleep-wake cycle, and is characterized by particular electroencephalographic patterns and by lowering of the metabolic rate. Healthy adults move their position 30–40 times per night.

Although sleep is a normal state, it can be difficult to distinguish from abnormal states of stupor or coma, and sleep can be deliberately simulated. It is not uncommon for nurses who are caring for sick and elderly people to be faced with the problem of distinguishing between normal sleep, incipient stupor, and feigned sleep. Indeed, if concern for the well-being of an elderly person is great, and doubt exists about the nature of his or her unresponsiveness, we almost reflexly resort to vocal or tactile stimuli to test the state of affairs — much to the annoyance of the 'sleeper'. However, sleep is a potentially dangerous (life threatening) state for some people, and the most common time of death is between 04.00 and 07.00 h.

Nurses have informally gleaned a wealth of information about the sleeping patterns of elderly people. We have observed the sick and frail elderly and to a lesser extent the healthy elderly in hospital and Homes. However, until the last few years we have had little scientific knowledge to back our hunches or inform our biases. Yet next to the elderly persons themselves and their families and friends we have the greatest vested interest in understanding the sleep of the elderly. Firstly, because our aim is to promote the optimal functioning of the elderly folk in our care and, secondly, because their sleep–wake pattern could have important implications for the 24-hour nursing workload and therefore for the way in which we choose to deploy the limited number of staff available in most geriatric nursing environments.

There are a number of beliefs about sleep which we and elderly persons are likely to hold. Some are philosophical and open to debate and others are scientific hypotheses which are open to testing by research. If we are to provide optimal care for elderly people we should examine the state of knowledge and our own beliefs and biases. The philosophical debate as to why or whether sleep is needed by humans rumbles on. Is sleep merely a hangover from evolutionary times when it was dangerous to move in the dark because of the risk of predators? Is it an essential means of energy conservation? Is sleep necessary for restitution of brain and body function? Individuals vary in their apparent need for sleep. Some people claim to and actually take very little sleep, others sleep longer than the normal 7–9 hours per day. However, the majority become concerned if they fail to sleep as long as is normal for them.

Two major propositions about sleep underlie the discussion in the remainder of this chapter. Efficient functioning of elderly people when they are awake is fundamentally dependent upon: 1. the quality and quantity of their sleep and 2. the pattern of their sleep–wake circadian rhythm. It is not possible to understand the particular problems of sleep in elderly people without examining the general state of knowledge about sleep.

NORMAL ADULT SLEEP

Most research on sleep has used young healthy adults as subjects. The physiological functioning of the brain, muscles, cardiac, respiratory and reproductive systems during sleep have been recorded, as well as the effects of total and selective sleep deprivation. Reviews of this research can be found in Colquhoun (1971, 1972), Minors and Waterhouse (1981) and Morgan (1987). Monitoring sleep classically uses scalp electrodes to measure electroencephalographic (EEG) and electroocculographic (EOG) changes, plus body electrodes and thermisters to record muscle (electromyographic), respiratory, cardiovascular and temperature changes. Hormone, electrolyte and other chemical levels in the blood can be monitored by the use of venous catheterization. The print-outs of this monitoring are termed polygraphic records.

SLEEP STAGES

Findings from this monitoring of sleep have led to a distinction between two major types of sleep, orthodox and paradoxical, defined by the EEG and EOG pattern. Sleep begins at stage 0, resting with eyes shut, and with alpha rhythms (8–12 cycles per second) on EEG. This is followed by orthodox, or non-REM (rapid eye movement), sleep which has four stages. As a person passes from stage 1 to stage 4 EEG rhythms become progressively slower, until large slow waves 0.5–3 cycles per second and 5–10 times the amplitude of wakefulness occur. Stage 1 has characteristic waveforms called 'sleep spindles' and 'K complexes'. Stages 3 and 4 slow waves are called delta waves and these stages are referred to as slow wave sleep (SWS). The person becomes more deeply asleep as they pass from stage 1 to stage 4. Paradoxical, or

Table 15.1 Types of sleep. *Adapted from Koreorgos, (1980).*

	Non-REM Orthodox	REM Paradoxical
Electroencephalogram (EEG)	Slow waves, 0.5–3 cycles/second plus sleep spindles and K complexes	Low voltage, desynchronized waves
Eye movement Electro-oculogram (EOG)	Absent, or slow rolling	Rapid eye movements
Muscle tone	Reduced	Abolished
Heart and respiratory rate Blood pressure Metabolic rate	Steady, regular, slow Lowered Lowered	Increased, irregular Raised Raised, relative to non-REM
Penile erection Vaginal blood flow	Rarely Lowered	Yes Increased
Growth hormone	Increased	No change
Dreaming	Infrequent	Frequent, vivid
Response to external stimuli	Reduced as pass from stage 1 to stage 4	Less responsive than stage 4. Very difficult to awaken or awakens spontaneously

REM, sleep occurs from time to time. This is a qualitatively different type of sleep in which the EEG appears similar to that of wakefulness (low voltage desynchronized). Rapid eye movements occur beneath closed lids and skeletal muscle tone is lost.

The distinction between orthodox and paradoxical sleep is important. It becomes progressively more difficult to arouse someone as they pass from stage 1 to stage 4. During paradoxical sleep, when skeletal muscles are functionally paralysed, the sleeper is variably responsive to external stimuli; she may awaken spontaneously, or may be very difficult to awaken. The main differences between these types of sleep are summarized in Table 15.1.

A major hypothesis is that both types of sleep are needed for restitution of body and brain function. It can be seen from Table 15.1 that orthodox sleep seems to be dominated by the activity of the parasympathetic nervous system. As growth hormone levels are high it has been suggested that anabolic processes of growth and tissue repair occur optimally during this stage (Beck et al 1975). Some of the evidence supports this view, although Horne (1980) disputes this hypothesis and says

that the peak in human 'growth hormone found during non-REM sleep' (Takahashi et al 1968) may not facilitate optimum protein synthesis and mitosis since nutrient levels may be low during night-time fasting. A potential danger to life may result from the lowered metabolic rate and hypothermia during SWS.

Paradoxical sleep, on the other hand, appears to be dominated by sympathetic nervous system activity. Indeed, cardiac output, heart rate and blood pressure can surpass waking levels, and angina and ventricular arrhythmias can occur during this stage. Respiration may mimic Cheyne-Stokes patterns, and apnoeic attacks may occur (Guilleminault & Dement 1978). However, it is a stage of sleep thought to be crucial to the maintenance of mental–emotional equilibrium.

In a typical night it has been found that adults pass through a complete cycle of stages approximately every 90 minutes, or 4–6 times per night. One complete cycle is illustrated in Figure 15.1. The length of time spent in each stage during the night differs such that more orthodox sleep occurs in the early part of the night and more paradoxical sleep in the early morning.

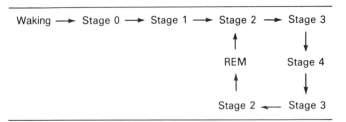

Fig. 15.1 Sleep cycle. *Source*: *Sanford (1982).*

SLEEP OF ELDERLY PEOPLE

SLEEP LENGTH AND SLEEP CYCLES

So far we have been discussing the sleep of adults in general. Does the sleep of the healthy elderly person differ? Is it normal for elderly people to sleep less well at night than younger adults?

Questionnaire survey findings support the view that elderly people are generally dissatisfied with their sleep and indeed the use of sedative-hypnotic medication appears to increase with age. McGhie and Russell (1962) conducted a survey of 2466 subjects in Britain of all age groups. They found that there was a significant increase in the proportion of people over 65 years who claimed to sleep less than five hours per night. Twenty to 30% of these , elderly people reported frequent night awakenings, 15% waking before 05.00 h; 25% of men over 65 years and 40% of women over 45 years described themselves as light sleepers. In this and similar studies complaints of sleeping difficulties tended to be higher for females than males. However, when objective measurements of sleep are taken, many research studies have found that elderly men have more disturbed sleep than elderly women (Dement et al 1982a, Webb 1982). Coleman et al (1981) monitored the sleep of 83 people aged over 60 years and compared their sleep with that of 423 younger adults. They found that the total amount of sleep was less for the elderly people although the number of daytime naps increased. The elderly were more frequently awake and awake for longer periods during the

night after the initial sleep onset. Webb and Swinbourne (1971) observed 19 people aged 66–96 years over 24 hours and found that although they spent 11–12 hours in bed they only averaged 8.5 hours sleep, including daytime naps. Their findings suggest that the sleep of the elderly is not less than that of younger people but is more variable in distribution throughout the 24 hours.

So although some early studies such as Feinberg (1968) state that the total sleep time declines with age, more recent studies report that the amount of sleep per 24 hours and the need for sleep does not decrease with age. Dement et al (1982b) state categorically that 'fragmented sleep in persons of advanced years is not the result of decreased sleep need' (p. 31). According to Dement et al (1982b) great individual variability in sleep has been found and significant ageing trends are rarely demonstrated. As with other age groups, elderly individuals cannot automatically be assumed to follow the general trend. On the whole, however, it seems that old people spend more time lying in bed at night without attempting to sleep, and more time unsuccessfully trying to sleep than younger folk. They also spend more time in bed in the daytime resting or napping, but their total sleep time is not usually increased compared with the young, and it may be reduced.

The major changes in sleep stages with age are summarized in Table 15.2. There is an increase in light sleep and decrease in deep sleep stages 3 and 4. The relative amount of paradoxical or REM sleep is found to persist until extreme old age, although a decline in the proportion of REM sleep seems to correlate with reduced intellectual functioning and organic brain syndrome. Many

Table 15.2 Sleep pattern and age. *Adapted from Feinberg (1968).*

	REM	Stage 1	Stage 2	Stages 3 and 4	Total
Infant — Newborn — 1 Year	50% 20–30%				14 — 18 hours
Young, active, healthy adult	25%	5–10%	50%	15–20%	6–9 hours
Elderly	20–25% (Decline associated with impaired intellectual functioning)	Increased	Unchanged	Decreased	Total variable — unchanged or reduced and fragmented

sleep is more evenly distributed throughout the night than in younger adults.

studies of REM sleep have shown that there is a change in the circadian rhythm such that REM

THE RELATIONSHIP BETWEEN NIGHT-TIME SLEEP AND DAYTIME BEHAVIOURS

According to Dement et al (1982b), and in agreement with common belief, 'it is axiomatic that there is a relationship between sleep at night and the way we feel during the day' (p. 30).

Most of us have felt the general effects of lack of sleep, including tiredness, headache or sensation of a tight band around the head, eye problems, such as 'prickling' or heavy lids, lack of muscle co-ordination, maybe even affecting speech (dysarthria), decreased facial expression and difficulty in maintaining attention. However, many of the symptoms attributed to lack of sleep in young folk are labelled as part of the ageing process in the elderly. Amongst these, Dement et al (1982b) include

losses of abilities to perform highly skilled tasks in a rapid fashion, to resist fatigue, to maintain physical stamina, to unlearn or discard old techniques, and to apply the rapid judgement needed in changing and emergency situations (p. 30).

Only those studies which cover the whole 24 hours can elucidate the relationship between night-time sleep and daytime naps. Many sleep researchers support the view that the daytime sleepiness of elderly people is the direct conse-

quence of night-time sleep deprivation. Johns (1975) found that not only did the amount of time awake after initial sleep onset increase with age, but that night-time wakefulness was associated with increasing amounts of sleep during the day. His conclusion was that daytime naps were compensating for broken night-time sleep.

Some studies have used a standard measure of daytime sleepiness termed 'sleep latency'. This is the speed of falling to sleep as measured by EEG polygraphic recordings. This sleep latency can be measured at any time of the day or night and is a more valid and reliable measure of sleepiness than naturally occurring naps. Measurement is precise and objective, and the opportunity and environment for sleeping is controlled. In a study of healthy, elderly subjects who were in bed for 10 hours per night, seriously fragmented and interrupted sleep was found (Carskadon et al 1982). About 60% of the subjects had more than 100 brief or prolonged arousals during the night's sleep. The number of brief arousals per hour of nocturnal sleep was predictive of daytime sleepiness, as measured by sleep latencies. The sleep latency scores suggested that a substantial number of elderly persons are pathologically sleepy in the daytime even when they do not complain of sleep problems.

CAUSES OF SLEEP PROBLEMS IN ELDERLY PEOPLE

If we aim to promote sleep in elderly people we

need to examine all possible causes for sleep abnormalities. We stand little chance of making logical decisions or taking helpful action unless we attempt to answer the following question: Are elderly people who appear sleepy, inattentive, un-co-ordinated and resistant to change, suffering from the inevitable effects of ageing, sleep deprivation, drug intoxication or specific disease?

BIOLOGICAL RHYTHMS, AGEING AND SLEEP

Disorders of the sleep–wake schedule are said to occur if this rhythm is out of phase either with other internal rhythms or with society's expectations of sleep–wake time.

One view of the ageing process is that it is characterized by the disorganization of biological rhythms. The sleep–wake activity pattern is a circadian rhythm (around a day) but all bodily functions display rhythmicity with peaks and troughs occurring at intervals of seconds, minutes, hours, days, months or years. Health and well-being is dependent upon these rhythms being synchronized with one another, and this synchronization is affected not only by internal events but also by external cyclic inputs (Zeitgebers) such as light–dark and socially determined rest activity cycles and eating times (Reinberg 1966). The regular alternation of sleep–wakefulness is regarded as a fundamental biological rhythm which in normal circumstances is able to entrain (synchronize) other circadian rhythms.

Samis ·and Capobianco (1978) in a book on ageing and biological rhythms stated in their introduction:

Senescent deterioration in form and function may be due, at least in part, to alterations in an organism's ordering among processes in time, with the result that the organism's adaptive capacity and vigor decreases and consequently its probability of death increases. If with advancing age, the circadian temporal organisation of an organism becomes altered, either by becoming more rigid and consequently less amenable to adaptive changes, or becomes disorganised in time, the consequences could have a profound influence on vigor and adaptive capability.

Shock (1977) suggests that internal desynchronization may be part of the general breakdown of regulatory mechanisms accompanying normal ageing. One interesting hypothesis put forward by Winget et al (1972) suggests that prolonged bed-rest may cause desynchronization of circadian rhythms. Dement et al (1982a) speculate that postural change alone — presumably prolonged lying — may in itself cause some of the changes in rhythms found in the elderly. Prinz et al (1982) studied the sleep of people with dementia of the Alzheimer type, and found that compared with healthy old people, they achieved considerably less deep sleep (stages 3 and 4) and REM sleep, were twice as likely to awaken during the night and 20 times more likely to sleep (nap) during the day.

It is obvious that the sleep–wake circadian rhythm of some elderly people remains virtually unaltered with age. But other elderly people have grossly changed patterns of sleeping. There are two main theories put forward to explain this change. One is that the sleep pattern of the elderly is a reversal of day and night (Armstrong-Esther & Hawkins 1982). The other is that elderly people revert to the childhood pattern of multiple sleeping time in 24 hours. Further research is needed to test these hypotheses, but since social cues are extremely important in maintaining a 24-hour rhythm of sleep–waking, all sorts of bizarre sleep–wake cycles can and do occur in elderly people. Winfree (1982) stated that

some sightless individuals, some recluses and some older people living indoors with little social contact, sometimes retire and rise later and later every day like the tides — eventually pursuing their solitary interests by night and sleeping by day, 180° out of phase with surrounding society; they drift still later into synchrony again after another two weeks or so (p. R200).

Isolation studies have demonstrated clearly that bereft of time cues, internal desynchronization occurs in about one fifth of young people, but in all older people.

When we first meet such elderly isolated folk they could be in any phase of their disrupted or drifting sleep-wake pattern, including a reversal of day and night. Many elderly people living with their families, or communally in hospital or

Homes, seem to shift their sleep rhythms to earlier times, being drowsy in the evening and 'larks' in the morning. A breakdown in the biphasic pattern of sleep and wakefulness and a return to the polyphasic alternations of infancy are well documented (Webb 1982). It should be noted that old people do not follow infancy patterns in all respects. They do not return to sleeping 14–18 hours per day, nor does the high proportion of REM sleep found in infancy return.

The picture of changes of other circadian rhythms with age is not fully explored, but alteration in urinary electrolytes (Lobban & Tredre 1964) and cortisol (Serio et al 1970) rhythms have been documented. A reduction in the peak of growth hormone, as stages 3 and 4 sleep are reduced, has been found. The latter finding suggests that night-time sleep may be less restorative to body tissues in the aged than in the young. One interesting finding by Wessler et al (1976) was that institutionalized elderly patients had a high order of circadian regularity and synchronization, and they concluded that the strict institutional regime was probably beneficial. There is some anecdotal evidence that a regular lifestyle plays a part in longevity and health. However, we should perhaps be wary of abruptly imposing a particular regime of sleep–waking on elderly people since their cycles are likely to be less adaptable and more easily disrupted than those of younger people (Preston 1973) and they need time to adapt to an unfamiliar regime. It may well take a couple of weeks or even months to nudge them into synchrony. Settling them for sleep one hour later each 24 hours would be a logical ploy to try. Forcible walking or awakening such elderly persons from daytime sleep would be both cruel and unlikely to achieve the aim of restoring a normal sleep–wake pattern. This is not to deny that some elderly folk nod off by day with sheer boredom. A routine of daytime activities including both physical and mental stimulation undoubtedly helps to maintain a healthy normal sleep–wake schedule for those whose rhythms are in synchrony, but abruptly enforced daytime activity will not help either the sleep deprived or the desynchronized elderly person.

SLEEP DEPRIVATION

Sleep deprivation has been studied in young rather than elderly adults. The effects of total sleep deprivation on performance and mood can be dramatic. Apart from the tendency to fall asleep and perform simple well-learned tasks, such as walking, in a semi-automatic way, subjects tend to become irritable and disoriented, to slur speech, and even become deluded, paranoid and hallucinated. An apparently analagous phenomenon in sleep-deprived seriously ill patients has been described as the intensive care syndrome (Helton et al 1980, Sanford 1982). Williams et al (1967) selectively deprived healthy subjects of different stages of sleep. Those who were prevented from having orthodox sleep complained of physical discomfort and were withdrawn and concerned over vague physical complaints or changes in body feeling. Those who were deprived of paradoxical sleep became anxious, insecure, withdrawn and some showed signs of confusion.

It seems possible, if not probable, that many of the complaints and problems of elderly people could be a result of sleep deprivation. Some elderly people including the healthy may lack all stages of sleep. Others, especially those taking hypnotic drugs and those with organic brain syndrome, may lack paradoxical sleep. Elderly people in particular risk losing out on sleep length when their time in bed is constrained if night-time sleep efficiency (time in bed/total sleep time) is reduced.

The finding that many healthy old people spend much of their sleeping time in light stages of sleep from which they awaken either momentarily or for long periods certainly suggests that unless daytime naps are obtained many of them lack sleep. It is not uncommon for night nurses and elderly patients to give very different accounts of the amount of sleep obtained. We should perhaps take heed of the finding that as many as 100 transient arousals per night (10 seconds or less) showed up on polygraphic records of 60% of healthy elderly people. Many or all of the brief arousals would not be visible to the observer.

ENVIRONMENTAL CAUSES OF SLEEP DISTURBANCE

There are a number of aspects of the environment in which we care for elderly people which may increase their sleep disturbance and deprivation.

Hospital or institutional admission

Research on the effect of hospitalization on the sleep of elderly people has compared institutional and home sleeping patterns. Pacini and Fitzpatrick (1982) investigated the sleep of 38 elderly people (average age 69 years), half at home and half during the first seven days of admission to medical/surgical wards. The hospitalized patients did not undergo surgery and were mainly cared for in private or semi-private rooms. The findings from self-kept sleep charts and sleep pattern questionnaires were that nocturnal sleep time was reportedly shorter in hospital. This was attributed to being woken for recording of vital signs, medication or venesection. More daytime sleep occurred in the hospitalized and they went to bed and were awakened earlier. However, the reported levels of anxiety, provoked by new medication and concern about impending investigations and discharge dates were higher in hospital and health and fatigue status was lower. So poor nocturnal sleep was not attributed solely or even primarily to the hospital environment, but to a significant extent to the status and anxiety levels of the person admitted. People in long-term institutional care, on the other hand, may adapt to the pattern of life and sleep well, especially if they are neither acutely sick nor insecure. As mentioned earlier, Wessler et al (1976) thought the strict institutional regime beneficial.

Many environmental factors, including boredom, social isolation, and physical confinement, are likely to result in excessive sleepiness, whereas heat, cold, light, movement and noise are liable to disturb sleep.

Noise effects on sleep

Auditory threshold awakening from stage 4 (deep)

sleep has been found to be lower in old people so that they are more easily aroused from sleep than younger people (Roth et al 1972). Gress et al (1981) observed the nocturnal behaviour of 11 elderly (60–97 years) persons in an institution between 23.00 h and 07.00 h on three nights. Their main findings were that sounds seemed to be amplified at night. Loud conversation, laughter and careless handling of supplies and equipment were observed to disturb some patients. Three subjects slept solidly each night, but the remainder were awake or up at least once. It seemed that 04.00 was the only hour at which all patients were in bed on all three nights, and 02.00 h was the most wakeful time.

Ogilvie (1980) compared the noise levels in a 'nightingale' ward and a cubicle 'race-track' ward. The patients were elderly. The nightingale ward was noisier than the cubicle but in both wards noise levels at night were comparable to 'a living room by day', and the average of noise levels on both wards consistently exceeded the recommended level of 35 decibels (dB(A)) (a standard measure of intensity of sound) for a bedroom at night often by as much as 15 dB. People — staff and patients — were the most frequent source of noise, but the loudest noises came from equipment such as telephones, trolleys, doors.

Confused patients and conversations with the hard of hearing can pose considerable problems when attempting to reduce noise at night. Indeed, increasingly high dosages of sedatives are sometimes requested for noisy patients in the hope that this will allow the other patients to sleep at night and reduce the night nurses' stress levels. This is an understandable reaction, but other solutions and detailed assessment by both nurses and doctors should be undertaken before 'stoning' the apparently demented even further out of their minds. Can the physical condition of the patient be improved such that they are less liable to nocturnal confusion? Would a reduction in sedation be more efficacious than an increase? If the noisy patient's behaviour is intractable, what is the bed position in which they will cause least disruption? Should more staff be on night duty so that such persons can be 'specialed'? Where an institution has many such night-awake and noisy patients, should we have a special ward for them (Armstrong-Esther & Hawkins 1982)?

Night staff are not alone in shouldering the responsibility for reducing noise and other environmental irritants at night — although it is axiomatic that they should be vigilant about their own noise making. Footfall, talking, and nursing procedures should be as quiet as possible and we should remember that being out of sight, in the kitchen, duty room or office does not make noise 'out of sound'. However, the day staff have infinitely more resources available to them than the night staff. Oiling door hinges and trolley wheels, fixing windows, lights, heating, etc. can be accomplished by day. The services of administrators, carpenters and electricians may all need to be used to reduce the problem. It would not be beyond our wit to identify the major noise sources in our area and remove or reduce many of them. Patients themselves would readily supply a list of disturbances for us, as Sue Hopkins did (1980).

Dietary effect on sleep

Dietary habits seem to be important determinants of sleep patterns. People who are gaining weight tend to sleep more and have a higher proportion of REM or paradoxical sleep, whereas those losing weight and anorexic persons sleep less and have disturbed sleep. An article by Beecham Foods Nutrition Information Centre (1978) discussed how diet affects our sleep. This article reviewed research on the complex effects on sleep of amino acids such as tryptophane and levels of the brain transmitter serotonin. Serotonin is known to have effects upon mood regulation, pain sensitivity and sleep.

Horlicks® was for a long time advertised as promoting sleep. In one study, sleep following Horlicks® was found to be less interrupted than sleep following either hot milk or a soya and egg drink. However, it would seem that the continuance of a person's normal eating habits is more crucial than any particular food or drink. Volunteers in another study were given either a food drink or an inert capsule at bedtime. 'The subjects who normally took a bedtime snack slept better after the food drink, while those who usually had

no food in the late evening slept better after the placebo' (p. 35). This suggests that it is important in promoting good sleep to provide nourishment at the time the elderly person would usually take it and not assume that everyone should have the same regime. It is probable that the supper meal is too early for many people both in hospital and in institutional care. We may need to provide snacks later in the evening and ones which are similar to those which the person would take at home.

Research on sleep following coffee found sleep to be disturbed within the first three hours and slow wave (orthodox) sleep reduced, although the total length of sleep was unchanged. More than 10 cups of caffeine beverages per day results in dependence and tolerance. Early morning drowsiness owing to caffeine withdrawal and the obligatory cup of coffee to wake up is a widespread phenomenon for all age groups, including the elderly. The sleep disrupting effect of caffeine greatly increases with age (Karacan et al 1976). Adam (1980) states that two cups of coffee at bedtime cause very disturbed sleep in elderly people.

Anxiety and sleep

Any acute emotional arousal or conflict caused by a loss or perceived threat can result in brief periods of sleep disturbance. Causes include bereavement of person or places, abrupt change in lifestyle such as illness, hospital or institutional admission or discharge, and intense positive feeling such as may result from the birth of a grandchild, or the security of being cared for after a struggle to manage alone.

The majority of people respond with difficulty in falling asleep, intermittent awakening during the night and early morning arousal. They may lose a substantial amount of sleep but are not truly sleepy by day, feeling fatigued, aching and 'washed out' but unable to nap. Some people respond with excessive difficulty in remaining awake, tending to stay in bed longer than usual and returning to bed frequently during the day to nap.

Both reactions to stress can be adaptive. The first maintains vigilance to cope with the new situation, the second conserves energy. They represent different coping styles which are likely to be typical of the individual. After a few weeks the emotional reaction resolves and sleep returns to normal. As the lives of many elderly people are strewn with major and minor losses and threats, we should expect to see these sleep disruptions fairly frequently.

More persistent periods of sleep disturbance may arise from chronic tension-anxiety states. Sleep disturbance seems to be conditioned to chronic anxiety and the sleep problem and tension mutually reinforce one another. Such elderly people may stay in bed longer in an effort to resume sleep and try to nap with little success. High muscle tension may result in complaints of back and headache and pulse rates may be fast. They may complain of worried thoughts and anxious dreams, exhibit restless vigilant behaviour, and regard tension as normal for themselves. Sometimes these people sleep better in a new or strange environment which has no conditioned associations with the sleep problems. Changing factors such as smells, furniture and bedroom routines may help. Other people are conditioned to internal factors and 'trying to fall asleep' results in central nervous system arousal. These people fall asleep when doing such things as reading, watching television, etc. but become fully alert when lying in bed trying to sleep. Less commonly, the persistent tension results in chronic weariness and excessive sleeping, bed-rest and napping. Such fatigue-prone patients learn to 'take to bed'. The term 'neurasthenia' has been applied to such people. They are liable to develop a disorder of their sleep–wake circadian rhythm. They may be in a state of chronic despair or mild depression and concerned about somatic illnesses and symptoms. Their sleep problem is sometimes further confounded by taking sedatives for 'nerves'.

DRUGS ASSOCIATED WITH SLEEP DISORDERS

Most CNS stimulants and depressants have a more dramatic effect on functioning of elderly people and so are more disturbing to their sleep patterns (Coleman et al 1981), and to their daytime ef-

ficiency (Morgan 1987). The effects of these drugs are well documented and are summarized below.

Central nervous system (CNS) depressants

These include: sedatives, hypnotics, tranquillizers, anticonvulsants, antihypertensives, anti-depressants, antihistamines, beta adrenergic blockers, alcohol.

Sustained use

Elderly people in particular are liable to develop excessive somnolence when these drugs are used therapeutically in moderate to high doses. In addition to sleepiness they feel groggy, depressed, unstable, shaky, agitated and may even have episodes of amnesia or paranoia. Regestein (1982) states that 'the chronic use of sedatives impairs the already diminished cortical functioning of the elderly, rendering the elderly insomniac patient worse rather than better' (p. 167). Use of large bedtime doses may result in alveolar hypoventilation.

Tolerance and withdrawal

With sustained use CNS depressants become ineffective in inducing sleep, leading to physical and psychological dependence, increasing dosage, plus intermittent attempts to reduce or withdraw the drugs. The person who has become tolerant to sedatives — including barbiturates and non-barbiturates such as glutethimide, chloral hydrate, methaqualone, antihistamines, bromides, benzodiazepines and alcohol — develops long (more than five minutes) and frequent periods of wakening from sleep, especially during the second half of the night. The time to fall asleep also gets longer as the person becomes used to the drug. If the drug is omitted sleep latency may be several hours. Residual (hangover) effects during the day include sluggishness, poor co-ordination, ataxia, slurred speech, visual problems, and in the late afternoon restlessness and nervousness. Gradual withdrawal from sedatives results in an improvement in sleep for many people, though after long habituation the individual may not return to an absolutely normal sleep pattern. Rapid reduction or abrupt withdrawal of CNS depressants almost completely disrupts sleep. REM sleep is suppressed by these drugs and REM rebound can precipitate terrifying nightmare attacks. Withdrawal symptoms of nausea, muscle tension, aches, restlessness and nervousness are likely to occur in the succeeding days and sleep-related myoclonus may appear.

Morgan (1987) suggests that the effect of hypnotics on the daytime performance of elderly people has not yet been adequately studied. His comparison between shorter-acting (lormetazepam 1 mg) and longer-acting (nitrazepam 5 mg) hypnotics on 12 people aged between 75 and 96 years after 7 consecutive nightly doses revealed a greater performance decrement following nitrazepam than lormetazepam. He concluded that residual effects following repeated dosages are less likely if short-acting hypnotics are used, but when a short-acting drug is withdrawn the rebound insomnia and anxiety will occur more quickly and may even occur between doses, i.e. during the day.

CNS stimulants

These include amphetamines, methylphenidate, sympathomimetic drugs, analeptics and caffeine. Apart from drug abusers, the majority of stimulants are prescribed to treat medical conditions, e.g. appetite suppressant drugs for weight reduction, sympathomimetic drugs for asthma and chronic obstructive airway disease, analeptics for mood elevation of the depressed, stimulants for patients with somnolence, especially narcolepsy.

Sleep onset is delayed and total sleep time declines. To overcome the resultant daytime sleepiness more stimulants may then be taken. Sudden episodes of sleepiness by day — the 'crash' of the stimulant-dependent individual — occurs from time to time. The person may also be anxious and irritable, have difficulty concentrating and even become severely depressed and suicidal.

Sustained use or withdrawal from other drugs

Many drugs interfere with sleep. Two lists are par-

ticularly mentioned in the classification of sleep disorders, some of which are recognized for their psychotropic action, others not.

Group 1 includes antimetabolites and other cancer chemotherapeutic agents, thyroid preparation and anticonvulsants such as phenytoin, monoamine oxidase inhibitors (MAOI), adrenocorticotrophic hormone (ACTH), alpha-methyldopa, propranolol and many others. Sleep onset is delayed by the drugs in group 1, and they also result in interrupted sleep and early awakening. The severity of the effect depends on the drug dosage.

Group 2 includes diazepam, the major tranquilizers, sedating tricyclics and sometimes MAOI, marijuana, cocaine, phencyclidene, opiates and even aspirin-containing drugs. Sleep is improved during the use of group 2 drugs, but sleep disturbance occurs during withdrawal in the same way as withdrawal from other CNS depressants.

ILLNESS AND SLEEP DISTURBANCE

The majority of illnesses result in sleep disruption and further confound the sleep problems of elderly people. The sleep problem will only improve when the underlying medical condition is alleviated or cured.

Psychiatric illnesses

Psychiatric disorders which are associated with sleep problems include phobic, obsessive-compulsive and other neurotic disorders. Patients with psychotic depression generally fall asleep readily, but have difficulty in maintaining sleep and wake early in the morning feeling fatigued, achy and 'washed out'. Patients in the depressed phase of manic-depressive psychosis and those with mild depressive disorders tend to be excessively sleepy by day. Mania or hypomania results in difficulty in falling asleep and short sleep time. Such people may wake refreshed after as little as two or four hours sleep. It should be noted that the more elderly the patient with depression the greater the sleep loss in the second half of the night. Schizophrenia and schizoaffective disorders can result in partial or complete inversion of the day–night sleep cycle, and extreme agitation in the first half of the night. The extent of sleep disruption will depend on the severity of the illness.

Physical pathologies

Conditions of the central nervous system are particularly liable to disrupt the quantity and quality of sleep. Many cause pain, parasthesia and abnormal movements. Some fundamentally alter the state of consciousness.

Lesions of the brainstem and hypothalamus and cerebral atrophy may disrupt sleep onset and maintenance, whether they are due to neoplasms, vascular disorders, CNS infections, trauma, toxicity or degenerative changes. Roffwarg (1979) states:

> The confusional pattern at night in patients with organic mental disorders should be differentiated from the very brief episodes of nocturnal confusion often experienced by elderly patients subject to a new environment. However, it is not known to what extent degenerative changes in the CNS are responsible for symptoms of insomnia in otherwise apparently normal elderly people (p. 47).

Daytime somnolence is associated with many CNS pathologies. Raised intracranial pressure from any cause, including tumours (especially those of the pineal and posterior hypothalamus and any which impinge on the third ventricle), subdural and subarachnoid haemorrhage and hydrocephalus, all cause hypersomnolence. Severe daytime somnolence may develop gradually 6–18 months following head injury. Many toxic and infectious conditions, whether fungal, viral or bacterial, result in excessive sleepiness, including neurosyphilis, encephalitis lethargica and trypanosomiasis.

Brain surgery for intractable pain, Parkinsonism and psychiatric disorders sometimes produces abnormal sleep patterns and somnolence. Peripheral nerve and muscular diseases such as peripheral neuritis, fibrositis and myotonic dystrophies are also catalogued as causes of sleep disruption.

Almost all major endocrine and metabolic diseases result in sleep disruption and/or excessive daytime sleepiness, including Addison's disease, Cushing's syndrome, diabetes mellitus and hypo-glycaemia, hyper- and hypothyroidism. Renal failure and uraemia result in excessive sleepiness. Hepatic failure is often accompanied by nocturnal delirium. Gastrointestinal disease, especially ulceration and sleep-related dyspepsia, interferes with sleep.

Poor cardiac and respiratory function tends to deteriorate further during sleep resulting in angina, palpitations, cardiac arrhythmias, myocardial incompetence, coronary artery insufficiency, nocturnal dyspnoea and hyperpnoea, and worsening of Cheyne-Stokes respirations. The incidence of asthmatic attacks is highest at about four hours before the mid-point of the subject's nocturnal sleep span. Respiratory impairment during sleep can be a major problem for elderly people.

Sleep apnoea (Sleep-related cessation of breathing)

This may be either central (CNS) apnoea in which no respiratory effort occurs or upper airway obstructive apnoea in which respiratory snoring increases until a loud choking inspiratory gasp occurs when the patient's respiratory effort overcomes the occlusion, or a mixture of both. Respiration is normal during the waking state. More than 100 apnoeic attacks may occur per night. Although sleep apnoea syndrome may occur at any age the frequency seems to be high in elderly people over 60 years. The ratio of men to women is 30:1.

In most cases no anatomical defect is apparent, though sleep apnoea syndrome, especially of the obstructive variety, tends to be associated with a short thick neck with or without obesity. Acromegaly, hypothyroidism and nasal polyps may cause secondary mechanical airway problems. Forty per cent of people with this syndrome have hypertension and the severely affected may have heart failure consequent to sleep apnoea.

Those suffering from sleep apnoea usually fall asleep quickly, but waken several times during the night, sometimes gasping for air or with a sensation of choking and anxiety. The obstructive apnoeic patient, although noisy and exceedingly restless during attempts to breathe may be totally unaware of the difficulty which has awakened him from sleep. Sufferers do not become fully awake every time an apnoeic attack occurs, even though they repeatedly become hypoxic and hypercapnic. Cardiac arrhythmias occur and the obstructive apnoeic is particularly at risk of sudden death during sleep as a consequence. Excessive daytime sleepiness is the major complaint of obstructive or upper airway sleep apnoea. Many patients have headaches and a degree of disorientation on waking, and some have drenching night sweats.

Drug treatment and even weight reduction are not always effective though Tirlapur and Mir (1982) advocate weight loss for the obese patient. According to Parkes (1981) surgery for obstructive apnoea can be highly effective in relieving the problem, including tonsilectomy and thyroidectomy where relevant — and tracheostomy may be accepted as a permanent cure by some sufferers.

Alveolar hypoventilation

Tidal volume decreases during sleep, resulting in hypercapnia and hypoxaemia without apnoeic attacks. There is a failure of ventilation to respond to chemical control. Causes in adults include massive obesity, chronic obstructive pulmonary disease, scoliosis, cordotomy and neurological lesions of respiratory control centres, poliomyelitis, myotonic dystrophy and narcolepsy.

Nocturnal sleep is disturbed for those who have actual or potential signs of daytime alveolar hypoventilation. Some complain primarily of sleep disturbance, others primarily of daytime sleepiness. An important finding by Calverley et al (1982) was that, of patients with chronic obstructive airway disease, 'blue bloaters' who have daytime hypoxaemia and hypercapnia have significantly more hypoxaemic episodes during sleep than 'pink puffers'. Giving continuous oxygen (O_2) at night reduced the number of hypoxaemic episodes and increased the amount of deep orthodox sleep. Wakefulness was reduced so that the sleep of 'blue bloaters' taking O_2 was similar to that of healthy normal people.

Sleep-related leg movements

These symptoms are predominantly seen in middle-aged and elderly persons. Nocturnal myoclonus involves repetitive and highly stereotyped leg muscle jerks, occurring about every 20–40 seconds for a few minutes or an hour in episodes of 30 or more jerks. The contraction always consists of extension of the big toe plus partial flexion of the ankle, knee and sometimes hip. These movements only occur during sleep, and are always followed by partial arousal or awakening. The jerks are not linked with whole body movements and are often not visible to the observer nor consciously perceived by the sleeper, but recorded by electromyography (EMG). People with nocturnal myoclonus complain of frequent nocturnal awakening, unrefreshed sleep and daytime sleepiness. The incidence of leg cramps, disruption of bedclothes and falling out of bed is generally higher than in the rest of the population.

'Restless leg' syndrome

This is an extremely disagreeable deep sensation of creeping inside the calves whenever sitting or lying down, resulting in an almost irresistable urge to move the legs. The aetiology is unknown, though inadequate circulation, motor neurone disease or inheritance may be implicated. Almost all patients with 'restless leg' syndrome also have nocturnal myoclonus, though not vice versa. It results in difficulty in maintaining unbroken sleep periods, with consequent complaints of insomnia by night and somnolence by day. The 'restless leg' syndrome becomes more severe with age and is exacerbated by sleep deprivation. Some people can gain relief by vigorous leg exercises.

Parasomnias (undesirable physical phenomena associated with sleep) may be exhibited by the old as well as the young. Sleep-walking in elderly people is more likely to be due to psychomotor epilepsy, fugue states or sleep drunkenness than to true somnambulism. Nightmares are more prevalent at times of emotional stress and during REM rebound from drug withdrawal. Elderly persons with sleep-related inadequacy in swallowing saliva are at risk of respiratory aspiration, and sleep-related gastrointestinal reflux may result in oesophageal stricture or aspiration pneumonia. The primary sleep disorders such as narcolepsy and idiopathic CNS hypersomnolence persist into old age, so may be occasionally seen. The habitual long and short sleepers will also continue this pattern into old age.

CONCLUSIONS

Sleep research has gone a long way toward helping us understand the sleep problems of elderly people. We can use this knowledge to assess, care for, teach and sympathize with the people in our charge. It may help us and the elderly people to overthrow the prejudice that 'sleeping by day is a sin'.

There is possibly greater variability in the sleep of elderly people than in that of the young adult, and sleep–wake cycles may be more easily disrupted in the elderly (Preston 1973). Increased dissatisfaction with sleep is generally supported by objective (EEG) evidence of reduced duration, depth and continuity of sleep (Morgan 1987). Many current sleep researchers consider elderly folk to need the same amount of sleep as younger people and to be at risk of becoming seriously sleep-deprived if they are not given lengthened opportunities to sleep compared with those of the young. All seem to agree that the potential causes of insomnia increase in old age, that the primary sleep abnormalities do not remit, that secondary sleep abnormalities increase and that hypnotic overuse is endemic in the elderly population with all its deleterious side-effects.

Gledhill (1985), in a questionnaire survey of 109 elderly people who were living in the community either in sheltered accommodation or attending a day centre, found that 53% reported a moderate or severe sleep problem (insomnia) which they attributed primarily to worry, or pain and discomfort, or lack of physical exercise. The most common causes of awakening reported by sleep observers of elderly people are: sleep apnoea; nocturnal myoclonus (Carskadon et al 1982); physical discomfort, especially distended bladder and urinary urgency (Webb & Swinbourne 1971); pain; 'restless legs'; and dyspnoea.

According to Roffwarg (1979), the most common causes of sleep disturbance for adults include

chronic pain (especially due to rheumatism and arthritis), nocturnal dyspnoea, nocturnal discomfort from pruritis, peripheral neuritis, enforced positions, strangury, dyspepsia, cerebral degeneration, abnormal movements, secondary disturbance of the circadian sleep–wake cycle and the environmental factors associated with hospitalisation (p. 49).

The most important and consistent finding regarding sleep problems for elderly people is the number and length of periods of awakening after sleep has started. However, as in all age groups, there are considerable individual differences. Research findings may reveal statistically significant differences between the sleep of the young and the old, but we can never assume that the individual elderly person in our care conforms to a trend. Detailed assessment is essential before we plan our care.

ASSESSMENT OF SLEEP

The initial assessment of sleep or lack of it by both medical and nursing staff relies heavily on the subjective report of the sleeper. Deeper analysis of the sleep problem is possible. Nurses have the inestimable advantage of being present night and day to assess the objective sleep and wake behaviour of individuals, whereas doctors and sleep researchers are able to undertake polygraphic recordings of internal events such as neurological and cardiovascular responses.

There are a number of potential problems which face us when assessing the quantity and quality of patients' sleep. To what extent do the person's subjective complaints about sleep correspond to objective measurable sleep problems? The correspondence is not absolute by any means. From some of the research discussed earlier it is obvious that some elderly people who have no sleep complaints in fact have multiple micro-arousals during their night's sleep and spend much of their sleep in light stages of sleep. Micro-apnoeic arousals and even nocturnal myoclonic attacks will not generally be visible even to the most observant night nurse, but the aftermath of daytime sleepiness and complaints of poor sleeping will be genuine. On the other hand, some elderly (and younger) people who complain of poor sleep do not exhibit EEG abnormalities when monitored in sleep laboratories.

An important distinction should be made between the person who is fatigued but tense and although longing to sleep is rarely able to do so, and the person who is tired and suffering from sleep deprivation who if given the opportunity will be able to make up the sleep lack by spending a longer time in bed at night and taking daytime naps. Severely sleep-deprived persons will eventually fall asleep whatever the surrounding activities, whereas the fatigued tense person is likely to be vigilant of all that is happening.

What about the person whose circadian rhythms are out of phase with surrounding society — wanting and able to sleep for long periods by day and having difficulty in sleeping by night? A detailed assessment of their sleep–wake patterns and social responses over the weeks before we meet them, plus a 24-hour diary of sleeping should be kept day after day before we can be certain of this diagnosis. We should not expect to be able to reverse the situation 'overnight'. We should obviously be wary of dismissing complaints about poor night-time sleep. Apart from any other consideration it is important that the elderly person feels she has slept well, that we are willing to listen and do all in our power to provide an environment in which she has the opportunity to sleep. Table 15.3

Table 15.3 Measurement tools for assessing sleep.

Objective

1. Polygraphic recordings, EEG, EOG, EMG, HR, RR, T Oxygen levels in blood or ear oxymetry
2. Movement — pressure transducers on bed
   — accelerometers on arms/legs
3. Observation of sleep–wake timing and behaviour using sleep charts

Subjective

1. Self-report or questionnaire, or sleep diaries

Assessment of fatigue and hypnotic drugs

1. Choice reaction time and critical flicker fusion threshold
2. Observation of person's behaviour and appearance
3. Rating scales of subjective feelings and questionnaires

illustrates some of the methods of sleep assessment used by researchers. Further discussion of nursing assessment of patients' sleep problems can be found in Fordham (1988).

When caring for elderly people, nurses are usually confined to observations of patients' sleeping and waking behaviours and subjective reporting by the elderly person and her relatives. The areas which should be assessed by the nurse or carer and the type of questions which can be used are shown in the following assessment of sleep.

SLEEP ASSESSMENT FORMAT

Name
Age
Sex
Medical diagnosis
Investigations
Admission
Discharge.

Major areas to be assessed

1. Normal pattern of sleep in health.
   Sleep pattern during periods of stress in life.
   Current sleep pattern — including day and night:

   (a) night and day nurse's (carer's) report of sleep pattern plus possible causes of sleep problems
   (b) patient's opinion of cause of problems and patient's views of what would solve the problems.

If elderly person, relative or carer, identifies a sleep problem then the following areas should be assessed in depth:

2. Drugs, especially narcotics, hypnotics, stimulants and sympathomimetics.
3. Nutritional status especially hyperphagia, anorexia, starvation, gaining or losing weight.
4. Normal eating and drinking habits. Special diets, recent changes, pre-sleeping food and drink.

5. Emotional state such as anxiety or depression, plus possible causes.
6. Daytime and night-time symptoms — awake and asleep, e.g. pain, discomfort, nocturia, incontinence, cough, dyspnoea, night sweats, snoring, disorientation.
7. Waking activities. Postural or other constraint on movement.
8. Sleeping environment — ward, institution, home, especially noise, light, cold, nursing/medical procedures interrupting sleep.

Sleep questionnaires (Malasanos et al 1977)

Using a selection of the following items will give the nurse comprehensive information about a patient's sleep pattern and problems with respect to:

(a) Normal pattern
(b) Since admission/illness.

1. How well do you normally/recently sleep?
2. What time do you usually/recently go to bed? Prepare to sleep?
3. Do you fall asleep right away — normally/recently? *or* How long does it take you to fall asleep?
4. Do you wake up in the night?
5. What wakes you once you have fallen asleep?
6. What (if anything) helps you get back to sleep?
7. What time do you normally/recently wake in the morning?
8. Do you normally take naps in the day? If yes — when, for how long?
9. How do you feel (rested?) when you wake up?
10. Do you dream at night?
11. Has anyone ever told you that you:
    — grind your teeth at night
    — walk or talk
    — snore?
12. How much sleep do you think you should have to stay healthy?
13. Have you had any worries recently?
14. What activity/work do you normally do in the daytime?
15. What do you normally do in the hour or so before night-time sleep — watch television, read, bath?

Preparation for sleep:

1. What do you do just before going to bed to sleep
   — lock up house, let cat out, wash face, clean teeth, say prayers?
2. Do you eat before going to sleep? If Yes — what?
3. Do you drink before going to sleep? If Yes — what?
4. Do you take any medicines to help you sleep?
5. Are you taking any other medicines at all?

Sleeping environment:

1. Do you need special bedding to help you sleep?
2. How many pillows do you use?
3. Do you sleep with lights on/off?
4. Does a light bother you?
5. Do you need absolute quietness to sleep?
6. Do noises keep you awake, or wake you up?
7. Do you need the bedroom cold/warm to sleep?
8. Do you sleep with the window open at night?

Pre-sleep tiredness questionnaire (Porter and Horne 1981):

1. Do you feel you have gone to bed — too early, at the right time, too late?
2. Has your day been — enjoyable, normal, upsetting?
3. Have you fallen asleep during the day? If Yes, when and for how long?
4. How sleepy have you felt in the last $\frac{1}{4}$ hour? Alert _____ Sleep onset soon
5. How tired have you felt in the last $\frac{1}{4}$ hour? Not tired _____ Very tired

Post-sleep questionnaire:

1. At what time did you:

(a) fall asleep last night?
(b) wake up this morning?
(c) get out of bed this morning?

2. Which of the following phrases do you consider best describes the quality of your sleep last night?

| Much better than normal | Better than normal | Normal | Worse than normal | Much worse than normal |

3. If you did not sleep well, please give reasons, if any, e.g. cramp, noise, not tired, hungry, full bladder.
4. What woke you this morning, e.g. alarm, person, light, bladder?
5. If you could, would you have liked to have slept longer this morning?

Assessment of sedative giving/withdrawal:

1. Leeds sleep evaluation questionnaire (Hindmarch 1980)

   (a) Ease of getting to sleep
       Extremely difficult _____ Extremely easy
   (b) Ease of awakening
       Extremely difficult _____ Extremely easy
   (c) Quality of sleep
       Excellent _____ Extremely poor
   (d) Extent of 'hangover' following awakening
       Severe _____ None

2. The following words produced a significant difference in response between those who had received diazepam and those who had received a placebo (Weber et al 1975). Those on diazepam were more likely to mark the line close to the right-hand (sleepy) words.

Strong	_____	Weak
Refreshed	_____	Tired
Energetic	_____	Lazy
Vigorous	_____	Exhausted

Awake	_____	Sleepy
Stimulated	_____	Sedated
Efficient	_____	Inefficient
Attentive	_____	Distracted
Able to concentrate	_____	Unable to concentrate

PATIENT GOALS/OBJECTIVES REGARDING SLEEP

1. The elderly person will sleep at the normal times and for the normal length for her.
2. The elderly person will have undisturbed sleep at night.
3. The elderly person will have rest-time during the day.
4. The elderly person will feel and appear rested.
5. The elderly person will understand the use of sedatives and analgesics.
6. The elderly person will be able to plan her return to a healthy sleep–wake activity pattern.

The exact goals and the priority for intervention will depend upon the findings of the assessment.

NURSING INTERVENTION TO PROMOTE SLEEP

1. Management of environment, e.g. position of beds, oiling door hinges and trolley wheels, ventilation, lighting, reduction of staff noise at night.
2. Planning 24-hour sleep–activity patterns suitable for the individual.
3. Helping patient to achieve pre-sleep rituals as near as possible to her normal pattern.
4. Provision of nutrition and fluids at times normal for that patient.
5. Organization of nursing, medical and other intervention to give patient undisturbed periods of time (90 minutes at least for one complete sleep cycle).
6. Relief of physical symptoms which interrupt sleep, e.g. pain, frequency, dyspnoea, cough.
7. Discussion and relief of psychological distress.

8. Review of the dosages and effects of sedatives and stimulants.
9. Patient teaching regarding sleep habits.
10. Treatment of any underlying medical/surgical condition.

The area of intervention over which nurses have most control are the sleeping environment and nursing interruptions of sleep. However, the total management of factors likely to disrupt sleep patterns requires discussion, decisions and action to be undertaken jointly by nurses, medical, paramedical and administrative staff, as well as help from engineers and porters.

Alternatives to hypnotic drugs for elderly insomniacs is well discussed by Morgan (1987). Gledhill (1985) in his review of the sleep of elderly people makes a strong plea for the use of psychological techniques in the treatment of insomnia. The two methods which he describes are stimulus control and relaxation. Stimulus control involves altering the sleep pattern or timing and strengthening the environmental and behavioural cues which are associated with sleeping. Relaxation techniques may involve either muscular tensing and relaxing, or mental focusing. Gledhill suggests that the latter may be more appropriate to the many elderly people who have pain or discomfort from musculoskeletal disorders such as arthritis.

There is a tendency for the sleep problems of elderly people to be regarded as intractable; techniques which would be tried for the young adult are often not even considered for old people. Nurses are in a position both to use and teach these interventions and to evaluate their efficacy.

REASSESSMENT OR CONTINUING ASSESSMENT OF SLEEP

This requires the repeated assessment of all the factors which were originally assessed.

The primary question which is being asked in reassessment is: Have the patient's goals been achieved or not? If not, why not? Have we or the patient failed to carry out the planned intervention?

Were the goals unrealistic? For example, we and the patient may have to accept disturbed night sleep as an intractable problem if the patient has irreversible CNS pathology. Were we trying to push the elderly person into a pattern of sleep which suited our needs rather than hers?

FINALLY, A WORD ON LONELINESS

Could we be more adventurous and enable institutional care to be more like home — where possible, allowing family members to settle their elderly folk for the night, and spouses (or partners) to sleep together if they wish?

Many elderly folk have had the physical comfort and warmth of a spouse in their bed for decades and either owing to bereavement or to hospital or institutional admission or both have to face the night in solitude. Some have substituted their pets as bed companions whilst at home. Others may be in a state of mental regression in which they long once more to hold their children and babies in their arms or even to be held again in their own mother's arms. Goodman, a poet in her seventies, wrote of the need to be mothered:

Sleeping pills

The light within me clicks
Who put out the light?

It is dark
I am alone, afraid,
Mother, Mother,
I can't sleep.

My mother does not come,
My mother is dead.

One pill,
Two pills,
Three pills,
Mother me, pills.

Night nurses often have a closer relationship with wakeful patients than day nurses. The comfort of a person who will listen to the troubles and anxieties at the end of the day and give a loving touch or hug may be the best tanquillizer in the world.

REFERENCES

Adam K 1980 A time for rest and a time for play. Nursing Mirror 150(10): 17–18

Armstrong-Esther C A, Hawkins S C H 1982 Day for night. Circadian rhythms in the elderly. Nursing Times 78(30): 1263–6

Beck U, Brezinova V, Hunter W et al 1975 Plasma growth hormone and slow wave sleep increase after interruption of sleep. Journal of Clinical Endocrinology and Metabolism 40(5): 812–815

Beecham Foods Nutrition Information Centre 1978 How diet affects sleep. Nursing Mirror 147(20): 32–35

Calverley P M A, Brezinova V, Douglas N J, Catterall J R, Fenley D C 1982 The effects of oxygenation on sleep quality in chronic bronchitis and emphysema. American Review of Respiratory Disease 126(2): 206–210

Carskadon M A, Van den Hoed J, Dement W C 1982 Insomnia and sleep disturbances in the aged. Sleep and daytime sleepiness in the elderly. Journal of Geriatric Psychiatry 13(2): 135–151

Coleman R, Miles S L, Guilleminault C 1981 Sleep–wake disorders in the elderly: a polysomnographic analysis. Journal of the American Geriatric Society 29: 289–296

Colquhoun W P (ed) 1971 Biological rhythms and human performance. Academic Press, New York

Colquhoun W P (ed) 1972 Aspects of human efficiency: diurnal rhythm and sleep loss. English University Press

Dement W C, Miles L E, Carskadon M A 1982a Changes in the sleep and waking EEG's of non-demented and demented elderly subjects. Journal of the American Geriatric Society 30(2): 86–93

Dement W C, Miles L E, Carskadon M A 1982b 'White Paper' on sleep and ageing. American Geriatric Society Journal 30(1): 25–50

Feinberg G I 1968 The ontogenesis of human sleep and the relationship of sleep variables to intellectual function in the aged. Comprehensive Psychiatry 9: 138–147

Fordham M 1988 Sleep disturbance. In: Wilson-Barnett J, Batehup L 1988 Patient problems. Scutari Press, London

Gledhill K 1985 Sleep and the elderly: some psychological dimensions and their implications for treatment. In: Butler A (ed) Ageing: recent advances and creative responses. Croom Helm, London

Gress L D, Bahr R T, Hassanein R S 1981 Nocturnal behaviour of selected institutionalised adults. Journal of Gerontological Nursing 7(2): 86–92

Guilleminault C, Dement W C 1978 Sleep apnoea syndromes and related sleep disorders. In: Williams R L, Karacan I (eds) Sleep disorders: diagnosis and treatment. Wiley, New York, p 9–28

Helton M C, Gordon S H, Nunnery S L 1980 The correlation between sleep deprivation and the intensive care syndrome. Heart and Lung 9: 465–468

Hindmarch I 1980 Calling time on hypnotic drugs. Nursing Mirror 150(11): 37–38

Hopkins S 1980 Silent night? In: Redfern S J, Fordham M (eds) Nursing 20 Sleep and Comfort 870–873

Horne J A 1980 Sleep and body restitution. Experientia 36: 11–13

Johns M 1975 Factor analysis of subjectively reported sleep habits and the nature of insomnia. Psychological Medicine 5: 83

Karacan I, Thornby J I, Anch A M et al 1976 Dose response effects of coffee on the sleep of normal middle aged men. Sleep Research 5: 71

Koreorgos J 1980 Sleep and sleep disorders. Practitioner 224: 717–721

Lobban M, Tredre B 1964 Diurnal rhythms of renal excretion and of body temperature in aged subjects. Journal of Physiology 170: 29

McGhie A, Russell S 1962 The subjective assessment of normal sleep patterns. Journal of Mental Science 108: 642

Malasanos L, Barkauska V, Moss M, Stoltenberg-Allen K 1977 Health assessment. Mosby, St Louis

Minors D S, Waterhouse J M 1981 Circadian rhythms and the human. Wright, Bristol

Morgan K 1987 Sleep and ageing. Croom Helm, London

Ogilvie A J 1980 Sources and levels of noises on the wards at night. Nursing Times 76(31): 1363–1366

Pacini C M, Fitzpatrick J 1982 Sleep patterns of hospitalised and non-hospitalised aged individuals. Journal of Gerontological Nursing 8(6): 327–332

Parkes J D 1981 Day-time drowsiness. The Lancet 2: 1213–1218

Porter J M, Horne J A 1981 Exercise and sleep behaviour: a questionnaire approach. Ergonomics 24(7): 511–521

Preston F 1973 Further sleep problems in airline pilots on world-wide schedules. Aerospace Medicine 44: 775

Prinz P N, Peskind E R, Vitaliano P P et al 1982 Changes in sleep and waking EEGs of nondemented and demented elderly subjects. Journal of the American Geriatrics Society 30: 86–93

Regestein Q R 1982 Insomnia and sleep disturbances in the aged: sleep and insomnia in the elderly. Journal of Geriatric Psychiatry 13(2): 153–171

Reinberg A 1966 Circadian rhythms. (Letter.) Journal of the American Medical Association 196: 108

Roffwarg H P (ed) 1979 Diagnostic classification of sleep and arousal disorders. Sleep 2(1): 1–137

Roth T, Kramer M, Trinder J 1972 The effects of noise during sleep on the sleep patterns of different age groups. Canadian Psychiatric Association 17: 197–201

Samis H V, Capobianco S 1978 Ageing and biological rhythms. Advances in Experimental Medicine and Biology 108. Plenum Press, New York

Sanford S 1982 Sleep and its implications for intensive care nursing. International Intensive Care Nursing Conference. Proceedings p 73–77

Serio M, Romano M, DeMagistris L et al 1970 The circadian rhythm of plasma cortisol in subjects over 70 years of age. Journal of Gerontology 25: 95

Shock N 1977 Biological theories of ageing In: Birren J, Schaie K (eds) Handbook of the psychology of ageing. Van Nostrand Reinhold, New York

Takahashi Y, Kipris D M, Daughaday W H 1968 Growth hormone secretion during sleep. Journal of Clinical Investigation 47: 2079

Tirlapur V G, Mir M A 1982. (Letter.) Lancet 1: 163–164

Webb W B 1982 Sleep in older persons: sleep structures in 50 to 60 year old men and women. Journal of Gerontology 37: 581–586

Webb W B, Swinburne H 1971 An observational study of sleep of the aged. Perceptual Motor Skills 32: 895–898

Weber A, Jermini C, Grandjean E P 1975 Relationship between objective and subjective assessment of experimentally induced fatigue. Ergonomics 18: 151–156

Wessler R, Rubin M, Sollberger A 1976 Circadian rhythm of activity and sleep-wakefulness in elderly institutionalised patients. Journal of Interdisciplinary Cycle Research 7: 333

Williams R, Agnew H, Webb W 1967 Effects of prolonged stage 4 and 1-REM sleep deprivation EEG task performance and psychologic responses. US School of Aerospace Medicine Report

Winfree A T 1982 Circadian timing of sleepiness in man and woman. American Journal of Physiology 243(3): 193–204R

Winget C, Vernikos-Danellis J, Cronin S 1972 Circadian rhythm asynchrony in man during hypokinesis. Journal of Applied Physiology 33: 640

CHAPTER CONTENTS

What is sexuality? 263

Sexuality in Western societies 263
Myths and stereotypes 263
Double discrimination 264
The experts' prejudices 265
Sex can be good for you 265

Sexuality and elderly people 265
Physiological aspects 265
Psychosocial aspects 266
Ill health, disability and sexuality 267
Treatments and sexuality 268

Roles for nurses 269
Nurses as educators 269
Nurses as advocates 269

Conclusion 270

16

Expressing sexuality

Christine Webb

WHAT IS SEXUALITY?

Sexuality is much more than physical acts of sex. It encompasses

the quality of being human, all that we are as men and women . . . encompassing the most intimate feelings and deepest longings of the heart to find meaningful relationships (Hogan 1980, p. 3).

Sexuality and sensuality go to make up our self-concept and how we see ourselves and are seen by others. Our sexual self-concept, like all other parts of our personality, is a social phenomenon. We learn through living in a culture what are its expected and approved forms of behaviour, and if we do not live up to these norms we may experience guilt and feelings of inadequacy.

SEXUALITY IN WESTERN SOCIETIES

MYTHS AND STEREOTYPES

Sexuality in Western societies is tied to youth and physical attractiveness, and we are bombarded with media portrayals of beautiful young women and handsome young men virtually 24 hours a day in advertisements on television, in public transport, on billboards and in magazines. Feminine delicate features and slim bodies or masculine rugged, sporty leanness are what we are urged to strive for. No advertising executive would dream of using images of elderly people with thinning, receding, greying hair and sagging breasts or abdomens to create an image of beauty and desirability. Mellowed, comfortable pictures of older people may sell thermal underwear or storage heaters, but there is nothing sexual or sensual about these. Very much to the contrary, older people are generally assumed to be sexless. It is thought that libido and sexual needs decline along with loss of the culturally valued outer signs of beauty or handsomeness, and that at the same time sexual capacity fades too. Social usefulness is defined for men by productiveness at work and retirement from work may be associated in people's minds with retirement from sexual life as well (Kuhn 1976). For women the menopause is widely believed to herald this sexless, useless phase. People are declared obsolescent and are cast aside as if they were a worn-out washing machine or broken-down car. This social devaluation is further signified and realized in the form of low old-age pensions.

Studies of attitudes of professional carers towards sexual expression by elderly people offer conflicting evidence. Szasz (1983) carried out a survey of attitudes of nursing home staff in the USA, and found that 'acceptable sexual behaviours identified by staff were limited to hugging and kissing on the cheek'. However staff also said that residents probably needed 'more intimate touching and affection'. Damrosch (cited in Allen 1987) studied American nursing and medical students' attitudes and concluded that they were favourably disposed towards sexuality in elderly people.

DOUBLE DISCRIMINATION

Even within this discrimination against elderly people there is yet further discrimination. Men who still show signs of sexual activity are labelled 'dirty old men', but there is a 'good public relations' side to this (Sontag 1978). Men are supposed to maintain their 'manhood' for longer than women, and society lends approval and even celebrity to those who father children at an advanced age. Charlie Chaplin and Pablo Picasso were two of these famous fathers. But there are no lauded

'dirty old women'. Signs of wanting a sexual relationship, 'flirting', and dressing like lamb when one is really mutton are viewed as unseemly and distasteful or even disgusting in a woman. Older men may be described as handsome but older women are never beautiful (de Beauvoir 1973, Sontag 1978).

Balding in men is often said to be a sign of increasing virility, and greying hair denotes a distinguished man. Women's thinning hair is never seen as enviable, however, and certainly not as an indication of increased sexuality. Rather, women often colour-rinse their greying hair to make it more 'attractive'. It is noteworthy that the English language has no parallel term for virility to describe high levels of sexuality in women — the phenomenon is not supposed to exist and so a name is not needed (Webb 1983).

The bad faith involved in these two sets of double standards for the old and young and for women and men (Sontag 1978) is further evidenced in jokes. A Dr Palmore has studied jokes related to ageing and sexuality and found that in general they reveal a hostile and negative view of ageing. However, jokes about women were negative in 77% of cases while this was true of only 51% of jokes about men (Puner 1974). Other cultural myths about sexuality in old age promote the idea that it is acceptable for older men to marry younger women. Indeed this is a cause for congratulation and envy of the man. Older women should not marry younger men, and such an act on the part of the woman would lead to accusations of cradle-snatching as well as to doubts about the motives or psychosexual adjustment of the man (Kuhn 1976). Marriage or remarriage by old people is generally frowned upon, and Trimmer (1978) considers this to be due to links between sexuality and procreation in our culture. Thus, once procreation is no longer possible all sexual activity should cease.

These myths and stereotypes act as self-fulfilling prophecies for elderly people (Kuhn 1976). They are told that they are sexually unattractive, unwanted and useless and this information rebounds on their self-concept and adds to their negative self-view (Weg 1983). As a result, when they experience sexual urges they think these are abnormal and feelings of guilt, shame and embarrassment ensue.

THE EXPERTS' PREJUDICES

Even among the 'experts' there are prejudices to be found. Sexual relations may be discussed in textbooks only in terms of marital relations, implying that there is no place for sex unless people are married. Masturbation may be seen as acceptable in the absence of a marital partner but not as an activity which anyone might partake of by choice, as in the articles written by Costello (1975) and Puner (1974). Scully and Bart discovered in 1973 that few of the findings of Masters and Johnson's famous and extensive studies of sexual behaviour had worked their way through into current textbooks in the 10 years following their publication. They found a widespread belief among medical writers in the 'normality' of vaginal orgasm and little reference to clitoral orgasm. Today, over 15 years later still, the same observations can be made of the literature on ageing and sexuality. The clitoris and its function are rarely mentioned, and marital sex is used as the standard for discussion of other forms, which are only of importance in the absence of a marital partner. This confirms a view of vaginal intercourse as the norm for women and the only way for men to achieve sexual satisfaction. Homosexuality and bisexuality are rarely discussed.

SEX CAN BE GOOD FOR YOU

After all this pessimism and simple inaccuracy it is a refreshing relief to learn that sex is good for elderly people. In a study of 70-year-old women and men in Sweden, Persson (1980) found that men who continued to have sexual intercourse slept better, had better mental activity and a more positive attitude towards sexual activity in old age. Similarly, women who continued to have sexual intercourse retained their former levels of emotional stability, had low levels of anxiety, had better mental health, felt generally more healthy and had a positive attitude towards sexual activity in old age.

Sexual activity has been said to help arthritis,

reduce physical and psychological tensions and promote a good physical condition (Butler & Lewis 1973, quoted in Robinson 1983 & Kuhn 1976). Taking the wider concept of sexuality, too, the value of continuing to take account of this dimension of humanity into old age is sympathetically expressed by Weg (1983) when she says,

The intimacy and warmth often associated with sexual expression have significance beyond the pleasurable release of sexual tension — an important assertion and commitment of self and a reaffirmation of the connection with life itself (p. 45).

On that positive note, myths and stereotypes will be left behind in order to consider the realities of sexuality and elderly people.

SEXUALITY AND ELDERLY PEOPLE

PHYSIOLOGICAL ASPECTS

Physiological changes occurring with ageing have a relatively small part to play in sexual function.

In older women, vaginal lubrication is slower, vaginal expansion and contraction of the uterus are depressed, the labia are no longer elevated and the fat under the mons veneris is much reduced. The clitoris remains relatively unaltered but low levels of oestrogen may cause vaginal soreness, painful clitoral stimulation and uterine spasms during orgasm (Berman & Lief 1976, Trimmer 1978, Masters & Johnson 1981). Women remain capable of multiple orgasms and may experience an increase in sexual desire after the menopause, when androgens are minimally opposed by oestrogens (Weg 1983) and fear of unwanted pregnancy is gone (Puner 1974). Regular sexual activity by women will usually help to maintain sexual capacity, but masturbation is less effective than coitus in counteracting vaginal dryness and irritation (Blackman & Leiblum 1981).

Masters and Johnson (1981) report that men over the age of 60 years take longer to achieve full penile engorgement, and may have a decrease in expulsive pressure and a reduction in the volume of ejaculatory fluid expelled. Also, although levels of sexual interest may remain, the subjective desire for ejaculation may be reduced. Erection is more rapidly lost after ejaculation than in the earlier years. Men may be affected by 'performance anxiety' if they are unaware that these changes are normal and do not herald the termination of sexual activity. Women, too, may feel threatened if their partners do not ejaculate (Hendricks & Hendricks 1978).

Contrary to popular mythology, both elderly women and men report that factors in the man usually lead to the cessation of sexual activity, rather than disinterest on the part of the woman (Hendricks & Hendricks 1978). The most common of these male factors are illness, lack of interest, and inability to have an erection (impotence). Berman and Lief (1976) also consider lack of knowledge about normal sexual function and a poor marital relationship to be important influences. There is wide agreement that psychosocial factors have a much greater impact on sexuality in elderly people than physiological factors (Hendricks & Hendricks 1978, Sontag 1978, Masters & Johnson 1981, Corby & Zarit 1983, Weg 1983).

PSYCHOSOCIAL ASPECTS

Past sexuality is the best predictor of levels of sexual activity in elderly people (Persson 1980, Masters & Johnson 1981). People who are at present in the elderly age groups were brought up as young people in a period of strict religious morality (Comfort 1977). They were taught that sex was an activity to be confined to the marital relationship and for purposes of procreation, at least for women. Thus sex outside marriage and sexual activity for simple pleasure, such as after the menopause or by masturbation, were sinful (Kuhn 1976, Weg 1983).

Women's tendency to live longer than men and therefore to be left without a marital partner, the earlier decline in sexual function in men already noted, and the cultural prescription that men should take the initiative in sexual relations make women's position more unsatisfactory. Nevertheless, studies report that increasing numbers of women in the 50 to 70 age group masturbate, suggesting that social mores are becoming more flexible (Hendricks & Hendricks 1978).

Single elderly people face particular problems

according to Corby and Zarit (1983) because they are not thought to have a legitimate right or need for sexual privacy, whether at home or in institutions. Frequently, sexual expression is discouraged in institutions by the physical segregation of the sexes, and this may be because of fears of 'inappropriate' sexual behaviour or of complaints from relatives who find the elderly person's sexuality anxiety-provoking. Corby and Zarit report on a study by Silverstone and Wynter in 1975 in which a 'heterosexual living space' was introduced in an institution. Better social adjustment followed, seen for example in improved grooming and less swearing by men, greater use of privacy by closing doors when dressing, and overt sexual contacts.

Homosexuality in relation to elderly people has been little studied, but the problems faced by older homosexual women and men are probably little different from those of heterosexuals, in that the major one is finding suitable partners (Weg 1983). Homosexual men may be damaged by stereotypes similar to those applied to heterosexuals, because generalizations are usually based on a youth-oriented perspective and the assumption that all homosexual men are alike. For older lesbians life may be easier because the number of eligible partners may be larger and because of a commitment to longer-term relationships (Weg 1983).

In a comparative study of literature available about 106 cultures, Winn and Newton (1982) found that in 70% of the cultures studied there were expectations of continued sexual activity by men as ageing advanced. The comparative figure for women was a higher 84%. A majority of these references were to women's changed reproductive role after menopause and a consequent lessening of inhibitions in sexual behaviour, conversation, humour and gestures. Overall, however, many references were found to negative attitudes to the sexual desirability of older people.

Psychosocial factors, then, play a greater role in influencing sexuality and sexual function in elderly people — as indeed they do at other stages of adult life. Availability of a suitable partner, physical health, past sexual activity and living accommodation are among the strongest factors involved.

For women, continuing sexual activity is positively related to a warm and socially approved relationship with a man, while for men boredom, fatigue, illness, overindulgence in food and drink, and fear of performance failure are reported to inhibit satisfactory sexual activity (George & Weiler 1981). Above all, it should be emphasized, to quote Weg again, that

there is no one way to love or to be loved; there is no one liaison that is superior to another. No one lifestyle in single-hood or marriage, heterosexual or homosexual, will suit all persons. Self-pleasuring, homosexuality, bisexuality, celibacy and heterosexuality are all in the human repertoire (Weg 1983, p. 76).

ILL HEALTH, DISABILITY AND SEXUALITY

Any illness or disability can disturb a person's self-concept, and the sexual self-concept is no exception (Weinberg 1982). General bodily disturbances, weakness, tiredness and malaise occur to varying degrees in all illnesses. The result is that there is less energy for investing in self-care, clothing, appearance, and for home, leisure, social and sexual activities. This leads to a rebound effect on self-esteem; energy levels fall further, and the vicious circle goes round again. In relation to sexuality, a further complication arises because it is known that old people are less likely than younger people to restart sexual activity after a period of cessation, such as a break due to illness (Berman & Lief 1976). Over and above these generalized effects, each illness or disability has its own unique repercussions for sexuality, in the broad sense of the term. Certain medical conditions and physiological changes are more common among elderly people than in the rest of the population and, although there is not space to go into detail about every possible condition, some important effects on the main body systems will be outlined.

Cardiovascular conditions, especially myocardial infarctions, are a great source of anxiety in relation to sex, especially for men. Hendricks and Hendricks (1978) state that 'actually sex requires no more exertion than taking a brisk walk or climbing a flight of stairs' (p. 69), and Comfort agrees that

'sex is a highly undangerous activity. Stopping it unwillingly is far more dangerous than a little exertion' (Comfort 1977, p. 193). Sudden death during or after intercourse is rare and the benefits of intercourse, including a sense of well-being, less depression, gentle exercise, and reduction of tension outweigh the risks (Weg 1983).

Respiratory disorders can cause shortness of breath, cough, recurrent infections, chest deformity and orthopnoea, with obvious implications for sexual acts and perhaps less obvious ones for the sexual self-concept. Inability to perform sexual activity without breathlessness will lead to feelings of inadequacy. Coughing and expectoration of large amounts of purulent sputum or being unable to adopt certain positions will cause embarrassment, if they do not make sexual intercourse impossible.

Musculoskeletal conditions and changes associated with ageing may cause weakness, limitation of movement, deformity and pain. Chronic pain such as that of arthritis can be extremely depressing and debilitating, and lead on to loss of interest in sex as well as decreased possibilities of performing satisfying sexual acts. On the positive side, sexual activity increases adrenal corticoid production, which may relieve arthritic symptoms (Weg 1983).

Nervous system changes in old age may affect perception and sensation, and thereby inhibit sexual response. Eyesight, hearing and touch all play a part in sensuality as well as in actual sex acts. More spectacularly, a stroke with its possible paralysis, loss of speech and continence, loss of independence and perhaps depression will have potentially devastating effects on all aspects of life, including sensuality and sexuality. There is a higher incidence of impaired sexual function, notably decreased libido and potency, in men who have suffered a right hemisphere stroke, because this area is dominant for sexual function (Costett & Heillmann 1986). Parkinson's disease too may have a very damaging outcome for self-confidence and self-concept, so that the sufferer feels sexually undesirable.

Common endocrine disorders occurring in old age are hypothyroidism and diabetes mellitus. People with hypothyroidism may be lethargic and lacking in interest in themselves, their surroundings and others, and may gain weight and lose hair. These may make them feel unattractive to others, which will further decrease the likelihood of partaking in sexual activities. Diabetes mellitus can cause specific complications both for women and men. For women, vaginal lubrication is delayed and scant even when oestrogen levels are adequate. There is therefore an increased susceptibility to vaginal soreness and infection, which is a disincentive to sexual activity. For men, retrograde and/or premature ejaculation may occur and as many as 50% of sufferers cannot have an erection. The cause may be changes in the arterial bed or neuropathy, but no satisfactory treatment has been found (Weg 1983). The multiple complications of diabetes, including cardiovascular disease, renal damage and neuropathy also have effects on sexuality and sexual function.

Genitourinary conditions in women and men have perhaps the most obvious link with sexual activity and sexuality. Men widely believe that prostatectomy means the end of sexual activity but this is not so in the majority of cases. Simple prostatectomy rarely affects potency (Mallett & Badlain 1987). Suprapubic and perineal operations lead to impotence more commonly than transurethral resection, but with the latter retrograde ejaculation may be distressing (Weg 1983). Comfort (1977) recommends all men to discuss sexual activity specifically with their surgeon prior to prostatectomy and make it clear if they wish to continue to have intercourse afterwards. Incontinence, urinary infections and atrophic vaginitis involve local pain or discomfort which may inhibit feelings and responses as well as making the person feel unclean or unattractive.

Cessation of sexual activity has been attributed to ill-health, particularly by men, but illness and disability do not necessarily mean that an active sex life is impossible or that sensuality and sexuality are compromised. Self-concept and confidence may be low and the sufferer may fear rejection, but desires and feelings continue (Costello 1975, Hogan 1980, Weg 1983). Reference has already been made to the effect that institutionalization, including hospitalization, may have on clients' or patients' opportunities for sexual expression. The role of the nurse in minimizing these disturbances and promoting healthy sexuality will be discussed in the concluding sections, after considering some aspects of the treatment of illness.

TREATMENTS AND SEXUALITY

People sometimes joke about the treatment being worse than the disease, but with regard to sexuality this may be no joke: it can be the devastating truth. Any surgical operation, for example, causes temporary disturbance of health which can also disrupt sexual activity. Particular operations, however, can have permanently destructive effects because they change the body image and the person's self-concept as an intact and sexually desirable being. Mastectomy, amputation and stoma formation are instances of this (Webb 1982) but other operations can in a less visible way have a similar effect, as Wilson-Barnett found with coronary surgery (Wilson-Barnett 1981).

Many drugs, both social and medically prescribed, affect sexual function, either as part of their desired mode of action or by causing debilitating side-effects. An example of a social drug which compromises sexual activity is alcohol, which has a depressant effect on the central nervous system with resulting impotence. Cigarettes cause respiratory illnesses and dysfunction as well as a halitosis which hardly adds to sexual appeal. As a Health Education Council poster said 'Kiss a non-smoker and taste the difference!'

Narcotics, tranquillizers, sedatives and anxiolytic drugs depress the central nervous system and suppress libido. Numerous antihypertensive drugs such as chlorothiazide, hydrallazine and methyldopa have the same effect, and tricyclic and monoamine oxidase inhibitor antidepressants can cause impotence. Other common drugs occasionally reported to have adverse effects on sexuality include cimetidine, which can cause impotence and gynaecomastia, and propranolol, which can lead to impotence (Hogan 1980, Weinberg 1982, Weg 1983).

The situations described in the two previous sections on ill-health, disability and treatments assume even greater importance when it is remembered that elderly people may be experiencing multiple pathology and concomitant multiple medications and treatments. Nurses can do much to help patients and clients in these circumstances to express their sexuality in the way they themselves choose as most appropriate. Weinberg (1982) proposes that nurses should function as educators and advocates in relation to sexuality and the needs of elderly people, and these two roles will be discussed in the concluding sections.

ROLES FOR NURSES

NURSES AS EDUCATORS

The primary need of elderly people is for information regarding sexuality. Myths and stereotypes should be stripped of their credibility and replaced with accurate information about sexual functioning and sexuality. Knowledge of how anatomy and physiology evolve with ageing would do much to dispel anxieties and shame in an age group which often feels that its sexual feelings are manifestations of over-sexuality or sinfulness (Burnside 1976, Renshaw 1981). The subject of sexuality and sensuality should be tactfully raised when taking a nursing history, and this also provides the first opportunity for education about normal functioning. Subsequently, when carrying out nursing care or working with clients, nurses should be alert to cues pointing to covert requests for information or to knowledge deficits, and should discuss these in an open, accepting and informative style. In this way elderly people can come to accept and feel comfortable with their own thoughts, feelings, fantasies and urges. Whether they wish to be sexually active or not they may have insecurities which need to be brought out into the open. This may equally apply to their families, whose own anxieties may cause or add to those of elderly people themselves and nurses can therefore assist by giving information to relatives of elderly people. Comfort (1977) suggests that staff who are unwilling to do this have sexual problems of their own which they are projecting on to elderly people.

It is just as important to take account of sexuality with those who do not wish to be sexually active. Whilst it would be undesirable to upset them by pressing them to behave in ways which others find liberating, sexuality is a much wider matter than sexual acts, as we have discussed. People who are sexually inactive, whether by choice or circumstances, are still sexual beings in this broader sense and have needs which nurses should try to meet (Comfort 1977, Robinson 1983, Weg 1983).

In emphasizing the value of a holistic approach to sexuality and ageing, Butler and Lewis (1976) advocate giving elderly people 'practical guidelines for nutrition, fitness, rest and personal appearance.' They suggest that exercise could include a daily programme of stretching and walking, as well as exercises to maintain the tone of abdominal, thigh, back and pelvic muscles. Poor nutrition can lead to depression and anxiety, which will affect sexuality, and nutrition education should focus particularly on prevention of anaemia and the inclusion of adequate fibre in the diet to reduce constipation and potential associated urinary problems including infection and incontinence.

NURSES AS ADVOCATES

The advocate role includes speaking for patients when they are not able to influence the situation themselves and working to provide services and facilities which they require. Nurses, whether working in clients' homes or in institutions, are in a potentially strong position to influence the care elderly people receive and to contribute to meeting their needs in relation to sexuality.

Elderly people in health and illness have the same needs in relation to sexuality as every other adult. Acts of intimacy and warmth, companionship and love, self-respect and the respect of others help to maintain an intact self-concept at this stage of life as at any other. Indeed, close friendships may be more important because relationships with family and friends grow fewer as some of them die, and work and social roles are curtailed with retirement and decreased mobility (Weg 1983). Physical appearance and dress are fundamental and highly visible ways of expressing sexuality and individuality. Maintaining a dignified style of dress and presentation is essential to self-respect but this may not be as easy as it used to be for people who have a lower income than during their working lives and cannot so easily get about to make purchases and launder their clothes. Full individually owned clothing, including under-wear, with washing facilities should be an obligatory provision. Impaired mobility and eye-sight may make it difficult to keep hair clean and groomed. Attractive and comfortable dentures, spectacles and hearing aids are a necessity for el-derly people, and functionality is not the only consideration required. Help with keeping up ap-pearance may be needed by elderly people, who will feel that this is not an added refinement or the 'icing on the cake', but is their basic right as human beings.

Privacy, too, is something we all need at times, whether to give an opportunity for quiet thinking, to attend to personal hygiene and grooming, or to carry out sexual acts. When elderly people live with their younger families or in institutions this need is easily forgotten. Doors may be left open routinely and people may enter the room without knocking and waiting for permission to enter. Pri-vacy is virtually absent where a room is shared with another resident or the old person sleeps in a downstairs room which the family uses as a living room during the daytime.

In the USA, federal nursing Home regulations make it obligatory for married residents to have privacy during their spouses' visits and for married couples who are both residents to share a room (Branzelle 1987). The same consideration of residents' rights should surely be afforded to non-married couples and friends, whether their re-lationship is a heterosexual or homosexual one.

As well as assisting people to satisfy their needs in these respects, nurses may have opportunities to influence medical treatment in relation to sexu-ality. For example, an elderly woman suffering from atrophic vaginal changes will benefit from using oestrogen cream. An elderly man is unlikely to need hormonal treatment because hormonal in-sufficiency appears to have little effect on male sexual potency (Finkle 1971). Nurses may be the first to notice that a drug is adversely affecting a patient's sexuality or, through closer knowledge of individual patients or clients, may be able to draw

a doctor's attention to the effect an illness or handicap is having in this respect.

CONCLUSION

All nurses cannot and should not be sex therapists. This is a role which requires extensive specialist training (Hogan 1980, Weinberg 1982). But all nurses should be able to identify problems, inter-vene appropriately by teaching or counselling within the limits of their knowledge, or by refer-ring patients or clients to specialists for help. Our cultural norms and values in the realms of sexual-ity have changed enormously in this century and particularly in the last 25 years (Robinson 1983). Our future clients and patients are likely to be in-creasingly assertive of their needs and rights in relation to sexuality. It is our responsibility as pro-fessionals to ensure that we are educated and equipped with the knowledge and skills to fulfil our obligations to them.

REFERENCES

Allen M E 1987 A holistic view of sexuality in the aged. Holistic Nursing Practice 1(4): 76–83
Berman E M, and Lief H I 1976 Sex and the aging process. In: Oaks W W, Melchiode G A, Ficher I (eds) Sex and the life cycle. Grune and Stratton, New York
Backman G, Leiblum S 1981 Sexual expression in menopausal women. Medical Aspects of Human Sexuality 15(10): 96B–96H
Branzelle J 1987 Ensuring residents' rights to sexual desire and expression. Provider October 30: 33
Burnside I M (ed) 1976 Nursing and the aged. McGraw-Hill, New York
Butler R, Lewis M 1976 Sex after sixty. Harper & Row, New York
Comfort A 1977 A good age. Mitchell Beazley, London
Corby N, Zarit J M 1983 The unmarried in later life. In: Weg R B (ed) Sexuality in the later years: roles and behavior. Academic Press, New York
Costello M K 1975 Sex, intimacy and aging. American Journal of Nursing 75(8): 1330–1332
Costett N B, Heillmann K M 1986 Male sexual function: impairment after a right hemisphere stroke. Archives of Neurology 43: 1036–1039
de Beauvoir S 1973 The coming of age. Warner Paperback Library, New York
Finkle A L 1971 Sexual function during advancing age. In: Rossman I (ed) Clinical geriatrics. Lippincott, Philadelphia

George L K, Weiler S J 1981 Sexuality in middle and late life. Archives of General Psychiatry 38: 919–923

Hendricks J, Hendricks C D 1978 Sexuality in later life. In: Carver V, Liddiard P (eds) An ageing population. Hodder and Stoughton/The Open University, Sevenoaks, Kent

Hogan R 1980 Human sexuality. A nursing perspective. Appleton-Century-Crofts, New York

Kuhn M E 1976 Sexual myths surrounding the aging. In: Oaks W W, Melchiode G A, Ficher I (eds) Sex and the life cycle. Grune and Stratton, New York

Mallett E C, Badlain G H 1987 Sexuality in the elderly. Seminars in Urology 2: 141–145

Masters W H, Johnson V E 1981 Sex and the aging process. Journal of the American Geriatrics Society 29(9): 385–390

Persson G 1980 Sexuality in a 70 year old urban population. Journal of Psychosomatic Research 24: 335–342

Puner M 1974 To the good long life. Macmillan/The Open University, London

Renshaw D C 1981 Sexuality in older women? Journal of Clinical Psychiatry 42(1): 3–4

Robinson P K 1983 The sociological perspective. In: Weg R B (ed) Sexuality in the later years. Roles and behavior. Academic Press, New York

Scully D, Bart P 1973 A funny thing happened on the way to the orifice. American Journal of Sociology 78: 1045–1049

Sontag S 1978 The double standard of ageing. In: Carver V. Liddiard P (eds) An ageing population. Hodder and Stoughton/The Open University, Sevenoaks, Kent

Szasz G 1983 Sexual incidents in an extended care unit for aged men. Journal of the American Geriatrics Society 31(7): 407–411

Trimmer E 1978 Basic sexual medicine. Heinemann, London

Webb C 1982 Body image and recovery from hysterectomy. In: Wilson-Barnett J, Fordham M (eds) Recovery from illness. Wiley, Chichester

Webb C 1983 Words fail me. Nursing Times Volume 27 (6 July): 62–66

Weg R B (ed) 1983 Sexuality in the later years. Roles and behaviour. Academic Press, New York

Weinberg J S 1982 Sexuality. Human needs and nursing practice. Saunders, Philadelphia

Wilson-Barnett J 1981 Assessment of recovery: with special reference to a study with post-operative cardiac patients. Journal of Advanced Nursing 6: 435–445

Winn R L, Newton N 1982 Sexuality in Aging: a study of 106 cultures. Archives of Sexual Behavior 11(4): 283–298

CHAPTER CONTENTS

Nature of pain 273
Acute and chronic pain 274

Is pain any different if you are old? 275
Sensory dimensions 275
Affective/evaluative dimensions 277

How can you manage pain? 278
Your own feelings 278
Assessing pain 279
Planning/intervention 283
Evaluation 285

Conclusion 285

17

Pain and elderly people

Kate Seers

NATURE OF PAIN

Pain is a common experience and caring for patients in pain is often a central part of the nurse's role. Pain has been described, however, as 'one of the most challenging problems in medicine' (Melzack & Wall 1988 p. ix). This applies equally to nursing. Part of this challenge lies in the complexity of the pain experience. Pain is more complex and dynamic than purely a response to stimulation — it includes the interaction of physiological, psychological and social factors and thus each person's experience of pain is individual and unique. Since others cannot directly measure this experience, pain is also subjective.

The multifactorial nature of pain was highlighted by Melzack and Casey (1968) who described sensory, motivational and cognitive determinants of pain. Syrjala (1987) restated these and described the sensory dimension as including qualities such as burning, stabbing, pressure or tingling. Motivational or affective terms can describe how the pain affects the person; for example, it may be perceived as unpleasant and/or exhausting. Cognitive appraisal or evaluating the pain experience can include thinking about the meaning of pain. Although described separately, all these dimensions are interrelated and can all influence behaviour, including both verbal and non-verbal expressions of pain.

The description of pain as consisting of more than a purely sensory dimension (the sensation of pain) provides a framework that allow variables such as mood, culture, anxiety, the meaning of pain and past experiences of pain, amongst many other things, to influence the experience of pain.

The modulation of pain sensation by factors other than the actual potentially painful stimulus can be explained conceptually by the Gate Control Theory of pain, stated by Melzack and Wall (1965) and updated by Melzack and Wall (1988). There are many discussions and disagreements about the exact neurophysiology involved, but the theory provides a way of understanding how pain can be influenced by factors other than the sensory stimulus.

Basically, Melzack and Wall propose that there is a gating mechanism in the substantia gelatinosa in the dorsal horn of the spinal cord. If the gate is shut, pain impulses can go no further. If it is partially or completely open, pain impulses can pass through the gate and ascend to the brain. The position of the gate can be influenced by activity in both the peripheral and central nervous systems. Thus potentially painful impulses can be modified by fibres descending from the brain. Ascending messages to the brain can also influence descending controls. For example, anxiety/fear could open the gate, thus increasing pain, whereas by reducing anxiety and closing the gate, pain may be relieved.

Many factors can act to open or close the gate, and this explains why the relationship between injury and pain is 'highly variable' (Melzack & Wall 1988 p. 165). Since there are so many potential influences on the experience of pain it follows that the response of each individual will be unique. The physiology of pain has been described in detail by Bullingham (1985), Thompson (1984) and Meinhart and McCaffery (1983), and will not be considered further in this chapter.

The role of endorphins (the body's own morphine) in pain and pain relief is complex and an area in which much work is currently being undertaken. However, Melzack and Wall (1988) state, 'their roles in pain and analgesia are poorly understood and their practical implications for pain therapy are uncertain'. (p. 286).

It is difficult to define pain. If pain has several dimensions and can be influenced by many things, how can it be defined? This complexity of pain

was summed up by the National Institutes of Health Consensus Development Conference (1987):

Pain is a subjective experience that can be perceived directly only by the sufferer . . . . Pain does not occur in isolation but in a specific human being with psychosocial, economic, and cultural contexts that influence the meaning, experience, and verbal and non-verbal expression of pain. (p. 36).

This definition emphasizes the subjective and individual nature of pain and complements McCaffery's 1972 definition, 'Pain is whatever the experiencing person says it is, existing whenever he says it does.' (p. 8).

ACUTE AND CHRONIC PAIN

A distinction is made between acute and chronic pain since what may normally work to control the pain of a patient in acute pain may not necessarily be so effective or appropriate for those with chronic pain (Fordyce 1978). Whereas anxiety is often associated with acute pain, depression is more commonly associated with chronic pain.

Acute pain

This refers to pain usually associated with trauma or disease and is of short duration or recent onset. Examples are stubbing your toe, or the pain of a myocardial infarct. Acute pain usually serves as a warning signal to stop further damage and/or make the person in pain seek help. Melzack and Wall (1988) describe the characteristics of acute pain as 'the combination of tissue damage, pain and anxiety'. (p. 35). The anxiety could, for example, centre on worries about future consequences of the injury.

Chronic pain

This is usually defined as lasting for 6 months or more (McCaffery & Beebe 1989), although they point out that there is disagreement over how prolonged pain should be before it is called chronic. Chronic pain persists long after it can serve as a useful warning signal. Sternbach (1987) points out that the difference between acute and chronic pain is much more than duration of pain. He argues that chronic pain is not a symptom or a warning signal or a need-state for rest, but a syndrome. By implication this syndrome could be treated in its own right.

IS PAIN ANY DIFFERENT IF YOU ARE OLD?

The acceptance that pain and old age go together seems widespread. Certainly many disorders common in elderly people produce pain. Kwentus et al (1985) outline certain types of pain common in elderly people, such as trigeminal neuralgia, diabetic peripheral neuropathy, arthritis, cancer, degenerative disc disease and residual neurological insults. Other pains, such as those caused by rheumatic diseases, temporal arteritis, herpes zoster, ischaemia, surgery and gout are mentioned by McKenzie (1985), and Matteson and Mc-Connell (1988) add coronary artery disease, peripheral neuropathy, post-herpetic neuralgia, osteomyelitis, osteoporosis, depression and constipation to this list.

Elderly people may have more than one pain from multiple pathology and their pain may be chronic, acute or both. Liebeskind and Melzack (1987) felt that 'Pain in the elderly is often dismissed as something to be expected and hence tolerated' (p. 1). There is, however, a growing body of opinion that pain is not an inevitable part of ageing, but demands diagnosis and treatment as it does at any age (Butler & Gastel 1980). Harkins et al (1984) state that 'Pain, discomfort and suffering are not natural consequences of growing old' (p. 112). Kwentus et al (1985) highlighted the need to understand age-related changes in how pain presents and how the older person perceives and tolerates pain. Pain in elderly people has been described by McCaffery and Beebe (1989) as a neglected area and they add that there are many gaps in our knowledge. Butler and Gastel (1980) remind the reader that the pain of elderly people is not others' pain but our own as more of us survive into old age. Elderly people are not well represented at pain clinics according to Wells (1989),

and he wonders if this is due to their complaining less, and to doctors assuming that their pain is acceptable in view of their age. From his experience he concludes that old people are more, not less, likely to experience chronic pain, especially neurological pain.

Although sensory, motivational/affective and cognitive/evaluative dimensions of pain all overlap, these categories will now be used to examine whether pain for elderly people is any different from pain for other age groups.

SENSORY DIMENSIONS

There is much debate over whether pain thresholds change in elderly people. Pain threshold is '[T]he least experience of pain which a subject can recognize', and pain tolerance is '[T]he greatest level of pain which a subject is prepared to tolerate' (International Association for the Study of Pain [IASP] 1986 p. S220–S221). Pain tolerance has also been defined as 'the duration or intensity of pain that a person is *willing* to endure' (McCaffery & Beebe 1989 p. 15). Clark and Mehl (1971) felt that age differences in pain were partly due to the tendency of elderly people to endure more noxious stimulation before reporting it as painful. Woodrow et al (1972) administered a pain tolerance test to over 41 000 subjects. They found pain tolerance decreased with increasing age for both sexes. In my own study of 80 post-operative patients, I found no significant difference in pain scores after surgery between patients aged 18–55 and those aged 56 or more (Seers 1987). Davitz and Davitz (1981) found that age of patients (65 years or more compared with younger adults) had little influence on nurses' inferences of physical pain or psychological distress. This view was supported by Harkins and Chapman (1976, 1977) who argued that perception was similar but that elderly people were less accurate in discrimination and less willing to label a sensation as painful. Charlton and Buckley (1984) described the comparisons of young and older subjects' pain threshold and tolerance data as conflicting. Harkins et al (1984) described results from laboratory studies as unclear, showing thresholds/tolerances as increasing, decreasing or remaining unaltered. They argued that these contradictions could be due to differences in inducing and assessing pain. They concluded that age-related changes in pain sensitivity and perception are difficult to document and may be of little significance. If elderly patients have pain, there is usually a physical and/or psychological pathology deserving attention. Harkins et al (1984) also point out that if you assume elderly people are less sensitive to pain, then their quality of life may be reduced. Although according to Kwentus et al (1985) there are sensory changes with ageing, such as a reduction in auditory and visual acuity, 'assertions of age changes in pain sensation should be viewed with caution' (p. 50).

There is debate about the differences in pain experienced by elderly compared with younger patients in some specific conditions. A small selection of these conditions will now be discussed.

Myocardial Infarction (MI)

Over an 11-year period, Pathy (1967) studied 387 patients with acute MI aged 65 years or more. Excluding 31 patients whose sudden deaths meant a history of pain was unavailable, 73% denied presence of chest pain. After a further 51 who were confused were excluded, there was still a 60% incidence of painless MI. In a study by Aronow (1987), which included 87 patients with acute MI aged 62 years and over, 72% did not present with chest pain. The prevalence and symptoms of MI in geriatric long term care patients were studied by Wroblewski et al (1986). They found that intense dyspnoea, syncope and weakness were more common than chest pain and that there was low diagnostic accuracy of acute MI in elderly people. Cocchi et al (1988) concluded that the clinical diagnosis of acute MI was more commonly missed in elderly patients with ageing, atypical presentation and the coexistence of several diseases accounting for most of the unrecognized acute MI.

The high incidence of painless MI in elderly people reported by Pathy (1967) and Aronow (1987) has not always been supported by other studies. MacDonald et al (1983) studied 296 patients admitted to a coronary care unit who were aged less than 60 and 317 aged 70 or more. They found 77% of the younger group, as compared to

61% of the older group, had pain as the main presenting symptom. Thus in the majority of the 70-plus age group, although chest pain was less common, it was still the commonest presenting symptom. MacDonald et al concluded that the incidence of painless MI had been overestimated in the past. This supported the work of Konu (1977), who found that chest pain was the most common symptom in over 65% of a sample of 226 MI patients aged 65 or over.

It has been found that atypical presentations of MI in elderly patients are associated with impaired mental scores on admission (Black 1987), and Kwentus et al (1985) argued that an MI may present atypically if patients are confused or have communication difficulties.

Other studies have suggested that the presentation of MI may be different in very elderly people. Bayer et al (1986) studied the symptoms associated with acute MI in 777 patients aged between 65 and 100 years. They reviewed discharge summaries and looked at original records, and found that the spectrum of presentation changed with increasing age. Although chest pain was still common, it became less frequent with increasing age. Chest pain was common and present in almost 70% of those aged 65 to 84. However, it tended to become less common with increasing age and the incidence of syncope, stroke and acute confusion increased. After age 84, shortness of breath was the most common symptom, present in 43%, and pain was the second most common symptom, present in 37.5%.

These findings were supported by Day et al (1987), who found atypical presentation was common in 100 patients aged 85 years or more. They found 69% of those aged 65–84 had chest pain compared to 41% of those aged 85-plus. Those aged 85 years or more were significantly more likely to be acutely confused. Only 2% in the 65–84 and 4% in the 85-plus group had a silent or symptomless MI. However, whilst this study supports that of Bayer et al, it appears to be based on essentially the same sample of patients, extended by two years. Thus it can be regarded only as an extension, rather than a replication of Bayer et al (1986). It is important to note that atypical presentation of acute MI can also occur in younger patients. MacDonald (1984) concluded that about 40% of elderly patients will present in a non-classical manner, as compared to about 25% of younger patients.

It seems that whilst reports of the incidence of painless MI in elderly people may have been over-estimated, the findings of Bayer et al (1986), extended by Day et al (1987), suggest that about 30% of those aged 65–84 and around 60% of those aged 85-plus who have an acute MI may present without chest pain.

Appendicitis

McCallion et al (1987) studied 30 elderly patients (average age 72) and 30 younger patients (average age 23) who presented with a confirmed diagnosis of appendicitis. They found that all the elderly patients had abdominal pain and the presentation was broadly similar between the two groups. The elderly patients had symptoms for significantly longer before they presented than the younger group and there was a longer delay between admission and surgery. Although presentation was similar, only 54% of the older compared to 90% of the younger group were correctly diagnosed before surgery. This may partly explain the delay to surgery. Their finding of a similar presentation between the two age groups was not supported in a multicentre, international survey of acute abdominal pain by Telfer et al (1988). They investigated patients with acute appendicitis and found 366 patients aged over 50 (who were termed elderly) presented differently from 1970 patients aged less than 50 years. Amongst other things they found that the 'elderly patients' were more likely to have general pain. The finding that pain was of a longer duration in the elderly group did support McCallion et al (1987).

It seems that appendicitis in elderly people is associated with pain. This conclusion differs somewhat from that of a study which investigated elderly patients with a peptic ulcer.

Peptic ulcer

Clinch et al (1984) compared the presentation of peptic ulcer in 132 patients aged 60 or more with that of 67 younger patients aged 20–50. They found that abdominal pain was not present in a third of the elderly group. Thirty five per cent of the elderly group, as compared to 8% of the younger group, had no abdominal pain at the time of referral or during the previous 6 months — a difference which was significant. Clinch et al speculated that this may be due to decreased cutaneous pain sensitivity, decreased visceral sensitivity or an increase in the use of non-steroidal anti-inflammatory drugs (NSAIDs) by the elderly patients.

AFFECTIVE/EVALUATIVE DIMENSIONS

What pain means and the effect it has is a crucial part of the pain experience for all age groups. We should recognize the sort of questions pain may raise in the sufferer. Illich (1977) outlines some of these questions: 'What is wrong? How much longer? Why must I/ought I/should I/can I suffer? Why does this kind of evil exist, and why does it strike just me?' (p. 149). Baken (1968) adds the question, 'Does this pain mean I will die?' Those questions may or may not be articulated. Some people may see some value in some pain some of the time, for religious or self-testing/self-growth reasons. Questions like this are very much part of the experience of pain.

Needless pain and suffering impoverish quality of life for patients and their families (Liebeskind & Melzack 1987). Ghose (1987) argues that socioeconomic factors, housing problems, social isolation and loneliness are all likely to influence pain sensitivity in elderly people. In an effort to minimize pain, activities of daily living can become time and energy consuming (Matteson & McConnell 1988). Pain may mean that the ability for self-care is reduced, and mobility is restricted; it may become difficult to go out independently and enjoyment of life can be limited. The ability to cope with pain is important. Harkins et al (1984) suggest that the negative social/psychological aspects of ageing may reduce the elderly person's capacity to respond successfully to the negative consequences of chronic pain. The results of a study by Walker (1989) suggest the sort of factors that influence ability to cope. She studied 190 elderly patients in the community with painful conditions and found that factors such as 'having regrets,' 'being occupied,' 'pain under control,' having 'personal problems' and 'feeling informed' were the best predictors of mood and coping. Walker suggested that all these predictors be included in pain assessment and intervention. The importance of ability to cope has also been emphasized by Wachter-Shikora and Perez (1988), who argued that elderly people reported pain less frequently or stated that they felt less pain since they knew what to expect and how to cope with their pain.

A report of pain may have wider implications and involve more than may be immediately apparent. Increasing age may be associated with loss of physical health, loss of loved ones, decreased economic resources and lowered social status, and complaints of pain may be seen as an acceptable attempt to elicit some caretaking (Kwentus et al 1985). Symptoms such as poor concentration, attention and memory dysfunctions can be ascribed to pain (Harkins et al 1984), as can behavioural changes such as confusion or restlessness, or nonspecific symptoms such as fatigue or anorexia (Butler & Gastel 1980). Moore and Whanger (1983) outlined how it is not uncommon for atypical pain to be the main, if not the sole symptom of depression. Many studies have found an association between chronic pain and depression (Doan & Wadden 1989, Kramlinger et al 1983), although the percentage reported to be depressed varies. There is also debate concerning the extent to which people are depressed because they are in chronic pain, or whether chronic pain is a manifestation of depression. Melzack and Wall (1988) argue that it is unreasonable to ascribe chronic pain to neurotic symptoms and whilst psychological processes contribute to pain, they are only one factor influencing the complex experience of pain.

The effects that chronic pain can have on behaviour have been utilized by Fordyce (1978). He argued that people often receive positive reinforcement for having pain. For example, complaints of pain may elicit sympathy from family/friends and allow the avoidance of activities the person in pain would not normally want to do. Thus they receive rewards for having pain and this reinforces the pain behaviour. Fordyce argues that these people can be retrained by stopping rewards of pain behaviour and reinforcing only 'well' behaviours. This is known as operant conditioning. However, this technique has been the subject of much discussion. Melzack and Wall (1988) question whether it means the patient feels less pain, or simply, for example, complains less. They also question whether this operant conditioning is any better than a placebo effect.

McCaffery (1983) highlights points to consider when using this technique, including that it be used only for *selected* patients in chronic pain, with their informed consent; that it has no place in the care of patients in acute pain; that learning to use pain for certain benefits does not occur on a conscious level; and that occasional use of pain to obtain certain benefits is not unusual and does not warrant any special treatment. Miller and Le Lieuvre (1982) used an operant conditioning approach in a small pilot study with four elderly residents in a nursing Home. They found attention and praise reduced the required medication, pain behaviour and self-reports of pain, but they were unable to show an increase in the number of activities in which residents engaged.

So, knowing that pain is sometimes dismissed in elderly people as an inevitable consequence of ageing, that many disorders common in the elderly produce both acute and chronic pain, and that pain can reduce quality of life, it is how pain in old people is *managed*, as Eland (1988) argues, that influences the degree of activity, social isolation and the quality of life for the elderly person.

HOW CAN YOU MANAGE PAIN?

YOUR OWN FEELINGS

Before you assess pain with any patient or intervene to help reduce her pain, it is important that you examine your own feelings about pain and pain relief. Some factors to consider include whether you think patients/clients should put up with some pain, and if so, how much? What are your own feelings about taking or giving pain-killers — both narcotic and non-narcotic? How do you decide whether a patient/client is in pain?

The first step towards offering effective pain control is knowing about a patient's pain. To do this you must assess the pain, but this is not always easy.

ASSESSING PAIN

Misconceptions

McCaffery and Beebe (1989) outline ten areas of pain assessment where misconceptions may exist that hamper assessment by causing us to doubt the patient's pain. An outline of these misconceptions follows. The interested reader is referred to the original reference, where each misconception is discussed in detail.

1. The first misconception concerns who is the authority about the patient's pain. McCaffery's 1972 definition, 'Pain is whatever the experiencing person says it is, existing whenever he says it does' emphasizes that the patient or client should be believed. McCaffery says this belief covers both verbal and non-verbal pain behaviours. It is the patient, not the health professional, who knows how much pain she has, as well as the effectiveness of any pain relief measures. Although we all probably make some inferences about pain, Mc-Caffery emphasizes that we do not necessarily see the situation as the patient does. In my own study (Seers 1987) I found that nurses consistently rated patients' pains as less severe than did the patient. We should be aware of the inferences we do make. Davitz and Davitz (1981) studied the effects of patient characteristics on nurses' inferences of physical pain and psychological distress. They concluded that stereotyped beliefs about the experiences of others in pain were bound to obscure individual differences.

2. The second misconception that can hamper pain assessment is a reliance on personal values or intuition to judge whether a person is lying about her pain. McCaffery and Beebe (1989) point out that whilst we may use this in our social life, it is not a professional approach.

3. That pain is largely an emotional/psycho-logical problem is the third misconception. However, reacting to pain with emotion does not mean the pain was caused by an emotional problem.

4. Lying about pain or malingering is regarded as common, whereas McCaffery and Beebe argue that this happens rarely and is thus a misconception. They emphasize the importance of avoiding inaccurate labelling of patients as malingerers.

5. The fifth misconception outlined is that patients who get benefits because of their pain are not in as much pain as they claim. However, using pain to one's advantage is not the same as malingering and it is not always easy to assess what does and what does not constitute using pain for advantage.

6. Another misconception is concerned with pain of unknown cause; if there is no obvious physical cause for pain, the existence of pain may be doubted. McCaffery and Beebe correct this by saying all pain is the result of both physical and mental events. The point is that whatever the cause of pain, the person still feels the pain.

7. The idea that pain is accompanied by reliable physiological and/or behavioural signs which can verify the existence and severity of pain is a misconception because physiological signs such as an increase in blood pressure and pulse can quickly adapt. Behavioural cues, such as cries, moans, wincing, guarding and so on can be unreliable and might not be present in cases of milder pain (Stewart 1977). Moreover, lack of pain expression does not necessarily mean a lack of pain. Patients/clients may take pride in self-control and may minimize their expression of pain in order to be a 'good' patient. Jacox and Stewart (1973) found 41% of the 31 surgical patients they studied said they would remain outwardly calm when in pain. McCaffery and Beebe also point out that sheer fatigue can reduce expressions of pain.

8. The predictability of duration and severity of pain in different people is the eighth misconception. There is not an invariant relationship between stimulus and perception of pain. There can be large variations between individuals after, for example, identical operations (Seers 1987). So, severity and duration of pain cannot be predicted with certainty.

9. The ninth misconception is that patients/ clients should have a high tolerance of pain. But how much pain 'should' a patient tolerate? Pain tolerance can differ between individuals and in the same individual at different times. Since pain is subjective and unique, tolerance to pain is likely to follow a similar pattern. Health professionals may tend to encourage a high tolerance. This in turn can encourage the patient to reduce her expression of pain in order to conform to these expectations.

10. The final misconception is that if a patient obtains pain relief from a placebo this must mean that her pain is not real. However, McCaffery and Beebe point out there is no evidence for this and that using a placebo in this way raises legal and ethical questions and may destroy the patient's trust in the health professionals.

Once you have considered the misconceptions that may hamper pain assessment and have thought about your own feelings concerning pain and pain relief, it is important to think how you are going to assess pain.

Suggestions for assessing pain

Purely physiological/behavioural cues can be misleading. These signs may suggest the patient/client is in pain, but it is important to verify these impressions with the person in pain. McCaffery (1972) argues that patients in pain should be believed, so it makes sense to ask them about their pain. To obtain a comprehensive picture of any person in pain, you should ask several questions in order to examine different aspects of the pain experience. These include:

1. How would she describe the pain? For example, is it burning/stabbing/throbbing/ sharp/aching and so on?
2. When did the pain start? Is it recent, or has it been there for months/years? What does the patient feel causes the pain?
3. How long does it last — is it intermittent or constant?
4. Where is the pain? There may well be more than one painful area, even if you think the site is obvious. The site of the pain may

vary. A body outline (see Fig. 17.1) could be a useful tool here.
5. How intense/severe is the pain? A pain scale (see Figs 17.2–17.4) could be useful.
6. Does anything make the pain better or worse?
7. What impact does the pain have on the person's life? Does it affect activities of daily living such as mobility, concentration, sleeping, eating and socializing?
8. How does the pain make the person feel? Is she anxious, depressed, angry?

Latham (1987) also recommends that the management and effectiveness of previous attempts at pain relief should be noted.

Assessing pain is more than asking 'Any pain?' You should sit down and discuss pain with the patient/client. You may not need to do a complete assessment of pain at every report of pain. McCaffery (1983) recommends that patients be asked to elaborate on any changes/difference in order to conserve time and energy, and to avoid an undue focus on pain.

Pain assessments should be documented, to provide a record which the patient and other health professionals can consult. How do you go about recording an assessment of pain? Pain history forms and pain charts can be useful tools. These scales/charts should be explained to the patient to make sure she understands what you are asking her to do before she starts to use them. Whenever possible, the patient rather than the nurse should complete the scale/chart, with help as necessary.

Pain scales

1. Verbal rating scale (Fig. 17.2)

With this scale the patient is asked to make a cross on the line where her pain is now, and each category can be scored 0, 1, 2, 3, or 4 to give a pain score. The advantage of this scale is that it is easy to use and understand.

2. Numerical rating scale (Fig. 17.3)

Again the patient marks on the line with a cross where her pain is, but other than the words at either end, there are numbers rather than words

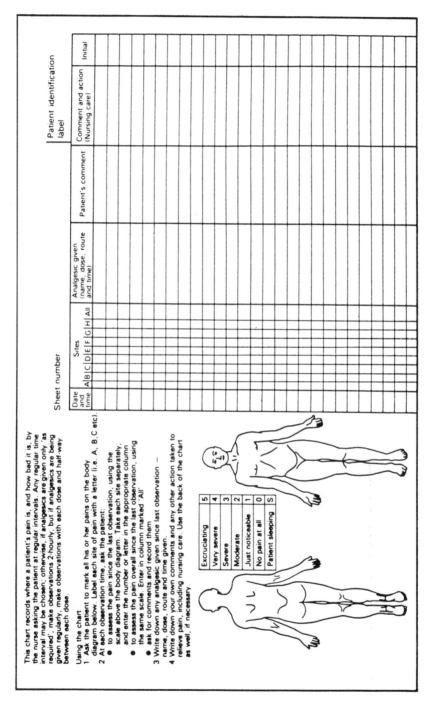

Fig. 17.1 The London Hospital pain chart
Source: Raiman (1981). Reproduced by permission of Jennifer Raiman, The London Hospital, Department of Pharmacology and Therapeutics, and Nursing Journal.

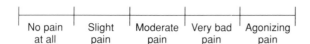

Fig. 17.2 Verbal rating scale.

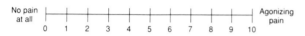

Fig. 17.3 Numerical rating scale.

along the scale. This can be useful if patients feel they need a greater choice of categories than the verbal rating scale allows. The pain score can be taken either as the nearest number to the mark, or by measuring along the line from the left hand side. Bourbonnais' (1981) pain scale incorporated elements of the verbal and numerical rating scales.

3. Visual analogue scale (Fig. 17.4)

As with other scales, the patient marks on the line with a cross where her pain is now. The pain score is derived by measuring to the mark from the left hand side. The drawback of this scale is that it can be difficult for patients to rate their pain on a line with no guideposts. Kremer et al (1981) found 11% of patients were unable to complete this scale, especially if they were elderly.

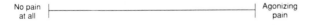

Fig. 17.4 Visual analogue scale.

Some patients/clients have difficulty with these lines. Drawings of faces — usually 8 faces from 'happy' to 'sad' may be useful (Wong & Baker 1988, p. 11). With some patients it may only be possible to elicit whether pain is there or not there, or is bad or not too bad. It important to be flexible and use a scale or chart that means something to the patient/client.

With all pain scales like these, the question of whether you can reduce the complex experience of pain to a single number on a scale is an issue for debate, but at least such scales are a start toward

understanding the needs of the patient. Any of these scales could form the basis of a pain assessment chart.

Pain charts

There are several charts that can be used, for example:

1. The London Hospital Chart. As Figure 17.1 shows, this chart, designed by Raiman (1981) for patients with chronic pain, includes not only a rating scale but also a body outline and space in which to note analgesics given, patient comments and nursing care given. This is especially useful if there is more than one pain. Instructions for use are on the chart. McCaffery and Beebe (1989, p. 27) also give an example of a pain chart (which they call a flow sheet).

2. Sofaer's post-operative pain chart (adapted from the London Hospital chart; see Sofaer 1984, p. 48 and 49). A chart based on Sofaer's has also been used with orthopaedic patients by Davis (1988).

3. A diary or home recording card can be used for patients/clients in the community (see McCaffery & Beebe 1989, p. 30).

In using these charts, it is important to return to the patient and evaluate the effect of any intervention.

An overview of some assessment tools has been presented. Matteson and McConnell (1988) point out that it is important to be familiar with a range of assessment methods, since choosing the right tool for the right person is the key to successful pain management. It is worth bearing in mind that a chart or scale is only a tool to help with assessment, planning and care evaluating care. The information on it has to be used for it to make a contribution to the effective management of pain.

Special considerations with elderly people

Assessment tools and research examining special considerations for elderly people are lacking, as McCaffery and Beebe (1989) point out. So really we don't have much information at present which can help highlight specific tools/strategies that are appropriate specifically for the elderly. McCaffery and Beebe (1989) argue that active elderly people who have little or no memory/cognitive problems may be assessed in the same way as younger adults. If the patient/client has problems in communicating, or if she is confused or demented, then family and/or friends may be able to tell you the signs they use to tell them that their relative/friend is in pain. It is a particular challenge to assess pain with these patients/clients since we lack answers to many questions. McCaffery and Beebe (1989) argue that, based on your knowledge of physical pathology, on what other patients have experienced and on non-verbal cues, you can guess the patient's pain in these cases, but it is only a guess. They suggest that if self-reports of pain are unclear, a trial dose of analgesics, the effects of which are monitored, could be considered.

Sight and hearing loss may cause problems. Ensure any glasses and hearing aids are to hand. The pain scales could be enlarged to enable them to be seen clearly. The verbal rating scale can be read out and a category chosen, or a number from 1 to 10 chosen if the patient/client has very poor or no sight. If hearing loss is a problem, as with all communication with that patient, sit so she can see your face and don't rush. If her concentration span is short try using a simple tool, like the faces or the verbal rating scale.

PLANNING/INTERVENTION

Is what you do about pain for elderly people any different from your approach with younger patients? For patients of all ages, basic considerations are very similar. When nursing care of a person in pain is planned, what is the aim of that care? Is complete relief or partial relief of pain the aim? Is the nurse's aim the same as the patient's? Davis (1988), working to assess pain with patients in an orthapaedic ward, found the aim of using pain assessment charts was to control pain 'to a level acceptable to the patient' (p. 326). The level acceptable to the patient should be reassessed regularly, since it can vary over time. What a person may be able to tolerate when there are the distractions of, for example, visitors, may be in-tolerable in the middle of the night when she is trying to sleep.

The plan should take into account usual methods of coping with pain. You may be able to help patients utilize and build on strategies that have worked in the past, as well as introducing them to new strategies.

Once pain has been assessed and the aim of pain relief decided, what are you going to do to achieve that aim? Pharmacological and/or non-pharmacological approaches may be used, and team-work and good communication among all health professionals is important. The National Institutes of Health (1979) recommended a multidisciplinary approach to the treatment of pain in elderly people.

Pharmacological approaches

These can consist of analgesics and possibly antidepressants and anticonvulsants which are effective for some types of pain. A knowledge of onset and duration of drug action as well as of likely side-effects is important. This area has been reviewed by McCaffery and Beebe (1989) and Latham (1987). When managing pain in elderly people, an awareness of their sensitivity to opiates and the margin between toxic and therapeutic doses of non-steroidal anti-inflammatory drugs should be part of planning and evaluating care.

Kwentus et al (1985) described elderly people as more sensitive to the pain relief effects of narcotics due to alterations in receptors, changes in plasma protein and prolonged renal clearance. They are thus more likely to develop narcotic side-effects such as a reduction in respiration rate, suppression of coughing, changes in level of consciousness and constipation. The studies in this area appear to corroborate this statement. Kaiko (1980) in a study involving 947 post-operative cancer patients found that after intramuscular morphine, older patients (aged 70–89 years) obtained more pain relief for longer than did younger patients (aged 18–29 years). Whereas half the older group no longer obtained pain relief 5 hours after the injection, half the younger group no longer obtained pain relief 3 hours later. This supported the earlier work of Bellville et al (1971), who found that older patients obtained more post-operative pain relief from intramuscular narcotics than did younger patients. They felt this was not purely the result of differences in absorption, distribution, metabolism and elimination of the drug, since the sedative side-effect did not correlate with age. In a study of 200 post-operative patients, Donovan (1983) found that dissatisfaction with pain relief was commoner in younger than in older patients. Whether this was due to differences in pain threshold, pain tolerance, or to the drugs being more effective or given more often to elderly patients is not known.

Studies looking specifically at plasma level and excretion of narcotics in younger compared to older patients have tended to use small samples, and so results should be interpreted with caution. Berkowitz et al (1975) used intravenous morphine 10 mg/70 kg for 11 patients aged less than 50 years and for nine who were 50 years or older. In the older patients, serum morphine was increased compared to levels for the younger group at two and five minutes after administration, although it was only slightly elevated at ten minutes. Berkowitz et al suggested that the rapid entry of morphine to the brain after intravenous injection may explain why old people are sensitive to morphine, since initial serum levels are higher than in younger patients. Metabolism and excretion of pethidine were examined by Odar-Cederlof et al (1985). They studied nine old (70–83 years) and seven young (18–29 years) patients. Pethidine 1 mg/kg was given intravenously. Excretion of the drug was similar in the two age groups, but its metabolism was slower in the older group because there was a slow disappearance of an active metabolite of Pethidine® from the plasma due to slower renal clearance of this metabolite. The authors concluded that the presence of pharmacologically active metabolites will increase and prolong the response to medication and possibly increase the risk of side-effects. Portenoy and Farkash (1988) argue that when using opioid analgesics for the elderly, there is a combination of a diminished volume of distribution, a longer half-life, and reduced clearance — leading to high peak or a more prolonged plasma level after a dose. They report few data for

non-steroidal anti-inflammatory drugs, but suggest a similar phenomemon for at least some of these drugs. Kwentus et al (1985) also state that the margin between toxic and therapeutic doses of NSAIDs in the elderly is reduced.

It is thus necessary to be vigilant for side-effects from any of these drugs, and the differences in metabolism and clearance in elderly patients should be borne in mind when assessing appropriate dosages. McCaffery and Beebe (1989) argue that this does not mean that the potential side-effects of narcotics make them too dangerous to use to relieve pain in elderly patients; these drugs may be used safely if response to medication is carefully monitored and the pharmacokinetics are recognized.

Non-pharmacological approaches

Other techniques are available to complement pharmacological treatments for pain. Health professionals such as nurses, physiotherapists, occupational therapists, clinical psychologists and doctors, amongst others, may be able to provide advice with these techniques. Techniques include positioning, exercise, deep breathing, relaxation, distraction, imagery, heat/cold, massage, and transcutaneous electrical nerve stimulation (TENS). These techniques have been reviewed in detail by McCaffery (1983), Gollop (1983) and Carey (1985). They all involve helping the patient to cope with pain. Patients or clients may already use some of these techniques and the nurse can help the patient build on past successful coping strategies. These techniques can help patients to have some control over their pain. The importance of this control had been emphasized by Walker et al (1989), who argued that to cope with pain the patient has to 'gain or maintain control over it even though the pain itself may persist' (p. 242).

The key to successful management of pain is to use a variety of techniques and to persist with these since a technique may require practice and may not work to its full potential on the first attempt.

There is much to learn about whether and how

demented or confused patients can use some or all of these non-pharmacological approaches.

EVALUATION

The effectiveness of any pain relief intervention should be evaluated with the patient whenever possible. If communication is problematic, changes in behaviour may suggest that pain has been reduced. Lekan-Rutledge (1988) emphasizes that you should ask yourself what advantage, if any, has the patient gained from the intervention to relieve discomfort. Good pain control can improve comfort, mobility and independence. This is important for all patients. Portenoy and Farkash (1988) emphasize that the goals of pain therapy to be evaluated include improved mood, normal sleep, reduction in isolation and better nutrition.

CONCLUSIONS

Pain relief is affected by the complexity of nurse–patient and nurse–nurse relationships as well as by workload and organizational setting (Fagerhaugh & Strauss 1977). Understanding the individual nature of pain and pain relief, making and recording thorough assessments and giving pain relief a high priority in care will go some of the way towards providing adequate pain relief.

Principles of care for patients in pain are similar for most adult age groups, but we lack a great deal of information about assessing and reducing the pain of elderly people. If nursing care is delivered that takes account of the patient as a person, the specific problems and pains that an elderly person may have will be included in this assessment as they would for any patient/client. A thorough and systematic assessment and documentation of pain and its treatment can lead not only to the reduction of pain but also to an improved quality of life. This will go some way to building up our knowledge of elderly people in pain. As Liebeskind and Melzack (1987) say, 'By any reasonable code, freedom from pain should be a basic human right, limited only by our knowledge to achieve it' (p. 1).

REFERENCES

Aronow W S 1987 Prevalence of presenting symptoms of recognised acute myocardial infarction and unrecognised healed myocardial infarction in elderly patients. American Journal of Cardiology 60: 1182

Baken D 1968 Disease, pain, sacrifice: toward a psychology of suffering. University of Chicago Press, Chicago

Bayer A J, Chadha J S, Farag R R, Pathy M S J 1986 Changing presentation of myocardial infarction with increasing old age. Journal of the American Geriatrics Society 34: 263–266

Bellville J W, Forrest W H, Miller E, Brown B W 1971 Influences of age on pain relief from analgesics. Journal of the American Medical Association 217: 1835–1841

Berkowitz B A, Ngai S H, Yang M D, Hempstead B S, Spector S 1975 The disposition of morphine in surgical patients. Clinical Pharmacology and Therapeutics 17: 629–635

Black D A 1987 Mental state and presentation of myocardial infarction in the elderly. Age and Ageing 16: 125–127

Bourbonnais F 1981 Pain assessment: development of a tool for the nurse and patient. Journal of Advanced Nursing 6: 277–282

Bullingham R E S 1985 Physiological mechanisms in pain. In: Smith G, Covino B G (eds) Acute pain. Butterworths, London

Butler R N, Gastel B 1980 Care of the aged: perspectives on pain and discomfort. In: Ng L K Y, Bonica J J (eds) Pain, discomfort and humanitarian care. Elsevier, New York

Carey K W 1985 Pain: nursing now. Springhouse, Pennsylvania

Charlton J E, Buckley F P 1984 The management of chronic pain. In: Grimley-Evans J, Caird F I (eds) Advanced Geriatric Medicine 4. Pitman, London

Clark W C, Mehl L J 1971 Thermal pain: a sensory decision theory analysis of the effect of age and sex on various response criteria and 50% pain threshold. Journal of Abnormal Psychology 78: 202–212

Clinch D, Banerjee A K, Ostick G 1984 Absence of abdominal pain in elderly patients with peptic ulcer. Age and Ageing 13: 120–123

Cocchi A, Franceschini G, Inclazi R A, Farina G, Vecchio F M, Carbonin P U 1988 Clinico-pathological correlations in the diagnosis of acute myocardial infarction in the elderly. Age and Ageing 17: 87–93

Davis P S 1988 Changing nursing practice for more effective control of post operative pain through a staff initiated educational programme. Nurse Education Today 8: 325–331

Davitz J R, Davitz L L 1981 Inferences of patients' pain and psychological distress. Studies of nursing behaviors. Springer, New York

Day J J, Bayer A J, Pathy M S J, Chadha J S 1987 Acute myocardial infarction: diagnostic difficulties and outcome in advanced old age. Age and Ageing 16: 239–243

Doan B D, Wadden N P 1989 Relationships between depressive symptoms and descriptors of chronic pain. Pain 36: 75–84

Donovan B D 1983 Patient attitudes to postoperative pain relief. Anaesthesia and Intensive Care 11: 125–129

Eland J M 1988 Pain management and comfort. Journal of Gerontological Nursing 14: 10–15

Fagerhaugh S Y, Strauss A 1977 Politics of pain management: staff patient interaction. Addison Wesley, California

Fordyce W E 1978 Learning processes in pain. In: Sternbach R A (ed) The psychology of pain. Raven Press, New York

Ghose K 1987 Pain and the elderly. In: Ghose K (ed). Drug management of pain in the elderly. MTP Press, Lancaster

Gollop S M 1983 Patient teaching: pain and pain control. In: Wilson-Barnett J (ed) Patient teaching: recent advances in nursing 6. Churchill Livingstone, Edinburgh

Harkins S W, Chapman C R 1976 Detection and decision factors in pain perception in young and elderly men. Pain 2: 253–264

Harkins S W, Chapman C R 1977 The perception of induced dental pain in young and elderly women. Journal of Gerontology 32: 428–435

Harkins S W, Kwentus J, Price D D 1984 Pain and the elderly. In: Benedetti C, Chapman C R, Moricca G (eds) Advances in pain research and therapy, vol 7. Recent Advances in the Management of Pain. Raven Press, New York

Illich I 1977 Limits to medicine. Medical nemesis: the expropriation of health. Pelican Books, London

International Association for the Study of Pain Subcommittee on Taxonomy 1986 Pain terms: a current list with definitions and notes on usage. Pain 27: S220–S221

Jacox A, Stewart M 1973 Psychosocial contingencies of the pain experience. University of Iowa, Iowa

Kaiko R F 1980 Age and morphine analgesia in cancer patients with postoperative pain. Clinical Pharmacology and Therapeutics 28: 823–826

Konu V 1977 Myocardial infarction in the elderly: a clinical and epidemiological study with one year follow-up. Acta Medica Scandinavica Supplement 604: 7–68

Kramlinger K G, Swanson D W, Maruta T 1983 Are patients with chronic pain depressed? American Journal of Psychiatry 140: 747–749

Kremer E, Atkinson J H, Ignelzi R J 1981 Measurement of pain: patient preference does not confound pain measurement. Pain 10: 241–248

Kwentus J A, Harkins S W, Lignon N, Silverman J J 1985 Concepts of geriatric pain and its treatment. Geriatrics 40: 48–57

Latham J 1987 Pain Control. Austen Cornish in association with Lisa Sainsbury Foundation, London

Lekan-Rutledge D 1988 Gerontological nursing in long term care facilities. In: Matteson M A, McConnell E S (eds) Gerontological nursing: concepts and practice. Saunders, Philadelphia

Liebeskind J C, Melzack R 1987 The International Pain Foundation: meeting a need for education in pain management. Editorial. Pain 30: 1–2

McCaffery M 1972 Nursing management of the patient with pain. Lippincott, Philadelphia

McCaffery M 1983 Nursing the patient in pain. Lippincott Nursing Series. Adapted for the UK by B Sofaer. Harper and Row, London

McCaffery M, Beebe A 1989 Pain. Clinical manual for nursing practice. C V Mosby, St Louis

McCallion J, Canning G P, Knight P V, McCallion J S 1987 Acute appendicitis in the elderly: A 5 year retrospective study. Age and Ageing 16: 256–260

MacDonald J B 1984 Presentation of acute myocardial infarction in the elderly — a review. Age and Ageing 13: 196–200

MacDonald J B, Baille J, Williams B O, Ballantyne D 1983 Coronary care in the elderly. Age and Ageing 12: 17–20

McKenzie G J 1985 Pain. In: Cormack D F (ed) Geriatric nursing: a conceptual approach. Blackwell Scientific, Oxford

Matteson M A, McConnell E S 1988 Gerontological nursing: concepts and practice. Saunders, Philadelphia

Meinhart N T, McCaffery M 1983 Pain: a nursing approach to assessment and analysis. Appleton Century Crofts, Norwalk

Melzack R, Casey K L 1968 Sensory, motivational, and central control determinants of pain: a new conceptual model. In: Kenshalo D R (ed) The skin senses. Thomas, Springfield

Melzack R, Wall P D 1965 Pain mechanisms: a new theory. Science 150: 971–979

Melzack R, Wall P D 1988 The challenge of pain, 2nd edn. Penguin Books, London

Miller C, Le Lieuvre R B 1982 A method to reduce chronic pain in elderly nursing home residents. Gerontologist 22: 314–317

Moore J T, Whanger A D 1983 Functional psychiatric disorders. In: Cape R D T, Coe R M, Rossman I (eds) Fundementals of geriatric medicine. Raven Press, New York

National Institutes of Health 1979 Pain in the elderly: patterns change with age. Journal of the American Medical Association 241: 2491–2492

National Institutes of Health Consensus Development Conference 1987 The integrated approach to the management of pain. Journal of Pain and Symptom Management 2: 35–44

Odar-Cederlof I, Boreus L O, Bondesson U, Holmberg L, Heyner L 1985 Comparison of renal excretion of Pethidine (meperidine) and its metabolites in old and young patients. European Journal of Clinical Pharmacology 28: 171–175

Pathy M S 1967 Clinical presentation of myocardial infarction in the elderly. British Heart Journal 29: 190–199

Portenoy R K, Farkash A 1988 Practical management of non-malignant pain in the elderly. Geriatrics 43: 29–47

Raiman J 1981 Responding to pain. Nursing. 1st series 31: 1362–1365

Seers C J 1987 Pain, anxiety and recovery in patients undergoing surgery. Unpublished PhD thesis, University of London

Sofaer B 1984 Pain: a handbook for nurses. Harper and Row, London

Sternbach R 1987 Mastering pain: a twelve step regimen for mastering chronic pain. Arlington Books, London

Stewart M L 1977 Measurement of clinical pain. In: Jacox A K (ed) Pain: a source book for nurses and other health professionals. Little, Brown, Boston

Syrjala K L 1987 The measurement of pain. In: McGuire D B, Yarbro C H (eds) Cancer pain management. Grune and Stratton, Orlando

Telfer S, Fenyo G, Holt P R, De Dombal F T 1988 Acute abdominal pain in patients over 50 years of age. Scandinavian Journal of Gastroenterology 23: 47–50

Thompson J W 1984 Pain: mechanisms and principles of management: In: Grimley-Evans J, Caird F I (eds) Advanced Geriatric Medicine 4. Pitman, London

Wachter-Shikora N, Perez S 1988 Unmasking pain. Geriatric Nursing 3: 392–393

Walker J 1989 The management of elderly patients with painful conditions. Nursing Times 85: 53

Walker J M, Akinsanya J A, Davis B D, Marcer D 1989 The nursing management of pain in the community: a theoretical framework. Journal of Advanced Nursing 14: 240–247

Wells J C D 1989 If you prick them, do they not bleed? Geriatric Medicine 19: 65–70

Wong D L, Baker C M 1988 Pain in children: comparison of assessment scales. Pediatric Nursing 14: 9–17

Woodrow K N, Friedman G D, Siegelaub A B, Collen M F 1972 Pain tolerance: differences according to age, sex and race. Psychosomatic Medicine 34: 548–556

Wroblewski M, Mikulowski P, Steen B 1986 Symptoms of myocardial infarction in old age: clinical case, retrospective and prospective studies. Age and Ageing 15: 99–104

CHAPTER CONTENTS

Introduction 289
The future framework of nursing practice 290

Psychiatric morbidity in the elderly population 291

Emotional well-being in old age 292

Nursing principles for multidisciplinary practice 294

Identification 295
Screening 295
Case finding 296

Assessment 297
The process of assessment 297
The assessment protocol 297
Methods of assessment 298
Components of the total assessment 300

Biographical approaches to assessment 303
Organizing and analysing the data 304

Planning interventions 304
Aims and objectives 304
Nurses as key workers 305
'Nursing process' or 'care process'? 305
Conclusion 306

18

Mental health problems of elderly people: assessment and planning

Ian J. Norman

INTRODUCTION

Stereotypes of old age encourage an exaggerated view of mental health problems experienced by elderly people. Whilst a minority suffer the impact of mental illness, public preoccupation with conditions such as dementia leads to the common error of generalizing from this minority to the majority.

Older people consistently display much higher rates of expressed satisfaction with their lives than do younger people (Hunt 1978; Palmore & Kivett 1977). Moreover, large studies of life satisfaction and living circumstances (Abrams 1978) and of adjustment to bereavement (Bowling & Cartwright 1982) demonstrate that whilst some experience depression and show signs of maladjustment, a great many old people come to terms with their losses. Whilst these findings may reflect, at least in part, the particular stoical and accepting attitudes of recent older generations, they also suggest that we should reconsider the commonly held preconception of old age as a particularly problematic time of life which threatens our mental health (Coleman 1988).

There is in one sense a contradiction between these opening remarks on the one hand and the remainder of this chapter and the two which follow on the other, for whilst a majority of elderly people enjoy good mental health, these chapters focus to a large extent on the minority who do not. Elderly people with mental health problems live in a wide variety of settings; in residential Homes, in hospital wards, with their families and in their own homes. These three chapters (18, 19 and 20) are written for all nurses who are engaged in the day-to-day care and support of these people and their families. Throughout these chapters the term 'client' is preferred to 'patient' and the term 'resident' is used to refer to elderly people in long-term institutional care.

THE FUTURE FRAMEWORK OF NURSING PRACTICE

The approach adopted in these chapters has been influenced by the long-awaited response by the government to the Griffiths report (Griffiths 1988) on community care (Secretary of State for Health, Social Security, Wales and Scotland 1989). The main objective of the new proposals is that, wherever possible, elderly people and other client groups will be cared for in their own homes and will be assessed by a multidisciplinary team which will then plan an individually tailored package of care based on need. With respect to elderly people with mental health problems a community focus for care is entirely appropriate. The nature of mental disorder is such that investigations in hospital are rarely necessary and there is little to gain from admission; old people are integrated into social networks which should be maintained; institutional care is expensive and in short supply; and hospital care has well-recognized disadvantages (Hemsi 1982). This is not to deny that there may be genuine conflicts of interest between the mental health of elderly people and the rights and sometimes even the mental health of other family members; thus the exercise of individual choice may necessarily be limited. However, this does not invalidate the principle of home-based care and indicates that admission to an institution should never be considered as an early option.

The transition to a local domestic health service has many implications for nurses caring for elderly people with mental health problems. For example, it is likely to blur the traditional distinction between hospital and community nursing as new appointments are made to the 'service' rather than to the 'hospital' in order to ensure flexibility of response and to enable nurses to work in hospi-

tal and community settings, wherever their skills are most required. Thus it is likely that nurses will be required to move from hospital to community as the old mental and geriatric hospitals are closed down.

The government has accepted Griffiths' central proposal that local authorities should in future be primarily responsible for the care of elderly and disabled people living in the community. The new system seems to be based upon Griffiths' controversial split between 'health and medical' and 'social' care. Nurses working in the community are expected to remain employees of the health authority and as such will only be expected to provide the 'health and medical' component of care while 'social' care will be provided by an auxiliary workforce based in the local authorities.

With respect to elderly people with mental health problems this administrative distinction between 'medical' and 'social' aspects of care is nonsense. Whilst mental disorders in elderly people may create specific health problems, these are intimately tied to the individual's social situation and to factors such as housing, economics and education. Moreover, the administrative separation of trained nurses and auxiliaries is likely to reduce the accountability of untrained to trained nursing staff and may raise questions of quality and safety.

The future framework of care will require nurses to work closely with social services departments and professionals from a wide variety of health care disciplines in assessing the needs of elderly clients and their families. The status of nurses within these multidisciplinary teams is uncertain. Moreover, the artificial separation of aspects of care raises the serious threat that nurses may be marginalized and forced back into a 'medical model' style of practice.

This chapter, and Chapters 19 and 20, are written in the belief that if nurses are to be a positive force within the multidisciplinary care teams of the future they must be prepared to challenge the distinction between 'medical' and 'social' aspects of care, adopt a broad perspective on the nursing role, use a variety of explanatory models and think in social and interactional terms. Accordingly, these chapters have abandoned the traditional clinically and physically orientated approach to the care of elderly people with mental health problems in favour of a perspective that highlights psychosocial aspects of care and sets the nurse's contribution within a multidisciplinary teamwork approach to health care provision. The focus of this chapter is upon the role of the nurse within the primary health care team but the issues discussed are relevant to all nurses caring for elderly people with mental health problems in a variety of institutional and non-institutional settings.

The first part of this chapter focuses on issues of general relevance to nurses concerned with the mental health of elderly people. A consideration of epidemiology is followed by a consideration of emotional well-being in old age which highlights the importance of physical health, social and cultural factors and developmental influences on the ageing process. The remainder of the chapter touches upon some aspects of multidisciplinary teamwork and specifically considers the processes of identification, assessment and planning. Chapters 19 and 20 discuss nursing interventions in relation to some of the more common mental health problems affecting elderly people

PSYCHIATRIC MORBIDITY IN THE ELDERLY POPULATION

The growth of numbers of very old people in the population suggests that there will be more old people with mental health problems in the future. However, giving a precise picture of the incidence of specific psychiatric conditions is problematic. A large number of studies have investigated the mental health status of the elderly population, but since very few studies of 'incidence' (the proportion of the population in which new cases of a disease occur over a particular time period) and 'prevalence' (the proportion of the population who are affected by a disease at one particular time) have been carried out on the same population sample over time, it is simply impossible to say for sure whether the incidence of particular mental health problems are increasing or decreasing.

The now-classic study by Kay et al (1964) of psychiatric disorders in a large sample of people over 65 living in Newcastle-upon-Tyne indicated that one in four had some kind of psychiatric disorder. The results of more recent epidemiological studies related to mental health problems in old age are summarized below:

Dementia

The prevalence of definite dementia rises with age. Overall, about 5% of those aged over 65 are affected (Brayne & Ames 1988). However, when broken down, this figure is 2.3% in the under-75 age group and rises to 20% in the over-80s (Pitt 1988). Encouragingly, there is some evidence that there is a decline in the incidence rate (Hagnell et al 1983), but this has yet to be confirmed.

Many studies fail to differentiate the prevalence of different types of dementia, but it would appear that senile dementia of the Alzheimer type (SDAT) is the most common form in the UK. SDAT may be less common in men than in women, and multi-infarct dementia (MID) less common in women than in men. In the Newcastle study (Kay et al 1964), 5.5% of the sample were assessed as possibly demented but this rate is suspect given the difficulty in distinguishing mild dementia from low performance for other reasons.

Confusional states

Since these are transient and often associated with medical conditions, epidemiological studies are rare (Liston 1982). Lipowski (1983) reports that 10–15% of the over-65s develop confusional states following surgery, and 16–25% admitted to general medical wards are confused on admission or develop a confusional state over the next month. In geriatric units the rate is higher, with 35–80% being confused on admission or developing a confusional state subsequently (Eastwood & Corbin 1985). These figures should be treated with caution since they may be distorted by the problems of comparing data from different studies and the fact that many studies exclude clients who are quiet and co-operative or asleep! Thus these figures may be an underestimate of the true incidence and prevalence in hospitalized elderly clients.

Studies of elderly clients with hip fractures (Williams et al 1979, 1985) suggest a relationship between confusional states and increasing age, but this relationship has not been substantiated (Foreman 1986).

Depression

The variety of methods of assessment and rating scales used in surveys makes it difficult to arrive at accurate figures. Approximately 10–12% of people over 65 have a clinical syndrome of depression, with a minority suffering a severe form (Eastwood & Corbin 1985, Copeland et al 1987). Depression would seem to be more common in females than in males (Maule et al 1984), is often unnoticed and undetected in elderly general hospital populations (Bergmann & Eastham 1974) and is particularly common in elderly people living in residential care. It is disturbing to note that in a survey of 12 Homes in one London borough, 38% of the elderly residents were found to be in a 'significantly depressed state' (Mann et al 1984).

Schizophrenia and paranoid states

Schizophrenia is a comparatively rare but important mental disorder in old age which has an estimated lifetime prevalence of about 0.9% (Shields & Slater 1975). Paraphrenia is the name given to a form of schizophrenia with its onset in late life.

Other mental health problems

Conditions not discussed in these chapters include neuroses, personality disorders, and alcohol and drug abuse. The epidemiology of neuroses and personality disorders is an under-researched field and suffers from lack of agreement between researchers on definitions. A series of European studies reviewed by Neugebauer (1980) indicate a range of prevalence for neuroses in the over-60s from 1 to 10%, and from 7 to 18% when personality disorders are added. Reported rates for women are higher for neuroses whilst men have higher rates of personality disorders.

It is difficult to make a reliable estimate of alcohol and drug abuse in the elderly due to marked variation in reported prevalence rates and difficulties in differentiating substance abuse from inadvertent misuse of prescribed drugs (polypharmacy).

For further information, readers are referred to recent reviews of epidemiological studies of mental disorders in old age by Eastwood and Corbin (1985) and Brayne and Ames (1988).

EMOTIONAL WELL-BEING IN OLD AGE

In general, successful ageing is characterized by continuity between late life and earlier periods. Thus emotional well-being is most likely to be maintained if the individual can sustain into late life her self-image and her own idiosyncratic pattern of relationships, values, activities and living arrangements that have been built up over a lifetime, and which she regards as normal (Johnson 1988). In old age there are an increasing number of threats to an individual's established pattern of living.

Older people are at greater risk of developing physical ill health; this has been identified as one of the strongest sources of distress and dissatisfaction in all age groups (Stoudemire & Blazer 1985; Flanagan 1978). It is particularly implicated in the aetiology of depression and this is discussed in detail in Chapter 20. A review of 81 empirical studies of physical status and subjective well-being suggests that whilst greater weight should be given to 'perceived' as opposed to 'actual' health, both are directly and consistently related to mental status (Zautra & Hempel 1984). Chronic physical illness such as arthritis or heart disease which restrict activity and induce disability may promote a sense of dissatisfaction and diminished well-being in old people. Moreover, drugs prescribed for chronic physical illness may sap vitality.

However, the mechanism linking health and

emotional well-being is complex. The advent of physical illness means something different from one individual to the next. Individual responses to physical ill health vary; some old people will 'battle on regardless', whilst others may feel completely overwhelmed. In some cases the relationship between emotional well-being and physical health may run counter to the direction usually assumed, in that a sense of well-being and life satisfaction may be predictive of physical health (Zautra & Hempel 1984).

A longitudinal study in the USA involving a ten-year follow-up of survivors in a community survey concluded that socioeconomic factors are strong and consistent predictors of mental health and other aspects of functioning amongst the 'old-old' (Palmore et al 1985). This finding is supported by other studies which have found a strong tie between lower socioeconomic status and psychopathology in all age groups (Hirschfeld & Cross 1982; Romaniuk et al 1983).

The inverse relationship between socioeconomic status and mental disorder has been the subject of involved debate. Some contend that lowered socioeconomic status is secondary to mental disorder, since the latter results in a drift down the socioeconomic scale, and that this predisposition is maintained by associative mating (Godberg & Morrison 1963). Others argue that factors associated with low socioeconomic status — such as poor living conditions, money worries and limited opportunities for the exercise of autonomy and initiative — create high levels of distress and that this is manifested in higher rates of psychological disorder (Kohn 1976; Abrahamson et al 1982). Another approach suggests that people of low socioeconomic status form a distinct subculture and that intercultural differences mean that psychiatrists are more likely to label them as severely mentally ill. Still others propose that the response of society and health care professionals to people with psychological problems vary according to their socioeconomic status; thus those of lower status may receive inappropriate (or inadequate) treatment and responses which tend to be pejorative and perpetuate psychological difficulties (Schwab & Schwab 1978).

Clearly, these hypotheses are not all relevant to all elderly people with psychological difficulties, but they may help to explain why in the absence of material resources diagnosis of mental disorder — particularly depression — becomes more likely.

In general, rapid change of all kinds, particularly when the elderly person is unprepared for it, may have negative consequences for emotional well-being. Self-esteem, well-being and coping effectiveness depend in part on confronting familiar challenges and problems which have been overcome successfully in the past. Unfamiliar life events — retirement, bereavement, onset of physical illness — and developmental tasks of late adulthood may have a very negative impact on mental well-being in the absence of strong coping skills and social supports (Dohrenwend & Dohrenwend 1984).

Ageism in its manifest forms constitutes another threat to mental well-being. Impatient or patronizing social reactions to the generally slower responses or physical frailty of old people may stigmatize and reinforce small deficits. This may undermine the old person's confidence and sense of sociability and have a negative impact on her sense of well-being. Reduction of citizenship, or what Townsend (1981) has called 'structured dependency', arising from factors such as the low valuation of old people, their exclusion from decision-making bodies, lack of community resource facilities, and inadequate material resources can have a negative impact on the emotional well-being of all old people, particularly those in the older age groups beyond 75 years.

From the discussion so far, it is clear that some groups of old people are better placed than others to manage or avoid the threats to continuity associated with old age. One of the groups particularly at risk is composed of those old people from ethnic minorities who came to this country as adults, having grown up in another culture. These individuals may often live in areas where the quality of housing and public services are low. In such circumstances the losses which often accompany old age may be experienced as additional stressors and lead to a variety of stress-related mental health problems. These old people often suffer from what

Norman (1985) has referred to as the 'triple jeopardy' of old age, racial or cultural discrimination, and lack of access to suitable services. Studies suggest that they are particularly at risk of mental disorder in old age and are less likely than old people in the indigenous population to have such disorders recognized and competently treated (Rack 1982, Norman 1988). The reader is referred to Chapter 25 for further discussion on elders from ethnic minorities.

In sum, it seems clear that the emotional well-being of old people is heavily influenced not only by their physical health but also by their material and social environment. There is considerable evidence to suggest that individuals who are closely integrated into their family, neighbourhood and community live longer and express greater well-being (Mechanic 1982). Ageism makes elderly people feel redundant and prematurely limits their options for meaningful activities. Whilst improvements to the social environment would not eradicate mental health problems experienced by old people, it would alleviate the suffering associated with some of these problems and prevent others.

This section has drawn attention to broad influences on the emotional well-being of old people. However, as Johnson reminds us in Chapter 1 of this volume and elsewhere (Johnson 1988), old age cannot be separated from earlier stages of life. Whilst the transition from youth and young adulthood to mid-life may bring the individual positive benefits associated with maturity, there is little evidence of a similar process occuring with the transition to old age. We are likely to carry our full set of strengths and weaknesses into our later years and these will be manifest in our behaviour. As Johnson puts it, 'nice younger people will tend to become nice older people. Those who were cantankerous, intolerant, spiteful, mean, narrow minded, selfish or indolent will continue to be' (Johnson 1988 p. 143). A recognition that personality traits are likely to be preserved into late life is important if nurses are to avoid confounding awkward or unpleasant behaviour with early signs of mental disorder.

Old age is above all an individual, subjective experience which is profoundly influenced by past experiences. Some of these experiences are unique to individuals whilst others are common to old people who are members of an historical cohort. This highlights the importance of nurses developing an understanding of old people as members of social groups and of factors which threaten the emotional well-being of all old people; but it is equally important to recognize the differences between old people who live in similar circumstances and who confront similar difficulties. It is these differences which make individual old people unique and shape the way in which they respond to the threats and opportunities of late life.

NURSING PRINCIPLES FOR MULTIDISCIPLINARY PRACTICE

Nurses currently work as members of multidisciplinary teams in a variety of hospital and community settings and, as previously discussed, this approach to service delivery is likely to increase as the care of elderly people with mental health problems becomes increasingly centred in the community.

Multidisciplinary teamwork requires the nurse to work jointly with individuals from other disciplines to generate integrated programmes of care for individual clients and their families. Health care professionals and social workers will have different viewpoints and may not share common values. Thus, a problem for the nurse is how to ensure a team culture which is supportive of central nursing values and principles of practice. This is not an easy task — particularly in teams in which power is unevenly distributed and one professional culture (usually medicine, perhaps in future social work) predominates — but it is important in the interests of good client care.

One source of central nursing principles is provided by models of nursing care which have been developed over recent years in an attempt to help nurses make sense of what they do and should do. Stuart and Sundeen (1987) suggest that all models of nursing incorporate three common features: a holistic approach, a collaborative relationship with the client, and an emphasis on 'care' as distinct from, although complementary to, 'cure'.

The adoption of these three broad principles as tenets of teamwork practice in residential and community settings may relieve the professional strain sometimes experienced by nurses practising in multidisciplinary contexts, and should facilitate the provision of sensitive, individualized care for clients and their families.

In the care of elderly people with mental health problems it is essential that assessment and intervention take account of the 'whole person' in relation to her environment. Social, psychological and biological/biochemical systems interact; a change in one system is likely to affect others. Take, for example, the case of an elderly woman who loses a valued pet (social change). This event may induce a depressed mood (psychological change) and if this change takes place in the absence of a confiding relationship (social/psychological circumstance) (Murphy 1982), it may lead to a depressive illness with accompanying biochemical changes (biochemical/biological change). This may lead in turn to self-neglect (social change).

A holistic perspective also draws attention to the fact that experiences and adaptation to illness differ according to the psychological response of the individual client to her disability and the way in which others who make up her formal and informal social networks — relatives, neighbours, friends and professional carers — respond. This highlights the importance of assessing the dynamics of the client's situation and of making informed judgements as to the contribution of each factor to her behaviour.

There are two important practical implications of a holistic approach to assessment and planning. In the first place, that assessment should take place as far as possible within the context of the client's normal physical and social environment. Secondly, in planning, consideration should be given to the timing and co-ordination of interventions at different levels; thus, taking the above example, the elderly woman is unlikely to be able to co-operate with interventions designed to promote self-care prior to the instigation of antidepressant drug therapy and behavioural/cognitive work designed to relieve her depressed mood and raise her self-esteem. Furthermore, these interventions are unlikely to be successful in the long term unless steps are also taken to improve her level of social support.

Whilst the client should remain the prime concern of the multidisciplinary team, informal carers may also need help and support, if only to enable them to help the client should they wish to do so. Thus, in line with the central principles of nursing practice, it is important for the carer to create a collaborative relationship with the client and informal carers, within which all may contribute ideas and energy to the therapeutic process. (See Chapter 27 for further discussion on the responsibilities and experiences of informal carers.)

The mental health problems experienced by old people are often intractable or cannot be easily resolved; thus 'care' becomes as important, and is often more relevant than 'cure'. The centrality of 'care' to nursing practice places nurses at the centre of service provision to this client group.

IDENTIFICATION

Contrary to popular belief, mental health problems are not a natural and inevitable consequence of the ageing process. If detection is early, assessment thorough and intervention vigorous, many problems are reversible. In the case of irreversible conditions such as dementia, early detection can delay dependency and prevent premature admission of the client to long-term residential care (Bergmann 1979).

Mental health problems in elderly people often come to light when odd behaviour is reported to health care professionals by neighbours, friends, family or, sometimes, the police. By this stage these problems may often have reached serious proportions; had detection occurred earlier, more might have been possible to alleviate their effects. There is general agreement that early detection of affected individuals is important, but how this should be undertaken is a matter of debate.

SCREENING

Studies by Williamson and colleagues in the early 1960s (Williamson et al 1964) identified a high level of unreported health needs amongst people over 65. These researchers commented upon the particularly poor mental health of some elderly people and found that a high proportion of people had more than one disabling problem. These studies suggested that elderly people could not be relied upon to report their health care needs and that GPs should seek to keep in touch with their older patients through maintaining sex/age registers. Williamson et al (1964) advocated that health visitors should be closely involved in this screening process.

Some health care professionals have followed Williamson's suggestions and have established systems for screening people over a certain age for a range of potential health problems (Kiehn 1986, Stringfellow 1986). It is generally accepted that there are benefits to such schemes in terms of quality of life of clients, satisfaction with the service and increased job satisfaction on the part of health care professionals. However, the nature of these benefits means that they are difficult to quantify and measure.

Screening programmes also have disadvantages. They require time and resources and may be construed by some elderly people as an invasion of privacy. Responding to a request to visit the doctor requires effort and probably expenditure on travel and may bring to light health problems which cannot be alleviated and which only cause the elderly client to worry. If social rather than health problems are identified this may result in referral to other agencies but this does not guarantee that assistance will be forthcoming. It must also be remembered that possible benefits of a screening programme rely upon the quality and availability of the age/sex data base. In many GP practices these do not exist and in others they may be out of date.

Evaluation studies into screening have produced few clear policy implications. Vetter et al (1984) found that a yearly visit by a health visitor to a group of elderly people in Wales had a beneficial impact upon mortality and increased the utilization of domicilary services. Tulloch and Moore (1979) found that a group of screened elderly people were referred to other services more than those in a control group. The screened group had a higher overall admission rate to hospital but spent less time as inpatients. There was no appreciable impact on mortality. The reader is referred to Chapter 26 for further discussion on screening.

CASE FINDING

'Screening' refers to identifying health problems which are unrecognized by the elderly person. In contrast, 'case finding' refers to the identification of treatable health problems with symptoms which are recognized but accepted by the client who has resigned herself to live with them. The enormity of the task of screening all elderly clients within a GP practice has led to screening and case finding being combined in attempts to identify elderly people who are more likely than others to have a health problem.

Taylor et al (1983) tested 11 structural characteristics as 'at risk' indicators but found that none of these identified a group of elderly people with a particularly high level of unmet need. These researchers concluded that none of the indicators provided an acceptable basis for case finding. Barber et al (1980) developed a postal screening questionnaire designed to identify elderly people who would benefit from a home visit for detailed assessment. The questionnaire which consisted of nine items requiring yes/no answers was found to be more successful in identifying cases with low levels of well-being than structural 'at risk' indicators. Whilst postal screening seems to be a useful approach to identifying physical health problems, the efficacy of this method of follow-up in relation to mental health problems is uncertain.

The research evidence suggests that most elderly people — 93% of those over 75 (Williams 1984) — make contact with their doctor each year. In view of this, Freer (1985) suggests that case finding be focused on patients who visit their doctor, thus combining routine care with prevention. This is sometimes referred to as 'opportunistic case finding' (Itzin 1986).

'Opportunistic case finding' as a central strategy is supported by a finding by Ebrahim et al (1984) that those elderly people who do not consult their GP are a low-risk group with few problems. In any case, the number of non-consulters is relatively small and thus contact screening may be a manageable strategy for this group. If financial constraints make this impossible, an option may be opportunistic case finding for the majority and contact screening of those who have previously consulted their GP each year but then failed to do so.

Nurses and health visitors remain committed to screening and case finding but there is also some evidence of growing interest in health promotion for elderly people rather than screening. Luker (1982) argues that rather than seeking illness health visitors should think more positively, in terms of promoting 'effective health'.

ASSESSMENT

THE PROCESS OF ASSESSMENT

In general terms, assessment involves looking at individuals and their circumstances to gain an overall picture of their problems and positive attributes. More specifically, assessment describes the skills, assets and other positive features of the person as well as her handicaps, disabilities and dysfunctions.

The process of assessment has three main phases: collecting information about how the person functions at different levels and in specific situations; drawing the information together into an organized format; and judging the significance of the information in order to achieve an understanding of the nature and scope of the person's problems.

Assessments of elderly people seek to clarify what may be done for the person and involve an attempt to define need. More specifically, assessments may be performed with a view to possible hospital admission, discharge, or transfer, or for a variety of other purposes. Thus the question posed will indicate what particular aspects of the person's functioning should be the focus of attention and which methods of assessment may be employed.

Assessment as described here should not be confused with 'diagnosis'. Whilst diagnosis involves a 'diagnostic assessment' this has a narrow focus which seeks to identify the presence of certain problems or abnormalities and ignores those aspects of the person which are positive and functioning normally.

THE ASSESSMENT PROTOCOL

Nurses and other care professionals who work with elderly people in a variety of settings invariably want to begin their work by assessing them. Often, information obtained by one assessor indicates the need for referral to another professional group for further assessment.

Dant et al (1987) point out that the way in which elderly people are frequently assessed brings them into contact with many different people, all of whom ask similar questions. Thus the client may be confused about who these assessors are and what services they may be able to offer. Assessments are often determined by the professional interest of the assessor and thus it is often not an assessment of what needs to be done but of what the professional herself — doctor, nurse, health visitor, social worker etc. — might do to help the client. In spite of this, most initial assessments of elderly people contain much basic information which is common to all.

These problems in the assessment process may be alleviated by the government's proposal for 'key workers' or 'case managers' to be appointed 'where necessary' to take responsibility for assessment of need and co-ordination of individual care packages with different agencies (Secretary of State for Health, Social Security, Wales and Scotland 1989). More generally, it points to the need for multidisciplinary care teams to establish an assessment protocol which defines who is responsible for collecting specific information about a client. This helps to ensure that the assessment is comprehensive, minimizes overlap by different team members, and ensures that there is a system for sharing information within the team.

The assessment protocol should be determined through frank and open discussion among team members which takes account not only of disciplinary boundaries but also of individual training. It is important that team members are prepared to recognize areas in which skill and responsibility are unique as well as where these overlap; they should be prepared to accept each other's skills regardless of different training backgrounds.

METHODS OF ASSESSMENT

A wide variety of methods of assessment are available and should be selected according to the purpose of the assessment and the aspects of the person's functioning under scrutiny. A general distinction can be made between 'formal' approaches, which use a predetermined structure for collecting information (e.g. structured interviews, standardized rating scales), and 'informal' approaches in which information is collected in a less structured way (e.g. open-ended interviews, conversations). Formal methods are traditionally used in assessing aspects of biophysical functioning (e.g. taking pulse and blood pressure). With respect to psychosocial aspects the mix of informal/formal methods which are appropriate will be determined to some extent by the individual client. Where the client is able and anxious to communicate, the nurse may obtain much information from informal conversations and open-ended interviews, whereas more specific measures of behaviour may be more appropriate where the client is inarticulate or withdrawn.

A holistic approach to assessment requires that it be undertaken as far as possible in the client's own home. Confusion and disorientation can be engendered through the elderly person attending the hospital or health centre and this can give a falsely pessimistic picture of the client's mental functioning. A home visit allows the environment to be assessed as well as the client and also the interaction between the two in terms of the client's ability to function within her familiar environment. A home visit has the additional advantage of allowing the level of social support to be accurately assessed since neighbours and relatives are close at hand to give their version of the client's history and discuss the impact of the client's illness on their lives.

Nursing assessment interviews

Accurate assessment and effective intervention de-

pend upon the establishment of a warm and supportive relationship with the client. With elderly people, as with other client groups, this depends upon positive attitudes, relevant knowledge and effective communication skills.

When a home assessment is impossible and the client is initially seen in hospital the nurse should ensure a quiet environment free of distraction in which privacy and confidentiality are assured. A useful exercise is for the nurse to try to imagine herself as the old person and look at the environment through her eyes. What impression does the interview setting create? Is it friendly, informal, clinical, tatty, threatening? What can be done to help the client feel at ease?

Nurses are not immune to the tendency to stereotype elderly people and in fact may have less opportunity than members of the public to have general negative beliefs disproved. Holden and Woods (1982) suggest that staff attitudes should allow the old person individuality as an adult, dignity, self-respect, choice and independence. Achieving these attitudes is not an easy task. Dignity and self-respect are hard to maintain when help is needed to go to the toilet. Individuality is problematic when dementia has robbed the old person of some elements of her personality or when she is living in a Home with others. It is important that nurses submit their attitudes to constant critical scrutiny and assess the extent to which they allow clients to reach these objectives.

Assessment must start from a sound understanding of the parameters of normal ageing. During the assessment interview itself the nurse should draw upon her knowledge of the social, economic and cultural background of the client and promote effective communication by adapting her own behaviour to reduce the impact of age-related sensory changes; thus, for example, sensitive use of touch may be used to compensate for poor vision and clear, slow speech used to compensate for poor hearing. The nurse should sit at the same height and possibly at a slight angle to the client to minimize any sense of threat and facilitate rapport on equal terms. An individual approach can be conveyed by using the client's surname as a mark of respect until she expresses a preference for first names, and in giving the cli-

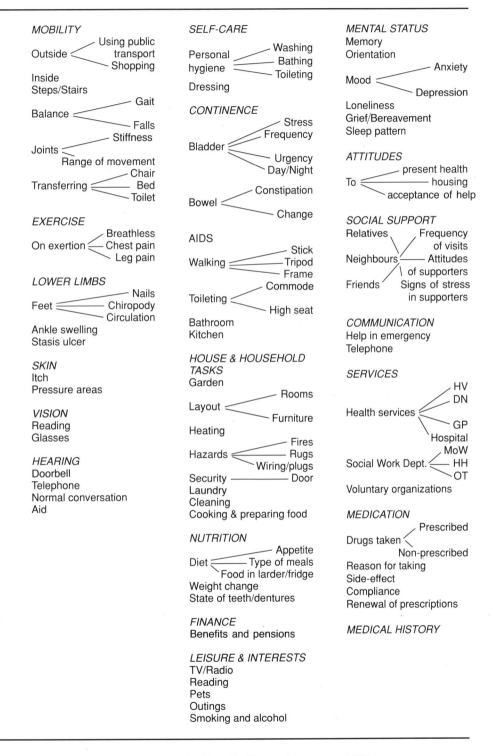

MOBILITY
Outside — Using public transport / Shopping
Inside
Steps/Stairs
Balance — Gait / Falls
Joints — Stiffness / Range of movement
Transferring — Chair / Bed / Toilet

EXERCISE
On exertion — Breathless / Chest pain / Leg pain

LOWER LIMBS
Feet — Nails / Chiropody / Circulation
Ankle swelling
Stasis ulcer

SKIN
Itch
Pressure areas

VISION
Reading
Glasses

HEARING
Doorbell
Telephone
Normal conversation
Aid

SELF-CARE
Personal hygiene — Washing / Bathing / Toileting
Dressing

CONTINENCE
Bladder — Stress / Frequency / Urgency / Day/Night
Bowel — Constipation / Change

AIDS
Walking — Stick / Tripod / Frame
Toileting — Commode / High seat
Bathroom
Kitchen

HOUSE & HOUSEHOLD TASKS
Garden
Layout — Rooms / Furniture
Heating
Hazards — Fires / Rugs / Wiring/plugs
Security — Door
Laundry
Cleaning
Cooking & preparing food

NUTRITION
Diet — Appetite / Type of meals / Food in larder/fridge
Weight change
State of teeth/dentures

FINANCE
Benefits and pensions

LEISURE & INTERESTS
TV/Radio
Reading
Pets
Outings
Smoking and alcohol

MENTAL STATUS
Memory
Orientation
Mood — Anxiety / Depression
Loneliness
Grief/Bereavement
Sleep pattern

ATTITUDES
To — present health / housing / acceptance of help

SOCIAL SUPPORT
Relatives
Neighbours
Friends
Frequency of visits
Attitudes of supporters
Signs of stress in supporters

COMMUNICATION
Help in emergency
Telephone

SERVICES
Health services — HV / DN / GP / Hospital
Social Work Dept. — MoW / HH / OT
Voluntary organizations

MEDICATION
Drugs taken — Prescribed / Non-prescribed
Reason for taking
Side-effect
Compliance
Renewal of prescriptions

MEDICAL HISTORY

Fig. 18.1 Prompt list for health assessment of elderly people, *From Buckley and Runciman (1985).*

ent clear choices; thus, for example, the nurse might ask permission to discuss particularly sensitive subjects, e.g., 'Do you mind if we discuss the death of your husband now, or would you prefer to leave it to another time?'

Since fatigue may contribute to diminished mental functioning in elderly people, assessment interviews should be kept fairly short and, wherever possible, conducted in the morning. To avoid tiring the client, information may be collected over two or three meetings. Communicating with elderly people is discussed in detail in Chapter 4.

A common misperception shared by clients and their relatives and applied particularly to psychiatrists and social workers is that they have come to 'put away' the client in the local institution or 'a Home'. Nurses are less likely to be perceived in this way and may often be best placed to openly acknowledge concerns, allay anxieties, and gain the trust and confidence of the client and her family. The sensitively conducted assessment interview may often form the foundation of a collaborative working relationship with the client and her family.

In order to facilitate an organized, systematic and structured approach to data collection a number of assessment schedules are available, mainly in the North American psychogeriatric literature (e.g. Wolanin & Phillips 1981). These schedules are comprehensive but generally complicated and time consuming. In the UK many hospitals have developed their own nursing assessment schedules for use with particular client groups — acute, continuing care, elderly, etc. — or have derived them from particular models of nursing. Whilst this works well in some cases, failure to develop the schedule in line with the agreed assessment protocol may make them unnecessarily repetitive.

An alternative to assessment schedules which is often preferred is a list of items which the assessor can use as a memory aid to ensure that adequate information is obtained to allow a comprehensive needs assessment. Buckley and Runciman (1985) developed a prompt-list which was found helpful by student health visitors in providing a mental framework for assessment. The areas covered are listed in Figure 18.1.

Other methods of assessment

There are various methods of assessment other than interviews; these include fairly loose self-report methods using logs and diaries, rating scales which may be used by clients or nurses, and tighter assessment methods using direct recording techniques. Discussion of these methods falls beyond the scope of this chapter, although some will be mentioned in relation to components of the total assessment. Readers are referred to Barker (1985) who does not specifically discuss elderly people but who gives an informed overview of assessment in psychiatric nursing.

Whichever methods of assessment are used, all information should be recorded clearly for the benefit of all team members. It is important when recording the history and presenting problems that everyone should avoid jargon and instead describe the situation and events precisely and accurately in ordinary words. For example, do not say that the client 'is aggressive' but that she 'hits her husband when he tries to help her to the toilet'; do not say 'she suffers from loss of recent memory', but that 'she cannot remember where she has put things and therefore keeps losing things and trying to find them'.

COMPONENTS OF THE TOTAL ASSESSMENT

Assessment of an elderly person should address the following components and levels of functioning.

The history

This includes the psychiatric history and an account of the client's previous life. Every informant involved with the client, starting with the client herself, is a potential source of history. Each will relate this history from her own perspective; no two histories will be identical, although there are likely to be correlations between accounts. If the client's mental state is abnormal her own version of her history will be affected by that abnormality and in some cases the reliability may be grossly impaired by severe intellectual impairment, depression or delusions. Whilst it is important to understand the client's viewpoint, in some cases persisting in attempting to gain a history from the client may only result in distress and time may be better spent gaining the 'facts' from others.

A sound knowledge of the biography and interests of the client is important if future nursing interventions are to be relevant to the client's needs and interests and reflect a holistic approach to care. The older person is more likely than her younger counterpart to have experienced loss in a variety of forms — loss of physical health, sensory abilities and significant relationships being common. Particular attention should be paid to these losses and to how the client has attempted to cope with them. Real-life difficulties will have an impact on the client's emotional state, and care must be taken to distinguish between realistic recognition of her limitations and emotional and cognitive distortions.

Mental state assessment

This is a way of organizing observational data covering all aspects of a client's mental functioning. It is usual to collect information under some or all of the following headings: general appearance and behaviour; speech — form and content; emotional state and mood; hallucinations and delusions; orientation; memory — recent and remote; comprehension; intelligence — reasoning, judgement, general knowledge and ability to calculate; abstract thinking; and level of insight (Brooking 1986, p. 243–244).

In some cases the client may be referred to the psychogeriatric team for a specialist opinion. For a full account of mental state examination of elderly people see Wattis and Church (1986).

Nurses may make use of simple scales to provide an objective assessment of the client's mental state and evaluate changes over time. The most widely known of these are Goldfarb's (1960) 10-point scale of cognitive impairment, Hamilton's (1960) depression scale completed by the nurse or doctor on the basis of observations of the client over time, and the depression inventory designed by Beck et al (1961) for use by the client. Psycho-

logical assessment is also discussed in Chapter 2 of this volume.

Physical examination

Mental health problems in old age are frequently associated with acute or chronic physical illness. The general practitioner may carry out a physical examination of the client at home assisted by the community nurse. In some cases it may be necessary for the client to attend the health centre or outpatient department or be referred to the specialist geriatric service.

An important part of this assessment is a consideration of all the drugs taken by the old person, including non-prescribed drugs and alcohol intake. Many drugs, for example digoxin, barbiturates, steroids and anti-parkinsonism preparations are reported to cause confusion in elderly people. In some cases these drugs are unavoidable and the advice of the geriatrician may be useful in rationalizing medication.

Everyday living skills

The ability to function emotionally and cognitively depends to a great extent on the client's overall physiological and psychosocial functioning. Thus it is important to assess the extent to which the client is independent in areas such as personal hygiene, safety, mobility and nutrition. This is best carried out in the client's usual environment by the community nurse or the occupational therapist.

This aspect of the assessment is useful in establishing baseline data on the client's potential for independence. It will indicate the level of support needed, identify where the use of aids and adaptations may be effective and act as a guide to nursing interventions.

A number of systems of assessment are available. The Everyday Living Skills Inventory (ELSI) (Barker 1985) was designed by nurses for use across a range of client groups and in a variety of care settings. An important feature of this system is its positive emphasis on the strengths of the client as well as her weaknesses.

Another widely used system is the Clifton Assessment Procedures for the Elderly (CAPE) (Pattie & Gilleard 1975) which provides a brief and simple method of assessing cognitive and behavioural competence. CAPE and similar systems enable the nurse to cover most potential problem areas in every assessment and provide a guide to the evaluation of change in overall levels of disability over time. However, it should be noted that they are of limited value in evaluating change in particular aspects of behaviour.

Assessment of everyday living skills is usually based upon observation or behaviour rating scale/scores. However, a number of objective tests have recently been developed — e.g. the Performance of Activities of Daily Living (PADL) test, (Kuriansky et al 1976) — and are reported to be useful (Huppert & Tym 1988). Functional assessment of the elderly person is discussed also in Chapter 28.

Behavioural assessment

Behaviour is the outcome of the interaction between the individual and her environment. Where neuropsychological deficits exist and these cannot be removed through medical or personal nursing care, as in the case with organic mental illness, the best hope of decreasing the individual's level of handicap may be to modify the environment; that is, both the physical environment and the way in which individuals in that environment interact with the client.

The importance of manipulating the environment to compensate for gaps in individual functioning has been recognized by nurses and so-called psychological approaches are assuming increasing importance in the nursing management of elderly people with mental health problems. The nurse should be able to undertake behavioural assessments and plan and implement psychological treatment programmes as an integral part of the nursing care programme. The clinical psychologist may be a valuable source of specialist guidance and support and should be called upon as required.

In some cases it may be considered helpful for the clinical psychologist to undertake a full neuro-psychological assessment to provide a detailed picture of the client's cognitive functioning — both her assets and deficits. In undertaking this assessment psychologists have largely abandoned measures of general intelligence and personality, since these are of little help in planning management or predicting outcome, and instead have turned to measures of more discrete but inter-related cognitive functions (Wattis & Church 1986).

In undertaking a behavioural assessment, nurses should make detailed recordings of any problems related to the client's behaviour. Holden and Woods (1982) suggest that the following issues be considered: the problem and who defines it as such; the frequency of its occurrence; the situation in which it occurs; the events preceding its occurrence which might act as a catalyst; the result of the behaviour in terms of the reaction of others; and losses and benefits to the client.

The most reliable method of gathering data for a behavioural assessment is direct observation of the client in the setting in which the behaviour occurs. If the client is already in hospital the nurse is well placed to make a detailed behavioural assessment over time. If the client lives at home, careful interviews with carers may elicit sufficient information.

There are a large number of standard scales available to assist in the evaluation of behaviour (Israel et al 1984) and many of these are usefully reviewed by Hall (1980).

Social assessment

This chapter has indicated that positive social support constitutes one of the more critical factors in determining the mental well-being of elderly people. As mentioned previously, a home visit has the advantage of allowing the nurse to assess social support networks at first hand by talking to neighbours and relatives. A frequent finding is that coping with the erratic behaviour of an elderly mentally ill relative has created intolerable tensions in the whole family; indeed the imminent collapse of the social support network around the client may have precipitated referral to the primary health care team.

BIOGRAPHICAL APPROACHES TO ASSESSMENT

An assessment of one human being by another can never be totally objective since assessments are inevitably shaped by the subjective interpretation of the assessor. However, most of the established assessment methods described so far attempt to present a more or less objective account of the client and her life situation. Critics suggest that in attempting (in vain) to be objective these methods of assessment fail to give sufficient weight to the unique qualities of clients as individuals and their particular viewpoints (Brost & Johnson 1982). By focusing on problems, many assessment methods may present an essentially negative picture of the client. Health care professionals may make the mistake of seeing the problem rather than the client first, and attempt to fit the client into existing treatment programmes and services rather than vice versa.

Establishing and valuing the views of clients and their relatives is fundamental to an understanding of the individual client and her unique situation. Sometimes the views of the client may be difficult to establish, as in the case of a seriously demented person who has difficulty in communicating. Where the client's views are known they may be in conflict with those of the relatives; or they may be difficult to comply with, as in a case where the old person with well-preserved insight says that she wants to die. These issues require careful consideration by the multidisciplinary team when planning interventions.

In an attempt to give prominence to the views of clients and promote the development of client-centred services, nurses and other professionals would seem to be increasingly interested in biographical approaches to assessment. One such approach has been developed by a research team at the Open University and has been applied in conjunction with an interview checklist to the assessment of elderly people living in community settings (Dant et al 1987, Johnson et al 1988, and see Chapter 1 of this volume). This biographical approach stresses the importance of the assessor getting to know the client, encouraging her to talk about her life history — her 'careers' (childhood,

family, work, marriage, leisure, retirement and health), 'life-events', and 'orientations' (values and beliefs). The client is encouraged to talk about her present in relation to her past, and the interview is given structure by the interviewer's understanding of the issues involved and a record sheet which is completed by the assessor following the interview/s. This sheet consists of a series of headings (basic personal details, life experience, support systems, social involvement and activity, health and social issues etc.) under which the information is summarized.

Dant et al (1987) acknowledge that the biographical approach may be time consuming but argue that it maximizes opportunities for the worker to establish a rapport with the client and to offer services based upon a detailed understanding of the client's needs rather than simply upon a knowledge of what is available.

The 'Getting to Know You' method is another biographical approach which has been described by Couchman (1987) in relation to the nursing assessment of confused elderly people in hospital. This method involves nurses getting to know the client through interviewing, observing, reading about and sharing time with the client so that her needs can be expressed in an autobiographical or story format, as if written by that person. This story is then used as a step towards detailed intervention plans or to complement other forms of assessment. This method of assessment seems to offer a means by which nurses may at least approach the perennial problem of how to collaborate with severely demented clients in planning individual care programmes. Whilst many of these clients may be unable to engage in this process directly, methods of assessment which help the nurse imaginatively to 'step inside the client's shoes' and see the world from her perspective would seem worthy of further development.

There is much within biographical approaches to assessment with which nurses will be familiar — for example, the creation of rapport and the search for the client's perspective. Biographical approaches to assessment highlight these aspects of good practice and emphasize the general point that information gained through all methods of assessment only becomes useful when it is set within the context of the client's individual biography.

ORGANIZING AND ANALYSING THE DATA

Information collected through assessment of an individual client may be pooled at a meeting of the multidisciplinary psychogeriatric team and is likely to be managed through a system of problem oriented records (PORs). PORs have been adapted for use in a variety of settings (Lowe 1975; Beattie & Cranshaw 1982, Hume et al 1984, Bracey & Wicikowski 1989). The POR provides a revisable database of client information, and may be used as an aid to planning and as a guide to clinical interventions.

A commonly used technique is to draw up a list of the problems experienced by the client and ensure that these are clearly defined. These problems may be experienced by the client 'directly', as in a case where the client wanders from the house at night without warning, thereby compromising her safety; or 'indirectly', as when the erratic behaviour of the client leads to a potential 'breakdown' in the family situation.

Sometimes problem lists will highlight areas for further assessment or more detailed observation; thus the list will change as old problems are resolved and new ones emerge. It is important that focusing on problems does not blind the mental health team to the client's positive assets and strengths. To avoid this possibility some teams prefer to focus upon the client's needs rather than her problems.

It is important for members of the multidisciplinary team to see the client's problems in the context of her overall history and to apply theory and draw upon relevant research findings to seek to understand how her problems arose. Alternative explanations of these problems may be generated and considered by the team. Whichever are selected may be used to prioritize problems, set appropriate aims of management, select appropriate interventions and plan the timing of them. Explanations of the client's individual set of problems may be modified or may be rejected and replaced as the team gains a clearer understanding

of the client over time; these changes will be reflected in the care process. The importance of generating and testing alternative explanations when planning interventions is not always fully appreciated in the nursing literature, which often relates nursing 'prescriptions' directly to client problems in a simplistic manner.

PLANNING INTERVENTIONS

AIMS AND OBJECTIVES

The multidisciplinary team should formulate two kinds of goals: the general aims of care and specific problem-oriented objectives.

It is first necessary to decide upon aims which are statements in broad terms of the purposes or goals of management. These are too general to guide specific interventions but largely determine the objectives appropriate to individual problems. Aims should be realistic in terms of the capacities of the client and resources available for her support. They should ensure that the client makes maximum use of her remaining capacities within the most normal possible social context and they should seek to improve the quality of her life. Wherever possible, aims should accord with the wishes of the client or her relatives, and should always be agreed upon through a process of negotiation.

Secondly, short- and long-term objectives should be set in relation to each problem. It may be impossible to work on all problems at once and consideration should be given to the priority of each problem in relation to the long-term aims.

There are a number of general issues which should be borne in mind when setting objectives and considering interventions appropriate to the older person. Perhaps the most significant issue is the client's physical health and the effect of medications. For example, client-centred counselling may be problematic with the elderly client who is almost deaf; as Woods and Britton (1985) point out, it is difficult to sound empathic if you shout. How far should an elderly agoraphobic client with gout be encouraged to walk outside? Or what effect are steroids having on an elderly person's mood? These are important issues to consider in setting objectives and are best considered within the multidisciplinary team, where a range of expertise may be brought to bear upon the case.

Another special consideration has been referred to by Emery (1981) as 'treatment socialization'. Thus most elderly clients expect medication or other physical treatments and not psychological interventions which rely upon talking. This may be to some extent a cohort effect and might not continue to be a special consideration with elderly clients of the future. In the meantime, Emery (1981) suggests that where psychological interventions seem appropriate an educational model may be used to socialize the elderly person into treatment.

NURSES AS KEY WORKERS

It is desirable for the team to designate a key worker who is responsible for the overall management of the case. The key worker will co-ordinate the contribution of other team members as required, act as a liaison between the client, the family and the health and social care services, encourage collaborative involvement of the client and the family in care, and update the individual care programme in the light of the client's progress. The ability of the key worker to gain the trust and confidence of the client and her relatives is often a crucial factor in the success of the care programme.

The confidence of the client and her family in the key worker depends, to some extent, on her ability to keep her promises and 'deliver the goods'. This requires that the key worker has a good understanding of the resources available and that she receives the full support of other members of the multidisciplinary team. No decisions regarding the client should be made without prior consultation with the key worker and conflicts between members of the team should be resolved through discussion and not by unilateral action.

Griffiths' (1988) artificial distinction between 'health and medical' and 'social' aspects of care is likely to exacerbate problems of service delivery to elderly clients living in the community and highlights the important co-ordinating role of the key worker. Community nurses have a sound knowledge of medical problems but operate from 'health' as opposed to 'illness', and 'social' as opposed to 'medical' models of care delivery. This unique position places able community nurses in an ideal position to act as key workers. Under the new administrative arrangements it is quite conceivable that local authority social service departments will arrange with health authorities for nurses to take on this important role if nurses express the desire and demonstrate the ability to do so.

If the client is admitted for long-term residential care in an NHS establishment, or in a Home run privately or by the local authority, it is sensible in most cases for a permanent member of the residential care staff to assume the key worker role since the propinquity in time and space between the nurse and the client holds the potential for the creation of a positive therapeutic relationship, and the quality of the client's life is to a great extent determined by good nursing care. In a residential setting the person who assumes the role of key worker is likely to provide much of the direct care for the client and will be referred to by a variety of titles — 'key nurse', 'primary nurse', 'primary carer', etc. — according to the setting. Supervision should be provided for the key worker in a form appropriate to the post that she holds and the setting within which she practises. Possible arrangements and strategies are discussed in detail elsewhere (Barber & Norman 1987).

'NURSING PROCESS' OR 'CARE PROCESS'?

A current problem for some multidisciplinary teams which have adopted problem-oriented records is that integration of nursing skills into the POR system may be undermined by the need for nurses to maintain their own system of client information, as with the nursing process. Bracey and Wicikowski (1989) advocate running both recording systems side by side. They point out that the nursing process record is up-to-the-minute and thus more accurate in reflecting the ever-changing nature of care, whereas the POR review is relatively fixed and constrained because the team may meet only every week or fortnight to discuss a particular client.

This seems to be a reasonable distinction but one that does necessitate a dual system of recording. An alternative may be one multidisciplinary 'care process' within which the client rather than any one professional group occupies the central ground. The importance of the nursing role may be best expressed through stronger advocacy of the nurse within the multidisciplinary team, and modification of the POR to ensure the clear identification of the nursing contribution rather than dogmatic retention of the nursing process.

CONCLUSION

This chapter has outlined the extent of mental health problems in the elderly population and has discussed aspects of multidisciplinary teamwork and service delivery. Early identification, thorough assessment and careful planning of individual care within a community-based approach to mental health provision are seen as important processes in alleviating the effects of mental health problems in elderly people.

REFERENCES

Abrahamson J H, Gofin R, Habib H et al 1982 Indicators of social class: a comparative appraisal of measures for use in epidemiological studies. Social Science and Medicine 16: 1739–1746

Abrams M 1978 Beyond three-score and ten: a first report on a survey of the elderly. Age Concern England, Mitcham

Barber J H, Wallis J B, McKeating E 1980 A postal screening questionaire in preventive geriatric care. Journal of the Royal College of General Practitioners 30: 49–51

Barber P, Norman I J 1987 An eclectic model of staff development: supervision techniques to prepare nurses for a process approach — a social perspective. In: Barber P (ed) Mental handicap . Hodder & Stoughton, London

Barker P 1985 Patient assessment in psychiatric nursing. Croom Helm, London

Beattie B L, Cranshaw M L 1982 Team approach to the problem orientated record in a long-term care facility. Journal of the American Geriatrics Society 30(2): 109–113

Beck A T, Ward C H, Mendelson M et al 1961 An inventory for measuring depression. Archives of General Psychiatry 4: 561–571

Bergmann K 1979 The problem of early diagnosis. In: Glen A I M, Whalley L J (eds) Alzheimer's disease: early recognition of potential reversible deficits. Churchill Livingstone, London

Bergmann K, Eastham E J 1974 Psychogeriatric ascertainment and assessment for treatment in an acute medical ward setting. Age & Ageing 3: 174–188

Bowling A, Cartwright A 1982 Life after a death: a study of the elderly widowed. Tavistock, London

Bracey R, Wicikowski D 1989 Apportioning care. Nursing Times 85(19): 49–51

Brayne C, Ames D 1988 The epidemiology of mental disorders in old age. In: Gearing B, Johnson M, Heller T (eds) Mental health problems in old age: a reader. Wiley in association with the Open University, Chichester

Brooking J I 1986 Dementia and confusion in the elderly. In: Redfern S J (ed) Nursing elderly people, 1st edn. Churchill Livingstone, Edinburgh

Brost M J, Johnson T Z 1982 Getting to know you; one approach to service assessment and planning for individuals with disabilities. Wisconsin Coalition for Advocacy, Wisconsin

Buckley E G, Runciman J 1985 Health assessment of the elderly at home. University of Edinburgh, Edinburgh

Coleman P 1988 Mental health in old age. In: Gearing B, Johnson M, Heller T (eds) Mental health problems in old age: a reader. Wiley in association with the Open University, Chichester

Copeland J R M, Dewey M E, Wood N et al 1987 Range of mental illness among the elderly in the community: prevalence in Liverpool using the GMS-AGECAT package. British Journal of Psychiatry 150: 815–823

Couchman W 1987 Getting to know you. Nursing Times 83(28): 57–58

Dant T, Carley M, Gearing B, Johnson M 1987 Identifying, assessing and monitoring the needs of elderly people at home. Care for Elderly People at Home, Project Paper 2. The Open University, Milton Keynes

Dohrenwend B S, Dohrenwend B P (eds) 1984 Stressful life events and their contexts. Rutgers University Press, New Brunswick, N J

Eastwood R, Corbin S 1985 Epidemiology of mental disorders in old age. In: Arie T (ed) Recent advances in psychogeriatrics, no 1. Churchill Livingstone, Edinburgh

Ebrahim S, Hedley R, Sheldon M 1984 Low levels of ill health among non-consulters in general practice. British Medical Journal 289: 1273–1275

Emery G 1981 Cognitive therapy with the elderly. In: Emery G, Hollon S D, Bedrosian R C (eds) New directions in cognitive therapy. Guildford, New York

Flanagan J 1978 A research approach to improving our quality of life. American Psychologist 33: 138–147

Foreman M D 1986 Acute confusional states in hospitalized elderly: a research dilemma. Nursing Research 35(1): 34–38

Freer C B 1985 Geriatric screening: a reappraisal of preventive strategies in the care of the elderly. Journal of the Royal College of General Practitioners 35(275): 288–290

Godberg E M, Morrison S L 1963 Schizophrenia and social class. British Journal of Psychiatry 109: 785–802

Goldfarb A I 1960 Psychiatric disorders of the aged: symptomatology, diagnosis and treatment. Journal of the American Geriatrics Society 8: 698–707

Griffiths R 1988 Community care: agenda for action. HMSO, London

Hagnell O, Lanke J, Rorsman B et al 1983 Current trends in the incidence of senile and multi-infarct dementia: a prospective study of a total population followed over 25 years; the Lundby Study. Archiv fur Psychiatrie und Nervenkrankheiten 233: 423–438

Hall J N 1980 Ward rating scales for long stay patients: a review. Psychological Medicine 10: 277–288

Hamilton M 1960 A rating scale for depression. Journal of Neurology, Neurosurgery and Psychiatry 23: 56–62

Hemsi L 1982 Psychogeriatric care in the community. In: Levy R, Post F (eds) The psychiatry of late life. Blackwell, Oxford

Hirschfeld R M A, Cross C K 1982 Epidemiology of affective disorders: psychosocial risk factors. Archives of General Psychiatry 39: 35–46

Holden U P, Woods R T 1982 Reality orientation: psychological approaches to the 'confused' elderly. Churchill Livingstone, London

Hume A, Barker P, Robertson W 1984 The individual patient profile. Nursing Times 80(26): 56–59

Hunt A 1978 The elderly at home. HMSO, London

Huppert F, Tym E 1988 Clinical and neuropsychological assessment of dementia. In: Gearing B, Johnson M, Heller T (eds) Mental health problems in old age: a reader. Wiley in association with the Open University, Chichester

Israel L, Kozarevic B, Sartorius N 1984 Source book of geriatric assessment. Karger, Basle

Itzin C 1986 Elderly screening project: conclusions and recommendations. Newham Health Authority Community Services Unit

Johnson M 1988 Biographical influences on mental health in old age. In: Gearing B, Johnson M, Heller T (eds) Mental health problems in old age: a reader. Wiley in association with the Open University, Chichester

Johnson M, Gearing B, Carley M, Dant T 1988 A biographically based health and social diagnostic technique: a research report. Care for Elderly People at Home, Project Paper 4, The Open University, Milton Keynes

Kay D W K, Beamish P, Roth M 1964 Old age mental disorders in Newcastle-upon-Tyne, Part 1: a study of prevalence. British Journal of Psychiatry 110: 146–158

Kiehn M 1986 A study of the elderly clients of Beech House general practice. Health Visitor 59: 300–302

Kohn M L 1976 The interaction of social class and other factors in the etiology of schizophrenia. American Journal of Psychiatry 133: 177–180

Kuriansky J B, Gurland J L, Fleiss J L et al 1976 The assessment of self-care capacity in geriatric psychiatric patients by objective and subjective methods. Journal of Clinical Psychology 32: 95–102

Lipowski Z J 1983 Transient cognitive disorders (delirium, acute confusional states) in the elderly. American Journal of Psychiatry 140(11): 1426–1436

Liston E H 1982 Delirium in the aged. Psychiatric Clinics of North America 5(1): 49–66

Lowe G R 1975 The problem orientated system in a multi-disciplinary psychiatric milieu. Canadian Psychiatric Association Journal 20(8): 585–593

Luker K 1982 Screening the well elderly in general practice. Midwife, Health Visitor and Community Nurse 18: 222–229

Mann A H, Graham N, Ashby D 1984 Psychiatric illness in residential homes for the elderly: a survey in one London borough. Age & Ageing 13: 257–265

Maule M M, Milne J S, Williamson J 1984 Mental illness and physical health in older people. Age & Ageing 13: 349–356

Mechanic D 1982 Disease, mortality and the promotion of health. Health Affairs 1(3): 28–32

Murphy E 1982 Social origins of depression in old age. British Journal of Psychiatry 141: 135–142

Neugebauer R 1980 Formulation of hypotheses about the true prevalence of functional and organic psychiatric disorders among the elderly in the United States. In: Dohrenwend B P, Dohrenwend B S (eds) Mental illness in the United States: epidemiological estimates. Praeger, New York

Norman A 1985 Triple jeopardy: growing older in a second homeland. Centre for Policy on Ageing, London

Norman A 1988 Mental disorder and elderly members of ethnic minority groups. In: Gearing B, Johnson M, Heller T (eds) Mental health problems in old age: a reader. Wiley in association with the Open University, Chichester

Palmore E, Kivett V 1977 Change in life satisfaction: a longitudinal study of persons aged 46–70. Journal of Gerontology 32: 311–316

Palmore E B, Nowlin J B, Wang H S 1985 Predictors of function among the old-old: a 10-year follow-up. Journal of Gerontology 40: 244–250

Pattie A H, Gilleard C J 1975 A brief psychogeriatric assessment schedule: validation against psychiatric diagnosis and discharge from hospital. British Journal of Psychiatry 127: 489–493

Pitt B 1988 Psychogeriatrics: an overview. Health Visitor 61: 247–250

Rack P 1982 Race, culture and mental disorder. Tavistock Publications, London

Romaniuk M, McAuley W J, Arling G 1983 An examination of the prevalence of mental disorders amongst the elderly in the community. Journal of Abnormal Psychology 92: 458–467

Schwab J J, Schwab M E 1978 The sociocultural roots of mental illness: an epidemiological survey. Plenum Press, New York

Secretary of State for Health, Social Security, Wales and Scotland 1989 Caring for people: community care in the next decade and beyond (White Paper). HMSO, London

Shields J, Slater E 1975 Genetic aspects of schizophrenia. In: Silverstone J, Barraclough B (eds) Contemporary psychiatry. British Journal of Psychiatry Special Publication 9.

Stoudemire A, Blazer D G 1985 Depression in the elderly. In: Beckman E E, Leber W R (eds) Handbook of depression. Dorsey Press, Homewood, Illinois

Stringfellow C et al 1986 Prevention for patients over 75: is it worth the bother? British Medical Journal 292: 1243–1244

Stuart G W, Sundeen S J 1987 Principles and practice of psychiatric nursing, 3rd edn. Mosby, St Louis

Taylor R, Ford G, Barber H 1983 Research perspectives on ageing. Age Concern, Mitcham

Townsend P 1981 The structured dependency of the elderly: creation of social policy in the twentieth century. Ageing & Society 1(1): 5–28

Tulloch A J, Moore V 1979 A randomized controlled trial of geriatric screening and surveillance in general practice. Journal of the Royal College of General Practitioners 29: 733–742

Vetter N J, Jones D A, Victor C A 1984 Effects of health visitors working with elderly patients in general practice: a randomised controlled trial. British Medical Journal 288: 369–372

Wattis J, Church M 1986 Practical psychiatry of old age. Croom Helm, London

Williams E I 1984 Characteristics of patients over 75 not seen during one year in general practice. British Medical Journal 288: 119–121

Williams M A, Holloway J R, Winn M C et al 1979 Nursing activities and acute confusional states in elderly hip-fractured patients. Nursing Research 28: 25–35

Williams M A, Campbell E B, Raynor W J Jr et al 1985

Predictors of acute confusional states in hospitalized elderly patients. Research in Nursing and Health 8: 31–40

Williamson J et al 1964 Old people at home: their unreported needs. Lancet 1: 1117–1120

Wolanin M D, Phillips L R F 1981 Confusion: prevention and care. Mosby, St Louis

Woods R T, Britton P G 1985 Clinical psychology with the elderly. Croom Helm, Beckenham

Zautra A, Hempel A 1984 Subjective well-being and physical health: a narrative literature review with suggestions for future research. International Journal of Aging and Human Development 19: 95–110

CHAPTER CONTENTS

Introduction 309

Organic mental disorders in old age 310

Confusional states 310
Factors predisposing to confusional states 310
Identified problems in acute confusional states 313
Chronic confusional states 314
Nursing care required by elderly clients suffering
from acute confusional states 315

Dementia 317
Classification of dementias 317
Conditions causing dementia 318
Alzheimer-type dementia (ATD) 318
Multi-infarct dementia 321
Pharmacological interventions in dementia 322
Identified problems in dementia 322
The multiple pathway model of behavioural
analysis 324

**Nursing management of the dementing
person** 326
Material aspects of the residential environment 326
Maintaining individuality and dignity 328
Promoting choice and opportunity 330
Maximizing activity and independent functioning 332

Conclusion 338

19

Confusional states and dementia

Ian J. Norman

INTRODUCTION

Chapter 18 focuses upon the processes of assessment and planning within a multidisciplinary framework. This chapter discusses nursing interventions appropriate to clients suffering from the more common organic mental disorders of old age — confusional states and dementia. The importance of clearly distinguishing between these conditions is emphasized and particular attention is given to the care of elderly people suffering from dementia and living in long-term residential settings.

The nature of these disorders is considered essential background information in the planning and implementation of nursing care and are discussed. Following Brooking (1986) a range of problems and behaviours that the nurse may assess is presented in relation to each mental disorder and classified according to cognitive, emotional, social and physical areas of functioning. Due to individual differences not all of these problems and behaviours will be observed in all clients and not all the interventions described will be appropriate. This chapter should therefore be viewed as a resource from which to glean appropriate information for use in each individual case. Timing, evaluation and revision of interventions specific to the client's specific situation is crucial and should be supplied by the responsible nurse in consultation with the client and members of the multidisciplinary team.

ORGANIC MENTAL DISORDERS IN OLD AGE

Mental disorders are broadly categorized by psychiatrists as 'organic' or 'functional' depending upon whether or not a definite organic cause is yet established. This distinction has been altered recently by the discovery of biochemical abnormalities in the brains of people suffering from depression and schizophrenia, which have generally been classified as functional disorders. However it is not yet clear whether these biochemical changes cause the mental disorder or are an associated finding.

Two of the more common organic mental disorders of old age are confusional states and dementia. Invariably, clients suffering from these disorders are described on nursing care plans as 'confused' and interventions are planned accordingly. This may have negative consequences for care. One problem is that the term 'confusion' is imprecise and subjective; it is used to describe people whose behaviour is seen as disordered and inappropriate to the occasion, and thus cannot be considered an objective description of behaviour (Wolanin & Phillips 1981). Secondly, the failure of some nurses to set the presenting problem against background factors, such as underlying disease processes, may lead in turn to a failure to differentiate between interventions appropriate to confusional states from those appropriate to dementia.

CONFUSIONAL STATES

The medical and nursing literature is peppered with multiple, overlapping, inconsistently used and defined terms. Pseudo-senility, clouded states, acute brain syndrome, confusion, reversible dementia, treatable dementia, acute confusional states and delirium, amongst other terms, are used interchangeably with confusional states.

In this chapter the term 'confusional states' is used to refer to conditions which are temporary; they always have a cause, and the potential exists

for reversal of the client's mental state back to its previous normal state if treatment is successful (Open University 1988). If treatment is not given, or is unsuccessful, the client may die or be left with permanent brain damage. She may then be described as suffering from non-progressive dementia.

FACTORS PREDISPOSING TO CONFUSIONAL STATES

Brooking (1986) points out that it is important for nurses to be aware of causes of confusional states in old age for three reasons. First, to enable the nurse to predict the pattern of problems likely to be experienced by the client, and to understand them. Secondly, to aid prevention through recognition of predisposing conditions in advance. Thirdly, because the main principle of treatment is to search for relevant causes and remove or reduce them.

Causes of confusional states in old age may be discussed under three broad categories: drugs, disease/disorders and psychosocial factors (Open University 1988).

Drugs

An acute confusional state is a common complication of drug therapy in elderly people. It can arise as a side-effect ·or a withdrawal effect and even quite small doses of some drugs may induce toxicity. Almost any drug can cause a chronic confusional state in an elderly person. In some cases the confusional state will persist as long as the drug is taken.

Certain common drugs deserve special mention. Digitalis and its derivatives may be toxic in elderly people, causing acute and chronic confusional states; because of this, drugs such as digoxin are often prescribed in doses comparable to paediatric doses. Drugs for the treatment of Parkinson's disease, such as carbidopa (Sinemet®), are also potentially toxic in relatively small doses in elderly people and some hypnotics, such as nitrazepam (Mogadon®), which persist in the body for a long time may cause drowsiness and confusion during the day. Other hypnotics, such as triazolam

(Halcion®), are shorter acting and may prove useful in inducing sleep for 6 to 8 hours in cases where sleeping tablets cannot be avoided altogether.

The treatment in cases of drug-induced chronic confusional states is to stop the drug altogether. The rate at which the drug is eliminated from the body will influence the rate of recovery.

Disease/disorders

This is a broad category which includes those conditions which cause direct damage to the brain and general disorders which interfere with brain function. Like drugs, almost any bodily disease can cause an acute confusional state. Typically, an old woman, normally lucid if a little forgetful at times, becomes confused and erratic over the course of a couple of days. She may possibly suffer from obstructive airway disease, with her sputum having recently become yellow and purulent. She may not appear ill but physical examination may reveal rapid breathing and pyrexia and radiological investigation may confirm a diagnosis of bronchopneumonia. In this case acute confusion is the consequence of anoxia and toxaemia, affecting both neurotransmitters and brain neurones.

A group of factors which are important to consider in relation to hospitalized elderly clients are those associated with surgery. In particular: prolonged anaesthesia, shock, pain, electrolyte imbalance, anxiety and major surgery — particularly to the heart, brain, eye, and reproductive organs.

There is a tendency for different groups of bodily diseases to cause acute and chronic forms of confusion and for neurological conditions such as epilepsy, strokes and dementia to increase the risk. Some diseases causing chronic confusional states in elderly people are shown on Table 19.1 alongside the treatment which may potentially arrest the disease process and other physical signs of the disorder. In all cases of confusion it is the physical signs which the person suffering from the disease or disorder may show which provide a clue as to the true nature of the confusional state.

Table 19.1 Some causes of chronic confusional states.

Type of Damage	Disease	Treatment	Other features
Infection	GPI (General Paralysis of the Insane)	Antibiotics	Tremors: face, hands Epilepsy Spastic legs Abnormal pupils Wassermann Reaction positive : blood, cerebrospinal fluid
Physical damage	Normal pressure hydrocephalus	Shunt operation	Urinary incontinence Unsteady gait
Nutritional deficiency	Pernicious anaemia	Vitamin B12	Polyneuritis Subacute combined degeneration of the spinal cord Anaemia
Endocrine disorder	Myxoedema	Thyroxine	Characteristic facial expression Slow pulse Constipation
Endocrine disorder	Hypoparathyroidism	Medical or surgical treatment	Tetany : phosphorus calcium
Toxic damage	Alcoholism	Stop drinking	Various
Toxic damage	Renal dialysis	Stop dialysis	Brain aluminium

Psychosocial factors

These are an important group of causal factors but should be considered last to ensure that treatable diseases or toxic drugs are not missed.

Moving from a familiar to an unfamiliar environment is one of the more common causes of confusion for elderly people. Moving house may entail loss of memory cues and resultant confusion and moving into hospital or into residential care may have a similar effect. Hospital wards are noisy, confusing places. Orientation aids (clocks, calendars) and familiar objects may be missing, the normal pattern of light and dark may be disrupted by bright artificial lighting, and general disturbance on the ward may disrupt sleep. These problems may be exacerbated by lack of sensory supports such as spectacles and hearing aids which enable clients to perceive their environment correctly; in some cases the elderly client may not have been assessed for sensory deficits for many years; more frequently, she has simply left her spectacles at home. Lack of visual accommodation may result in confusion or disorientation at night, known as 'sundown syndrome'.

Armstrong-Esther and Hawkins (1982) argue that admission to hospital may eliminate the social cues which elderly people need to maintain synchronization of circadian rhythms. Should this occur, the result may be confusion, sleep disturbance and incontinence.

The 'self-fulfilling prophecy' — described by Merton (1957) as a prophecy which is fulfilled solely because it was made — has been shown to be important in sustaining confusion in elderly clients who are labelled 'confused' through the behaviour of ward staff (Chisholm et al 1982). Confusion may also be sustained by nursing elderly clients in environments which lack orientation cues, or by ward staff assuming that what is in fact a reversible confusional state is dementia and can therefore not be treated (La Porte 1982).

There are many other causes of confusion which fall under the broad category of psychosocial factors. Confusion following the death of a spouse is quite common and related factors such as loss of control over events and self, social isolation, stress

Table 19.2 Some causes of acute confusional states. *After Jacques (1988 p. 45).*

Direct damage to the brain	Head injury Cerebrovascular accident (thrombosis, embolus or haemorrhage) Subdural haemorrhage after injury Epileptic fit (post-ictal) Post-operative Infection (meningitis, encephalitis) Sudden change in a brain tumour
General disorders which disturb brain function	Constipation (reason unclear) Infection (especially chest or urinary tract) Cardiac failure and other heart disorders Kidney failure (raised blood urea) Liver failure Respiratory failure (raised carbon dioxide) Vitamin deficiency (lack of thiamin — vitamin B1 — in alcoholics) Endocrine disorders (especially hyopoglycaemia in diabetics)
Drugs	Tranquillizers including alcohol Antidepressants Antiparkinsonism drugs Digoxin and other cardiac drugs Cimetidine (for peptic ulcers) and many others
Drug withdrawal	Alcohol (delirium tremens — DTs) Benzodiazepines (including diazepam and lorazepam) Barbiturates
Psychosocial factors	All forms of socioenvironmental change; e.g. bereavement, moving home, admission to hospital, etc. Acute confusion due to any cause is more likely to occur in young children, the elderly and dementia sufferers.

and anxiety can all precipitate a confusional state.

It should be emphasized that the factors precipitating a confusional state may sometimes be inextricably linked; thus, for example, poor social conditions (psychosocial factor) may lead to infection (disease factor) and an acute confusional state. This highlights the importance of comprehensive multidisciplinary assessment.

Some causes of acute confusional states in elderly people are shown in Table 19.2.

IDENTIFIED PROBLEMS IN ACUTE CONFUSIONAL STATES

Clients suffering from confusional states present a variety of behaviours or problems which vary between individuals and within individuals over time. However, there are distinctive differences between acute and chronic forms.

The onset of an acute (or subacute) confusional state may be over hours, days, weeks — *but not months* — and the best clue to diagnosis is the relatively short history of the client's deteriorating mental status.

Three variants of acute confusional state are sometimes identified: hypokinetic, hyperkinetic and mixed (Foreman 1986). In the hypokinetic variant, psychomotor activity, arousal and excitability are all characteristically reduced and the client seems apathetic and appears half asleep. In contrast, the hyperkinetic variant is characterized by psychomotor hyperactivity, marked excitability, and occasional hallucinations, illusions and delusions. The mixed variant involves fluctuation between the extremes of the other two over time. The variability in clinical features is reported to be the function of the client's environment, her personality and her cultural background; however Foreman (1986) points out that there is no research to indicate that the variants are either separate or expressions of the same clinical entity.

The following description of the main behaviours and problems experienced by elderly people suffering from acute confusional states has drawn upon a clear description of the symptomatology of organic disorders provided by The Open University (1988). The elderly person suffering from an acute confusional state may be assessed by the nurse under four areas of functioning: cognitive, emotional, social and physical.

Cognitive problems
Clouding of consciousness
The client slips back and forth from sleep and alertness and exhibits altered mental activity.

Poor concentration
Concentration is difficult and the client is easily distracted. In part this is a consequence of drowsiness, but even when alert the client's mind tends to wander.

Disorientation in time and space
The client loses track of where she is, and of the time and day. Memory is affected and confabulation can occur.

Misinterpretation of the environment
The client may experience illusions (i.e. misunderstanding of a real sensory stimulus) and visual hallucinations (i.e. a false perception occurring in the absence of a real sensory stimulus). Shadows may be misinterpreted and shapes misconstrued. As the day draws on and night-time falls, perceptual difficulties are exacerbated. Information and ordinary events may be misunderstood and the client may seem perplexed.

Emotional problems
Fear
Misinterpretation of the environment evokes feelings of apprehension, anxiety, fear and even terror. The client may feel that danger lurks everywhere and may react with suspicion and aggressive outbursts.

Social problems
Disruption of communication
The client's fluctuating alteration of mental activity may be reflected in talk which is vague, inconsequential or inappropriate. The client may

hardly say a word or her speech may be verbose, rambling and disorganized.

Physical problems

Many of these will arise from the cause of the confusional state and some clients will be very ill. Other problems include the following:

Restlessness

If the confusional state has come on gradually (subacute) the client is likely to be described as restless, pacing up and down aimlessly or engaged in an endless fruitless activity, for example trying to open non-existent drawers in her bedside locker.

Muscular excitability

There tends to be excitability of the bodily muscles. If in bed the client may pick constantly at the sheets or be constantly engaged in rolling the bedclothes into a ball. When approached or touched the client may jump out of bed taking the bedclothes with her. The client may sleep very little and have insufficient rest in spite of a level of consciousness fluctuating from drowsiness to alertness. This may lead to exhaustion.

Neglect of self care

Regular toileting habits as well as diet may be neglected due to general disorientation. This may lead to constipation, incontinence and loss of weight and strength. Inadequate fluid intake may lead to dehydration.

CHRONIC CONFUSIONAL STATES

This type of confusional state lasts much longer than the acute form and is also slower to develop, perhaps taking months or even years. The person may or may not feel slightly off-colour and will be able to walk about unless the underlying cause — for example, nerve damage — prevents this.

In contrast to clients suffering from acute confusional states, the chronically confused client will not experience clouding of consciousness; her main problems are likely to be difficulty in thinking clearly and in recalling events accurately in time and space. There may also be personality and behavioural changes in addition to features that relate to the effects on the body of the underlying cause. There is a likelihood that these problems and changes may be attributed to the ageing process (ageism) or that the client will be mistakenly thought to be suffering from dementia.

Confusional states have been defined in this chapter as temporary, always having a cause the treatment of which will potentially allow the client's former mental state to re-establish itself (Open University 1988). Chronic confusional states display all these characteristics but are sometimes classified as treatable or reversible dementias since they will follow the course of dementia as long as their particular cause is present. For example, the client with syphilis who develops general paralysis of the insane (GPI) will continue to decline mentally until antibiotic treatment is given. She may then recover well if the damage has not been too severe. Likewise, surgery for hydrocephalus or a brain tumour can halt the progress of dementia.

Clients who have treatable causes of mental decline may be reasonably described as 'dementing' while the cause continues to damage their brains progressively, and then as 'chronically brain damaged' if, following removal of the cause, the damage becomes static. However, the term 'chronic confusional state' is used in this chapter in preference to that of 'treatable (or reversible) dementia' to highlight the importance of clearly differentiating treatable conditions of mental decline from true dementia, which is untreatable and irreversible.

In all cases of confusion the main principle of treatment is to search for the cause and treat or reduce all precipitating factors. The important role of the nurse in ensuring accurate observations for diagnostic purposes cannot be overstated, since if a chronic confusional state is not recognized, or if it is mistaken for dementia it will be left untreated. If untreated (or if treatment is unsuccessful or the condition is only partially reversible) the client will die or will be left with permanent brain damage with resulting cognitive and personality deficits.

There are many similarities between chronic confusional states and dementia. The nursing care for both groups of clients is very similar, apart from the fact that in the case of chronic confusional states the nurse must take account of the features of the underlying disease. The care of dementing clients is discussed later.

NURSING CARE REQUIRED BY ELDERLY CLIENTS SUFFERING FROM ACUTE CONFUSIONAL STATES

In most cases, care is based on the expectation of reversing the psychopathology; the long-term aim is for the client to resume her former lifestyle, with appropriate changes as required to reduce the risk of further illness. Clearly, acute confusional states which are physical in origin demand nursing interventions different from those demanded by states which have a psychosocial cause, and care should be geared towards meeting the needs of particular individuals. Some of the major elements of care and issues relevant to the nurse's role are discussed below.

Prevention

Prevention of acute confusional states is the first priority. An understanding of the predisposing factors, combined with careful observation, may allow high-risk individuals to be identified so that supportive and orientating environments may be emphasized as part of their care. For example, a dry bed at night for an elderly client who is usually incontinent may indicate dehydration, which may not otherwise be noted until a confusional state is evident.

Few studies have focused specifically on identifying predictors of acute confusion in elderly clients. An exception is a study by Williams et al (1985), who identified a number of predictive variables, the most important of which were the pre-injury level of activity, age, and errors on a mental status test on admission. This study is useful but the findings must be interpreted cautiously since the identified predictive variables did not prove as sensitive as sound clinical judgment.

A recent prospective study of a small sample of 78 elderly surgical clients (Platzer 1988) found that clients receiving glycopyrronium bromide (Robinul®), an anticholinergic drug which does not cross the blood–brain barrier, were less likely to become confused postoperatively than those receiving similar drugs which cross the blood-brain barrier, such as atropine and hyoscine. It has been known for a long time (Longo 1966) that atropine and hyoscine can cause confusion and hallucinations and that hyoscine is more likely to cause mental disturbance in elderly clients. Atropine has usually been given in preference to hyoscine and, until recently, there has been no alternative. Platzer (1988) found that most medical and nursing staff she spoke to were unaware that atropine could cause confusion in elderly clients and were also unaware that Robinul® was less likely to cause confusion. Research to see how extensively atropine is still used for elderly surgical clients may highlight an area where prevention of acute confusion is possible.

Another area of interest is the link between postoperative analgesia and confusion. Platzer (1988) hypothesizes that elderly clients may have an atypical response to pain which may be confusion rather than complaining. She points out that it is often assumed that elderly clients have less pain than younger people, tolerate more pain or are particularly sensitive to the side-effects of analgesic drugs. In fact, only the latter assumption has been confirmed. She suggests that elderly clients may not actually receive adequate analgesia postoperatively and that confusion may result. No research is known that specifically addresses these issues. The analgesia needs of elderly clients would seem to be an area where further research is needed, to look specifically at attitudes and knowledge of health care professionals, current practice and the experiences of clients themselves in relation to postoperative confusion.

Physiological needs

In many cases the client will be gravely ill. She may be unable to attend to her physiological needs through disorientation and agitation and highest priority should be given to nursing interventions designed to maintain life.

Inadequate sleep and rest may exacerbate the client's confused state. Particularly in cases where the diagnosis has not been firmly established, the doctor may be reluctant to prescribe sedation. In such cases nursing measures such as a glass of warm milk and verbal reassurance may allow a mildly agitated client to fall asleep.

Where the client is agitated or restless and sedation is considered appropriate it should be used with caution and its effect closely monitored since it may add to the client's confusion. Thioridazine (Melleril®) is commonly used because it is safe and effective but chlormethiazole (Heminevrin®) may be preferred because it is shorter acting. Haloperidol (Serenace®, Haldol®) may be used to calm the agitated client without causing much drowsiness, but has unpleasant side-effects, such as muscular stiffness, which may necessitate the use of anti-parkinsonian preparations. Thioridazine, chlormethiazole and haloperidol may be conveniently administered in liquid form and haloperidol may also be given parenterally should this be necessary.

Anorexic clients require help and encouragement to take a light, nutritious diet; to prevent dehydration they should be offered frequent drinks. Sometimes nutrition and fluid balance may be maintained by intravenous therapy and the client may be so restless and agitated that restraints are required to keep the intravenous lines open. However, this can mean that the client will become even more agitated and frightened and these should only be used when absolutely necessary.

Acutely confused clients are best nursed in single rooms which are quiet and peaceful and in which the environment is kept constant to ensure familiarity. Since darkness is likely to increase confusion the client's room should be lit night and day but lighting should be concealed to promote rest. The room should contain orientation cues such as clocks and calendars, familiar objects (such as windows) and personal photographs. The client should be encouraged to wear her spectacles and hearing aid to support sensory perception. Background noise from the radio, television and conversations should be kept to a minimum since this constitutes random stimuli which may exacerbate the confusion.

Clients who are restless and wander require close observation within a safe and reasonably enclosed environment. However, restrictions should be kept to a minimum since they are likely to result in the client becoming frustrated and angry. Restraints should only be used as a last resort.

Hallucinations

Particularly if hallucinating, the acutely confused client may be unpredictable and may need to be protected from hurting herself or others. Sensible safety precautions such as ensuring the windows are secured and removing unnecessary furniture may be necessary and in extreme cases one-to-one observation may be required.

In an effort to reassure it may seem natural for the nurse to respond to the client's pleas to remove the hallucination by, for example, brushing the imaginery spiders from her bedclothes. This is unhelpful since hallucinations will persist and by her actions the nurse will only confirm that the spiders are real and thereby reinforce the client's fears. A more therapeutic response is to stay with the frightened client and continually orientate her to the fact that she is ill and in hospital and that she is safe. Touch may be used to reassure and prevent panic, e.g. 'I'll stay with you and hold your hand.'

Alleviating emotional distress

Effective communication skills are essential if the nurse is to reduce the client's psychological distress. Since confused clients are experiencing difficulty processing information they require statements and instructions delivered in a clear, calm, kindly and concerned manner, and plenty of basic information about what is going on around them. Choices should be kept to a minimum since the client will not be able to determine priorities and think of alternatives and this may generate anxiety. However, the use of relevant and timely closed questions requiring yes/no answers will allow the nurse to ascertain the client's individual needs and may give the client some sense of control over her chaotic perceptual world.

If possible, the same nurses should care for the client since familiar faces are likely to promote reassurance. Occasional lucid moments may be used to establish rapport. Whenever possible, members of the client's close family should be included in her care since this will introduce another familiar element into the client's perceptual world. Explaining the reasons for the client's confusion will increase the family's ability to cope and by role-modelling how to interact with the client the nurse will increase the family's ability to participate in the plan of care. This may in turn decrease the family's feelings of helplessness.

Research

Nurses are in a strategic position to research acute confusional states since they have continuous contact with the client and are thus able to monitor changes in her mental state from admission throughout her period of treatment and hospitalization. They may also be able to assess the client's preadmission mental state through liaison with nurses who have cared for her in the community and through obtaining a relevant history from relatives and friends.

One problem facing researchers is how to define acute confusion in operational terms. Whilst many tests are used to assess confusion in elderly people (see for example, Folstein et al 1975, Hodkinson 1973, Pfeiffer 1975), these are of limited usefulness for research purposes. Elderly people have been noted in many research studies to have a low tolerance for batteries of formal mental tests and repeated questioning (Platzer 1988). Confused clients may refuse to answer questions, thus making it impossible to include a confused client in a study about confusion! Furthermore, formal mental tests have been shown to produce similarly low scores for both confusion and depression; this lack of discrimination is important because seriously ill clients may well be depressed (Platzer 1988).

In order to arrive at an operational definition of acute confusion for research purposes it is preferable to assess confusion through observation of certain behaviours. In a study of elderly clients in surgical wards Williams et al (1985) used four categories of observable behaviour to develop a score for confusion. They had previously found that these behavioural measures correlated with scores on formal mental tests (Williams et al 1979). The four behaviours were: a) verbal or nonverbal manifestations of disorientation to time, place, or persons in the environment; b) inappropriate communication or communication unusual for the person, such as nonsensical speech, calling out, yelling, swearing, and/or unusual silence; c) inappropriate behaviour such as attempting to get out of bed, pulling at tubes, dressings, and/or picking at bedclothes; d) illusions or hallucinations (Williams et al 1985, p. 33).

Studies investigating the nursing care of acutely confused elderly people are scarce. The study on prediction by Williams et al (1985) has been mentioned earlier. Other studies have examined the effectiveness of nursing interventions that manipulated psychological and environmental variables thought to affect confusion (Budd & Brown 1974, Chatham 1978). These studies found that nursing interventions reduced the incidence and symptomatology of acute confusional states. However, confusion persisted at significant levels and further research is needed if effective nursing management protocols are to be developed.

DEMENTIA

Dementia may be defined quite simply as 'an acquired global impairment of intellect, memory and personality without impairment of consciousness. It is almost always of long duration, usually progressive and irreversible' (Working Party on Care of the Dementing Elderly 1988, p. 127).

CLASSIFICATION OF DEMENTIAS

There are three main ways in which dementia may be classified. First, according to origin; thus, a 'primary' dementia develops from the start as a dementia, whereas a 'secondary' dementia develops from a confusional state (usually chronic) which is unresolved, and in which permanent brain damage occurs. Secondly, according to whether or not the condition is treatable.

'Treatable' or 'reversible' dementias are the conditions which have been referred to in this chapter as 'chronic confusional states'. Thirdly, according to age; thus dementias are termed senile or pre-senile, according to the age of onset — before or after 65 years.

An increasing number of authorities are questioning the value of the pre-senile and senile dementia division, arguing that it is of little clinical significance (Pearce 1987). The pattern of symptoms and decline exhibited by clients who develop dementia in their 50s is very similar to that shown by those who develop it in their 70s. Attempts to distinguish the genetics of the two categories have so far been inconclusive and, even more significantly, it has been impossible to distinguish between the pathological changes in the brains of the two groups (Jacques 1988). Moreover, the psychogeriatric services frequently provide support to clients in both categories, in the absence of sufficient alternative provision for clients with pre-senile dementia, and through admission of some clients to psychogeriatric wards some years after the original diagnosis.

The distinction between senile and pre-senile dementia is further muddled by the loose use of the term 'senile dementia'. When a person is described as senile it is unclear whether she is suffering from the commonest cause of dementia — senile dementia of Alzheimer's type (or, less clumsily, Alzheimer-type dementia) — or whether it is merely being stated that she is over 65 and 'dementing'. Jacques (1988) points out that the word 'senile' is much misused in common speech and may be used pejoratively. It may mean old, physically decrepit, more likely to happen to older people, mentally infirm or plain unwanted.

CONDITIONS CAUSING DEMENTIA

Every bit of the cerebral cortex is not damaged equally in all forms of dementia but what has been called the 'law of mass action' seems to apply (Jacques 1988). This law states that where there is widespread damage to the cerebrum there is proportionate damage to general functions, such as intelligence, thinking and understanding. The conditions causing dementia are thus mainly conditions which result in gradually increasing cerebral damage. Major conditions resulting in dementia are shown in Table 19.3.

This chapter focuses on the two main conditions causing dementia in all age groups, Alzheimer-type dementia (ATD) and multi-infarct dementia (MID). These conditions account for up to 95% of all cases of dementia in the over 65s (Kellett 1987). Further details of these and rarer conditions causing dementia may be found in Jacques (1988), which provides a clear (although unreferenced) account of pathological aspects and current theories and has been a useful source for the following sections.

ALZHEIMER-TYPE DEMENTIA (ATD)

ATD is characterized by an insidious onset with continuous downhill progression with death following some 2–8 years after onset. It has a bimodal distribution with peaks at ages 40 to 54 and 70 to 84 (Katzman et al 1978). Death is usually attributed to accompanying disorders, such as pneumonia, vascular disease, cancer, or accidental trauma rather than ATD itself.

Pathology

A definitive diagnosis of ATD can be made only on autopsy, where the distinctive neurological changes in the brain can be noted. Shrinkage and loss of weight of the cerebral hemispheres of the brain are noted in younger clients and may be displayed by brain scanning using computerized tomography (CT scanning), but in old people there is more variability in brain size and shrinkage is less easily demonstrated.

Certain areas of the brain are damaged more than others in ATD; particularly affected areas are the temporal and frontal lobes and, to a lesser extent, the parietal lobes. Damage to the temporal lobe includes the hippocampal region, an area specifically involved in short term memory.

In all these areas loss of brain cells has been demonstrated but of even more significance is evidence that the endings and connections of neurones are degenerating. Microscopic examination reveals widespread distribution of 'senile'

Table 19.3 Some causes of dementia*.

Type of damage	Disease	Brief details
Transmitter defects, plaques and tangles	Alzheirmer-type dementia (ATD)	Accounts for about 65% of cases of dementia in the over-65s (Kellet 1987)
Multiple infarcts	Multi-infarct dementia (MID)	Accounts for about 30% of cases of dementia in the over-65s (Kellet 1987)
Transmitter defects	Parkinson's disease	About 20% of parkinsonism sufferers will also suffer dementia (Jacques 1988) Anti-parkinsonism drugs do not help the dementia
Genetic disorder	Huntington's chorea	Develops mainly in people in their 40s and 50s Dementia is combined with chorea — i.e. dancing, jerky movements of the limbs
Infections	Creutzfeldt-Jacob disease	Very rare; caused by a virus or a 'prion'
White matter damage	Multiple sclerosis	Dementia is usually fairly mild. It may be first noticed in the sufferer's flat emotional response to her progressive disabilities
White matter damage	Binswanger's disease	A variety of vascular dementia but without the infarcts of MID
Trauma	Head injury	A head injury may result in a one-off loss of brain cells and a 'non-progressive dementia'.
Various	Chronic confusional state	The underlying cause of a chronic confusional state may go on to cause dementia if treatment is unsuccessful or does not occur e.g. syphilis causing General Paralysis of the Insane (GPI) Vitamin B12 deficiency

* Pick's disease is sometimes referred to as a form of dementia. Although progressive and irreversible it is a localized disorder. Damage is mainly to the frontal lobes and the main effect is a progressive decline in the sufferer's personality without any intellectual or memory loss.

plaques and neurofibrillary tangles which are characteristic of ATD. There is some overlap between these changes and those seen in the normal ageing brain, but there are qualitative as well as quantitative differences and ATD would not seem to be an exaggerated form of normal ageing.

Neurotransmitter deficits

In the early 1980s it was demonstrated that enzymes related to the neurotransmitter acetylcholine were greatly reduced in the brains of ATD sufferers. It was postulated that ATD was the result of a failure of acetylcholine nerve cells to pass electrical and chemical messages, so interfering with the general functioning of the brain. However, this simple theory has been modified by further research which has revealed many other neurotransmitters to be affected in ATD — although not all, and not to the same extent.

In sum, current thinking suggests that ATD, which was once thought of as shrinking of the brain, is in fact a disorder involving several types of neurone. However, the exact site of the damage is unclear (Jacques 1988).

Causes

Research into the cause of damage to the particular types of neurone implicated in ATD has revealed several possibilities:

Genetic factors

In a small number of cases there is a family history with a clear inherited tendency. However, in the majority of cases genetic influences are less well demonstrated. The present conclusion is that there is some genetic contribution to ATD although the nature of this contribution is uncertain.

Infection

An infective aetiology for ATD has been considered in view of the known transmission of Creutzfeldt-Jakob disease. However, according to Lishman (1987) the evidence so far is slender and the conclusion must be that transmissibility in ATD has not been demonstrated.

Chemical damage

Older neurones are known to build up toxic chemicals, presumably produced by internal processes, which cannot be disposed of. It is possible that these toxins are damaging to nerve cells. Poisons from the outside environment — for example, substances like lead and aluminium — are also known to damage nerve cells and it seems possible that one of these poisons may build up in the neurones. There has been considerable interest in the relationship between aluminium toxicity and dementia since aluminium levels were found to be above normal in autopsy and biopsy specimens from cases of ATD (Crapper et al 1976). The presence of aluminium in the senile plaques of ATD sufferers (Candy et al 1986) may possibly be explained by excess aluminium in the diet but, according to Jacques (1988), is more likely to be due to failure to eliminate normal amounts of aluminium from the brain.

Chromosome damage

A surprising finding is that many people with Down's syndrome (mongolism) who survive into middle age exhibit the typical pathological changes and neurotransmitter losses of ATD. This is paralleled by intellectual deterioration and it seems possible that the majority of Down's syndrome sufferers would develop ATD if they lived long enough (Ellis et al 1974, Ball & Nuttal 1980). This, combined with the recent finding of defective genetic material on chromosome 21 in familial ATD (St George-Hyslop et al 1987), supports the idea that damage to chromosomes provides the link which explains how any of the above factors may impair the function of nerve cells; thus, for example, a genetic factor may increase the vulnerability of the DNA to damage from a chemical or infective agent.

'Young-old' and 'old-old' ATD

The value of retaining the distinction between senile and pre-senile dementia is further questioned by the emergence of a dividing line between groups of ATD sufferers at a greater age. Jacques (1988) suggests that ATD might be divided into two varieties: a malignant, early or 'young-old' dementia mainly affecting people in their 60s and early 70s and a more benign 'old-old' dementia affecting people in their 80s and 90s. The early onset variety is associated with rapid intellectual decline. Individuals in the older age group, who are mainly women, suffer from a less profound memory disorder and would seem to have a more normal lifespan than younger sufferers. Table 19.4 sum-

Table 19.4 A comparison of 'young-old' and 'old-old' ATD. *Source: Jacques (1988, p. 22).*

	Younger patients (onset below 75 years)	Older patients (onset above 75 years)
Life expectancy	Shortened	Less shortened or normal
Damage to cerebral cortex cells	More widespread More severe	More localized Less severe
Neurotransmitter losses	More transmitters affected More widespread damage	Mainly acetylcholine More like normal age changes

marizes the main differences between these two forms.

This emergent division suggests that an increasing number of very old people will suffer from dementia and that many of these will have a near normal lifespan. This, in turn, has important economic implications for health and social services for elderly people.

MULTI-INFARCT DEMENTIA

Next to ATD the most common form of dementia in all age groups is multi-infarct dementia (MID), a vascular condition characterized by an abundance of large and small infarcts all over the cerebral cortex, causing diffuse, irregular, asymmetrical regions of cerebral softening.

Causes

This form of dementia is linked to arteriosclerosis and many patients will show evidence of this disease in other parts of their body — heart disease, poor circulation in their legs and in particular, hypertension. Previously it was thought that arteriosclerosis actually caused dementia by reducing the blood flow to the brain as a whole and gradually damaging its functions; thus the disease was termed arteriosclerotic or vascular dementia. It is now known that infarcts rather than arteriosclerosis itself constitute the crucial factor.

Diet and genetic factors would seem to play a part in the development of generalized arteriosclerosis. However, the blockage of particular blood vessels at particular times causing damage to parts of the cerebral cortex is yet to be fully explained. Only when emboli have migrated from other arteries is the cause of MID obvious (Jacques 1988).

Pathology

A knowledge of the pathology of MID is particularly helpful to nurses, since this may be reflected in the nature of the patient's problems. The 'law of mass action' seems to apply; thus, the large number of small infarcts act as if they are one general injury and the total area of cerebral softening

is directly proportional to the degree of intellectual impairment. The result of this is that many patients who experience small cerebral infarcts over many years will exhibit a pattern of gradual intellectual decline which mimics ATD. In fact it is often difficult to distinguish between the two disease processes in clinical practice — a task made more difficult by the fact that a considerable proportion of patients suffer from both conditions. One estimate is that for every 60 ATD cases there are 20 MID cases and 20 mixed (Jacques 1988).

Against this background of gradual intellectual decline, patients with MID may experience acute cerebral episodes — sudden defined strokes or transient ischaemic attacks (TIAs) which may result in a marked change in the patient's mental state. Following these episodes the patient may become disorientated and experience clouding of consciousness, ranging from drowsiness to coma, as a result of oedema around the infarct and general disruption of brain function. This confusional state will persist for hours or even weeks and only when it has lifted will the extent of the damage become apparent. Thereafter there may be a period of relative stability or even improvement as the brain seeks to compensate for the damage that has occurred. However, further infarcts are likely to follow and the pattern of progressive mental decline will be resumed. Thus mental deterioration in MID is sometimes described as 'stepwise' or 'irregular'.

The 'patchy' nature of damage to the cerebral cortex in MID may also result in the patient experiencing decline in very specific functions whilst the decline in general abilities is less marked. Thus, for example, the patient may experience temporary or permanent difficulties with speech, vision or movement whilst retaining general assets such as personality, insight and the ability to respond emotionally. Moreover, at any stage in her illness the patient may suffer the effects of disorders of other arteries, such as a heart attack or a major stroke. As a result of these pathological changes MID may often be more distressing to the sufferer than ATD, in which insight and emotional responses are lost as part of the patient's general decline.

For purposes of research the distinction between

Table 19.5 Hachinski's score for the diagnosis of MID. *Adapted from Hachinski VC et al (1975). Source: Jacques (1988, p 28).*

Abrupt onset	2
Stepwise deterioration	1
Fluctuating course	2
Nocturnal confusion	1
Relative preservation of personality	1
Depression	1
Somatic complaints	1
Emotional liability	1
History of hypertension	1
History of stroke	2
Evidence of arteriosclerosis elsewhere	1
Focal neurological signs	2
Focal neurological symptoms	2
Total score possible	18

A score of more than 7 is said to favour the diagnosis of multi-infarct dementia.

the two major types of dementia in old age is important. The Hachinski Score (Hachinski et al 1975) is one commonly used method of drawing this distinction and, incidentally, provides a useful summary of the major features of MID (Table 19.5).

PHARMACOLOGICAL INTERVENTIONS IN DEMENTIA

Pharmacological approaches to dementia are related to theories about the causes of the disorder. When impairment of acetylcholine action was established in ATD there followed attempts to find a substance which might replace the deficit. So far, clinical trials have yielded few hopeful results. Substances to promote the production of acetylcholine have been found ineffective. Arecoline has proved toxic as a substitute for acetylcholine. Drugs to decrease the breakdown of acetylcholine or stimulate neurotransmitter action have been investigated (Pajk 1984). Such treatments, even if effective, would of course only delay the decline since they address the effects of nerve damage and not the damage itself.

Many drugs have been tried to improve cerebral circulation in cases of MID. Drug trials have been contradictory in their results and as yet no particular drug has been found effective in reducing the

progress of MID (Jacques 1988). A more hopeful approach has been the widespread use of aspirin, dipyridamole and other substances to reduce the formation of small emboli and thus prevent transient ischaemic attacks. If drugs can be developed to reduce the small strokes characteristic of MID the progress of the disease may be reduced or even halted.

Demented individuals may be given tranquillizers, antidepressants or sedatives as symptomatic treatment.

IDENTIFIED PROBLEMS IN DEMENTIA

The main behaviours and problems of an elderly patient suffering from dementia may again be assessed by the nurse under four areas of functioning: cognitive, emotional, social and physical.

Cognitive problems

Memory impairment

Memory problems, in particular short term memory impairment, is a marked feature of dementia and can vary in degree of severity. Confabulation may occur.

Disorientation

Closely linked with memory is the typical disorientation with regard to time experienced by most sufferers. As with memory impairment, this can occur to various degrees; thus a dementing person may know the month, but not the date or even the year. Disorientation with regard to time may commonly lead to such problems as forgetting that it is the middle of the night and disturbing relatives and neighbours.

Disorientation with regard to place may develop. Thus a moderately demented patient may know that she is in hospital but not know its name. A severely demented patient may not be able to give any information about the function of her surroundings. Later, disorientation with regard to persons may occur and the demented person may be unable to recognize members of her own family. This may cause great distress to relatives.

Understanding

The dementing person is likely to experience increasing difficulty in making sense of what is going on around her. Her judgement may be poor and her evaluation of events impaired; she may misinterpret what she sees and hears. This may sometimes lead to behaviour problems such as outbursts of aggressive behaviour.

Emotional

Personality change

The characteristic response of the demented patient to events may alter to the extent that relatives may often say that the sufferer seems like a different person from the one they had known. The personality change may take the form of an exaggeration of the patient's usual self so that a previously quiet individual hardly utters a word, or sometimes a dramatic reversal of previous characteristics, so that a quiet and reserved individual becomes garrulous and boisterous. Some sufferers exhibit a diminished emotional response to situations and events, or emotional lability, that is, instability with rapid and inappropriate emotional changes.

Emotional distress

Dementia must be a very bewildering experience to the sufferer. Many individuals react to the disease by becoming anxious, irritable or depressed. This reaction may be so severe that the person may develop an anxiety state, a depressive illness or psychotic features such as delusions and hallucinations. The sufferer may become suspicious or paranoid. Combined with forgetfulness this may lead to accusations of theft against relatives and professional carers which can be distressing to those accused.

Lack of insight

Many dementing individuals may fail to recognize that they are ill. In some ways this may be a blessing but it can cause practical problems for carers.

Social

Decline in social competence

Social competence typically declines when the dementia is more than mild. This may lead to difficulties with shopping, cooking, dressing and keeping clean. If the sufferer has little insight she may be unable to appreciate the decline in her abilities and attempts by well-meaning carers to compensate for these deficits may be resented.

Desocialization

The dementing individual experiences progressive difficulties in coping with environmental demands and the tendency is to restrict these in order to maintain control. As the disease progresses the sufferer may give up her interests, become increasingly reluctant to meet people or even to leave the house for fear of getting lost.

Restriction of interests and regression

The patient's range of thought may diminish until it becomes restricted to a total concern with immediate considerations — eating a piece of cake or smoking a cigarette. Performing activities of daily living — dressing, washing, going to bed — may become haphazard or be forgotten completely. Eventually the picture becomes one of withdrawal, self-neglect and social isolation.

Behavioural disorders

Dementia sufferers may exhibit a range of behavioural problems which arise from conscious decisions taken under conditions of memory loss, misinterpretation and poor understanding of what is going on around them.

Restlessness and wandering are common and may often be seen in those individuals who have been used to leading an active life. Other behavioural problems include incontinence, aggression, noisiness and stripping off clothes.

Communication difficulties

Speech often deteriorates in dementia, becoming anecdotal, repetitive and ultimately irrelevant and disjointed. This may be an early or a late feature of the disease. If an early sign, the extent of the person's disability may be overestimated. Alternatively, what is in fact an early sign of dementia may be mistakenly seen as a language disorder.

Stress of caring

The 24-hour nature of the problems of dementia imposes a considerable strain on relatives and carers at home. The ways in which these people may be supported are discussed in Chapter 27. The importance of support systems for nurses and other professional carers is not always fully appreciated.

Physical

Most patients experience general physical deterioration and loss of self-care capacities. A variety of physical deficits may emerge as a result of focal brain damage in some forms of dementia but not in all.

THE MULTIPLE PATHWAY MODEL OF BEHAVIOURAL ANALYSIS

Differences in pathology will result in slightly different clinical features of dementia and age of onset will affect the particular problems experienced by individual sufferers and their families. Moreover, since dementia of all types is progressive, nurses will work with people at different stages of the dementing process. Those mildly affected will experience problems with complex tasks and with time constraints. At the other extreme some individuals will be totally helpless and dependent. The three main phases of ATD which are commonly distinguished illustrate the range of problems which may be experienced over the course of the disease (Table 19.6). As previously

Table 19.6 Phases of ATD.

Stage 1
Failing memory
Loss of initiative and interest
Subtle personality changes
Disorientation in time and sometimes in space
Insidious onset which may be hard to discern in older clients.

Stage 2
More rapid intellectual and personality deterioration
Impaired cognition and abstract thinking
Inappropriate social behaviour
Impaired judgement
Restlessness, wandering and agitation
Decrepit and shrunken posture
Slow and shuffling gait
Repetitive futile behaviour
Dysphasia, apraxia, agnosia
Inability to carry out activities of daily living

Stage 3
Body wasting — indifference to food
Inability to communciate
Urinary and faecal incontinence
Seizures

noted, there would seem to be differences in progression between 'young-old' and 'old-old' forms.

Underlying pathological processes are important but provide an oversimplified explanation for the changes exhibited by dementing persons and may engender a sense of therapeutic pessimism amongst carers. The 'multiple pathway model' (Stokes 1989) indicates that behaviour is influenced by biogenic, psychogenic and environmental factors and that these should be considered in turn to help explain why a dementing person behaves in the way she does or exhibits an intellectual deficit. The model is a useful aid to assessment and planning since it helps the nurse to understand how dementing behaviour may arise and how it may be maintained (Fig. 19.1).

Organic pathway

This acknowledges the importance of investigating not only brain pathology but also the impact of possible physical and sensory handicaps, ill health and pain. Some severely demented individuals may be unable to express the effects of these fac-

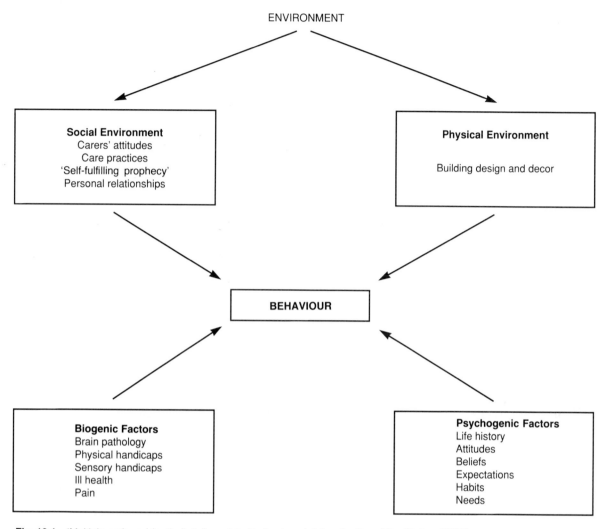

Fig. 19.1 'Multiple pathway' (or 'holistic') model of behavioural determination. *After Stokes (1989).*

tors and nurses should be mindful of the more subtle indicators of pain or ill health.

Psychosocial pathway

This incorporates a consideration of the client's life history and personality from which has arisen an established pattern of attitudes, beliefs, expectations, habits and needs. Thus, for example, aggressive or resistive behaviour following admission to hospital may be the outcome of enforced disruption of long-established routines.

Social environmental pathway

This incorporates factors such as relationships with family and friends, attitudes of carers and care practices. A number of examples illustrate the impact of these factors on behaviour. For instance, increased dependency and disruptive behaviour may be the result of care practices — regimented bathing, toileting, etc. — which fail to consider individual needs. A further example is the 'self-fulfilling prophecy' which has been identified as relevant to dementia by Macdonald (1973) and

Libow (1978). Nurses may *expect* 'senility' and foster it by treating clients as 'senile'; other mechanisms are those previously discussed in relation to confusional states.

A final example within this category is Grimley Evans' (1982) description of how dementia may remain hidden within families for long periods without being recognized. Families may collude, may accept deterioration as a normal part of ageing, or may fail to notice the change due to the concrete or superficial nature of interaction within the family. Alternatively, the sufferer may restrict her lifestyle to conceal deficiencies. If a disruption occurs within the family — for example, moving house, the death of a spouse or a family holiday — the mechanisms which conceal the dementia may break down and the true extent of the family member's disability become obvious. Dementia arising in this way may be referred to as 'revealed dementia'.

Physical environmental pathway

This includes a consideration of features such as the design and furnishing of the individual's environment. For example, behavioural deterioration may arise from socially isolating or uncomfortable physical surroundings. Again, as Stokes (1989) observes, incontinence may arise from a race between legs and bladder across excessive distances between chair and toilet.

As Stokes (1989) acknowledges, the 'multiple pathway model' is complex, but it seems to offer the potential for positive therapeutic intervention.

NURSING MANAGEMENT OF THE DEMENTING PERSON

Effective management requires the nurse to recognize that in the face of gradual decline most dementing individuals retain some abilities. Social and non-verbal skills — for example, use of eye contact, responsiveness to tone of voice, facial expression — develop early in life and are preserved in many cases (Hussain 1984, Church & Wattis

1988). These preserved abilities are important. If fostered they will help the sufferer to compensate for deficits. Furthermore, they may provide the channel through which the nurse is able to establish a trusting relationship, which may be used to provide emotional support to the resident during frightening periods of her illness.

The term 'management' is used purposely to indicate that it is not cures for dementia which are considered but long-term strategies for working with a person who is likely to experience a progressive decline in her level of abilities. The general aim should be to maintain the person's functioning at the highest possible level for as long as possible and to promote her overall 'quality of life'. More specifically, attention should be given to the following objectives:

- the maintenance of individuality and dignity
- the promotion of choice and opportunity
- the maximization of activity and independent functioning.

We are grateful for the excellent publication by Norman (1987a) on which we have drawn in discussing the nursing management of elderly dementing people. Norman has criticized nurses caring for elderly dementing people in long-stay residential care for having, 'a somewhat clinical and physically orientated approach to their work' and for failing to take full account of the psycho-social needs of both staff and residents (Norman 1987a p. 82). This section seeks to meet this criticism by placing particular emphasis on psychosocial aspects of care and focusing upon general issues of principle and practice in the management of dementing people related to the objectives of care identified above.

The following discussion is centred around the care of elderly people living in residential care settings and specific attention is paid to the material aspects of that environment. However, many of the points raised are relevant to the care of people living with relatives or in their own homes.

MATERIAL ASPECTS OF THE RESIDENTIAL ENVIRONMENT

The general feeling amongst care staff in residential facilities is that 'small is beautiful' in that it is considered easier to provide individualized and personalized care in small (6–8 residents) domestic units than in larger facilities (Norman 1987a). This arrangement is generally thought to enable greater socialization and to create opportunities for autonomy and control. It also relies upon the interaction among residents to encourage independence and self help. Holden and Woods (1982) cite a number of studies which report correlations between small living units of 8–12 and residents being more vocal and active and having reduced levels of disorientation and incontinence.

Good facilities and high-quality furniture and furnishings say something about the value of the work of caring for dementing people. Comfortable surroundings are an important aspect of the living environment for residents and promote quality nursing care through boosting staff morale. Free-standing furniture may be moved from room to room as required to make space for personal items which reinforce the resident's individuality. Communal areas, such as the lounge and dining room should allow safe mobility in relative freedom by limiting furniture and providing non-slip floors.

If well-planned, the dining room may be used as a valuable activity area between meals. It is wise to allow smoking only in designated areas and to keep an unobtrusive eye on residents who are smokers and may pose a serious fire risk. Bathrooms and toilets should be spacious and suitable for use by very disabled people.

A communal area found to be particularly popular with elderly residents in long-term care facilities (Norman 1987a) was the entrance hall or 'hotel foyer' which provides the chance to observe lots of coming and going and presents natural opportunities for social contact. Another much appreciated aspect of design was found to be a large, attractive accessible staff office which was not 'defended' against residents. Norman (1987a) suggests that interaction between staff and residents on staff territory is an important indicator of the style of management of the residential establishment.

Orientation aids (signs, colours) are useful but, in excess, may create an institutionalized atmosphere. A recent exploratory study (Netten 1989)

suggests that features which promote orientation may differ according to the overall design of the residential facility; thus, for example, many doors along a long corridor may promote orientation in one type of setting but not in another. There would appear to be associations between design features of residential facilities and factors such as orientation, dependency of residents and social atmosphere. These associations seem to be complex and are best considered on an individual basis from one type of facility to the next.

Common sense dictates that stairs and corridors should be well lit for reasons of safety. Recent research suggests that lighting may have a significant impact on orientation (Netten 1989) and behaviour. For example, Ford et al (1986) found that subdued lighting in a unit caring for dementing clients led to a decreased frequency of confused and agitated behaviours and that these behaviours increased when fluorescent lighting was reintroduced. Staff themselves also reported feeling calmer with low-level lighting. The need for study to examine the effects of light upon client and staff behaviour is acknowledged.

In some cases, dementing individuals may feel more settled sharing a bedroom, as for example where an elderly person had become accustomed to sharing a room with her now deceased spouse. However, as Norman (1987a) points out, privacy is a feature of being a free and responsible adult and is the strongest argument in favour of most dementing residents having their own rooms suitably personalized with photographs and selected furniture and possessions. Norman found that the provision of single rooms allowed residential facilities to be flexible in their response to resident need. Residents with a wide range of mental disabilities are more easily catered for and respite and assessment services may be offered alongside long-stay care with the minimum of disruption and distress. Moreover, it seems that staff are more likely to perceive dementing residents who have their own rooms as individuals deserving of privacy and respect (Norman 1987a).

General issues of design and furnishings are discussed in greater depth by Norman (1984), who makes a number of observations of relevance to the above discussion.

MAINTAINING INDIVIDUALITY AND DIGNITY

One of the best indicators of quality nursing care is the extent to which the individuality of dementing residents is respected and care strategies assist residents to maintain their dignity, personality and personal relationships. Factors relating to these issues include the provision of individualized care plans, the maintenance of personal contacts, communication and social interaction and staff attitudes.

Individualized care plans

The importance of these and the role of the 'key worker' has been discussed in Chapter 18. Individual care plans rely upon nurses having a sound knowledge of the resident's unique and personal biography. In cases of severe dementia this may be obtained from relatives who may be asked as a matter of course to provide a written (possibly illustrated) personal history of the resident on admission.

Maintaining personal contacts

Continued contact with family and friends is important for residents and should be encouraged through totally flexible visiting hours. Relatives and friends should be involved in the life and activities of the unit — for example, in parties, outings and fund-raising events. Relatives may wish to become involved in the day-to-day care of residents — for example, by assisting them at mealtimes. This may make them feel of practical use and may strengthen family ties. Some relatives may be prepared to accept a regular evening telephone call from their relative. In many cases this will promote orientation at a time of day when residents are often most disorientated, and may reassure the resident prior to retiring.

At times, visiting may be difficult for relatives, particularly if the resident does not recognize them or becomes distressed when they are about to leave. Nursing staff have an important role in supporting relatives and helping them to see the positive benefits of visiting. A Relatives' Group for regular visitors to the unit may provide a valuable source of peer support.

Norman (1987a) found that volunteers in residential homes for dementing people were conspicuous by their absence. The difficulties in attracting volunteers to befriend residents who may fail to remember them from one visit to the next must be acknowledged. However, once committed, volunteers are valuable in supporting activity and stimulation programmes as well as in relating to particular individual residents who share similar interests or skills.

Whilst nurses who have looked after a resident for some years may have a good understanding of her individual needs, they are perhaps not in the best position to stand back and take a critical look at the care they themselves provide. This suggests the need for formal systems of advocacy which lie outside the residential care establishment. It also highlights a possible role for volunteers as advocates helping to strengthen the voice of elderly residents, particularly those without family or friends, at case conferences and reviews. Advocacy is a valuable role which should not be seen as implying criticism and confrontation, but rather, as giving an opportunity for partnership to ensure the highest possible quality of life for the resident.

Communication and social interaction

The need to communicate and establish relationships is important for us all and dementing residents are no exception. Even at very severe levels of disability at which verbal interaction has ceased in any recognizable sense partnerships may become established between residents which may only be recognized when they are separated — through, for example death, or ward transfer — and one or both begin to exhibit signs of distress.

It is well established that relatively simple environmental changes, such as placing chairs in small groups around coffee tables rather than in traditional placement around the walls, has been shown to increase social interaction among elderly residents (e.g. Peterson et al 1977). However, research has established that other strategies for promoting social interaction among residents may be successful. Examples include small group work, involving the use of prompts, social reinforcement and positive feedback (Linsk et al 1975, Gray & Stevenson 1980) and shared tasks. In one study (Melin & Gotestam 1981) residents were given an opportunity for increased choice and independence through replacing a system for serving afternoon coffee (by which coffee was brought to residents at their seats with sugar and cream already added) with a system that involved the residents in laying out coffee, cups, sugar, cream and cake without staff being present. The increase in social interaction among residents was marked.

Whilst the importance of interactive skills is emphasized in the nursing literature, most studies of communication reveal inadequate or inappropriate communication between nurses and clients (Altschul 1972, Galliard 1978, Lipman et al 1979) and the relatively few communication studies involving dementing clients are consistent with these general findings. A study of female clients in a geriatric ward (Armstrong-Esther & Browne 1986) found that nurses spent only 10.7% of their time interacting with clients. Moreover, they spent a significantly greater amount of time interacting with lucid as opposed to confused/demented clients: 15% as against 5.6%. For all clients the interactions took the form of statements and instructions rather than questions.

Other studies (e.g. Baltes et al 1984) indicate that staff spend more time talking to one another than to elderly clients, in spite of the relatively small numbers of staff compared to clients on the ward. It has been suggested that low level nurse-client interaction is reinforced by a task-centred approach to nursing care in which the clients' physical care and the ward routine are seen as of primary importance and the psychological and social needs of individual clients are very much in second place.

Low level social interaction between nurses and dementing residents is worrying, given the importance of interaction in promoting individuality, in psychological and physical rehabilitation and in decreasing client dependency. The observation by Sommer and Ross (1958) that health professionals make strangers of their clients, who become silent observers of ward activity, would seem to be as true of some wards today as it was 30 years ago.

Nurses may need to be creative in their attempts to communicate with dementing residents whose problems of dysphasia or asphasia or disorientation may make it difficult for them to respond (Bleathman 1987). The use of pictures and drawing and writing things down may be tried; simple guidelines designed to help carers compensate for communication deficits may be adhered to — for example, the sensitive use of closed questions, demonstrating actions beforehand, telling the sufferer what is happening and what is going on next, etc. Advice on how to communicate with dementia sufferers is available from a number of sources (see for example, Phillips 1987).

Staff attitudes

The principle of 'normalization' which has had considerable impact on the lives of mentally and physically disabled people is also relevant to dementia (Woods 1987). This principle does not mean forcing people to do 'normal' things or conform to an approved pattern. Rather, it emphasizes the importance of social values which support individual characteristics and personal experiences and behaviour.

The resources devoted to the care of dementia sufferers and aspects of the daily routine and staff behaviour towards residents are good indicators of the extent to which the principle of normalization is being applied. There are, however, more subtle indicators — for example, constant TV at high volume may indicate that staff are unconcerned about what captive residents are subjected to. Again, language used by staff when talking to or about residents can be very revealing in indicating infantilizing and denegrating attitudes and names applied by staff to residents merit careful consideration.

Positive staff attitudes to residents may be fostered by positive attitudes of managers towards staff. Opportunities for the exercise of initiative and responsibility, access to professional training courses, staff support groups, direct involvement of staff in developing a coherent philosophy of care, a career structure, adequate financial rewards, recognition of the skilled and difficult nature of the work and above all ensuring adequate staff numbers are amongst many factors which are important in creating a climate for good practice. Of particular note is the need for sensitive supervision arrangements to foster personal and professional growth and this is an area for development particularly in residential care facilities. Aims and strategies for supervision are discussed in detail elsewhere (Barber & Norman 1987a, 1987b).

PROMOTING CHOICE AND OPPORTUNITY
Issues of safety and security

There is growing awareness that elderly people have the right to take risks as a part of everyday normal living, and that because they are 'in care' they should not be deprived of this right (Norman 1987b). In the case of residents who are dementing this principle raises particular problems, since many may be unaware of the risks that they are running and have lost the ability to make rational choices. Thus nurses are forced to make choices between liberty and danger on a daily basis.

One of the more dramatic problems which highlights this issue is 'wandering'. Nurses are often fearful that wandering residents will come to harm and may find the apparent searching activity of some wanderers upsetting. Indeed an analysis of the problem may indicate that wandering may be more of a problem for staff than for the resident (Bleathman 1987). Some wards and residential establishments have locked exit doors and staff take it for granted that their responsibility to protect residents from physical harm outweighs the right of residents to come and go as they please. Others keep exit doors unlocked as a matter of principle (Norman 1987a). The Royal College of Nursing (1987) suggests the use of individualized assessment and planning as an alternative to security doors or so called 'baffle locks' and provide guidelines for good practice. Stokes (1986) considers these issues in detail.

Some residential establishments have tagging systems in which residents who wander have tags attached to their clothes which activate a buzzer if they leave. These systems have mechanical problems and concern has been expressed that health authorities and social services departments may opt for electronic tagging rather than address other issues such as staffing levels (Gaze 1989). However, they do seem to offer some solution to the problem of containment of wanderers whose safety is at risk. More generally, it is clear that building designs in which observation and proper supervision can only be achieved at the cost of restricting access to personal space are unsatisfactory.

Tagging may be helpful with some residents but it does not offer a solution to the problem of those who do not want to stay in the ward or refuse to return. If coaxing fails, nurses may be tempted to lie to the resident to persuade her to return to the ward. This goes against the ethics of nursing education and is, speaking practically, unhelpful since it may in some cases destroy the resident's trust in her carers and store up management problems for the future.

Few dementing residents are subject to compulsory care or treatment provisions under the law. Under the mental health acts which cover the UK a nurse of the prescribed class may exercise holding powers to detain residents whose safety is at risk, but this is generally impractical and considered inappropriate with this client group. Clinical experience suggests that an honest, gentle explanation pitched at the resident's level of understanding may reduce distress. A subsequent offer of a realistic alternative may be acceptable since many dementing residents have a limited attention span and are distractable. Failing this the nurse may accompany the resident on a walk which finally leads 'back home'. If all else fails the nurse may exercise her duty of care under common law to prevent the resident from coming to harm. In all cases the nurse should be able to give good reasons for her actions.

The exercise of choice in daily living

The exercise of choice and self-determination in daily living is one of the hallmarks of good quality care. Routine and order are important to dementing residents since they increase the predictability of events and thus allow residents more control over their lives. However, because dementing people often experience difficulty expressing their wishes they are particularly at risk if care routines become inflexible and fail to respond to individual needs and preferences. In general it is useful to allow the dementing resident to establish her own daily routine and then support this through a structured and dependable programme to which changes are introduced slowly and only after careful preparation. The remainder of this section will discuss choice and opportunity in relation to rising and going to bed, clothing and personal appearance, meals and the use of money.

Rising and going to bed

Norman (1987a) found most residential establishments to have flexible regimes. Residents may be given the opportunity to get up early or rest in bed until 10.00 or 11.00 h according to their personal preference. An uncooked breakfast may be made available when residents are ready for it. If cooked breakfasts are provided, waiting may be made more pleasant by offering tea, making TV and radio available in other rooms or providing personal earphones and, more generally, by ensuring that residents have pleasant surroundings to wait in.

If residents are busy and active during the day, night sedation is less likely to be necessary. For some, an alcoholic drink may be the best sedative. A short nap after lunch may be customary and may restore energy for evening activities.

Clothing and personal appearance

There seems to be a general awareness of the need for residents to have personal clothing, clearly marked and properly laundered, although in many NHS settings communal nightclothes are still used (Norman 1987a). Mildly or moderately demented residents may be able to express choice at point of sale. With more severely disabled residents it may be important to consult relatives or look for non-verbal expressions which indicate whether or not items of clothing suit their personal taste. It is also important to offer choice at point of dressing and

to take steps to ensure that residents are able to follow customary habits with respect to make-up and jewellery etc. Whatever clothing is preferred, nurses should be aware of the risk of hypothermia in elderly people — even in those who are ambulant — and should take steps to ensure that the resident keeps warm.

The necessity of protective clothing, particularly at mealtimes, results in a wide array of bibs and aprons being used for this purpose (Norman 1987a). Care should be taken to ensure that whatever protective clothing is used should be effective, and as non-infantilizing as possible.

With respect to the continuing debate about the appropriateness or otherwise of staff uniforms it is interesting to note that Norman (1987a) found that even severely demented residents noticed, appreciated and commented with pleasure upon the ordinary day clothes worn by nursing staff. As she rightly points out, in a situation where contact with the 'ordinary' world is limited, such practices should be encouraged.

Meals

Flexibility of response to individual need and preferences should be one of the aims of catering facilities in residential care settings. This is not easy to achieve since the timing of meals is often the product of other factors — working hours of domestic and catering staff, the routine of the main kitchen and other administrative constraints.

Dementing residents may be involved in planning menus through careful questioning to disclose preferences; this may be supplemented by information from relatives. Involvement in cooking and washing-up is a normal part of daily life and may be encouraged.

Staggering the serving times of uncooked breakfasts and the availability of snacks night and day may go some way towards meeting individual preferences. This may be achieved through the provision of a pantry/kitchen in all new buildings (Norman 1987a) and through nursing staff becoming directly involved in some aspects of food preparation.

Eating is a complex process which involves the resident understanding the situation, being motivated and having certain psychomotor skills. Particularly in later stages of dementia, residents may experience eating problems (Sandman 1986, Athlin & Norberg 1987) due to lack of concentration, agnosia and apraxia (Vitaliano et al 1984, Cogan 1985, Foster et al 1986). In the final stages of the illness the resident may require a liquidized diet or be unable to swallow.

Modifications to cutlery and crockery may assist residents with psychomotor problems to feed themselves. Regular monitoring of weight is important, as is ensuring adequate hydration with a wide selection of preferred drinks.

Choice, meal environment and the presence or absence of staff have been shown to be important in affecting behaviour and communication in dementing elderly residents at mealtimes. One study illustrating this (Melin & Gotestam 1981) has already been mentioned. Another study (Sandman et al 1988) involved video-recording a small group of five institutionalized dementing clients at mealtimes. It showed that if nurses were absent social interaction within the small group increased. Two of the least demented clients became caregivers in the group and helped the three other demented clients to eat. Significantly, this role was dropped when nurses rejoined the group. These and other studies suggest that mealtimes may be a natural setting for reorientating and reactivating dementing residents. They also suggest that residents may have more self-care skills than they are given the opportunity to display.

Use of money

Most dementing residents will be unable to manage their personal allowance and many may be unable to express their views on how it should be spent. Where funds are managed by the providing authority it often falls upon nurses to spend it for the maximum benefit of the resident. Nurses are often faced with difficult decisions, such as when money should be legitimately spent on communal enjoyments rather than individual needs, or how to distinguish between appropriate use and expenditures which should be the responsibility of the providing authority.

MAXIMIZING ACTIVITY AND INDEPENDENT FUNCTIONING

A study by Barton et al (1980) showed that dependent rather than independent behaviour tends to be reinforced by staff in long-stay institutions. A feature of this is that elderly residents become increasingly inactive. One observation study (Armstrong-Esther & Browne 1986) found that, on average, clients on a geriatric ward spent 88.5% of the time sitting and only 9.1% standing or walking. The level of inactivity was most pronounced amongst confused and demented clients. Whereas lucid clients spent 30.5% of the observed time in some purposeful activity (e.g. self-care, eating, drinking, craft work, reading etc.), confused/demented clients spent only 18% of time on such activities.

This study supports Galliard's (1978) conclusion that clients are likely to spend their time sitting in armchairs or wheelchairs mostly uninterrupted by nursing staff, unless they are sufficiently active or motivated to either maintain their mobility or seek assistance. These findings are important and worrying, given the fact that immobility may lead to increased client dependency, and nursing workload and client inactivity may lead to boredom and demoralization.

The provision of purposeful organized activity can make an important contribution to the quality and quantity of activity and can promote social interaction in residential care settings. In turn, this may enhance the residents' levels of confidence, responsibility and self-esteem and may help to maintain existing skills.

Independent functioning can be promoted by outings and holidays, and by 'in-house' activities, with varying levels of therapeutic purpose, for individuals and groups. Independent functioning may also be encouraged through behavioural approaches designed to reduce behaviour problems and improve self care skills.

Outings and holidays

Outings to the shops or the surrounding countryside and more ambitious trips to the seaside or the zoo are stimulating for residents and help to keep them in touch with the outside world. However, they are expensive in terms of staff time and material resources, e.g. funds for hiring a mini-bus or taxi fares. They also require much organization, skill and good public relations. Volunteers and old friends offer the possibility of outings for individual clients to old haunts and accustomed activities — a favourite pub, a cricket match. These outings may have the effect of reactivating memories of a previous lifestyle, and can be regular events.

A common belief is that holidays are disorientating for dementing residents and stressful for staff due to the constant requirement to prevent anti-social behaviour. Certainly holidays may be demanding on staff — however, even severely demented residents have been reported to respond positively to the increased social demands of holidays undertaken in small well-staffed groups (Norman 1987a). Chalets are perhaps the most suitable form of accommodation, since they allow a daily living pattern to suit the needs of the particular group of residents and their small scale limits disorientation (Norman 1987a).

In-house activities

In-house activities can take many forms, including small group games (e.g. snakes and ladders, dominoes, quizzes); music and movement (taking a variety of forms); crafts and skills (e.g. singing, dancing, painting); individual therapy or small group sessions (e.g. reality orientation, reminiscence therapy, validation therapy). Maintaining activities and interests of old people in institutional settings is discussed in some detail in Chapter 7.

The amount of organized activity in residential care facilities for elderly dementing people varies a great deal (Norman 1987a). The constant flicker of the television and the drone of recorded music may give the illusion of activity but is more likely to indicate the reverse.

Concern about the empty days and empty lives of long-stay residents has prompted some elderly care units based in hospitals to appoint an 'activity nurse' to co-ordinate organized activities and to build them into the residents' daily programme.

An alternative approach is to make each member of the staff, including domestics, nursing auxiliaries and porters, responsible for organizing in-house activities during particular periods in the week. This relies upon adequate resources being made available to support staff. However, it may have the positive effect of committing staff to the activities which they themselves arrange, as well as giving them a sense of being valued for their individual talents.

The organization of activity programmes requires that nurses address certain issues of principle (Norman 1987a) — for instance, how far residents should be pushed into activities which they might once have found childish and demeaning. At times activities may be of more benefit to staff than residents by giving the staff alone the feeling of purposeful activity; this may sometimes be legitimate, given the difficulties of the nursing task and the importance of maintaining staff morale.

More generally, staff might consider ways in which activities can be made more 'adult'. For example, hanging the products of art therapy where residents can see them or turning 'music therapy' (elderly residents banging tamborines and hitting triangles) into a sing-along music hall evening.

Groupwork

At first glance there would seem to be many reasons why groupwork, particularly with severely demented individuals, may be impossible. Problems of dysphasia and deafness, behaviours such as wandering and shouting, short attention span and defective recent memory may impede or disrupt communication and prevent the formation of a sense of group identity.

In spite of these difficulties the pioneering work of Burnside (1976) showed that even severely demented individuals may be responsive to groupwork which is skillfully handled and which makes use of techniques such as touch. Burnside was able to increase appropriate verbal communication and eye contact in groups of dementing residents by encouraging 'affective touch'. This took the form of shaking each client's hand at the beginning and end of group meetings, placing her hand on the client's shoulder when speaking, and encouraging hand-holding within the group.

Clinical experience suggests that whatever form the groupwork takes success is more likely if groups are small, have clear goals, and have increasingly active therapists as the level of handicap of the members increases. Generally, members should be carefully selected in order that the activities of the group be structured towards a particular level of ability. However, in some circumstances a mixed ability group may provide opportunities for more able residents to help their less able peers, thereby having positive benefits in terms of increasing social interaction and self-esteem.

The following three sections discuss particular forms of small group therapy with dementing residents — reality orientation, reminiscence therapy and validation therapy. It is important to note that these therapies may also be undertaken on a one-to-one basis. A final section outlines what has recently been termed 'resolution therapy'.

Reality orientation

Disorientation is to some degree an inevitable consequence of dementia and is a major focus for nursing intervention. Most of the research comes from studies of reality orientation (RO), which has received much attention in recent years and has come to symbolize a whole philosophy of care rather than a set of particular techniques.

Two forms of RO are usually described. RO group sessions involve a small number of selected residents meeting with staff for between 20–60 minutes at least twice a week. The setting varies. In some establishments an RO classroom may be used, complete with stimulating material (posters, pictures of food, animals, plants, etc.) and perhaps a board clearly displaying orientating data — such as the day, date, weather and the next meal. Elsewhere, social aspects are emphasized and a more informal approach is taken — to the extent of holding sessions in the local pub. The content of RO group sessions vary according to the interests and abilities of participants, but will usually in-

volve discussion of current events, making links with past well-known knowledge and drawing upon visual and auditory aids as appropriate. Whichever format is chosen, relieving tension and pressure and eliminating fear of failure is important if individual performance is to be maximized (Woods 1987).

The second form is 24-hour RO, which is intended to be a continuous informal interactive technique which involves all staff and participating relatives 'orientating' or discouraging disorientation at every interaction. This is reinforced by memory aids — clocks, signposts, calendars, etc.

Two aspects of orientation may be identified. Verbal orientation (being able to answer questions related to time, place and person correctly) and behavioural orientation (being able to go from one place to the next without getting lost). Woods (1987) points out that early studies led to hopes that improvements in verbal orientation might result in behavioural changes mediated through increased self-esteem. This early optimism has not been supported by subsequent studies. It is now clear that generalizing improvement from one area of functioning to the next is not straightforward; whilst improvements in verbal orientation have been demonstrated by a number of studies (e.g. Hanley et al 1981, Johnson et al 1981, Zepelin et al 1981), other behavioural changes have been reported much less frequently (Brook et al 1975, Reeve & Ivison 1985).

Some studies consider both forms of RO, others only RO group sessions (Woods 1987). Few studies have sought to evaluate the relative contribution of each form to client outcome, although Reeve and Ivison (1985) suggest that the efficacy of 24-hour RO may be increased by RO group sessions.

Some studies have sought to isolate particular aspects of RO. Thus, for example, Hanley et al (1981) found that ward spatial orientation increased through using a simple training procedure as part of a 24-hour RO programme focusing upon activities of daily living rather than verbal orientation in time, place and person. Ward spatial orientation seems to improve by signposting the ward, pointing the signposts out to clients and using them in orientating the client to the ward. Signposts alone seem to have little effect (Hanley et al 1981, Gilleard et al 1981).

In addition to benefiting residents, several writers suggest that RO, and in particular 24-hour RO, has positive benefits for nursing staff in terms of bringing about closer nurse-client relationships (Merchant & Saxby 1981), improving morale, discouraging institutionalized and custodial work practices and promoting individualized care (Powell-Proctor & Miller 1982).

In spite of recent critiques (Burton 1982, Schwenk 1981, Powell-Procter & Miller 1982) it is probably fair to say that RO can make a valuable contribution to the overall management of some dementing residents and may promote a more positive approach by nurses to the care of mentally frail elderly people. However, uncritical adoption of RO is ill-advised and it is important that the limitations of the approach are acknowledged.

RO seems to be based upon the assumption that relief of disorientation will in turn alleviate the emotional distress experienced by the dementia sufferer. For many severely demented clients clinical experience suggests that quite the reverse may be true. Providing orientating data for these individuals may leave their level of orientation quite unaffected but may increase levels of emotional distress and dependency through sudden, short-lived insight into their intolerable situation. Thus RO may be of most benefit to mildly and moderately demented residents and of no benefit at all to more severely demented residents. It may even be true that its greatest value does not lie with the management of residents with organic disorders but those whose disorientation arises from an impoverished institutional environment (Powell-Procter & Miller 1982).

Reminiscence therapy

Reminiscence therapy, like RO, is undertaken on an individual basis or, more commonly, in groups. Broadly, it consists of employing a range of audio-visual aids — old photographs, music, mementoes from the past etc. — to encourage old people to recall the past, or to reminisce. The assumption is that this has positive benefits in itself or that the stimulation of long-term memory will in turn stimulate short-term memory. Since reminiscence therapy is discussed in Chapter 7 of this volume, this section is restricted to a brief consideration of its application to the management of individuals with dementia.

The traditionally held view that reminiscence contributes to mental deterioration has been overturned, to be replaced with the belief that it may in fact help to preserve mental functioning in old age (Coleman 1986). As a result, reminiscence therapy has been introduced into a wide variety of settings for elderly mentally ill people. The therapy has theoretical and emotional appeal, since reminiscence is a normal activity of late (and earlier) life which reverses the normal power differential between nurse and resident; the dementing resident is placed in the role of expert — she was there whereas the nurse was not (Woods 1987). Moreover, it allows staff to see beyond the shell of dementia and to place the person within the context of her whole life.

Studies of the effects of reminiscence therapy on dementing residents are scarce, most of the literature taking the form of anecdotal or descriptive accounts (Kiernat 1979, Lesser et al 1981, Norris & Abu El Eileh 1982, Cook 1984). However, it is consistently considered as a positive activity promoting improvements in many areas of functioning. These include increased levels of communication among residents, increased socialization before and after the group therapy sessions, improved self-esteem and improvements in behaviour. Benefits for staff in terms of closer relationships with residents and increased job satisfaction have also been reported.

Comparison with the enthusiastic claims made for RO come quickly to mind and Woods and Britton (1985) warn future researchers to learn the lessons now emerging from previous RO studies. Thus, for example, research attempting to measure the effects of reminiscence therapy on cognitive and behavioural factors may be of limited value. Instead it may be more appropriate to consider the potential of the therapy to generate spontaneity and enjoyment in group sessions or to facilitate psychological adjustment (Coleman 1986).

Validation therapy

Disillusionment with RO, in particular with its potential for increasing the distress levels of some severely demented residents, led Feil (1972, 1982) to devise an alternative interactive technique known as validation therapy. This approach aims to reduce distress and maximize self-esteem through communicating with disorientated residents in whatever reality they are in rather than through attempting to orientate them to reality. Like RO, validation therapy can form the basis of individual or small group work.

The philosophy which underpins validation therapy appears to be strongly influenced by psychodynamic theory. This is reflected in the assumptions behind the technique which are summarized by Van Amelsvoort Jones as follows:

. . . that all behaviour has meaning; that early learned emotional memories replace intellectual thinking in the disorientated old-old; and that the disorientated old-old return to the past for the purpose of trying to resolve unfinished conflicts by expressing feelings hidden in youth, in order to relive past pleasures, to restimulate sensory memories, and to relieve boredom and stress by retreating from painful feelings of uselessness and loneliness (Van Amelsvoort Jones 1985, p. 21).

The aim of therapy is to facilitate and encourage this process. In practice, this entails the nurse 'validating' what has been said in order that meaningful conversation can take place on subjects which are important to the individual or members of the small group.

Whilst validation therapy is in widespread use in North America it seems to have only recently appeared in British nursing practice through the work of Bleathman and Morton (1988, 1989), two charge nurses at the Maudsley Hospital, London. Results of their study of the verbal interaction among members of a small validation therapy group have not yet been fully analysed. However, the researchers have been struck by the ability of severely demented residents, who usually display a near-total lack of meaningful interaction, to maintain and discuss themes and issues for 45 minutes and longer within a validation therapy group. These results are encouraging and suggest the need for further research to identify the specific benefits of the therapy for particular groups of residents.

Resolution therapy

In a recent paper, Goudie and Stokes (1989) express reservations about the philosophical under-pinnings of validation therapy and its relevance to the care of dementing people. They argue that psychodynamic theory is an unhelpful basis for counselling techniques with this client group since it deflects the attention of the counsellor away from the underlying content and feelings which may be obscured by the confused message. Moreover, it inappropriately attributes to the dementing individual intellectual powers for abstract reasoning, fantasy development and the use of defence mechanisms when confronted by distressing emotions.

Goudie and Stokes (1989) argue that, particularly when dementia is advanced, confused messages are more likely to reflect attempts by the client to make sense of 'the here and now' and express her needs rather than escape from painful reality. They advocate that nurses seek to understand and acknowledge these here-and-now feelings of demented clients and then explore ways to help the client cope with them, rather than interpret them in psychodynamic terms. They advocate what they call 'resolution therapy', which would seem to be a form of one-to-one counselling during everyday social interaction, drawing upon Rogerian (Rogers 1951) counselling principles. The practical applications of resolution therapy have yet to be examined.

Reducing behaviour problems

A substantial body of applied research suggests that, by altering appropriate situational variables, we may help individuals to learn new adaptive behaviours and unlearn those which are maladaptive (Rimm & Masters 1974). Dementing residents may exhibit a variety of behaviour problems — for example, wandering, screaming, shouting, and many others. Dealing with these requires a thorough analysis of the problem — its intensity, frequency and duration, its precursors and consequences, and the situations in which it is more or less likely to occur. It also requires an understanding of how the reaction of nurses or others may unwittingly 'reinforce' or encourage the problem behaviour and a recognition that 'common sense' explanations may not always apply. To take a simple example, common sense suggests that reprimanding a dementing resident for spitting at another should reduce the reoccurrence of the behaviour, since a reprimand is normally regarded as a punishment. A behavioural approach suggests that quite the reverse may be true, in that a reprimand may in fact reward or reinforce the behaviour and thus encourage repetition.

It is important to bear in mind that elimination of the problem behaviour is usually insufficient and that emphasis should be placed upon building up appropriate behaviour to replace it. This requires the nurse to adopt a perspective which sets the problem behaviour within the context of broad situational and biological variables; this may be done through, for example, the multiple pathway model (Stokes 1989). It also points to the importance of identifying residents' remaining abilities, which may then be drawn upon to encourage new adaptive behaviour (Barrowclough & Fleming 1986).

One of the particular problems of behaviour modification with dementing residents is the difficulty of finding effective rewards. For example, Birchmore and Clague (1983), in reducing the frequency of shouting of a blind elderly resident, tried several reinforcements when she was quiet before finding touch — rubbing the person's back — to be the most effective. In this instance, behavioural analysis of the problem had suggested that the shouting was a form of self-stimulation in the absence of adequate sensory inputs. However, shouting may occur for other reasons, for example, pain, anxiety, desire for staff contact, and thus alternative interventions may be appropriate.

An important lesson which has emerged from studies of behavioural approaches to the manage-

ment of dementing clients is that they are unlikely to be successful, at least in the long term, unless the sources of reward and satisfaction for carers are taken into account in the initial assessment. Godlove et al (1980) has shown that care staff in residential settings may prefer dependent rather than independent residents, possibly because their behaviour is easier to predict and manage. This points to the need for the promotion of positive attitudes amongst nurses towards residents and a philosophy of care which values individual case management and work directed at the achievement of small, attainable goals.

Promoting self-care

A common complaint from nurses is that helping dementing residents with self-care tasks takes so long that there is often little time for other kinds of intervention. Whilst many residents do need help to carry out their activities of daily living the temptation for the nurse is to do more and more and thereby inadvertently encourage dependence. As previously indicated, staff attitudes are important in creating an atmosphere within which residents are not treated as sick, inactive, dependent 'patients' but are expected to make best use of their remaining abilities.

Behavioural approaches discussed in the previous section seem to offer the hope of improvement in self-care abilities for some residents. Self-care activities of bathing and toileting provide useful examples.

Rinke et al (1978) studied the effects of prompting and reinforcing separate elements of 'self bathing' — undressing, soaping, rinsing, drying and dressing — in four dementing nursing Home residents. A marked improvement occurred in all four residents as against two controls, although it is unclear what level of intervention would have been required to maintain the improvement. In this study prompting was both physical (handing the resident a towel) and verbal (giving direction). Reinforcements included a wall chart for visual feedback on progress, verbal praise and a choice of pleasant toiletries on achievement of a set level of achievement.

Clearly there are cases where a behaviour programme may be inappropriate — for example, with certain cases of severely demented people in which the potential of increasing self-care skills to any noticeable degree is negligible. In such cases self-care may still be encouraged but other objectives should take priority, such as deriving as much enjoyment as possible from the bathing process.

Loss of continence is a major problem in the care of dementing people and exerts a strong influence on placement decisions and general quality of life. Reports of behaviour programmes with this client group are mixed (Woods 1987). A number of complex skills must be mastered to achieve independent toileting. These include dressing, undressing, mobility, finding and recognizing the toilet and planning ahead. The complexity of independent toileting highlights the need for a detailed behavioural analysis of the particular individual's toileting difficulties (see Hodge 1984, and Ch. 12 of this volume) which takes into account institutional and environmental features and relevant medical and nutritional factors.

In some cases independent toileting may be a feasible objective but in many cases of severe disability the goal may be to increase the proportion of successful visits to the toilet and to minimize accidents. The rapid success of some toileting programmes indicates that incontinence may sometimes be due to nursing staff failing to respond to requests rather than residents failing to issue them (e.g. Schnelle et al 1983).

With respect to night-time incontinence, urinary sheath systems have been found to offer the possibility of a dry undisturbed night for some male residents. Catheterization should be a last resort.

A clear and detailed description of the principles and practice of behaviour modification is given by Woods and Britton (1985). The more specific area of memory rehabilitation for dementing people is discussed by Wilson and Moffatt (1984).

CONCLUSION

This chapter has indicated important differences between confusional states and dementia and has suggested that nurses be mindful of these when planning care. A variety of therapeutic interventions and aspects of management have been discussed. It is hoped that this will discourage therapeutic pessimism, which is possibly the single greatest threat to the quality of care delivered to confused and dementing people.

REFERENCES

Altschul A T 1972 Patient-nurse interaction: a study of interaction patterns in acute psychiatric wards. Churchill Livingstone, Edinburgh

Armstrong-Esther C A, Hawkins L H 1982 Day for night: circadian rhythms in the elderly. Nursing Times 78: 1263–1265

Armstrong-Esther C A, Browne K D 1986 The influence of elderly patients' mental impairment on nurse-patient interaction. Journal of Advanced Nursing 11: 379–387

Athlin E, Norberg A 1987 Caregivers' attitudes to and behaviour of severely demented patients during feeding in a patient assignment care system. International Journal of Nursing Studies 24: 145–153

Ball M J, Nuttal K 1980 Neurofibrillary tangles, granulovacuolar degeneration, and neurone loss in Down syndrome: quantitative comparison with Alzheimer dementia. Annals of Neurology 7: 462–465

Baltes M M, Barton E M, Orzech M J, Lage D 1984 Behaviour mapping in a nurses home: observations of elderly residents and staff behaviours. Zeitschrift Fur Gerontologie 16: 18–26

Barber P, Norman I J 1987a An eclectic model of staff development: supervision techniques to prepare nurses for a process approach — a social perspective. In: Barber P (ed) Mental Handicap. Hodder & Stoughton, London

Barber P, Norman I J 1987b Skills in supervision. Nursing Times 83(2): 56–57

Barrowclough C, Fleming I 1986 Goal planning with elderly people, making plans to meet individual needs. A manual of instruction. Manchester University Press, Manchester

Barton E M, Baltes M M, Orzech M J 1980 Etiology of dependence in older nursing home residents during mourning: the role of staff behaviour. Journal of Personality and Social Psychology 38: 423–431

Birchmore T, Clague S 1983 A behavioural approach to reduce shouting. Nursing Times 79 (20 April): 37–39

Bleathman C 1987 The practical management of the Alzheimer's disease patient in the hospital setting. Journal of Advanced Nursing 12: 531–534

Bleathman C, Morton 1 1988 Validation therapy with the demented elderly. Journal of Advanced Nursing 13: 511–514

Bleathman C, Morton 1 1989 Validation; a search for a therapy. Paper presented to a symposium on the 'Uses and applications of research in advanced clinical practice' at the Institute of Psychiatry, 7 July, unpublished

Brook P, Degun G, Mather M 1975 Reality orientation, a therapy for psychogeriatric patients: a controlled study. British Journal of Psychiatry 137: 566–571

Brooking J I 1986 Dementia and confusion in the elderly.

In: Redfern S J (ed) Nursing elderly people, 1st edn. Churchill Livingstone, Edinburgh

Budd S, Brown W 1974 Effect of a reorientation technique on postcardiotomy delirium. Nursing Research 23: 341–348

Burnside I M 1976 Nursing and the aged. McGraw Hill, New York

Burton M 1982 Reality orientation for the elderly: a critique. Journal of Advanced Nursing 7: 427–433

Candy J M, Oakley A E, Klinowski J et al 1986 Aluminosilicates and senile plaque formation in Alzheimer's disease. Lancet 1: 354–357

Chatham M A 1978 The effect of family involvement on patients' manifestations of postcardiotomy psychosis. Heart & Lung 7: 995–999

Chisholm S E, Deniston O L, Igrisan R M, Barbus A J 1982 Prevalence of confusion in elderly hospitalised patients. Journal of Gerontological Nursing 8(2): 87–96

Church M, Wattis J 1988 Psychological approaches to the assessment and treatment of old people. In: Wattis J, Hindmarch I (eds) Psychological assessment of the elderly: behavioural and clinical aspects. Churchill Livingstone, London

Cogan D C 1985 Visual disturbances with focal progressive dementing disease. American Journal of Opthalmology 100: 68–72

Coleman P G 1986 Ageing and reminiscence processes: social and clinical implications. Wiley, Chichester

Cook J B 1984 Reminiscing: how it can help confused nursing home residents. Social Casework: The Journal of Contemporary Social Work (Feb): 90–93

Crapper D R, Krishnan S S, Quittkat S 1976 Aluminium, neurofibrillary degeneration and Alzheimer's disease. Brain 99: 67–80

Ellis W G, McCulloch J R, Corley C L 1974 Presenile dementia in Down's syndrome: ultrastructural identity with Alzhimer's disease. Neurology 24: 101–106

Feil N 1972 A new approach to group therapy, research findings. Unpublished paper presented to the 25th Annual Meeting of the Gerontological Society in San Juan. Puerto Rico

Feil N 1982 Validation: the Feil method. Edward Feil Productions, Cleveland, Ohio

Folstein M F, Folstein S E, McHugh P R 1975 'Mini-mental state': a practical method for grading the cognitive state of patients for the clinician. Journal of Psychiatric Research 12: 189–198

Ford M, Fox J, Fitch S, Donovan A 1986 Light in the darkness. Nursing Times 83(1): 26–29

Foreman M D 1986 Acute confusional states in hospitalized elderly: a research dilemma. Nursing Research 35(1): 34–38

Foster N L, Chase T N, Patronas N J, Gillespie M M, Fedio P 1986 Cerebral mapping of apraxia in Alzheimer's disease by positron emission tomography. Annals of Neurology 9: 139–143

Galliard P 1978 Difficulties encountered in attempting to increase social interaction among geriatric psychiatry patients — clean and sitting quietly. Paper presented to the British Psychological Society Annual Conference, York University

Gaze H 1989 An invisible leash. Nursing Times 85(25): 22–23

Gilleard C J, Mitchell R G, Riordan J 1981 Ward orientation training with psychogeriatric patients. Journal of Advanced Nursing 6: 95–98

Godlove C, Dunn G, Wright H 1980 Caring for old people in New York and London: the 'nurses' aide' interviews. Journal of the Royal Society of Medicine 73: 713–723

Goudie F, Stokes G 1989 Understanding confusion. Nursing Times 85(39): 35–37

Gray P, Stevenson J S 1980 Changes in verbal interaction among members of resocialisation groups. Journal of Gerontological Nursing 6: 86–90

Grimley Evans J 1982 The psychiatric aspects of physical disease. In: Levy R, Post F (eds) The psychiatry of late life. Blackwell, Oxford

Hachinski V C, Iliff L D, Zilkha E, Du Boulay G H, McAllister V L, Marshall J, Russell R W R, Symon L 1975 Cerebral blood flow in dementia. Archives of Neurology 32: 632–637

Hanley I, McGuire R J, Boyd W D 1981 Reality orientation and dementia: a controlled trial of two approaches. British Journal of Psychiatry 138: 10–14

Hodge J 1984 Towards a behavioural analysis of dementia. In: Hanley I, Hodge J (eds) Psychological approaches to the care of the elderly. Croom Helm, London

Hodkinson H M 1973 Mental impairment in the elderly. Journal of the Royal College of Physicians London 7(4): 305–317

Holden U P, Woods R T 1982 Reality orientation: psychological approaches to the confused elderly. Churchill Livingstone, London

Hussain R A 1984 Behavioural geriatrics. In: Herien M, Eiser R M, Miller P M (eds) Progress in behaviour modification. Academic Press, London

Jacques A 1988 Understanding dementia. Churchill Livingstone, Edinburgh

Johnson C H, McLaren S M, McPherson F M 1981 The comparative effectiveness of three versions of 'classroom' orientation. Age and Ageing 10: 33–35

Katzman R, Terry R D, Bick K L (eds) 1978 Alzheimer's disease: senile dementia and related disorders. Raven Press, New York

Kellett J 1987 Psychiatry of old age. The Practitioner 231 (June): 855–861

Kiernat J M 1979 The use of life review activity with confused nursing home residents. American Journal of Occupational Therapy 33: 306–310

La Porte H J 1982 Reversible causes of dementia: a nursing challenge. Journal of Gerontological Nursing 8: 213–216

Lesser J, Lazarus L W, Frankel J et al 1981 Reminiscence group therapy with psychotic geriatric inpatients. The Gerontologist 21: 291–296

Libow L S 1978 Senile dementias and pseudo-dementias: clinical diagnosis. In: Eisdorfer C, Friedal R D (eds) Cognitive and emotional disturbance in the elderly. Year Book Medical Publishers, Chicago

Linsk N, Howe M W, Pinkston E M 1975 Behavioural group work in a home for the aged. Social Work 20: 454–463

Lipman A, Slater R, Harris H 1979 The quality of verbal interaction in homes for old people. Gerontology 25: 275–281

Lishman W A 1987 Organic psychiatry, 2nd edn. Blackwell, Oxford

Longo V G 1966 Behavioural and EEG effect of atropine and related compounds. Pharmacological Reviews 28: 965

Macdonald M L 1973 The forgotten Americans: a sociopsychological analysis of ageing and nursing homes. American Journal of Community Psychology 3: 272–292

Melin L, Gotestam K G 1981 The effects of rearranging ward routines on communication and eating behaviour of psychogeriatric patients. Journal of Applied Behavioural Analysis 14: 47–51

Merchant M, Saxby P 1981 Reality orientation — a way forward. Nursing Times 12: 1442–1445

Merton R K 1957 Social theory and social structure, rev. edn. Free Press, Illinois

Netten A 1989 The effect of design of residential homes in creating dependency among confused elderly residents: a study of elderly demented residents and their ability to find their way around homes for the elderly. International Journal of Geriatric Psychiatry 4: 143–153

Norman A 1984 Bricks and mortals: design and lifestyle in old people's homes. CPA Reports no 4, Centre for Policy on Ageing, London

Norman A 1987a Severe dementia: the provision of longstay care. Centre for Policy on Ageing, London

Norman A 1987b Risk or restraint. Nursing Times 89(30): 31

Norris A D, Abu El Eileh M T 1982 Reminiscence groups. Nursing Times 78: 1368–1369

Open University (Department of Health & Social Welfare) in association with the Health Education Authority 1988 Handbook of mental disorders in old age. Open University Press, Milton Keynes

Pajk M 1984 Alzheimer's disease inpatient care. American Journal of Nursing 84(2): 216–224

Pearce J M S 1987 Dementia. Medicine International: 1956–1960

Peterson R F, Knapp T J, Rosen J C, Pither B F 1977 The effects of furniture arrangement on the behaviour of geriatric patients. Behavior Therapy 8: 464–467

Pfeiffer E 1975 A short portable memory status questionnaire for the assessment of organic brain deficits in elderly patients. Journal of the American Geriatrics Society 23(10): 433–441

Phillips A 1987 Clearing a path to communication; dementia — how you can help. Geriatric Nursing & Home Care (November): 16–18

Platzer H 1988 A study into the causes of post-operative confusion in the elderly. Unpublished MSc Thesis, King's College, London

Powell-Proctor L, Miller E 1982 Reality orientation: a critical appraisal. British Journal of Psychiatry 140: 457–463

Reeve W, Ivison S 1985 Use of environmental manipulation and classroom and modified informal reality orientation with institutionalized, confused elderly patients. Age and Ageing 14: 119–121

Rimm D C, Masters J C 1974 Behaviour therapy: techniques and empirical findings. Academic Press, London

Rinke C L, Williams J J, Lloyd K E, Smith-Scott W 1978 The effects of prompting and reinforcement on self-bathing by elderly residents of a nursing home. Behaviour Therapy 9: 873–881

Rogers C R 1951 Client centred therapy. Houghton, Mifflin, Boston

Royal College of Nursing 1987 Focus on restraint. RCN, London

Sandman P O 1986 Aspects of institutional care of patients with dementia. Medical dissertation, new series no 181, University of Umea, Sweden

Sandman P O, Norberg A, Adolfsson R 1988 Verbal communication and behaviour during meals in five institutionalized patients with Alzheimer-type dementia. Journal of Advanced Nursing 13: 571–578

Schnelle J F, Traughber B, Morgan D B, Embry J E, Binion A F, Coleman A 1983 Management of geriatric incontinence in nursing homes. Journal of Applied Behavior Analysis 16: 235–241

Schwenk M A 1981 Reality orientation for the institutionalised aged: does it help? Gerontologist 19: 373–377

Sommer R, Ross H 1958 Social interaction on a geriatric ward. International Journal of Social Psychology 4: 128–132

St George-Hyslop P H, Tanzi R E, Polinsky R J et al 1987 The genetic defect causing familial Alzheimer's disease maps on chromosome 21. Science 235: 885–890

Stokes G J 1986 Wandering. Winslow Press, Bicester Oxon

Stokes G J 1989 Hospital structure bars quality care in dementia. Geriatric Medicine (July): 58–61

Van Amelsvoort Jones G M M 1985 Validation therapy: a companion to reality orientation. The Canadian Nurse 81(3): 20–23

Vitaliano P P, Breen A R, Albert M S, Russo J, Printz P N 1984 Memory, attention, and functional status in community-residing Alzheimer type dementia patients and optimally healthy individuals. Journal of Gerontology 39: 58–64

Williams M A, Campbell E B, Raynor W J Jr, Musholt M A, Mlynarczyk S M, Crane L F 1985 Predictors of acute confusional states in hospitalized elderly patients. Research in Nursing and Health 8: 31–40

Williams M A, Holloway J R, Winn M C, Wolanin M O, Lawler M L, Westwick C R, Chin M H 1979 Nursing activities and acute confusional states in elderly hip-fractured patients. Nursing Research 28: 25–35

Wilson B A, Moffat N 1984 Clinical management of memory problems. Croom Helm, London

Wolanin M O, Phillips L R F 1981 Confusion: prevention and care. Mosby, St Louis.

Woods R T, Britton P G 1985 Clinical psychology with the elderly. Croom Helm, London

Woods R 1987 Psychological management of dementia. In: Pitt B (ed) Dementia. Churchill Livingstone, Edinburgh

Working Party on Care of the Dementing Elderly 1988 A review of published research and recommendations for future research priorities. Health Bulletin 46(2) (March): 127–137

Zepelin H, Wolfe C S, Kleinplatz F 1981 Evaluation of a year long reality orientation program. Journal of Gerontology 36: 70–77

CHAPTER CONTENTS

Introduction 341

Definition 342

**Theoretical explanations of late life
depression** 343
Physical disease and disability 344
Social causation: the impact of loss and social
support 346
Age-related neurophysical changes in the central
nervous system 347

Identified problems of depression in old age 347
Emotional 348
Physical 348
Cognitive 349
Social 350

Prevention of depression in old age 351

**Nursing care required by depressed elderly
people** 354
Counselling 354
Specific psychological interventions 358
Physiological interventions 360
Social and environmental considerations 364
The outlook for depressed elderly clients 365

**Research into the efficacy of nursing
interventions** 366

Suicide in old age 366

Conclusion 368

20

Depression in old age

Ian J. Norman

INTRODUCTION

The days of our years are threescore and ten; and if
by reason of strength they be fourscore years, yet is
their strength labour and sorrow (Psalms 90: 10)

Historically, old age has been seen as the season
of despair and sorrow. How far this perception
reflects reality or is a young person's pessimistic
view of the prospect ahead is difficult to judge.
Clinical experience suggests that many 'healthy'
old people experience a deep sense of sadness; Stevenson (1989) considers that some, particularly
those who reflect upon the multiple losses associated with old age, may experience a kind of
existential depression for which there is no
remedy.

By contrast, Murphy (1986) states that most elderly people do not feel depressed, unhappy or
unfulfilled and that the gloom that younger people
may feel about the future is mainly the result of
stereotyped misconceptions. She cites Harris'
(1975) finding that whilst one old person feels that
life in old age is worse than expected, a further
three consider that things have turned out better
than they had hoped.

For most of us, depression is part and parcel of
the 'human condition', to be endured and managed as best we can. Distinguishing between this
normal life experience and depression as a clinical
and disease entity is difficult. Lack of consensus
as to what constitutes a 'case' of depression makes
comparison between epidemiological studies
which employ different methodologies problem-

atic. When defined on the basis of complaints in surveys the highest prevalence of depression is found in the over-65s, whereas when diagnosed by psychiatrists mild depression is most common in the 35–45 year age group and severe depression amongst those aged 55–65 (Gurland 1976).

Overall, it would seem that depression is the most common functional mental disorder of late life (Brayne & Ames 1988), accounting for about 40% of all referrals to comprehensive district psychiatric services (Jolley & Arie 1976, Murphy 1986). Mild depression is probably five times more common than major depression in elderly people (Gurland et al 1983) but is frequently overlooked (e.g. Williamson et al 1964) or dismissed as an understandable and untreatable response to the vicissitudes of the final stage of life.

This chapter discusses theoretical explanations of depression in late life and outlines problems experienced by old people who may be clinically depressed or best described as just plain unhappy. Therapeutic interventions are discussed and particular attention is given to the nurse's contribution to care and treatment. This is followed by a brief consideration of the small number of research studies into the efficacy of nursing interventions. The chapter concludes with a discussion of the problem of suicide.

Not all problems described will affect all clients and not all the interventions described will be appropriate. This chapter, like the previous one, should therefore be viewed as a resource from which to glean information to apply, as appropriate, to individual cases. Timing, evaluation and revision of interventions specific to the client's situation should be supplied by the responsible nurse in consultation with the client and other members of the multidisdisplinary team.

DEFINITION

Depression is a complex phenomenon which may be viewed from a variety of perspectives. In clinical practice, definitions of depression suggest an emotion of deep unhappiness with a sense of worthlessness and hopelessness and loss of interest or pleasure in usual activities or pastimes. Lowered mood must be prominent and persistent but need not necessarily be the overwhelming feature and there may be other physical and behavioural changes.

Wilson-Barnett and Batehup (1989) point out that depression may be only one dimension in a set of negative emotions experienced at any one time; thus, for example, a person may be primarily anxious but also report feeling depressed and behave aggressively. Differentiating anxiety from depression and determining which emotion is dominant is thus problematic. Izard (1972) found that similar statements were used to describe both emotions, and Marks (1975) indicates that severe neurotic illness may generate both anxiety and depressed behaviour.

Some clinicians resolve these problems by grouping depression and anxiety together under the general heading of 'affective states', describing them both as anhedonic emotions, associated with stress and triggered by threats to self-esteem. Others suggest that anxiety reflects attempts to mobilize resources to cope with a threat, whereas depression reflects a sense of inevitability and passive despair (Becker 1974).

Another debate amongst clinicians is whether depression is best conceived of as essentially two separate conditions with different causes or as a single wide-spectrum disorder with forms that range from the mild to the severe (Kendell 1976). Zung (1973) argues that there is no qualitative difference between feelings of sadness and feelings of depression in a psychiatric illness. He maintains that depression is 'a ubiquitous and universal condition which as a human experience extends as a continuum from normal mood swings to a pathological state'. Thus the term may be used in several ways to describe 'an affect which is a subjective feeling tone of short duration'; a mood which is a state sustained over a long period of time; an emotion which comprises the feeling tones along with objective indications; or a disorder which has characteristic symptom clusters, complexes or configurations' (Zung 1973: 330). This view of depression is supported by Beck (1967), who claims that depressed people score higher than 'normals' on his inventory, which consists of items which are relevant to both groups.

In contrast to this model, the most influential classification schemes are those which contrast extremes of the phenomenon under such headings as cause, symptomatology and response to treatment. None of these schemes is wholly satisfactory. Perhaps the most influential are the psychotic/neurotic, and endogenous/reactive models.

The psychotic/neurotic model highlights the presence or absence of psychotic symptoms. Thus psychotic depression is severe and characterized by loss of insight, delusions, hallucinations, or thought disorder. In contrast, neurotic depression is less severe and the client displays none of these other features. In clinical practice, however, it is found that severe depression may occur without psychotic features but with marked physical or behavioural features.

The term 'endogenous' may be used to refer to severe forms of depression which seem to come 'out of the blue' in that they do not appear to have a precipitating psychological cause arising from the environment and are thus explained by a combination of genetic and biochemical factors. In contrast, 'reactive' depression is less severe and an environmental cause may be discerned. Reviews of the research literature by Kendell (1976) and Lader (1976) have cast doubt upon this dichotomy. Symptoms and aetiology are often very mixed (Lader 1976) and the majority of depressive illnesses would seem to be preceded by stressful events of one kind or another (Kendell 1976). In clinical practice the terms tend to be applied on the basis of severity alone.

In addition to the above classification schemes a distinction is often made between bi-polar and uni-polar depression. Bi-polar depression refers to severe depressed states experienced by a client who has experienced episodes of mania, whereas in uni-polar depression there have been no previous episodes of mania. Specific aspects of the nursing care of elderly people suffering from bi-polar disorder will not be discussed in this chapter. However, general aspects of care apply.

It is important that nurses have an understanding of the terms discussed above since they will come across them in clinical practice. However, for practical purposes, debates about appropriate systems of classification are sterile. They reflect the traditional clinical-somatic construction (or medical model) of depression, which encourages abstraction of the condition from the client. This model, which is still prominent in the British nursing literature (Barker 1989), may result in nurses discussing the disease as if it existed separately from the person experiencing it, so that the disease itself becomes the focus of the nurses' attention. It may also serve to relegate the client to the role of passive recipient of care and is thus particularly inappropriate in relation to depressed people whose active involvement in treatment is often vital to recovery.

Conceiving depression along a continuum from normal feelings of unhappiness to conditions which constitute serious psychiatric disorders allows the nurse to recognize signs of depression in her elderly clients and to alleviate suffering through the medium of her relationship with the clients and by instigating other appropriate nursing interventions.

THEORETICAL EXPLANATIONS OF LATE LIFE DEPRESSION

The existence of severe disturbances of mood, such as depression, have been explained by a variety of models or theories of causation which seek to identify predisposing and precipitating factors that may affect individual coping abilities and level of adjustment.

Biophysical theories stress the role of genetic, biochemical and constitutional factors. In contrast, sociological theories stress social factors as correlates of mood disorder. Psychodynamic theories tend to view depression as a severe mourning response to events symbolic or otherwise, which involve the loss of an important object. Learning theories often see depression as a lowered level of responsiveness arising from a reduction in reinforcement and activity. Specific and important models include aggression-turned-inward theory (Freud), object-loss theory (Bowlby), cognitive theory (Beck), and learned helplessness (Seligman).

These theories are complex and some are in conflict. They are not all applicable to each client and some are not supported by research. A detailed consideration of these theories falls beyond the scope of this chapter and readers are referred to textbooks of abnormal psychology (e.g. Davison & Neale 1986) and psychiatric nursing (e.g. Stuart & Sundeen 1987).

The following discussion will be restricted to a consideration of predisposing or 'triggering' factors and major explanatory hypotheses associated with the onset of depression in late life.

A starting point is the well-established finding that the genetic contribution to the aetiology of depression decreases with age (Stenstedt 1959, Kay 1959, Post 1962, Hopkinson 1964). Thus, in late life depression, ageing-related changes in the individual's internal/external environment would seem to assume increasing importance. We are grateful for a helpful paper by Meyers and Alexopoulos (1988) which identifies three main sources of such changes. These are: the development of physical disease and disability; social stressors involving loss; and ageing-related changes to the central nervous system.

PHYSICAL DISEASE AND DISABILITY

A number of physical illnesses have been found to be associated with depression and elderly people are at increased risk of developing many of these. If the physical illness is relieved the depression is also likely to lift. However, prolonged depression may impede physical recovery and may require specific attention. Both the illness itself and its treatment — drugs/surgery — may be associated with depression, separately or in combination. Examples of physical illnesses and drugs associated with depression are shown in Table 20.1.

In certain cases, causal connections between physical illnesses and depression are well established; for example, 50% of clients suffering from pancreatic carcinoma exhibit symptoms of depression prior to other clinical manifestations, which leads to the conclusion that depressive symptoms are caused by the specific illness (Fras et al 1967). However, in many other cases causal

Table 20.1 Examples of physical illnesses associated with depression. *After the Open University (1988).*

Body system	Disease	Notes
Various	Chronic ill health	May perpetuate depression in elderly people
	Carcinoma	
	Infections, e.g. influenza and herpes zoster (shingles)	Many infections may cause mental disorders
Vascular	Stroke	More likely to arise in a right hemiplegia (in a right-handed person) since the centre for spatial awareness is usually not disturbed and thus the client is aware of her disability
Nervous	Parkinson's disease	Be aware, however, that neurological changes may affect facial expression, giving an appearance of depression even when this does not exist
Sensory	Blindness in late life	Also associated with confusional states and paranoid disorders
	Deafness	
Endocrine	Myxoedema	
	Hyperparathyroidism	
Digestive	Pernicious anaemia	May also cause chronic confusion
Hepatic	Liver disease, e.g. acute/chronic hepatitis	

mechanisms are unclear. The bodily illness may be a physiological precipitant of depression; but, conversely, depression may be an emotional response to perceived loss of health or a consequence of persistent disability. These issues are well demonstrated by studies of post-stroke depression, which suggest that depression shortly following a stroke is often attributed to physiological factors, but if delayed may be seen as an emotional response to disability (Robinson et al 1985).

Since elderly people are particularly at risk of developing chronic incapacitating illness, the differential contribution of chronic disability and acute medical illness and the links between these is of particular interest.

Brown and Harris, (1978) concepts of 'provoking agents' (in the form of life crises) acting in combination with 'vulnerability factors' to produce depression was applied to elderly people by Murphy (1982). She found acute medical illness to be the most frequently occurring major life event and her study suggests that chronic health problems increase individual vulnerability. Poor physical health has also been found to be predictive of a poor outcome in treated cases (Murphy 1983, Baldwin & Jolley 1986).

A particular problem with respect to disabled elderly people who may also be depressed is how to avoid confounding one condition with the other — or, more specifically, how to distinguish somatic symptoms due to depression from those arising from chronic disability or an accompanying physical illness (Raskin 1979, Salzman & Shader 1978).

Clues to psychological distress are often not recognized within the context of physical care (Maguire 1985), with the result that signs of depression such as slowed activity, poor appetite, weight loss, disturbed sleep, fatigue, weakness and sexual indifference are likely to be attributed to the client's generally poor health. This is particularly likely when the disturbance of mood is not really evident ('masked' depression), as is quite often the case amongst elderly depressed people with coexisting physical illness (Cohen-Cole & Stoudemire 1987, Ouslander 1982).

Gurland et al (1988) point out that change, in the chronically disabled person's behaviour is the crucial clue that clinical depression has supervened. Unless a reliable informant is at hand, ad hoc consultations by a psychiatrist may be less likely to pick up diagnostically significant changes than careful observation and monitoring by nurses who have regular or, in the case of hospitalized clients, 24-hour contact. Warning signs of depression include an increase in demands and hypochondriacal complaints, sleep disturbance with bouts of brooding and wakefulness, indecisiveness, increased alcohol consumption, and increased social withdrawal (Gurland et al 1988). The elderly client who becomes 'awkward' should always be suspected of being depressed.

Indications that depression is not present in a physically ill client include an interest in things going on around them, a positive response to warmth and affection and maintenance of a sense of humour (Gurland et al 1988).

Certain scales for depression are thought to retain good diagnostic discrimination in the presence of physical illness (Yesavage et al 1983) but are no substitute for good nursing observation and monitoring change over time.

It should also be noted that depression may arise in association not only with physical disease but also with other mental disorders. It may occur, for example, along with paranoid disorders or as a consequence of or precedent to alcohol abuse.

Depression may also be a forerunner of dementia and quite often accompanies dementia, when it may be known as 'organic depression' (Pitt 1986). Roth (1983) considers that this is particularly common in multi-infarct dementia, with about a quarter of all cases being affected. Coexistence of the two conditions can make the assessment of depression difficult, since the symptoms are masked by intellectual impairment. One of the main dangers is that depression in an elderly person may be misdiagnosed as dementia and therefore not treated appropriately. Clinical experience suggests that if in doubt doctors may prescribe a course of antidepressants and monitor results.

Physical illness or chronic disability may result in hospitalization or admission to long-term residential care. The debilitating effects of some institutions are well documented. Care practices may deprive elderly people of a sense of power and control over their environment. Those who would like to have some control but feel that this is impossible may suffer from lowered morale and self-esteem and experience feelings of helplessness (Seligman 1975); this has been linked with depression and may contribute to withdrawal, physical disease and even death (Rodin & Langer 1977). Conversely, those elderly people who perceive that they have a degree of control report higher morale (Chang 1978, 1979, Ryden 1983). These factors illustrate the importance of nurses being aware of the expectations of their elderly clients and of the importance of interventions designed to maintain self-esteem and thus guard against the onset of a depressive illness.

In sum, there is an emerging consensus that health and psychological well-being are intimately related. Elderly people are at high risk of physical ill health and chronic disability and there are positive associations between these factors and clinical depression. However, Meyers and Greenberg (1986) found that 54% of physically well depressive clients had their first episode of depression after age 60. This study excluded individuals with chronic disability and those who had a history of physical illness around the time of the onset of depression. However, it does suggest the need for alternative explanations.

SOCIAL CAUSATION: THE IMPACT OF LOSS AND SOCIAL SUPPORT

The assumption of a causal link between stress and depression lies at the heart of explanations of the role of social factors in the aetiology of depressive illness. Pioneering work by Holmes and Rahe (1967) suggested that the degree of change experienced by individuals determines its degree of stressfulness. More recently, this suggestion has been challenged by researchers concerned with the meaning of changes to the particular individuals involved and with factors such as locus of control, the fatefulness of an event, desirability and lack of mastery (Dohrenwend et al 1978, Meyers & Alexopoulos 1988).

Paykel et al (1969) found that life events perceived as undesirable rather than overall life changes were frequent precipitants of depression and that 'exit' events which involved separation or

interpersonal loss had the greatest impact. This finding is supported by studies of bereavement, which have found that perhaps 35% of widows and widowers become clinically depressed within three months of their loss (Clayton et al 1972).

Gerner (1979) has described a 'social deprivation syndrome' characterized by withdrawal, apathy and pessimism which, he considers, arises from cumulative losses in old age of social contact, personal resources and meaningful activity. This syndrome may appear indistinguishable from clinical depression but the sufferer will respond to resocialization and structured activity. Thus, in the case of wards in which residents exhibit high levels of withdrawal and apathy, reviewing nursing care practices may prove a better starting point than treating individuals medically.

Brown and Harris (1978) hypothesize that social factors play such a crucial role in causing depression that irrespective of differences in constitutional predisposition, all individuals would become depressed if they lived long enough to be exposed to sufficient provoking agents. Murphy (1982) in applying this hypothesis to a sample of elderly people found a background of social disadvantage, such as housing problems and financial hardship, poor health and adverse life events, to be associated with depression in old age. However, the negative impact of these social losses would seem to be mediated by the individual's perceived social support. Thus Murphy (1982) found that old people with no intimate confiding relationship were three times more vulnerable than those who reported having an intimate confidante of some kind.

These findings are in line with other studies, which have found a relationship between social isolation and depression in old age; however, the nature of this relationship is complex. Lowenthal, in a series of studies in San Francisco (Lowenthal 1964, Lowenthal & Haven 1968), found that those who adapted negatively to the stresses of old age were not those who were life-long isolates by choice. Rather, they were those who had throughout life sought the intimacy of others but had failed. As for those who were previously socially integrated but had become socially isolated in old age, this was found more likely to be a consequence of mental illness rather than a cause.

Lowenthal (1964) found that those who had a good relationship but who lost it fared better; thus it seems that it is 'better to have loved and lost than never to have loved at all'.

Murphy (1982) found that old people with infrequent contact with a confidante, perhaps a child or a sibling, were as protected against depression as those who had a close relationship with a spouse. This suggests that it is the capacity for intimacy rather than the closeness or frequency of intimate contacts that provides a protective buffer against the social losses of later life. That this capacity for intimacy can be regarded as a personality trait is suggested by the fact that two thirds of those old people who reported not having a confidante could not remember having had one at any time in their lives.

In a helpful discussion of social factors in late life depression, Murphy (1986) concludes that those with a long-standing incapacity for close friendship and who are also most vulnerable to social misfortune are most at risk of becoming depressed in old age.

Meyers and Alexopoulos (1988) point out that theories of social causation owe much to studies involving samples covering a broad age range, and that the relevance of these to late onset depression is uncertain. Older individuals suffer more major losses than younger individuals (Palmore 1969) but may be more able than younger people to cope and adapt to these anticipated ageing-related events (Neugarten 1970). They may, however, be less able to cope with unanticipated events. Research evidence on these and other questions is lacking (Blazer 1982). Whilst social factors are clearly important, systematic testing of relationships between loss, physical health, perceived and real social support and emotional well-being is required if the role of social stress in the aetiology of late life depression is to be clarified (Blazer 1982, Meyers & Alexopoulos 1988).

AGE-RELATED NEUROPHYSICAL CHANGES IN THE CENTRAL NERVOUS SYSTEM

The so-called 'ageing brain hypothesis' emphasizes the central role of age-related neurophysical changes in late onset depression. The hypothesis is that at an undefined point of degeneration clinical depression will occur. The closer individuals come to this point the slighter the external stress required to precipitate a depressive illness. Thus in extreme cases of degeneration external stressors may not be involved and clinical depression may come 'out of the blue'.

Individuals who suffer depressive episodes from early adult life may be predisposed genetically to reach this degenerative threshold, whilst those who suffer late onset depression become vulnerable through the biological processes of ageing (Meyers & Alexopoulos 1988).

Research findings in this area are complex and conflicting. The present conclusion is that changes in the structure and function of the central nervous system which accompany ageing may act as predisposing factors for depression, perhaps especially in males (Philpot 1986). The mechanisms by which these biological factors interact with life events and physical illness remain speculative. However, Murphy's (1982) finding that between 15 and 20% of late life depressive illnesses 'come out of the blue' suggests that in a small proportion of elderly people depressive illness may have a purely organic basis. Further details may be found in Philpot's (1986) helpful review of biological factors in depression.

In recent years, useful attempts have been made to integrate theories of depression and produce unified models — see for example Akiskal & McKinney, (1973).

IDENTIFIED PROBLEMS OF DEPRESSION IN OLD AGE

The main behaviours and problems of an elderly depressed person may be assessed by the nurse with regard to emotional, physical, cognitive and social functioning. These problems will vary within individuals and from one individual to another. They will also vary, according to the severity of the condition, along a continuum — from mild to moderate to severe. The mildly depressed elderly person may be described as unhappy but may not be classified as clinically depressed until her degree of depression becomes moderate or even severe. The majority of elderly depressed people fall in the middle range of this continuum and are not easily 'pigeon-holed' into 'illness' or 'not illness' categories (Murphy 1985).

EMOTIONAL

Lowered mood

A problem experienced by all depressed elderly people is a lowering of mood and a general pre-occupation with gloomy thoughts. In mild depression these feelings may not persist all day but are always ready to come to the surface. As depression deepens the client may feel persistently low and experience diurnal variation, which often takes the form of feeling worse in the latter part of the day. The client may complain of feeling 'down in the dumps', 'blue', low, sad or of having 'a weight on her mind'. She will be aware that her mood is affecting her ability to maintain her normal pattern of activities and this will exacerbate her feelings of pessimism. She will cry easily, feel that no one can help her and believe that her position is hopeless.

Severely depressed people may not necessarily look sad and may not necessarily cry. Their mood may have gone beyond tears and they may see nothing ahead but darkness and suffering. Even when something good happens they may be unable to derive any pleasure from it. At all levels of depression, lowered mood may be reflected in suicidal thoughts and actions.

PHYSICAL

Somatic complaints

In younger clients lowered mood is often the main complaint, but in older depressed clients this is often not the case. Characteristically the elderly depressed person expresses her illness through complaints of bodily symptoms — especially constipation and abdominal pains. As the depression deepens, somatic complaints may become more widespread — muscular pains, headaches, palpitations — and these may be accompanied by

irritability, outbursts of temper and symptoms of anxiety.

De Alarcon (1964) found that almost two thirds of a sample of depressed elderly clients admitted to hospital had hypochondriacal complaints. In terms of identification, an important finding was that this was the first indication of depression in 30% of cases, preceding overt depression by two to three months. In only 20% of those with hypochondria was it a feature of their previous personality.

Pitt (1986) points out that complaints of a persistent pain may sometimes be the overwhelming presenting feature of depression in an elderly person. Typically, the patient provides an elaborate although imprecise description of the pain and is vague about its location. She is likely to request analgesia and hypnotics, although she complains that they are unhelpful and her pain becomes a total preoccupation which dominates all her conversation. Assessment may reveal that the pain has existed for a long time but has been exacerbated by depression, probably through lowered tolerance. Alternatively, it may have arisen along with other problems associated with depression, but these have receded and the pain has gradually taken over. According to Pitt (1986), these elderly depressed clients may often be found to have lapsed into a passive, dependent existence and require the attention of a close attentive relative to undertake daily activities, most of which they are capable of carrying out independently.

The expectation amongst doctors and nurses that older clients may have diverse physical ills means that somatic complaints, particularly in the mild to moderately depressed client may lead to the depression being missed altogether or to an undue delay in starting treatment.

The evaluation of somatic complaints in an elderly person known to be physically ill but who may also be depressed is particularly problematic. Pitt (1986) suggests that in such cases bodily complaints may have to be put on one side and other possible indications of depression considered.

Loss of appetite and weight

Appetite declines and there may be some loss of

weight. Constipation is a constant complaint and in severe depression life is threatened through starvation and dehydration. 'Comfort eating' and associated weight gain sometimes seen in young depressed patients is uncommon in elderly people, particularly where the depression is severe.

Decrease in sex drive

Sexual drive and interest is lost as the depressed state deepens, in line with loss of interest or pleasure in usual activities.

Loss of physical energy

In mild depression the elderly patient may complain of tiredness and having to make an effort to get through the day. In extreme cases the client may have so little energy that she can hardly drag herself around.

Psychomotor retardation or agitation

In severe depression psychomotor retardation shows itself in delayed speech to the point of total silence, slowed movements to the point of immobility (with consequent incontinence) and stupor with refusal of food and fluids. Pitt (1986) points out that severe retarded depression may not be recognized as a life-threatening condition in urgent need of treatment, but may be interpreted as the old person's evident wish to die; further, it may be felt that this wish should be respected.

In a less severe form, retardation manifesting itself in withdrawal, peevishness, and apathy may resemble the stereotype of 'crabbed age' (Pitt 1986) and may be misinterpreted as a severe form of the ageing process.

Rather than manifesting retardation the client may appear agitated and burn up physical energy in restlessness and unproductive activity. The classic late life depressive illness was considered to be 'involutional melancholia' (Stenstedt 1959), in which agitation and extreme nihilistic hypochondriacal delusions were the dominant problems. However, this combination may also be found in younger depressive clients.

Sleep disturbance

Sleep disturbance is common. Characteristically, elderly people with mild depression may have difficulty falling asleep and be restless during the night. More severely depressed clients typically fall asleep without difficulty but wake at least two hours before the usual time and are unable to fall asleep again. If concern with insomnia becomes the primary complaint, the doctor may feel pressured into prescribing higher and higher doses of hypnotics.

Hypersomnia may be seen in younger depressive clients but is uncommon in elderly patients.

COGNITIVE
Loss of concentration and motivation

Concentration declines and the client may find it difficult to settle to any task — reading, watching TV — for more than short periods. The client may complain that every little thing requires a major mental effort and may lose motivation to undertake almost any task.

In elderly clients, cognitive problems may give the appearance of dementia; this is called 'pseudo-dementia'. Various checklists of symptoms have been devised to differentiate pseudo-dementia from organic dementia (e.g. Wells 1979) but these conditions remain difficult to differentiate, particularly since depression may be a forerunner of dementia and may often accompany dementia in old age (Pitt 1986).

Negative thoughts

As depression deepens the elderly client may be self-reproachful, ruminating about having mismanaged her affairs, or having let herself down. She may look on the gloomy side of everything and complain that her life has been a complete failure. Sometimes these negative thoughts may be echoed by fleeting hallucinatory voices which berate the client.

The self-reproach and feelings of injustice of mild and moderate depression may take on a psychotic quality as depression deepens, assuming the form of delusions. These are usually mood-congruent, taking various forms in different people. Commonly they appear as delusions of guilt and self-blame ('I'm wicked'; 'I should be put in prison'), or of poverty ('I'm ruined'; 'I'm going to be evicted') or are nihilistic in nature ('I can't eat because everything's blocked up' 'I'm dead'). Occasionally, paranoid ideas surface, probably because the profoundly guilty person believes that others know of her misdeeds and are planning retribution.

SOCIAL
Social withdrawal and isolation

A combination of loss of interest, feeling 'down in the dumps' and fatigue results in social withdrawal. Particularly if the elderly client is also irritable or hostile, family and friends may feel alienated and be less inclined to visit.

Loneliness and social isolation may arise from abandonment but Pitt (1986) points out that it may also be a primary complaint of an old person who is in fact depressed. Factors such as failing health or memory or traumatic life events such as a fall or being mugged may generate understandable anxiety and a rational request for a place in a Home. However, if an elderly person who has lived alone for many years and who has been generally contented urgently seeks resettlement, depression should be suspected. In such circumstances Pitt (1986) warns against a hasty move into residential care which the elderly person may come to detest once her mood has lifted.

Family stress

This can be created by a variety of factors. Loss of sexual interest may create marital difficulties or relatives may become angry and frustrated with the patient, who they may see as making little effort to 'buck up'.

Behaviour problems

Drawing upon his clinical experience, Pitt (1986) identifies several behaviour problems of elderly depressed patients which often come to dominate all others and become the prime focus for therapeutic intervention. These are food refusal, incontinence, screaming and aggression to others.

Food refusal, possibly with regurgitation, and a marked loss of weight may at first appear to be linked to other problems such as despair, suicidal intent or somatic complaints. However, these may fade into the background so that food refusal becomes predominant. Parallels with anorexia nervosa in younger patients are superficial but, as in the latter condition, or as with children who will not eat, the result may be a battle of wills between the elderly depressed patient and the family and therapeutic team. This battle of wills may itself become part of the dynamics of the problem. According to Pitt (1986), many of these patients make little progress and die.

Incontinence of urine and faeces is not infrequently associated with depression in elderly people either as a causal factor inducing humiliation or, as previously mentioned, the outcome of lowered physical energy. However, Pitt (1986) claims that some elderly depressed inpatients will purposefully eliminate in the wrong place and may sometimes compound this by faecal smearing. This may be a form of angry regression; analogies with encopresis and enuresis in childhood are suggested and the fact that these clients are inpatients would seem significant.

A little less common is the depressed elderly person who starts to scream in the middle of the night, wakes neighbours and may continue to scream for a while if admitted to hospital. The elderly person is unable to give an adequate explanation of her behaviour and Pitt (1986) suggests that it may be interpreted as arising from disinhibited lonely despair.

The elderly patient who for no apparent reason kicks, scratches or bites the person who comes to help her will be only too familiar to many nurses. However, the fact that this patient may be depressed may often be overlooked.

All these behaviour problems would seem directed at others by elderly people whom Pitt (1986) describes as being in a state of resentful dependency. As indicated in the previous chapter, certain attitudes and behaviours of carers may reinforce dependency and these behaviour problems may sometimes be the outcome of care practices.

This section indicates that depression in old age may manifest itself as a variety of problems and suggests that the underlying mental state may be missed or dismissed. Old people who are unhappy and withdrawn are disinclined to visit their doctor and, even if they do, their complaints may be ascribed to a physical illness, interpreted as a reaction to getting older, or even seen as an integral part of the ageing process itself. Failure to recognize indications of depression may delay the start of treatment. This may lead to a deepening of depression, worsen the likely outcome (Pitt 1986) and, possibly, have fatal consequences.

PREVENTION OF DEPRESSION IN OLD AGE

Murphy (1985) suggests that preventability rests upon a thorough understanding of aetiology and points out that with respect to depression this has not yet been achieved. However, three groups of factors which help to explain depression in old age have already been discussed — neurophysical age-related changes in the central nervous system, physical disease and disability, and social factors. The following paragraphs draw upon Murphy's (1985) helpful paper in discussing the implications of these factors for nurses working with elderly people living at home.

As previously noted, the genetic component for depression in old age is small. However, there are age-related changes in the structure and function of the brain which may act as predisposing factors and some severe depressions in old age may have a purely organic basis. Causal mechanisms linking neurophysical changes and psychosocial factors are speculative, and in our present state of knowledge prevention of age-related biological changes is not possible. Thus a consideration of other causative factors is indicated.

The close link between physical disease and disability and depression has been noted and it seems possible that preventing physical illness and associated handicaps may reduce the occurrence of depression amongst elderly people. There is ample evidence that health hazards are higher in the elderly population and thus the usual economic objections to mass screening programmes do not apply. Modest screening programmes for the over-70s would offer the possibility of earlier detection and treatment of physical illness and it is unfortunate that the present patchiness of age/sex registers in general practice appear to impede their development (Stevenson 1989).

Nurses have opportunities to provide information on such issues as diet and smoking during their day-to-day contact with clients of all age groups and may thus help reduce the prevalence of cardiovascular disease. Such interventions may in turn reduce the occurrence of severe depression amongst elderly people associated with disabling health problems such as strokes and heart attacks. However the picture is more complex than it at first appears. As Murphy (1985) points out, the wide range of illnesses found in depression indicates that the meaning of the illness for the individual involved is more important than biological mechanisms. Thus, for example, loss of mobility may lead to a dependence on others to maintain social relationships, serious illness may generate fear and anxiety about the future, or chronic pain may reduce individual tolerance to life's irritations.

Murphy (1985) suggests that sensitive management of physically ill elderly people by members of the primary health care team opens up the possibility of a variety of preventive mental health strategies. Quality of life may be improved by the provision of appropriate physical aides and adaptations to assist the individual to maintain daily living activities and by direct nursing assistance with activities which the old person may find impossible to perform unaided, such as bathing, getting up and going to bed.

Lightening the load on family carers through the provision of practical help may make the old person feel less of a burden and generally improve family relationships and morale. Physical care may provide a vehicle for establishing a therapeutic relationship with the client and her family, which may be a source of psychological support. The future consequences of a serious illness or disability may often be frightening and the nurse may alleviate anxieties and fears by taking time to listen, providing information on the illness and advising on coping strategies. The nurse should be conscious of early warning signs of demoralization and depression and draw upon the advice and skills of the specialist psychogeriatric health care service as appropriate.

There is clearly much to learn about social influences on depression in old age and the implications for preventive strategies are unclear. However, the close association between social and economic deprivation and emotional distress is well established. Middle-class property-owning elderly people, whether disabled or otherwise, are able to choose to move house, take a holiday or employ domestic help. Other elderly people have no such choices. Murphy (1985) suggests that improving the financial status of elderly people would reduce the frequency of stressful class-related life events, promote a sense of psychological security, and give old people a sense of mastery over their future options. These are component elements of hope and it is perhaps the periodic renewal of hope which prevents feelings of depression and demoralization from becoming chronic.

The direct influence of nurses over the social and economic status of their client is limited. However, the close links between deprivation and poor health in all age groups suggests that nurses should seek to promote the welfare of disadvantaged social groups through active participation in the political process both as individual citizens and through the work of their professional associations.

The link between depression and precipitating severe adverse life events — bereavement, separations, illness and so on – is well established and the value of crisis intervention therapy in reducing distress and the possibility of a depressive reaction has been demonstrated. According to theorists, crises represent both a threat to previously successful coping mechanisms and an opportunity for personal growth. The need for a prompt response is highlighted by the belief that a person is psychologically less defended during the 4–6 week crisis period and is consequently more amenable to change (Caplan 1964, Baldwin 1988). The dis-

tress experienced during this period and the desire to alleviate it motivates the client to adopt new ways of dealing with problems and to engage with the nurse or another health care professional in a problem-solving partnership. The aim of crisis intervention is to re-establish the client's level of functioning to a pre-crisis level or better. However, this may not be realistic in the case of many elderly people, who may have fewer options than those who are younger. When faced, for example, by the loss of a lifelong partner a more realistic goal may be for the elderly person to maintain some hope for the future and avoid slipping into a state of melancholy and despair.

Various studies have identified factors which indicate high risk of developing an abnormal grief reaction following bereavement. These factors include an unsupportive family or social network, a particularly traumatic bereavement, a highly ambivalent relationship with the deceased and the presence of another major concurrent life crisis. Parkes (1980) in a review of studies of bereavement counselling (incorporating specific support for grief and the encouragement of mourning) concludes that counselling can reduce the risk of an abnormal grief reaction for a high risk bereaved person to that of a low risk person. He also concludes that a trained and experienced volunteer counsellor is able to provide this service at least as well as many professional workers. The implication is that bereavement counselling services offering a befriending and counselling service, ideally in the client's home, may help to prevent the onset of depression, particularly in cases of elderly bereaved people with poor social supports.

Murphy (1985) acknowledges the importance of bereavement counselling schemes and other counselling approaches which draw upon crisis theory, but questions whether those elderly people who are prepared to accept formal counselling are those at risk of developing a depressive illness. She points out that those who are most prepared to accept such a service are those who already recognize the value of support from others and the importance of talking about their problems. Paradoxically, it may be those elderly people who feel ill at ease and most likely to reject the offer of counselling who are at greatest risk. This indicates the importance of providing less formal opportunities to elderly people to discuss their losses, and again highlights the important role of the nurse, who is often best placed to develop a trusting relationship with her elderly clients whilst giving physical care and practical support.

Nurses who undertake bereavement counselling of a formal or informal nature require knowledge of the phenomenon of grief (see Parkes 1972) and counselling skills. Worden (1984) outlines ten principles of bereavement counselling — summarized in Table 20.2 — and provides a helpful description of how they may be applied.

Murphy's (1982) finding that a confidante may be a buffer between the elderly person and the social losses of late life raises the issue of providing alternative social supports for those who have the capacity for intimacy but have no close relatives. The popularity of day centres, luncheon clubs and hundreds of clubs and interest groups indicate the value of these in maintaining morale and hope for the future. However, the value of these formal organizations in protecting people from the impact of life crises will clearly differ according to the quality of relationships which they foster. A file of all local resources, services and agencies listing the names of local contacts and details of the referral method can be a valuable source of information for

nurses trying to establish a supportive social network for elderly clients.

Whilst formal facilities for meeting others are important for many old people, Murphy (1985) suggests that special clubs and residents' lounges in sheltered housing schemes are more likely to attract elderly habitual extroverts rather than those who are at most risk of depression. Perhaps of greater significance for elderly people living alone are informal social networks fostered or otherwise by features of the local environment. For example, Murphy (1985) points out that thoughtful town planning and co-ordinated planning of housing and social services can have a marked impact on the experience of old age. Feelings of loneliness and social isolation may be markedly reduced by cheap and convenient public transport and housing schemes and shopping facilities which provide opportunities for people to meet.

In sum, a general improvement in living standards and health care services are indicated as general measures which are most likely to prevent the occurrence of depression in old age (Murphy 1985). Whilst the promotion of mental health and the prevention of illness is the responsibility of all members of the multidisciplinary team the nurse is particularly well placed to monitor the emotional state of elderly clients and use the provision of physical care as a vehicle for the delivery of psychological support.

Depression, in common with many mental disorders, does not have a single identified precondition; causative factors seem to be multiple and interactive. This suggests the need for nurses working with depressed elderly clients to move away from a conception of primary prevention as the 'prevention of illness' to a more behavioural definition which stresses the 'prevention of problems and maladaptive responses'. Thus, for example, Hollister (1977) calls for the prevention of specific behaviours which are self-defeating or harmful to others (poor diet, smoking, blaming others); role failures (as a parent or spouse); relationship breakdowns (between spouses, between parents and their children); feeling overreactions (panics, anxieties in new situations); and psychological disabilities (falling into depression rather than experiencing normal grief). This perspective

---

Table 20.2 Principles of bereavement counselling. *After Worden (1984).*

1. Encourage the client to talk about the death and admit the loss.
2. Facilitate expression of the client's feelings — anger, guilt, anxiety, sadness, etc.
3. Utilize a problem-solving approach to explore life without the deceased.
4. Discourage emotional withdrawal and encourage new friendships.
5. Allow the client plenty of time to work through her grief.
6. Provide reassurance that 'strange' feelings and experiences are quite normal.
7. Do not expect all clients to grieve in the same way. There are wide variations.
8. Provide continued support over time. Be available at critical times — the anniversary of the death, etc.
9. Assist the client to examine her coping behaviours.
10. Be aware signs of 'pathology' which may require referral for specialist health care.

suggests that there are many agencies already operating within the community which may be defined as undertaking preventive work with elderly people and which should be supported and utilized by nurses in their clinical practice.

NURSING CARE REQUIRED BY DEPRESSED ELDERLY PEOPLE

Depression would seem to arise from the interplay of a multiplicity of genetic, developmental, chemical and interpersonal factors (Akiskal & McKinney 1973) and gives rise to a variety of behaviours and problems. This complexity indicates the importance of individual assessment and encourages an holistic perspective which highlights the importance of multifaceted intervention strategies.

The general aim of care is to increase the amount of pleasure and satisfaction which the depressed client derives from living and to enhance her ability to cope positively with the crises of late life. Specific goals depend upon the particular problems and needs experienced by individual clients. Timing and co-ordination of interventions are discussed in Chapter 18. These are important and should be negotiated by the key nurse in consultation with other members of the multidisciplinary team, the client's relatives and, if possible, the client herself. In considering the timing of interventions it is important to recognize the association between early identification and treatment of depression in old age and a positive outcome (Pitt 1986).

This section outlines some possible interventions in the care of depressed elderly people and draws particular attention to the role of the nurse. It also briefly discusses the outlook for elderly depressed clients who receive treatment.

COUNSELLING

In general terms counselling is the process of helping another person to come to terms with her life and tackle her problems and difficulties. More specifically, it involves the nurse helping her client to reflect upon her life, express her feelings, and develop new responses to her situation. Thus it is a process which begins with self-assessment, moves through increasing self-awareness, involves self-expression and may end in the client exercizing increased self-determination.

There are a variety of approaches to counselling, which are associated with different 'schools'. Arguments about theory may give the impression that counselling is a highly specialized skill requiring lengthy training and that it can only be undertaken by qualified practitioners. This impression is unfortunate because it obscures the fact that counselling involves qualities and techniques — warmth, empathy and good communication skills — which are used in everyday life for helping people with life problems. This is not to deny the importance of good training but it does suggest that the counselling role is available to all nurses who genuinely care about their elderly clients and who are prepared to reflect upon their practice.

Individual and group counselling

Counselling may take place on an individual basis or in groups. Whilst individual counselling is perhaps most common, depressed elderly people who are also lonely and socially isolated may find this difficult, particularly in the early stages. Being asked to consider their problems in isolation may make them feel even more hopeless and these people may often derive more benefit from counselling in groups of other people who face similar situations or share common difficulties. Group counselling may allow depressed, lonely elderly people to appreciate that their problems are not unique and to overcome their self-defeating attitudes and behaviour through adopting a counselling-type role for others. Group approval may also prove an important incentive for members seeking to take action on their own problems.

Family counselling or family therapy may also be indicated where the problems of the older person relates to other family members. Scrutton (1989) makes some suggestions as to how the techniques which have been developed to help families cope with bringing up children may be applied to help those who are experiencing difficulties caring for an ageing relative.

Forms of counselling in nursing

The nature of nursing work often demands a high degree of contact with clients over prolonged periods of time and involves a variety of interactive activities. In this context it is helpful to distinguish between 'structured' and 'unstructured' counselling. In the 'structured' form, counselling is the main task; in the 'unstructured' form, counselling is secondary to the delivery of another aspect of care. In addition to being structured or unstructured counselling may be 'planned' or 'unplanned'; the latter covers occasions when counselling is immediately required. Examples of these forms of counselling are given in Figure 20.1. In practice, the difference between structured and unstructured or between planned and unplanned counselling is one of degree rather than kind ; distinctions are often blurred.

A feature of present-day nursing, particularly in general nursing settings, is that most nurses caring for depressed elderly people have limited experience of structured/planned counselling and may

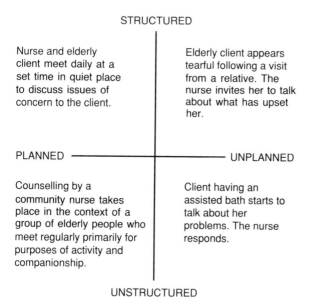

Fig. 20.1 Forms of counselling in nursing: some examples.

find it difficult to develop this aspect of their counselling role. Whilst no other health care professionals have the opportunities for informal counselling afforded to nurses it is important for nurses to distinguish between taking opportunities which arise during the course of nursing work and feeling trapped into a particular way of working.

The issue of ageism

Counselling elderly troubled people requires the nurse to have an understanding of the ageist creation of 'old age'. 'Ageism', which is discussed in detail in Chapter 31 of this volume, is increasingly recognized as contributing to a stereotype of old people which undermines their social status and has a negative impact on their self-esteem.

Scrutton (1989) points out that old people may accept this stereotype and resign themselves to social roles which are inadequate, unrewarding and unfulfilling. Other old people may struggle against the social forces which seek to confine them — but their strategies may be self-defeating. They may strike out at those who appear to represent those forces, such as professional carers. They may also turn on relatives and friends, who may respond with anger and bewilderment and the withdrawal of social support. Thus the old person may become isolated, and feel increasingly unhappy.

Social attitudes may result in old people failing to recognize the importance of social constraints and automatically attributing their troubles and feelings of unhappiness to personal inadequacy or, more commonly, to 'natural', 'inevitable' or 'irreversible' ageing. This may lead to the feelings of powerlessness and fatalism often experienced by depressed older people, which may in turn constrain their lives.

The inexorable processes of ageing affect us all but ageism may often result in these processes being prematurely and universally attributed to people of a prescribed age. In view of these issues the counselling task with many troubled elderly people may be to help them to distinguish between the *reality* of old age and old age as a *social construction* — that is, between factors which are clearly irreversible by the very nature of the ageing process and those aspects of old age that result from personal acceptance of social attitudes which limit the potential of elderly people to lead more fulfilling lives. When counselling elderly depressed people, nurses must consider certain issues, which may be broadly divided into issues of 'content' and 'process'.

Content

The nurse may combat the negative impact of ageism on older individuals by raising issues such as social attitudes within the counselling relationship and helping the client relate these to her own views and self-image. However, it is important to recognize the limitations of counselling in this respect. Counselling may be able to ameliorate the impact of ageism but cannot in itself change the social structures which produce it. Thus, for example, distress and depression may legitimately arise from inadequate finances and poor social conditions which may ultimately require political solutions. In other cases counselling may be helpful but insufficient; other interventions may be indicated — for example, where physical illness or disability causes chronic pain, or where the person is so low in mood that she is unable to respond.

Counselling people of all ages usually focuses upon the unpleasant emotions — low mood, despair, anger, frustration, anxiety, etc. However, the issues giving rise to these emotional states will vary. Scrutton (1989) points out that in the case of older people it is particularly important to determine whether these emotional problems are long-standing and rooted in the person's earlier history or reasonably recent and related to ageing. In the latter case counselling is likely to focus upon issues of loss — loss of friends and relatives, loss of status and roles, loss of physical abilities and of independence.

The counselling agenda may also focus upon late life tasks. Bergmann (1978) identifies four of these. In the first place, there is the problem of accepting the proximity of death. This may require the application of specific counselling techniques, which are discussed later in this section.

Secondly, there is the familiar problem experienced by many depressed elderly people of coping and coming to terms with physical disability and ill health. This may generate emotions associated with loss — guilt, anger and resentment — and these may be directed at the nurse. Woods and Britton (1985) point out that the elderly person may be consumed by a search for the cause of her disability (Why did it happen?) and that this quest is unlikely to be satisfied by the provision of rational information.

The third task is to achieve a rational dependence on various support systems — medical, social and familial — and to identify and exercize choices to achieve maximal satisfaction. Some elderly people cling desperately to what they see as independence and may find it difficult to accept that interdependence is the true reality.

The final task identified by Bergmann (1978) is that of sustaining mutually rewarding relationships with friends and family. Interpersonal conflict and dissatisfaction are common themes in the lives of unhappy elderly people: for example, marital tensions tolerable when partners were separated by work routines may suddenly erupt when retirement brings more time at home together; or unresolved conflicts with children may be reactivated by the elderly parent becoming dependent or having to move into the son or daughter's marital home. Family therapy may be useful in some cases.

Process

Three aspects of counselling should now be considered — the process of change, the nurse-client relationship and counselling skills.

The process of change refers to the elderly client's journey from self-assessment to increased self-determination. On this journey a number of steps and difficulties may confront the client and the counsellor. A knowledge of these will help the counsellor to recognize such difficulties for what they are and to monitor the client's progress. These are complex issues which cannot be discussed here. Interested readers are referred to Sherman (1981), who puts forward a model of counselling older people, and Scrutton (1989) who provides a useful overview of the change process and draws particular attention to the counsellor's response to ageist ideology.

The nature of the counselling relationship is vitally important since it will determine the quality of counselling offered. In Britain, the process of building therapeutic relationships with clients has only recently received attention (see Reynolds 1985). However, in the North American nursing literature there have been a number of attempts to define its components. Of particular influence has been the work of Rogers, who has identified components of 'client-centred counselling' (Rogers 1951). Scrutton (1989) summarizes these as a non-directive approach, non-judgemental attitudes, genuineness, trust and confidentiality, unconditional positive self-regard, and empathic understanding.

Establishing therapeutic relationships with depressed clients who defend themselves against involvement through withdrawal and non-responsiveness is a difficult task. The nurse may commonly experience anger, or resent the client's helplessness, or fear rejection. She may require supportive supervision designed to encourage patience and optimism, so that she can maintain the belief that the elderly depressed person is capable of growth and change and communicate this belief to the client.

In order for quality counselling to take place, nurses must also be skilled. Counselling has been described in this chapter as a special form of communication. Counselling skills are those which enable this process of communication to take place and the problems raised to be addressed. Many of the skills involved in communicating are discussed in Chapter 14 of this volume. Key counselling skills include active listening, establishing an atmosphere of psychological safety, assisting self-expression, interpreting what the client says, building a working hypothesis, focusing on difficult issues, facilitating the exercise of choice and decision-making and avoiding the temptation to give advice. These are discussed in detail in Scrutton (1989).

Whilst the skills employed in counselling older people are similar to those employed with younger age groups there are significant differences. Church (1983) reviews the evidence relating to changes in language, memory and abstract ability which accompanies the ageing process. He concludes that elderly people experience increasing difficulty with psychological approaches which are progressively verbal and interpretive in structure. These findings again cast doubt upon the value of traditional analysis for elderly people.

A number of writers have identified strategies designed to enhance therapeutic rapport with elderly people (Sparacino 1979, Mintz et al 1981, Sholomskas et al 1983, Wattis & Church 1986). Table 20.3 summarizes some of these strategies which nurses may wish to bear in mind when counselling the older client.

In a recent paper Barker (1989) identifies three central interventions which are prescribed in the British nursing literature for interactions between the nurse and the depressed client: the expression of sympathy, the expression of reassurance and the expression of general support and acceptance. What emerges from Barker's paper is that the rationales for adopting these different strategies are rarely explained and that authors have been insufficiently critical of the research base of prescribed care. In other words, the nursing literature informs the nurse of what she should do or say but rarely explains why she should do or say it and does not provide evidence that what she is doing is likely to have positive benefits. Research into the efficacy of particular interactions between nurses and depressed clients is required.

Table 20.3 Guidelines for maximizing therapeutic rapport with elderly clients

1. Be active rather than passive and be prepared to take the initiative.
2. Be aware of the interpersonal context of problems within families, institutions and so on.
3. Establish explicit, concrete goals within a time-limited contract.
4. Be aware of possible ageist attitudes within yourself and critically examine them.
5. Be aware of real social and physical limitations of the individual which may exacerbate 'psychological' problems. Mobilize supportive services where necessary.
6. Be aware of issues of dependence and attachment. It may be necessary to encourage these in the short term to give the client confidence to face her deficits and difficulties.
7. Be aware of the importance of the client having a sense of control within the relationship. This may combat feelings of helplessness and insecurity.
8. Anticipate and be prepared to discuss with your supervisor the particular transference and counter-transference problems which arise; for example grandparent–grandchild is not uncommon where the nurse is young.

SPECIFIC PSYCHOLOGICAL INTERVENTIONS

The previous section has discussed counselling of elderly depressed people in general terms. This section identifies specific psychological interventions which may be helpful to depressed elderly people and which are used increasingly by nurses within the context of the counselling relationship. Most of these interventions may be used with both individuals and groups. Further details may be found in Woods and Britton (1985).

Reminiscence and life review

A further late life task identified by Bergmann (1978) is accepting the proximity of death. Death may be a taboo subject in the client's social circle and may need to be discussed openly within the safety of the therapeutic relationship. The nurse may also assist the process of 'life review' (Lewis & Butler 1974), which entails the client surveying and reintegrating her life experiences. Successful reintegration can give meaning and perspective to life and aid preparation for death by relieving fear and anxiety. Life review has also been found useful in assisting preparation for life, as in the case of an elderly person who has been widowed (Westcott 1983).

The associated process of reminiscence was mentioned in Chapter 19 and is discussed in Chapter 7. Studies of the efficacy of reminiscence therapy with depressed elderly people have produced mixed results. Perrotta and Meacham (1982), in a study of mildly depressed elderly people, compared structured reminiscence with current events discussion and a no-treatment control group and found no changes in depression or self-esteem. Hanley and Baikie (1984) suggest that reminiscence with depressed older people may be counter-productive, since this client group may be inclined to recall negative events selectively. These authors advocate encouraging pleasant rather than unpleasant memories in order to enhance morale. This seems to be the rationale behind the popular 'Recall' package produced by Help the Aged (1981).

In contrast, Fry (1983) used reminiscence to focus specifically on unhappy memories. This study found that the expression of strong emotions and unresolved feelings and fears resulted in a significant reduction of self-reported depression and in increased self-confidence. The efficacy of reminiscence may depend upon how negative feelings are handled when they are expressed, but further studies are required before any firm conclusions can be reached.

Loss and grief work

Central to our understanding of unhappiness and depression in old age must be an appreciation of the impact of loss on the psychic state of old people. Individuals who do not engage in mourning may experience an abnormal grief reaction — i.e. one in which unresolved grief extends over perhaps a year or more. These depressed people may require nursing interventions to help them experience grief within the safety of a therapeutic relationship.

A variety of strategies may be employed. Clinical experience suggests that skilled nurses use cathartic interventions derived from Heron (1975). Hodgkinson (1982) and Mawson et al (1981) discuss the use of 'guided mourning' techniques. Thus the client may be exposed to stimuli such as old photographs and other reminders of the deceased and encouraged to talk about them. The aim of this approach is to facilitate a full emotional response which subsides in the presence of the stimuli as in 'flooding'.

The importance of bereavement counselling for elderly people at the time of bereavement or shortly afterwards to prevent abnormal reactions occuring has already been noted.

Cognitive behaviour therapy

The best known models are often the oldest and many nurses still equate behaviour therapy with stimulus–response psychology; that is, with operant and classical conditioning and the assumption that the principles and procedures acquired from conditioning experiments may be applied to lessen psychological distress in humans. This conception of behaviour therapy is misleading. Behaviour therapy today is characterized by open debates as to which of a range of conceptual models are appropriate and which therapeutic procedures are effective. In recent years behaviour therapy has 'gone cognitive'; many proponents are influenced by conceptual models which emphasize the importance of hidden events — thinking, fantasy, imagination — and pay attention to the world as it is perceived by the client. Thus a guiding principle of stimulus–response theory — that behaviour is the outcome of exterior factors which impinge upon us — has been modified by the recognition that the way in which people interpret the world affects their feelings and behaviour, and is in turn important in determining the nature of their problems. A range of cognitive therapies have developed which aim to help the client identify and change the inner processes which produce or maintain negative emotions.

Cognitive therapy for depression (Beck et al 1980) rests upon the assumption that depression arises from primary abnormalities of cognition — i.e., of judgement, reasoning and remembering. Thus the person may make incorrect assumptions about herself and those around her and have an irrational belief of worthlessness.

The therapy relies upon the therapist forming a collaborative relationship with the depressed client and working with her to define her distress as grounded in specific problems which are capable of resolution. The client may then be helped to subject her irrational and maladaptive beliefs to critical review; thus the client is not persuaded of the incorrectness of her interpretations but gradually comes to discover these for herself. To this end, cognitive and behavioural techniques may be used.

For example, a depressed person who fails at one task is encouraged to view the event as unfortunate but not to overgeneralize (a common cognitive error) and thus believe that failure in future tasks is inevitable. Or we might take the case of a person who is convinced that she constantly feels depressed and who feels even more depressed because of this belief. One behavioural technique which may be used is to encourage the client to record her mood at regular intervals during the day. These reports are likely to vary, in which case they can be used as evidence that life is not in fact always completely miserable. A change in thinking may in turn be used as a springboard for a change in behaviour, such as getting up in the morning or doing some jobs around the house.

Cognitive behaviour therapists recognize that the client's beliefs must be altered if a change in behaviour is to endure. However, perhaps the majority would hold the view that behavioural procedures are more effective than strictly verbal ones in affecting cognitive processes. Certainly behavioural strategies may be more appropriate than cognitive ones for elderly clients whose thinking processes are not intact.

There is substantial evidence that depressed older clients can benefit from psychological interventions. Gallagher and Thompson (1983) compared the impact of cognitive, behavioural and insight-oriented psychotherapy on elderly depressed outpatients who received one of the three therapies for 16 individual sessions over a three-month period. All three were found equally effective in alleviating depression at the end of the treatment period. Severely depressed clients benefited less than those who were less depressed, but some severely depressed clients showed improvement. Those receiving insight-oriented therapy tended to relapse more during the one-year follow-up period. Presumably, clients in the cognitive and behaviour therapy groups were continuing to apply the skills that they had learned.

The short-term nature of cognitive behaviour therapy and its problem-solving focus suggests that it may be suitable for older clients. It may be particularly useful for older depressed clients who are sensitive to medications or who may suffer from medical problems that contraindicate the prescription of psychoactive drugs.

Cognitive behaviour therapy is attractive to nurses since it involves notions of collaboration and partnership. Moreover, it provides a rationale for depressed clients to adopt a problem-solving approach as an alternative to passively waiting for the drugs to work or for something to come along to raise their mood. However, there is a need for research into the efficacy of cognitive behaviour therapy practised by nurses in relation to depressed elderly clients who experience different sets of problems.

There is strong evidence that nurses who are well trained can function as highly effective behaviour therapists (Marks et al 1977, Barker & Fraser 1985). Other nurses have voiced concern that training in behaviour therapy may result in nurses ceasing to be primarily carers, instead seeing themselves as technicians (Shanley 1984) or becoming psychologists' assistants (Wilson-Barnett 1976). These fears are not shared by nurse behaviour therapists themselves, who clearly do not view behaviour therapy as the sole property of psychologists and acknowledge the therapeutic importance of the interpersonal relationship between the therapist and the client (Barker 1982, Barker & Fraser 1985).

Social problem solving

Depression in some elderly clients may be seen as a reaction to problems for which they have no ready solution. One approach to this is training in Social Problem Solving (SPS), which seeks to teach the client skills which may be applied to a wide variety of problems which she may face in the present or future. SPS is essentially an educational therapy and is also an important component of cognitive behavioural therapy. SPS consists of teaching the client a number of steps, the first of which is to see her distress as a reaction to an unresolved problem. Subsequent steps involve teaching the client to define problems, generating alternative solutions through 'brainstorming', assessing the effects of each solution, choosing and implementing the favoured option and, finally, evaluating the solution. The client may have to return to earlier stages in the cycle if her initial solutions prove unsatisfactory.

A study of older depressed clients in a nursing Home found that those who underwent SPS training showed greater improvement than those who were given a more behaviourally based treatment (Hussain & Lawrence 1981). These researchers argue that SPS training may increase the clients' perceived control over their environment — a factor demonstrated to be related to higher levels of self-esteem and contentment (Reid et al 1977, Ziegler & Reid 1979).

Skills training

Skills training is another technique increasingly applied by nurses to enhance an elderly person's sense of control over her environment. A simple example adapted from Woods and Britton (1985) is of an elderly man whose wife dies and is subsequently seen by the community nurse. Since his wife always did the cooking, one 'solution' may be to provide meals-on-wheels. This solution, however, removes the elderly person's choice regarding meals. An alternative may be to arrange for the man to be taught to cook for himself, thus reducing his dependence and increasing his sense of control.

Sometimes the depressed client may require social skills training, which may be provided by nurses. Winefield's (1984) study of skills required to elicit satisfactory support is of interest because it suggests that standard social skills training may produce disappointing results when applied to depressed and lonely people. She suggests a model which in addition to teaching the client to reinforce or reward those who offer attention, incorporates an educational component to provide the client with a clear understanding of the social norms governing intimacy and reciprocation.

PHYSIOLOGICAL INTERVENTIONS
Drug therapy

Antidepressant drugs are of most benefit in moderate and severe depression. The tricyclic group (e.g. imipramine, amitriptyline, dothiepin) are well proven and are usually the drugs of first choice for depressed clients of all age groups. However, fears have been expressed that they may cause cardiac arrhythmias or precipitate infarction. These fears may have been exaggerated (Veith et al 1982), but these drugs are probably best avoided for clients with cardiac problems, many of whom are elderly.

In a study of the use of tricyclic drugs with a sample of depressed elderly people in the USA Richter et al (1983) found that one fifth of the sample reported side-effects and that half of these had to discontinue the drug. Side-effects were more frequent at higher dosage levels and most were the result of the sedative and anticholinergic properties of the drugs, which gave rise to a variety of complaints — in particular, dry mouth, postural hypotension and hesitancy.

Some tricyclic drugs have a marked sedative effect (e.g. amitriptyline) and are usually prescribed for depressed clients who are also anxious. Others, for example imipramine, are more suitable for clients who are slow or withdrawn. Usually the client is prescribed a small dose of 10–25 mg each night rising to 75–100 mg in regularly increasing doses. A dose of between 50–100 mg daily has been reported to be optimal (Richter et al 1983).

There are some newer tetracyclic compounds (e.g. mianserin, maprotiline) which are less proven and certainly seem no more effective than the tricyclics. However, they have the advantage of having fewer side-effects and of being safer for clients with cardiac problems.

There is a third main group of antidepressant drugs, the monoamine oxidase inhibitors (or MAOIs) — for example, tranylcypromine and phenealzine. These do not produce anticholinergic side-effects, but are rarely prescribed for elderly clients because of incompatibility with other commonly prescribed medications (e.g. antiparkinsonism drugs and decongestants) and the need for dietary control.

Elderly clients who are depressed may already be taking other psychotropic drugs for complaints such as anxiety or insomnia. These complaints are likely to be relieved by the antidepressants and other psychotropic drugs should be avoided wherever possible.

The responsibilities of the nurse with respect to antidepressant drugs prescribed for elderly people are similar to those regarding any other prescribed medication. However, there are particular issues to bear in mind. Compliance is crucial to successful treatment but, particularly with older clients, may be difficult to achieve. Many factors are involved (Burns & Phillipson 1986). These include forgetfulness; lack of comprehension of the drug regime; positive decisions by the client to either alter the dosage herself (even after understanding the regime) or to stop taking the drug; the client's

feeling that drug therapy makes no difference to her well-being or that it makes her feel worse. Alternatively, elderly clients with poor follow-up by the doctor or community nurse may continue to obtain repeat prescriptions and take the drug (along with others) forever.

To ensure that these problems do not go unrecognized the community nurse should allow time for ongoing discussion about the drug regime and negotiate the most appropriate strategy with the elderly client and her family. Packaging devices — such as calendar packs similar to those used for oral contraceptives — as memory aids have been found to improve drug compliance in all age groups (Linkewich et al 1974) and may be particularly useful for elderly clients with complicated drug regimes or memory problems. A directive client education group run by nurses has also been found effective in increasing compliance amongst psychiatric outpatients with disorders of mood (Youssef 1983). Alternatives are for a relative to be asked to administer the drug, for the community nurse to call each evening to give it herself, or even to admit the client to hospital.

The nurse should inform the client taking antidepressants and her relatives not to expect any improvement for at least seven days and perhaps up to three weeks after therapeutic doses have been established. Often the client will stop taking the drug once she feels better. Antidepressant drugs should be maintained for three to six months following improvement and then withdrawn gradually. Discontinuing the drug prematurely may precipitate a relapse.

The client should be informed of possible side-effects. These should be closely monitored and reported back to the doctor, since the occurrence of side-effects will guide the rate at which the dose may be increased.

A final factor for the nurse to bear in mind is that antidepressant drugs can be lethal to elderly people even in relatively small doses and are therefore most dangerous in the hands of the people who need them most — those tempted to suicide. This factor highlights the importance of good follow-up, of prescribing in moderate doses and of reviewing progress prior to repeat prescriptions.

Electroconvulsive therapy (ETC)

The main advantage of ECT over other physiological treatments is its speed of action. Suicide and death through self-neglect are very real dangers with elderly people who are moderately or severely depressed and swift and effective treatment may be necessary. Antidepressant drugs may not offer either of these advantages. They take time to act and are reported to be effective in a smaller proportion of clients than ECT (Medical Research Council 1965). They also have a range of unwanted side-effects and, as previously discussed, ensuring compliance may prove difficult.

Some authorities suggest that ECT should be the treatment of first choice with *severely* depressed elderly clients (Roth 1981, Sim 1984). However, drug therapy is more convenient and often more acceptable to the client and her relatives, and in practice the majority of clients treated with ECT will already have been treated with antidepressants. Thus ECT is generally considered by psychiatrists to be a second-line physiological treatment but first choice where the client's life is seriously threatened by a suicide attempt, serious weight loss or dehydration.

As a general rule, ECT is likely to be effective only when the elderly client is suffering from a true depressive illness in which she experiences a range of functional problems in addition to depressed mood. Fraser (1986) identifies the following clinical features as making for a good response in elderly people: 'pathological guilt, agitation, impairment of work and interests, subjectively depressed mood, psychic anxiety and greater overall severity'. He lists contraindications to ECT in elderly people, in descending order of importance, as follows: 'unfitness for anaesthesia, brain tumour, increased intracranial pressure, demyelinating disease, recent cerebrovascular accident or extensive cerebrovascular disease, and poorly controlled heart failure, atrial fibrillation or hypertension' (Fraser 1986, p. 130).

The two most common side-effects of ECT recognized by nurses are confusion in the immediate post-ECT period and longer term memory disturbance. Confusion may last for perhaps 15 minutes or in exceptional cases up to several hours. This period is significantly shortened if unilateral (as opposed to bilateral) ECT is given and this form is the one of choice for elderly clients and, especially, elderly outpatients (Fraser 1986).

The effects of ECT on the memory of elderly people are difficult to measure since there are few memory tests standardized for use with this age group, and other variables may intervene, such as the effect of the depression itself. Studies on clients of mixed ages suggest that they forget information, particularly that acquired before treatment (retrograde amnesia), and that this defect may persist. They also experience impaired learning following treatment (anterograde amnesia). Memory functions improve over time and may be expected to be back to normal within six months following the end of treatment (Weeks et al 1980, Frith et al 1983). A study of 29 elderly clients by Fraser and Glass (1980) found that, in general, memory functions improve as depression is relieved and that memory impairment was not detectable at three weeks following the end of the course. In this same study, elderly clients reported other side-effects which they rated as mild or moderate — notably ataxia (32%), headache (25%), drowsiness (10%), nausea (7%) and double vision (3%). Thirty-two per cent reported no side-effects.

The responsibilities of the nurse with respect to ECT involves physical and psychological preparation of the client, liaison with the family, preparation of the ECT equipment, safe management of the convulsion, and aftercare of the client. These issues are discussed fully in the Royal College of Nursing's guidelines for electroconvulsive therapy (Royal College of Nursing 1982). There are specific aspects of the nurse's role which are of particular interest. ECT is a frightening prospect for many clients and may also arouse strong emotions in nurses. The client and her family will probably have a negative and distorted mental image of the treatment inspired by the media and this may cause her to reject a potentially helpful form of treatment out of hand. In these circumstances the client and her family require factual information upon which to make a rational rather than an emotional decision and reassurance that she will be cared for during and following the treatments.

There is strong research evidence to suggest that ECT is an effective and safe treatment for depressed elderly clients if correctly prescribed. A frequently voiced criticism by nurses is that some psychiatrists prescribe ECT too freely and fail to take full account of more appropriate alternatives. This highlights the importance of nurses having the confidence to challenge clinical decisions as active members of the multidisciplinary team and to support their views with a sound knowledge of the research evidence. A paper by Fraser (1986) is a particularly helpful source of information on the subject.

Physical care and exercise therapy

In depression the client may neglect her physical care and become increasingly unable to look after herself as her depressed state deepens. It is helpful for the nurse to explain to the client that physical problems may be a feature of depression and are likely to be relieved as the depression lifts. Generally, nurses feel skilled and competent in monitoring and handling such problems as dehydration, malnutrition, constipation and insomnia. These problems are discussed elsewhere in this volume and only points relevant to the physical care of depressed elderly people will be mentioned here.

Sleep disturbances are common. In general it is helpful to plan activity in relation to the client's own rhythms; some may feel more alive in the morning, others in the evening. More specifically it should be noted that depressed people experience less stage III and stage IV sleep. These stages are dependent upon the period of wakefulness and for this reason frequent naps or staying in bed all day are likely to exacerbate sleep difficulties. However, a planned rest period may help the elderly client to recharge her batteries for evening activities.

It is well known that exercise promotes sleep, stimulates appetite and may relieve or prevent constipation if combined with adequate fluids. In addition, studies have suggested that exercise reduces anxiety and relieves depression, whether used in isolation or with other therapies, and that its effects are related to intensity and duration (Snyder 1985). Elderly depressed clients may be very reluctant to take exercise because of feelings of lethargy but should be encouraged to do so within their individual capabilities.

The client's movements may be slow and she may be unable to attend to self-care activities — such as skin care, dressing and grooming — which are important for physical comfort and emotional well-being. The nurse should support self-care abilities by giving positive feedback to the client and may provide assistance in activities of daily living when necessary.

The most appropriate response to somatic complaints will vary from one client to another; the approach taken should be discussed in the multidisciplinary team to ensure consistency. In all cases somatic complaints should be noted and properly investigated. In cases in which somatic complaints are closely tied up with depression it may be appropriate for the nurse to gently acknowledge the client's complaints, inform her of the negative results of investigations, discuss them in relation to depression and distract the client through the provision of an activity or another topic of conversation. In cases of severe depression where the complaints have a delusional quality the client may be unable to accept the explanations offered and continually return to her aches and pains in every conversation. In most cases persistence pays in combination with antidepressants or ECT.

Other physiological treatments

Research indicates that depriving some depressed clients of even one night's sleep may improve their condition (Bhanji 1977). However, the duration of improvement varies greatly and how sleep deprivation actually works is unknown. The treatment does not appear to be in widespread use.

Psychosurgery may be used in a tiny proportion of elderly depressed clients, predominantly those who suffer from severe, persistent or recurrent depression that fails to respond to properly admin-

istered ECT or adequate courses of antidepressants. There do not seem to be any recent
research studies of the effects of psychosurgery on
elderly people. The issue is briefly discussed by
Fraser (1986).

Finally, it may be noted that research is under
way to try to identify biological markers of depression. There is currently no foolproof way of doing
this but the Dexamethasone Suppression Test
(DST) is a promising development. This is a
straightforward, relatively inexpensive test with
minimal risks to the client. It seems most useful
in identifying those clients who do not show the
typical behaviours associated with depression but
who may well benefit from antidepressants or
ECT. It may also prove helpful in monitoring recovery. The relatively few reports on the use of
the DST with elderly clients are reviewed by
Philpot (1986).

SOCIAL AND ENVIRONMENTAL CONSIDERATIONS

In every case a decision must be made as to the
most appropriate treatment setting — at home, as
an outpatient, a day patient or an inpatient. This
decision will be influenced by the assessed risk of
suicide, the severity of the illness and its impact
upon the client's daily life, the client's support
systems and available treatment facilities.

Barker (1989) points out that the nursing literature stresses the fundamental role of the nurse in
creating a supportive social environment in which
there are opportunities for recreation, distraction
and social stimulation. In Chapter 19 these issues
have been discussed in relation to the care of
dementing elderly people living in institutions and
many general aspects of the physical and social
environment are also relevant to the care of chronically depressed elderly residents.

Activity

Depressed people of all ages often experience a
decrease in their previous level of activity. The implication drawn in many nursing textbooks is that
an increase in activity will relieve depression since,
as Stuart and Sundeen point out, 'inactivity pre-

vents the patient from obtaining satisfaction and
receiving social recognition . . . so in actuality it
serves to reinforce one's depressed state' (Stuart
& Sundeen 1987, p. 470).

Whilst nursing interventions which encourage a
gradual increase in activity and the provision of
structured activity programmes for severely depressed clients may be helpful within the context
of an overall treatment strategy, it is important to
recognize that activity alone is unlikely to significantly reduce depression in elderly clients.
Lewinsohn and Macphillamy (1974) found that,
unlike their younger counterparts, older depressed
clients did not report any loss of enjoyment in
pleasant activities which they had previously engaged in more frequently. Thus, for these older
clients, inactivity is not necessarily related to the
fact that they do not gain reinforcement from engagement in the activity. Furthermore, Simpson et
al (1981) in a study of residents in an old people's
Home found no relationship between levels of activity and depression. In fact, there was a strong
relationship between engagement in activities
which clients described as enjoyable and mild depression. Woods and Britton (1985) point out that
this study suggests that overt activity is therefore
not the only source of positive reinforcement for
old people and that hidden activities such as reminiscence may be more important in some cases.

The implications of this research for nurses is
that it may be more fruitful to work at a cognitive
level by exploring the significance of particular
activities for elderly depressed clients on an individual basis rather than seek to involve them in
indiscriminate activity programmes.

Opportunities for control

Assessment of the chronically depressed elderly
person living at home may often indicate that she
is lonely, has been neglected by friends and relatives and has no outside interests. The quality of
housing may often be poor and there may be evidence of malnutrition. This state of affairs may
have arisen in a variety of ways. A physical illness
may have precipitated depression which has in
turn led to self-neglect. Family members may have
become increasingly disinclined to visit, in re-

sponse to the elderly person's withdrawal, irritation or hostility. For elderly chronically depressed people living alone or in institutions, experiences of 'helplessness' and 'powerlessness' are integral to depression; thus, as previously mentioned, nursing interventions should seek to create a social environment which increases opportunities for 'control'.

Interventions designed to create opportunities for control will vary from one individual to the next. For the client who has become demoralized through the requirement for age-related retirement or through physical disability, voluntary clubs and organizations may offer opportunities for satisfying employment. For those clients who are fit but isolated, a luncheon club may provide opportunities to form new attachments. Chronically depressed clients living in institutions may derive a sense of control from having personal possessions (such as furniture), caring for plants (Langer & Rodin 1976) or pets, being provided with information (Glass & Grant 1983), or even being able to control or predict the frequency and duration of visits by volunteers (Schulz 1976). Whatever procedures are adopted it seems important that they encourage the client's control over a range of situations and events rather than over one specific event (Rodin & Langer 1977, Schulz & Hanusa 1978).

Whilst a sense of control seems important in mediating the effects of stress, Rodin (1983) points out that approaches to increasing control have limitations. Thus it is conceivable that with some clients efforts may be directed towards helping her give up futile attempts to control the uncontrollable.

Socializing with others may moderate the experience of depression for elderly people since it increases self-esteem through social reinforcers such as acceptance and recognition and is incompatible with depressive withdrawal. However, many elderly chronically depressed clients will be unwilling or unable to become involved with others. They may lack relevant interpersonal skills, in which case the nurse may work with them on improving their social skills and interpersonal style. More frequently the client may simply lack confidence or be self-absorbed and pessimistic and feel unable to avail herself of opportunities. In

these cases the relationship which the nurse may form with the elderly person is crucial in generating hope, encouraging change and motivating her to accept help. Sometimes the provision of practical assistance — such as meals-on-wheels and a home help or transport to and from the day centre — will help to raise morale and restore hope for the future.

The involvement of family and friends will often enrich the elderly person's social environment and the nurse may encourage this by explaining the nature of depression and its possible effects on behaviour to family members. Wherever possible members of the family should be involved along with the client in planning therapeutic interventions. It may sometimes be important for the nurse to examine the client's feelings of powerlessness and helplessness in relation to the family. Not uncommonly, friends and family may inadvertently reinforce depressive behaviours by being helpful, sympathetic or even annoyed in response to them or by ignoring the elderly person when she acts in non-depressed ways. It may be necessary for the nurse or another member of the multidisciplinary team to explore these issues with family members and help them to understand their contribution to the overall strategy.

THE OUTLOOK FOR DEPRESSED ELDERLY CLIENTS

As previously mentioned, depression is the commonest mental health problem in old age. However, most elderly people experience mild or moderate forms and either endure their discomfort, are treated by their GP or seek alternative remedies. Little is known about the outlook of this large group or their response to treatment.

As mentioned, there is evidence that depressed older clients can benefit from psychological interventions both in the short and long term (Gallagher & Thompson 1983). However, follow-up studies of the effects of psychological treatments are rare compared with those by psychiatrists on samples of more severely depressed elderly clients who may be hospitalized and are treated with ECT or antidepressants or both.

Millard (1983), in an analysis of Murphy's

(1983) study of a cohort of elderly depressed clients referred to psychogeriatric services, concluded that for depressed elderly people 'no matter what is done, a third get better, a third stay the same and a third get worse' (Millard 1983). Subsequent studies (Baldwin & Jolley 1986, Baldwin 1988) have suggested that the outlook is in fact less bleak than this summary suggests. Murphy (1985) states that the prognosis is influenced by three important factors: the initial severity of the depressive illness, continuing poor physical health, and adverse life events during the year in which they are followed up.

RESEARCH INTO THE EFFICACY OF NURSING INTERVENTIONS

In his review of the nursing literature on affective disorders, Barker (1989) found only one published nursing research study involving depressed people. This study (Gordon 1986) showed that mildly depressed women who attended group therapy sessions led by nurses showed a significant decrease in depression and an increase in self-esteem as against a control group who received no intervention. This study is important because it was well controlled and suggests that nurses can work effectively as group therapists. However, the relevance of these findings to elderly depressed clients is unclear.

The focus of Gordon's study on younger clients is reflected in research within other disciplines. For example, in a review of mainstream psychology journals Bender (1986) reported that only 10% of experimental papers included clients over 65 years old and only 4% of studies focused specifically on elderly people.

There is a need for nursing research to evaluate the impact of nursing interventions on elderly depressed clients. Whilst a variety of research designs may be useful, it is suggested that prospective researchers consider alternatives to simplistic designs which seek to apply different interventions to 'matched' groups. Groups are extremely difficult to match and one is never sure whether the change in one group rather than the

other was in fact due to the intervention or to another variable. This chapter and Chapter 18 have indicated that the problems experienced by depressed people and their reactions to those problems vary from one individual to the next and that this in turn has implications for the timing and co-ordination of interventions. In view of this, single case study designs may be considered an appropriate method for describing and evaluating these complex individual situations.

SUICIDE IN OLD AGE

Elderly people are more likely to commit suicide than are members of any other age group. In the UK, the incidence of suicides in men over 65 is approximately 20 per 100 000, which is three times higher than that in the 15–24 age group. In all age groups, women are less likely to commit suicide than men. Statistics suggest that female suicide peaks at about 11 per 100 000 in middle age and remains at this level into the eighties. Amongst the very old the suicide rate drops, perhaps because these survivors are the healthiest and most stable of their historical cohort (Lindesay 1986).

These suicide statistics are sobering but perhaps more so is the fact that they are probably an underestimate. Older people have more opportunities than younger people of 'letting go' by neglecting their diet or failing to take their medications and thereby committing suicide in a more passive fashion.

By and large, most elderly people who attempt suicide intend to be successful and use dangerous means. Hanging (more common in men), overdoses of drugs or poison (more common in women), and drowning are the most frequent methods and account for 85% of completed suicides in this age group (Lindesay 1986). Other methods are much less common, although Lindesay (1986) reports that there are increasing numbers of elderly men turning to exhaust fumes as a means of suicide.

Among elderly people most suicide attempts have a fatal intent, whereas in younger age groups, where suicide attempts are more common, they are more often an expression of distress. Sendbuehler and Goldstein (1977) suggest that failed suicide attempts in old age are often serious bids but fail because of confusion due to physical illness, over-medication and alcohol abuse. Their serious nature is indicated by the greatly increased rate of subsequent completed suicide. Compared to the general population, those with a history of attempted suicide have been found to complete suicide 18 times more often in the over-55 age group as against nine times more often in the under-55 age group (Gardner et al 1964).

Studies of attempted suicide in old age should alert nurses to the fact that there is little difference between those who die and those who survive. Thus all such attempts should be taken seriously and the individual should be thoroughly assessed for physical illness, psychiatric disorders and social stressors associated with growing old. These have been identified as antecedent factors in many studies of attempted and completed suicide in old age (Lindesay 1986).

A background of depression is a frequent finding in studies of attempted suicides and in retrospective examination of completed suicide in old age. Depression is very common in old age but only 0.5% of elderly depressed people kill themselves. This leads Lindesay (1986) to suggest that suicide risk is affected by the personal and cognitive context of the depression; thus the intensity of feelings of hopelessness seem to be a more important risk factor than the severity of depression (Beck et al 1975). The implication for nurses is that cognitive behavioural strategies designed to generate more positive attitudes may be an effective preventive measure amongst this high risk group.

Nurses caring for elderly people should be mindful of the possibility of suicide, especially if the client falls into a high risk group, such as those who are recently bereaved, those socially isolated, depressed, suffering from a physical illness or with a history of previous attempts. Studies suggest that elderly people contemplating suicide are less likely than their younger counterparts to tell anyone directly about their intentions or to seek appropriate help from organizations such as the Samaritans.

However, elderly people may communicate their suicidal intentions in more subtle ways. Activities such as putting their affairs in order, making a will or giving away possessions, may of course be quite innocent but should be noted by the nurse and evaluated in context, as should sudden interest in religion — which may involve loss of faith or the client's sudden conversion in preparation to meet her Maker. Perhaps of greater significance is impersonal talk of death and suicide through which the elderly person may be testing out the reaction of family and friends, or overt suicide threats — which should always be taken seriously. If the client lives at home with her family these signals may only be apparent to family members. However they may be unaware of their significance and teaching the family to be sensitive to them may be appropriate.

Whenever the nurse suspects suicidal intent by picking up signals or recognizing that the client is in a high risk group it is important for her (or him) to ask sensitively but directly about suicidal thoughts and plans. Some nurses may fear that in addressing these issues they may put the idea of suicide into the client's mind. These fears are groundless. High risk clients will already have suicidal thoughts and there is no evidence that raising the subject will precipitate a suicidal act. On the contrary, discussing these feelings may help the client to dispel them.

Interventions designed to reduce the risk of suicide will depend upon the nature of the client's underlying problems. In many cases detecting and treating depression will reduce the risk, as may swift referral to specialist psychogeriatric services in appropriate cases. Relieving physical problems such as pain or disability may also be necessary and this may in turn promote the client's sense of independence.

On a more general level, one way of reducing suicide in all age groups is to reduce the means available (Hudgens 1983). Thus the unavailability of guns in the UK means that relatively few people shoot themselves. Similarly, the decline in the suicide rate during the 1960s is usually attributed to the detoxification of domestic gas. The dangers of tricyclic drugs for elderly clients known to be at risk has previously been mentioned. 'Blister packs' have been suggested as an impediment to impulsive suicides since determination must be maintained over several minutes. These may prove helpful in reducing suicide in younger people but their effectiveness against the more determined attempts by older clients has yet to be demonstrated.

Murphy (1985) points out that in this society there is a tendency to see suicide in old age, but not at any other age, as somehow 'normal'. Butler and Lewis (1982) argue that suicide by older people is more likely to be a rational or philosophical decision than in younger people; thus it may reflect a deliberate choice by someone in constant pain, or who does not wish to live out the rest of her life as a burden on others, or who believes that life has no more to offer. This view of suicide as a normal response to the vicissitudes of old age is supported by studies of elderly suicides, which suggest that between 35% and 85% were suffering from serious physical illness (Sainsbury 1962, Barraclough 1971). However, it fails to take full account of the link between suicide and treatable mental health problems (particularly depression) or of the close connection between physical illness and depression; thus it may be unwise to attribute suicide in a physically ill elderly person to rational judgement without considering her mental state. It also fails to recognize the serious impact that suicide may have upon immediate relatives, who may be devastated by their inability to help someone close to them. Moreover, it is a sad reflection on our society that old people will kill themselves because they see themselves as a burden or simply feel that no one cares anymore whether they live or die.

Social attitudes towards suicide in old age may be subtly reflected in the attitude of nurses and other health care professionals, who are often younger and fitter, and may unwittingly try less hard to prevent an older client committing suicide than one who is younger. Whilst rational suicide may occur amongst isolated physically ill elderly people who know that their quality of life is unlikely to improve, it is important to remember that even elderly people are often grateful for another chance at living when the immediate crisis has passed.

CONCLUSION

This chapter has discussed problems commonly experienced by unhappy and depressed older people and has suggested a range of treatment strategies which may be employed to prevent or alleviate them.

Whilst we who are younger may have to accept that deep sadness is, at least for some people, an integral part of the experience of old age (Stevenson 1989), this is no reason for therapeutic pessimism. Depression in old age is neither inevitable nor irreversible and there is much that nurses can do to help older clients find new meaning and purpose in daily living and shift the balance in their lives from sadness towards hope.

REFERENCES

Akiskal H, McKinney W 1973 Depressive disorders: towards a unified hypothesis. Science 182: 20

Baldwin R C, Jolley D J 1986 The prognosis of depression in old age. British Journal of Psychiatry 149: 574–583

Baldwin R C 1988 Delusional and non-delusional depression in late life: evidence for distinct subtypes. British Journal of Psychiatry 152: 39–44

Barker P 1982 Behaviour therapy nursing. Croom Helm, London

Barker P, Fraser D 1985 The nurse as therapist: a behavioural model. Croom Helm, London

Barker P J 1989 The nursing care of people experiencing affective disorder: a review of the literature. Journal of Advanced Nursing 14: 618–629

Barraclough B M 1971 Suicide in the elderly. In: Kay D W K, Walk A (eds) Recent developments in psychogeriatrics. Headley Bros, Ashford, Kent

Beck A T 1967 Depression, clinical, experimental and theoretical aspects. Hoeber Medical Division, Harper and Row, New York

Beck A T, Kovacs M, Weissman A 1975 Hopelessness and suicidal behaviour — an overview. Journal of the American Medical Association 234: 1146–1149

Beck A T, Rush A J, Shaw B F, Emery G 1980 Cognitive therapy of depression. John Wiley, London

Becker J 1974 Depression: theory and research. Wiley, London

Bender M P 1986 The neglect of the elderly by British psychologists. Bulletin of the British Psychological Society, 30 November: 414–416

Bergmann K 1978 Neurosis and personality disorder in old age. In: Isaacs A D, Post F (eds) Studies in geriatric psychiatry. Wiley, New York

Bhanji S 1977 Treatment of depression by sleep deprivation. Nursing Times 73(15): 540–541

Brayne C, Ames D 1988 The epidemiology of mental disorders in old age. In: Gearing B, Johnson M, Heller T (eds) Mental health problems in old age. Wiley, Chichester

Blazer D G 1982 Social origins. In: Blazer D G (ed) Depression in late life. Mosby, St Louis

Brown G W, Harris T O 1978 Social origins of depression. Tavistock, London

Burns B, Phillipson C 1986 Drugs, ageing and society — social and pharmacological perspectives. Croom Helm, Beckenham

Butler R N, Lewis M I 1982 Aging and mental health: positive psychosocial approaches, 3rd edn. Mosby, St Louis

Caplan G 1964 Principles of preventive psychiatry. Basic Books, New York

Chang B L 1978 Generalized expectancy, situational perception and morale among institutionalized elderly. Nursing Research 27(5): 316–324

Chang B L 1979 Locus of control, trust, situational control and morale of the elderly. International Journal of Nursing Studies 16: 169–181

Church M A 1983 Psychological therapy with elderly people. Bulletin of the British Psychological Society 36: 110–112

Clayton P J, Halikas J A, Maurice W L 1972 The depression of widowhood. British Journal of Psychiatry 120: 71–78

Cohen-Cole S A, Stoudemire A 1987 Major depression and physical illness: special considerations in diagnosis and biological treatment. Psychiatric Clinics of North America 10(1): 1–17

Davison G C, Neale J M 1986 Abnormal psychology, 4th edn. Wiley, New York

De Alarcon R D 1964 Hypochondriasis and depression in the aged. Gerontology Clinic 6: 266–277

Dohrenwend B S, Krasnoff L, Askenasy A R et al 1978 Exemplification of a method for scaling life events: the PERI life event scale. Journal of Health and Social Behaviour 19: 205–229

Fras I, Litin E M, Pearson J S 1967 Comparison of psychiatric symptoms in carcinoma of the pancreas with those in some other intra-abdominal neoplasms. American Journal of Psychiatry 123: 1553–1562

Fraser M 1986 Physical methods of treatment for depression in the elderly. In: Murphy E Affective disorders in the elderly. Churchill Livingstone, Edinburgh

Fraser R M, Glass I B 1980 Unilateral and bilateral ECT in the elderly. Acta Psychiatrica Scandinavica 62: 13–31

Frith C D, Stevens M, Johnstone E C, Deakin J F W, Lawler P, Crow T J 1983 Effects of ECT and depression on various aspects of memory. British Journal of Psychiatry 142: 610–617

Fry P S 1983 Structured and unstructured reminiscence training and depression among the elderly. Clinical Gerontologist 1: 15–37

Gallagher D, Thompson L W 1983 Effectiveness of psychotherapy for both endogenous and non-endogenous depression in older adult out-patients. Journal of Gerontology 38: 707–712

Gardner E A, Bahn A K, Mack M 1964 The relationship between premature deaths and affective disorders. British Journal of Psychiatry 115: 1277–1282

Gerner R H 1979 Depression in the elderly. In: Kaplan O J (ed) Psychopathology of aging. Academic Press, London

Glass J C, Grant K A 1983 Counselling in the later years: a growing need. Personnel and Guidance Journal 62: 210–213

Gordon V 1986 Treatment of depressed women by nurses in Britain and the USA. In: Brooking J I (ed) Psychiatric nursing research. Wiley, Chichester

Gurland B J 1976 The comparative frequency of depression in various adult age groups. Journal of Gerontology 31: 283–392

Gurland B, Copeland J, Kuransky J, Kelleher M, Sharpe L, Dean L L 1983 The mind and mood of ageing. Croom Helm, London

Gurland B J, Wilder D E, Berkman C 1988 Depression and disability in the elderly: reciprocal relations and changes with age. International Journal of Geriatric Psychiatry 3(3): 163–179

Hanley I, Baikie E 1984 Understanding and treating depression in the elderly. In: Hanley I, Hodge J (eds) Psychological approaches to the care of the elderly. Croom Helm, Beckenham

Harris D 1975 The myth and reality of aging in America. The National Council on Aging Inc, Washington, DC

Help the Aged 1981 Recall. Help the Aged Education Department, London

Heron J 1975 Six category intervention analysis. Human Potential Research Project, University of Surrey

Hodgkinson P E 1982 Abnormal grief — the problem of therapy. British Journal of Medical Psychology 55: 29–34

Hollister W 1977 Basic strategies in designing primary prevention programs. In: Klein D, Goldston S (eds) Primary prevention: an idea whose time has come. Department of Health, Education and Welfare No (ADM) 77–447. National Institute of Mental Health, Rockville, Md.

Holmes T H, Rahe R H 1967 The social readjustment rating scale. Journal of Psychosomatic Research 11: 213–218

Hopkinson G 1964 A genetic study of affective illness in patients over 50. British Journal of Psychiatry 110: 244–254

Hudgens R 1983 Preventing suicide: editorial comment. New England Journal of Medicine 308: 897–898

Hussain R A, Lawrence P S 1981 Social reinforcement of activity and problem solving training in the treatment of depressed institutionalised elderly patients. Cognitive Therapy and Research 5(1): 57–69

Izard C 1972 Patterns of emotions. Academic Press, New York

Jolley D, Arie T 1976 Psychiatric services for the elderly: how many beds. British Journal of Psychiatry 129: 418–423

Kay D W K 1959 Observations on the natural history and genetics of old age psychoses: a Stockholm material 1931–1937. Proceedings of the Royal Society of Medicine 52: 791–794

Kendell R D 1976 The classification of depressions: a review of contemporary confusion. British Journal of Psychiatry 129: 15–28

Lader M 1976 Depression. Bethlem and Maudsley Gazette Summer: 12–15

Langer E J, Rodin J 1976 The effects of choice and enhanced personal responsibility for the aged: a field experiment in an institutional setting. Journal of Personality and Social Psychology 34: 191–198

Lewis M I, Butler R N 1974 Life review therapy: putting memories to work in individual and group psychotherapy. Geriatrics 29: 165–174

Lewinsohn P M, Macphillamy D J 1974 The relationship between age and engagement in pleasant activities. Journal of Gerontology 29: 290–294

Lindesay J 1986 Suicide and attempted suicide in old age. In: Murphy E (ed) Affective disorders in the elderly. Churchill Livingstone, Edinburgh

Linkewich J A, Catalano R B, Flock H L 1974 The effect of packaging and instruction on outpatient compliance with medication regimes. Drug Intelligence and Clinical Pharmacy 8: 10–15

Lowenthal M F 1964 Social isolation and mental illness in old age. American Sociological Review 29: 54–70

Lowenthal M F, Haven C 1968 Interaction and adaption intimacy as a crucial variable. American Sociological Review 33: 20–30

Maguire P 1985 Barriers to psychological care of the dying. British Medical Journal 291: 1711–1713

Marks I 1975 Modern trends in the management of morbid anxiety: coping, stress immunisation and extinction. In: Spielberger C D, Sarason L G (eds) Stress and anxiety. Hemisphere, New York

Marks I M, Hallam R S, Connolly J, Philpott R 1977 Nursing in behavioural psychotherapy: an advanced clinical role for nurses. Royal College of Nursing, London

Mawson D, Marks I M, Ramm L, Stern R S 1981 Guided mourning for morbid grief: a controlled study. British Journal of Psychiatry 138: 185–193

Medical Research Council 1965 Clinical trial of the treatment of depressive illness. British Medical Journal 1: 881–886

Meyers B S, Greenberg R 1986 Late-life delusional depression. Journal of Affective Diseases 11: 133–137

Meyers B S, Alexopoulos G 1988 Age of onset and studies of late-life depression. International Journal of Geriatric Psychiatry 3(3): 219–228

Millard P H 1983 Depression in old age. British Medical Journal 287: 375–376

Mintz J, Sener J, Jarvick L 1981 Psychotherapy with depressed elderly patients: research considerations. Journal of Consulting and Clinical Psychology 49(4): 542–548

Murphy E 1982 Social origins of depression in old age. British Journal of Psychiatry 141: 135–142

Murphy E 1983 The prognosis of depression in old age. British Journal of Psychiatry 142: 111–119

Murphy E 1985 Prevention of depression and suicide. In: Muir Gray J A (ed) Prevention of disease in the elderly. Churchill Livingstone, London

Murphy E 1986 Social factors in late life depression. In: Murphy E 1986 Affective disorders in the elderly. Churchill Livingstone, Edinburgh

Neugarten B L 1970 Adaption and the life cycle. Journal of Geriatric Psychology 4: 71

Open University 1988 Handbook of mental disorders in old age. The Open University Press, Milton Keynes

Ouslander J G 1982 Physical illness and depression in the elderly. Journal of the American Geriatics Society 30: 593–599

Palmore E 1969 Physical, mental and social factors in predicting longevity. Gerontologist 9: 103

Parkes C M 1972 Bereavement: studies of grief in adult life. Tavistock, London

Parkes C M 1980 Bereavement counselling. British Medical Journal 281: 3–6

Paykel E S, Myers J K, Dienelt M N et al 1969 Life events and depression. Archives of General Psychiatry 21: 753–760

Perrotta P, Meacham J A 1982 Can a reminiscing intervention alter depression and self-esteem? International Journal of Ageing and Human Development 14: 223–230

Philpot M P 1986 Biological factors in depression in the elderly. In: Murphy E (ed) Affective disorders in the elderly. Churchill Livingstone, Edinburgh

Pitt B 1986 Characteristics of depression in the elderly. In: Murphy E (ed) Affective disorders in the elderly. Churchill Livingstone, Edinburgh

Post F 1962 The significance of affective symptoms in old age. Maudsley Monographs 10, Oxford University Press, London

Raskin A 1979 Signs and symptoms of psychopathology in the elderly. In: Raskin A, Jarvik L F (eds) Psychiatric symptoms and cognitive loss in the elderly. Hemisphere, New York

Reid D W, Haas G, Hawkins D 1977 Locus of desired control and positive self concept of the elderly. Journal of Gerontology 32: 441–450

Reynolds W 1985 Issues arising from interpersonal skills in psychiatric nurse training. In: Kagan C (ed) Interpersonal skills in nursing: research and application. Croom Helm, London

Richter J M, Barsky A J, Hupp J A 1983 The treatment of depression in elderly patients. Journal of Family Practice 17: 43–47

Robinson R G, Starr L B, Lipsey J R et al 1985 A two year longitudinal study of poststroke mood disorders. Journal of Nervous and Mental Diseases 173: 221–226

Rodin J 1983 Behavioural medicine: beneficial effects of self control training in aging. International Review of Applied Psychology 32: 153–181

Rodin J, Langer E J 1977 Long term effects of a control relevant intervention with the institutionalized aged. Journal of Personality and Social Psychology 35: 897

Rogers C R 1951 Client-centred therapy. Constable, London

Roth M 1981 Treatment of depression in the elderly. Acta Psychiatrica Scandinavica Supplement 290: 401–433

Roth M 1983 Depression and affective disorders in late life. In: Angst J (ed) The origins of depression: current concepts and approaches. Springer-Verlag, New York

Royal College of Nursing 1982 Nursing guidelines for electro-convulsive therapy. Royal College of Nursing Society of Psychiatric Nursing, London

Ryden M B 1983 Morale and perceived control in institutionalised elderly. Nursing Research 33(3): 130–136

Sainsbury P 1962 Suicide in late life. Gerontologica Clinica 4: 161–170

Salzman C, Shader R I 1978 Depression in the elderly. I. Relationship between depression, psychological defense mechanisms and physical illness. Journal of the American Geriatrics Society 26(6): 253–260

Schulz R 1976 Effects of control and predictability on the physical and psychological wellbeing of the institutionalised aged. Journal of Personality and Social Psychology 33: 563–573

Schulz R, Hanusa B 1978 Long term effects of control and predictability-enhancing intervention: findings and ethical issues. Journal of Personality and Social Psychology 36: 1194–1201

Scrutton S 1989 Counselling older people: a creative response to ageing. Edward Arnold, London

Seligman M E 1975 Helplessness. Freeman, San Francisco

Sendbuehler J M, Goldstein S 1977 Attempted suicide among the aged. Journal of the American Geriatrics Society 25: 245–248

Shanley E 1984 Evaluation of mental nurses by their patients and charge nurses. Unpublished PhD thesis, University of Edinburgh

Sherman E 1981 Counselling the ageing: an integrative approach. Collier Macmillan, London

Sholomskas A J, Chevron E S, Prusoff B A et al 1983 Short term interpersonal therapy IPT with the depressed elderly: case reports and discussion. American Journal of Psychotherapy 37(4): 552–566

Sim M 1984 Re: the diagnosis of depression in old age. British Journal of Psychiatry 144: 101

Simpson S, Woods R T, Britton P G 1981 Depression and engagement in a residential home for the elderly. Behaviour Research and Therapy 19: 435–438

Snyder M 1985 Independent nursing intervention. Wiley, New York

Sparacino J 1979 Individual psychotherapy with the aged: a selective review. International Journal of Ageing and Human Development 9: 197–220

Stenstedt A 1959 Involutional melancholia. Acta Psychiatrica Scandinavica: Supplement 127

Stevenson O 1989 Age and vulnerability. Edward Arnold, London

Stuart G W, Sundeen S J 1987 Principles and practice of psychiatric nursing, 3rd edn. Mosby, St Louis.

Veith R C, Raskind M A, Coldwell J M 1982 Cardiovascular effects of tricyclic antidepressants in depressed patients with chronic heart disease. New England Journal of Medicine 306: 954–959

Wattis J, Church M 1986 Practical psychiatry of old age. Croom Helm, London

Weeks D, Freeman C P L, Kendell R E 1980 ECT: enduring cognitive defects. British Journal of Psychiatry 137: 26–37

Wells C E 1979 Pseudo-dementia. American Journal of Psychiatry 136: 895–900

Westcott N A 1983 Application of the structured life review technique in counselling elders. Personnel and Guidance Journal 62: 180–181

Williamson J, Stokoe I H, Gray S, Fish M, Smith M, McGhee et al 1964 Old people at home: the unreported needs. Lancet 1: 1117–1120

Wilson-Barnett J 1976 Talking point. Nursing Times 72: 962

Wilson-Barnett J, Batehup L 1989 Patient problems: a research base for nursing care. Scutari, London

Winefield H R 1984 The nature and elicitation of social support: some implications for the helping professions. Behavioural Psychotherapy 12: 318–330

Woods R T, Britton P G 1985 Clinical psychology with the elderly. Croom Helm, London

Worden J W 1984 Grief counselling and grief therapy. Tavistock, London

Yesavage J A, Brink T L, Terrence L R, Adley M 1983 The geriatric depression rating scale: comparison with other self-report and psychiatric rating scales. In: Crook T, Ferries S, Bartus R (eds) Assessment in geriatric psychopharmacology. Mark Powley Associates, Connecticut

Youssef F 1983 Compliance with therapeutic regimens: a follow-up study for patients with affective disorders. Journal of Advanced Nursing 8: 513

Ziegler M, Reid D W 1979 Correlates of locus of desired control in two samples of elderly persons: community residents and hospitalised patients. Journal of Consulting and Clinical Psychology 47: 977–999

Zung W W K 1973 From art to science: the diagnosis and treatment of depression. Archives of General Psychiatry 29: 328–337

CHAPTER CONTENTS

The use of drugs for treating elderly patients 374
Therapeutic drugs 374
Replacement drugs 374
Symptomatic relief 374

Prescribing patterns 374

The problems associated with drug use by elderly people 376

Changes in drug response with age 376
Changes in the ability to absorb drugs 376
The absorption of drugs from other sites 377
Changes in drug distribution 377
Changes in metabolism 378
Changes in excretion 378
Changes in receptor sensitivity 379
Adverse reactions 379

Compliance with treatment regimes 380
Refusal of treatment 380
Medication errors 381
Measures to improve compliance 381
Accurate administration 382

Self-medication 383
Problems associated with self-medication 384
Non-drugs 384

Where the nurse can help 385
On admission to hospital 385
Checklist for a drug history 385
During the hospital stay 386
On discharge from hospital 356

The drugs industry 387
Drug monitoring and limited drug lists 387
The drugs industry and health education 387

21

Drugs and elderly people

Jill A. David, Sally J. Redfern

As yet, no drug has been produced which can delay natural senescence. After all, age is not a disease even though many seek a 'cure'. With increasing age the likelihood that anyone will develop a chronic disabling condition increases; physiological ageing and the ravages of time make the body more susceptible to disease, accident or infection and reduce the ability to heal. Many of these conditions can be treated with drugs, allowing the elderly patient years of comfortable, independent living, while others can be relieved without drugs if adjustments of lifestyle are made. For example, the introduction of bran to the diet can reduce the need for aperients as gut motility decreases.

Symptoms of age-related diseases which in the past were suffered as 'part of life', are now treated and as a consequence elderly people expect more from doctors, nurses and the National Health Service, a situation which is both desirable and increasingly expensive. At the present time elderly people (over 65 years) make up approximately 15% of the population but consume 30% of the NHS drugs budget. Nurses can expect to care for more and more elderly patients as the years pass, more and more of whom will be taking drugs. In spite of this, how drugs act in the ageing body is not well understood. It is only comparatively recently that studies on drug handling have been attempted with elderly people and that an awareness of the problems which may be encountered by the patient in adhering to prescribed treatment has emerged. Although nurses are not responsible for diagnosis or the prescription of drugs, they are ideally placed where patients are concerned for observing the effects of drugs, administering the dose and monitoring progress. Their day-to-day contact allows them to assess patients' ability to take their own drugs and to educate patients about drug effects.

THE USE OF DRUGS FOR TREATING ELDERLY PATIENTS

Drug treatment for elderly patients may be initiated for any reason, with the obvious exception of contraception. The conditions most commonly treated are those which are associated with ageing. Those not related to the patient's physiological degeneration must also be treated, while taking into account other drugs used and the body's capability in dealing with drugs. Drugs prescribed fall into three main groups: therapeutic, replacement and symptomatic relief.

THERAPEUTIC DRUGS

These are prescribed for specific curable conditions and include antimicrobials for infection, iron for anaemia and antidepressants. The course is usually short, but may need to be repeated if the problem recurs. Where the body fails to combat the condition (e.g. infection) the condition may become chronic, leading to the continued use of antimicrobials together with anti-inflammatories.

REPLACEMENT DRUGS

These are chemicals, often endogenous substances, used to treat conditions where the chemical is reduced or absent because the body can no longer produce it. Many of these conditions, such as hypothyroidism or diabetes, occur often in elderly people and in such cases drugs can replace the lost chemical and allow the patient to lead a normal life. In parkinsonism, drugs can rebalance the acetylcholine/dopamine levels in the brain, allowing the patient relief from the symptoms. Drug replacement therapy does not, however, cure

the condition and drugs will usually have to be continued for life.

SYMPTOMATIC RELIEF

This can be given for many of the distressing symptoms which occur frequently with age, such as arthritis and rheumatism, cardiac failure, agitation and pain. Once initiated, treatment may need to continue for life and may, from time to time, require a change in dose. With long-term symptomatic relief there is always the problem of keeping a balance between desired comfort and the adverse effects of prolonged drug therapy.

PRESCRIBING PATTERNS

Initial diagnosis and treatment of elderly people is often made by the general practitioner (family doctor). The presentation of disease symptoms in the older patient may be unusual or confusing and current illness may be the culmination of a number of minor problems. Over the years the patient acquires more problems and consequently more drugs, which may themselves produce symptoms treated with more drugs.

The review of the literature on prescribing patterns by Burns and Phillipson (1986) reveals that three-quarters of the population aged 75 years and over receive prescribed drugs and one third of this group are prescribed between four and six drugs simultaneously. The number of prescriptions for elderly people has increased sharply and in greater numbers than the rise in the elderly population. In 1982, old people in the UK received 15.9 prescriptions per head, compared with 5.2 for younger people. Repeat prescriptions are particularly common for old people and are often given by ancillary staff, and so the patient is not seen by the general practitioner. This has led to an increase in the number of drug errors and adverse reactions.

A study made in a Southampton health centre showed that of the prescriptions written for patients over the age of 65, 25.6% were for cardiovascular drugs, 16.5% for analgesics and central nervous system (CNS) drugs, 16.2% for psychotropic and 13.5% for metabolic drugs (Freeman 1979). In a hospital in Dundee, neuroleptics topped the list (33%), chloral derivatives accounted for 32% and benzodiazepines 16%; other drugs prescribed included diuretics 29% and laxatives 27% (Christopher et al 1979). The most commonly treated conditions of elderly people in both hospital and community care are therefore those of the cardiovascular and central nervous systems. The use of antimicrobial drugs is lower than in the community at large (16% of all NHS prescriptions): in hospital only 12% of drugs for the elderly and in the community 8.6% were for antimicrobials. These figures support the belief that cardiovascular symptoms are common in old people and that infection plays a prominent role in hospital admission. The frequency with which laxatives are prescribed in hospital is not, one hopes, a reflection upon the hospital diet. A more likely explanation is the imposed change of routine and the institutional take-over of the patient's self-medication responsibilities.

Widespread overprescribing in nursing Homes is also common, particularly of hypnotics, psychotropic drugs and laxatives (Wade et al 1983). Burns and Phillipson (1986) refer to Bliss' (1981) assertion that the most common iatrogenic illness in elderly people requiring hospital admission is the result of cumulative toxic effects of tranquillizers (parkinsonism, postural hypotension, drowsiness, confusion, skin rashes, jaundice). Often, hospital geriatricians find that patients improve markedly when they discontinue their cocktail of drugs.

With the development of geriatric medicine, drugs emerged as the dominant method of treatment, resulting in a boom industry in the 1960s and onwards. By the mid-1980s, the annual NHS drugs bill had approached £2000 million. Demand for tranquillizers increased from the mid-1960s; for anti-hypertensives from the mid to late 1960s; and for non-steroidal anti-inflammatory drugs (NSAIDs) from the mid-1970s. By the 1970s, 20% of all elderly people were taking at least three medicines daily and 10% were taking four or more (Burns & Phillipson 1986).

Many factors contributed to the growth of drugs as the treatment of choice for elderly people (Burns & Phillipson 1986). Doctors were not encouraged to consider treatments other than drugs. With a few exceptions, such as the geriatrician, Ferguson Anderson and his GP colleague, Nairn Cowan in Scotland, there was a limited awareness amongst doctors and other health professionals of the role of preventive medicine and health education for older people. The dangers of drugs for elderly people were consistently ignored or underestimated. General practitioners relied heavily on the marketing propaganda of the pharmaceutical industry rather than on neutral sources or their own training. The lack of comprehensive facilities and resources for the care of the elderly prompted recourse to drugs. The policy of community rather than institutional care, though laudable in many ways, created new problems in that prescribing and administration of drugs could no longer be controlled. This has led to drug hoarding and the abuses of repeat prescribing common in the 1970s and 1980s. Very little health education was given to old people by health professionals with regard to, for example, the benefits of good nutrition, exercise and blood pressure control.

Professionals, it seems, preferred the power associated with sole ownership of knowledge (Burns & Phillipson 1986). Old people, therefore, were vulnerable to the seductive claims of drug companies in being able to provide instant and long-lasting cures. The physical dependence and harmful side-effects were played down.

The vulnerability to the inflated benefits of drug treatment is a particular problem for elderly women (Burns & Phillipson 1986). More elderly women than men are likely to visit their general practitioner, since two thirds of pensioners in the UK are women, and elderly women experience more health problems than elderly men. Most of the geriatricians and general practitioners in the UK are men, and women's health problems throughout life are often denigrated by doctors and by women themselves. Women's health problems may be dismissed as 'neurotic' or treated with antidepressant drugs. Furthermore, the deference women — particularly elderly women — show to their GP might conceal the real problem, such as the damaging effects of bereavement. Many GPs encourage deference and regard the ideal patient as passive, obedient, co-operative and un-complaining.

THE PROBLEMS ASSOCIATED WITH DRUG USE BY ELDERLY PEOPLE

The first problem related to drug use by elderly people is selecting the right drug, since symptoms of disease often differ from those seen in the young. Patients present with vague symptoms and unsuitable drugs may be used; patients treated for many years may develop new symptoms and these could require treatment with additional drugs. This can lead to interactions or even to a situation where one drug is used to treat the side-effects of another. The addition of more drugs to the patient's programme leads to confusion, mistakes, wrong reporting by the patient and, ultimately, hospital admission.

CHANGES IN DRUG RESPONSE WITH AGE

Many of the strange effects of drugs in elderly patients can be accounted for by the changes in drug handling which occur with increasing age. No two individuals are the same in their response to illness or drugs, and similarly they are not the same in the degree or sequence with which their organs age. The normal dose recommended and response expected of a given dose of a drug is calculated using the dose response of normal healthy young men; from these recommendations the prescribing doctor must estimate doses for young, old and sick patients. This situation has been remedied for some drugs by comparative studies of young and elderly volunteers, but as yet there are many areas in which the appropriate dose for elderly people has to be determined by trial and error, based on the theoretical changes in drug handling which might be a consequence of ageing.

CASE HISTORY

Mr M, aged 81 years, was admitted to hospital following a 'funny turn' which included inability to walk. A civil servant who retired at the age of 61 years with hypertension, he was prescribed at this time Decaserpyl® plus a reserpine alkaloid by his general practitioner, who suggested also a change of lifestyle (early retirement). Over the following years the patient moved house and transferred to a new general practitioner, who continued his drug by repeat prescription, in spite of the advent of beta-blocking drugs, and without regular check up. When the patient was 75 years old his wife complained of his unsteadiness, fidgety movements and withdrawal. During a hospital consultation Parkinsonism was diagnosed and Sinemet® (levodopa with carbidopa) was prescribed. Both drugs were then supplied on repeat prescription and no further consultation made until the present admission.

On Mr M's admission to hospital a cardiac monitor was set up and all drugs stopped. Blood pressure was only slightly raised and subsequently fell to within a normal range. No abnormality was detected and after 10 days the patient was discharged on a small dose of Sinemet® to reduce slight rigidity. At an outpatient follow-up the drug was withdrawn and the patient remains well and drug free.

This problem was due to both side-effects and interactions; first, reserpine alkaloids (Decaserpyl-plus®) deplete dopamine; secondly, the addition of the drug levodopa (Sinemet®) rectified the condition — one drug nullifying the effect of the other. The patient's 'turn' was most probably due to postural hypotension, a known side-effect of levodopa, and an increasing sensitivity to the drug.

CHANGES IN THE ABILITY TO ABSORB DRUGS

Most drugs are administered orally. Before they can reach the site of action they must be absorbed into the body, enter the circulation and be transported to that site. Changes in the gastrointestinal tract associated with ageing could account for differences in the amount and timing of drug absorption.

Reduced gastric acid secretion as shown by a reduction in basal gastric acid and histamine-stimulated secretion occurs in the elderly.

This could reduce the solubility of acidic drugs (aspirin) and could protect drugs (penicillins) destroyed by gastric acid.

Gut motility and the rate of gastric emptying are reduced. This increases the overall transit time of drugs to the site of absorption. A slower peak and prolonged overall absorption of the drug may result. In general this is of little consequence when drugs are given long-term, but if a speedy, high concentration is required (analgesia, antimicrobial, chemotherapy) the expected effect may not be achieved. Delayed emptying of the stomach may also result in excessive irritation from known gastric irritants (non-steroid anti-inflammatories and levodopa), causing non-compliance by patients. Reduced gut transit time may result in an overall increase in drug absorption, and so lower doses of drug can be given.

Actively absorbed drugs such as the amines (methyldopa, levodopa) may have reduced absorption because of a decrease in absorbing cells, resulting from the slower turnover of active cells with age. Most drugs are, however, unaffected since absorption is generally passive.

The destruction of drugs by gut metabolic enzymes is probably reduced as enzyme levels decrease, although where duodenal diverticula are present bacterial colonization may result in bacterial enzyme destruction of some drugs and so account for unpredictable treatment failure.

The effects of ageing on drug absorption are therefore subtle, variable and unpredictable and can only be proved by the assay of plasma drug concentrations during the absorption period. Even then, more than one change may occur and one may counter the other; for example, a reduced ability to absorb may be unnoticed because decreased transit time allows a prolonged period for the slow absorption to take place.

THE ABSORPTION OF DRUGS FROM OTHER SITES

Changes in drug absorption from other sites may also be affected.

Injected drugs rely on subcutaneous or muscular circulation to carry the drug into the body circulation. Reduction in muscle tone and inactivity can mean that the injected drug remains in a tissue depot for longer than usual. Bruising may occur because of increased fragility of blood vessels, so that a careful rotation of sites is important, when repeated injections are necessary.

Locally administered drugs instilled into the eye, nose or ear and applied to the surface of the skin, mouth or vagina are generally not absorbed into the circulation, but produce an effect locally. With age, the elasticity, moisture and turnover of the body's surface cells is reduced and repeated applications may, therefore, result in irritation, soreness or local breakdown of the surface. A check of the surface condition should be made prior to each application, particularly in less visible places (ear, mouth) and any discharge (vagina) or soreness reported before another application is made.

CHANGES IN DRUG DISTRIBUTION

The usefulness of any drug lies both in its specific action against the disease for which it is prescribed and in its ability to concentrate in the diseased organ. Alterations in the body's composition and physical activity which are the result of ageing can affect the distribution of drugs in the body.

The relative proportions of muscle and fat in the body change with increasing age. In young people, body fat represents 18% of tissue mass in men and 33% in women. By the age of 65 to 85 years these proportions are increased to 36% in men and 45% in women (Novak 1972). This increase in the proportion of fat to muscle means that there is a larger depot for fat-soluble drugs (barbiturates, anaesthetics, benzodiazepines) in elderly people. On administration the drug is rapidly taken up into the fatty tissue and subsequently released only slowly for metabolism and excretion. This accounts for some of the changes seen in elderly patients in their response to fat-soluble drugs — including prolonged confusion after anaesthetics and reduced neuromuscular responsiveness after sedation (Cook et al 1983).

A significant relationship was found between the anticholinergic drugs often used in premedication regimes before surgery (e.g. atropine, hyoscine) and post-operative confusion in elderly people (Platzer 1988). Platzer found significantly less post-operative confusion in elderly patients who received the anticholinergic drug Robinil® (glycopyrrolate), which does not cross the blood–brain barrier.

Body water reduces by as much as 15% between the ages of 20 and 80 years (Norris et al 1963). The reduction in fluid, with a parallel reduction in size, leads to the higher concentrations of some drugs recorded for elderly patients following a standard dose. This may result in unexpected signs of overdose following what is considered to be 'normal' dosage, particularly during long-term therapy.

Changes in plasma proteins occur in elderly people. Although the overall plasma protein concentration is not changed, a 19% reduction in albumin content has been recorded (Misra et al 1975). Albumin is the most plentiful protein in the plasma and acts as a vehicle for drug transport by binding drugs. Bound drugs are carried in the plasma and are not active or available for metabolism or excretion. A reduction in albumin may result in higher concentrations of unbound drug and increased drug action.

Changes in blood flow caused by reduced cardiac output have been reported in old people, the reduction being about 30% between the ages of 30 and 65 years. The consequent reduction in blood flow to the organs is not uniform, flow to the liver and kidney being more reduced than that to the brain, with little overall change to the circulation of the cardiac and skeletal muscle (Bender 1965). These changes are likely to reduce the speed of detoxification and excretion of drugs from the body.

CHANGES IN METABOLISM

Drugs entering and circulating in the body are generally treated as foreign substances. They are actively destroyed and made harmless, a process which usually renders them more easily excreted. The most active site of drug metabolism is the liver, where drugs absorbed from the gut are subject to breakdown and/or conjugation, which renders them inactive. A considerable amount of any drug dose may be lost during this 'first pass' through the liver before entering the general circulation, and the dose is calculated accordingly.

Theoretically, liver drug metabolism is reduced in old people by the combined factors of reduction in liver size (from 2.6% body-weight in middle age to 1.6% at 90 years), reduction in blood flow, and reduction in the capacity for enzyme production. Liver capacity is well in excess of requirements throughout life, and although studies have been made of the metabolism of some drugs in elderly people, little change in rate has been shown. With antipyrine, however, the drug usually used to test metabolic capacity, an increased half-life (the time taken for plasma concentration to reduce by 50%) and metabolic clearance has been demonstrated with age. It is therefore probable that the liver's capacity to metabolize drugs is impaired in elderly people, and that the normal response to repeated drug administration (i.e. an increase in the production of metabolizing enzymes) is sluggish or delayed. In the same way, the response of metabolizing enzymes in the gut and other tissues will be lower. Diminished overall metabolism would lead to an increase in drug concentration and a great risk of toxicity.

CHANGES IN EXCRETION

Renal excretion is the principal route for the removal of excess toxins and waste from the body. Changes in the kidney's capacity as measured by renal function are, therefore, an important pointer to both the concentration and rate of excretion of drugs and metabolites in the elderly. Although serum creatinine levels remain constant in healthy individuals throughout life, the rate of creatinine excretion as calculated by the creatinine clearance rate decreases steadily throughout life. For drugs that are excreted unchanged, creatinine clearance can be a direct indicator of the rate of drug excretion. As we have seen, it is doubtful that the passive absorption of drugs is reduced in elderly people. Any increase in the plasma levels of drugs principally excreted in the urine is therefore likely to be due to reduced renal clearance. For drugs (e.g. digoxin) which have only small differences between the concentrations that are therapeutic and toxic, and are excreted unchanged in the urine, any build-up of drug could be dangerous.

The elderly patient is therefore vulnerable to the

risk of unintentional overdose effects. Patients on long-term therapy will, as they grow older, become more at risk so that dose adjustment will be necessary. Many elderly patients regulate their drug intake themselves according to side-effects or unintentionally by forgetting the odd dose. When admitted to hospital the full prescribed dose will be administered, leading to the possibility of a toxic response.

Although the action, concentration and clearance of drugs metabolized before excretion will not be altered by reduced renal capacity, their metabolized products will be. As a consequence these metabolic products may accumulate in the body.

Other routes of excretion are possible. As with any other products of metabolism, excretion via the bile, skin, lung or body fluids may occur with drugs. These routes are only of major importance in cases of renal damage. For elderly people, a general decline in the efficiency of these other routes makes the consequences of renal failure even more disastrous.

CHANGES IN RECEPTOR SENSITIVITY

The changes in the physiology of the gut, skin, circulation and liver account for the variations of drug concentration seen in elderly patients and hence the unexpected symptoms of over- or under-dosage to a normal dose. For elderly patients a number of responses have been recorded which do not readily fit into the accepted categories of toxicity and which can only be explained as differences in sensitivity. For example, a single dose of a barbiturate can produce a whole range of responses, from restlessness to frank psychosis. Sensitivity may also be altered with diseases such as those of the vascular system where an increased sensitivity to warfarin can be expected. On the whole the unexpected symptoms of drug sensitivity are vague; rashes, dizziness, confusion and agitation are common symptoms, which may often be passed off as signs of 'getting old'.

ADVERSE REACTIONS

Elderly people suffer double the rate of adverse drug reactions compared with people aged under 50 years (Bossum and Dunn 1986 cited in Burns and Phillipson 1986). This is partly because more elderly people than young take drugs regularly and few are warned about side-effects of the drugs prescribed. Old people are also more likely to be taking several drugs (polypharmacy), which results from multiple symptoms. A number of the drug prescribed are known to cause problems because of side-effects (anti-inflammatories) or because there is only a small difference between the toxic and therapeutic drug concentration (digoxin). The drug-taking habits of elderly patients may make them vulnerable to adverse reactions. Where knowledge and understanding of the treatment is lacking and memory is needed to take the drugs effectively, mistakes are liable to occur.

Adverse reactions fall into three classes: dose-related, hypersensitivity and idiosyncratic.

Dose-related reactions are apparent as overdose symptoms. These are due either to exceeding the dose or to changes in the individual's handling or sensitivity to the drug.

Hypersensitivity reactions are due to genetic or immunological abnormalities. Genetic differences may not be discovered even for elderly patients if the drug has not been taken before.

Idiosyncratic responses may also result from a combination of genetic, disease and age-related causes. These reactions are bizarre, not being within the range of expected effects of the drug.

Drug-induced disease

Disease may result from either dose-related or hypersensivity reactions and there are individual variations in the presentation of disease from the same drug. Drug-induced disease usually develops with prolonged use of the drug. The likelihood of gastric ulcer during anti-inflammatory use increases with age. Nutritional defects are more likely with the prolonged use of drugs which dull the appetite or reduce absorption (digitalis, anticonvulsants, amphetamines), create malabsorption (mineral oil, phenolphthalin, phenytoin), increase urinary loss of ions (diuretics, cortisone, alcohol) or act as vitamin K (warfarin), vitamin B6 (levodopa) or folate (trimethoprim) antagonists.

The majority of deaths from adverse drug reactions are due to commonly used drugs such as digitalis, antimicrobials, insulin and diuretics, from overdosage, or from predictable side-effects. The most common adverse reactions reported for elderly people are shown in Table 21.1.

Table 21.1 Problem drugs for elderly people.

Drug group	Problems/symptoms
Cardiac glycosides	Overdosage easy — little difference between toxic and therapeutic dose. Overdose effects more common when combined with potassium depleting diuretics, hypercalcaemia and hypothyroidism. Adverse symptoms — nausea, vomiting, confusion, depression, gynaecomastia and acute abdominal syndrome. Any sort of arrythmia may occur.
Diuretics	Thiazides — potassium deficiency, digoxin toxicity. Frusemide and ethacrynic acid — homeostatic upsets, transitory or permanent deafness, impaired glucose tolerance.
Benzodiazepines	Reduced reaction time. Build-up of sedation with repeated dosage.
Antidepressants	Tricyclics — accentuated side-effects, dry mouth, hypertension, drowsiness. Many interactions possible. MAOIs — potential hazard due to interactions with food and self-administered drugs.
Anti-inflammatories	Age-related increase in incidence of gastric ulcer, bleeding and dyspepsia with both steroid and non-steroid drugs. Interactions with anticoagulants.
Phenothiazines	Induce parkinsonism, lethargy and hypotension. May cause cholestatic jaundice or reduce liver and thyroid function. Contribute to accidental hypothermia. Interacts with alcohol — effects enhanced.
Oral anticoagulants	Increased anticoagulant response (warfarin), possibly due to reduced clotting factor production. Unpredicted haemorrhagic complications. Possible interactions, non-steroid anti-inflammatories, steroids, barbiturates, quinadine, thyroxine.

COMPLIANCE WITH TREATMENT REGIMES

No drug can be effective unless it is taken. Non-compliance is therefore a major cause of treatment failure. True non-compliance (the complete refusal of treatment) is less common than repeated medication errors which can amount to treatment failure. In hospital it is the nurse's responsibility to ensure that drugs are administered correctly and that the patient actually receives the drug. Omissions do happen, the majority of which are due to the unavailability of either the patient or the drug (Bergman et al 1979). In addition, administration may prove difficult because the patient fails to swallow the tablet. The patient should be offered a full glass of, preferably, water with tablets and possibly more liquid if there are a number of tablets. Rushing does not help, if the patient fails to swallow, remove the tablet with a spoon, offer a drink, and start again. A drink of water should also be offered following liquid drugs as these are often sticky and leave an unpleasant feeling in the mouth. Injections may be difficult or even ooze out of flabby skin, and bruising commonly occurs with elderly patients. Such problems should be reported to the doctor so that, where possible, alternative routes of administration can be used on either a temporary or a permanent basis.

REFUSAL OF TREATMENT

Some patients will openly refuse treatment and where the situation is known it can be easily dealt with. In most cases explanation of the reason for treatment and the benefits to be expected, or the suggestion that the patient try the drug for a few days, will win confidence and get treatment started. If the patient dislikes the drug because of its taste or form, a change may be possible and should be made. Often the reason for refusal is this simple and seeing the patient's point of view makes all the difference. In other instances the refusal of drugs may be legitimate, for example when analgesics are given and there is no pain or when the patient knows of or is suffering side-effects.

The reason for refusal may appear to be for a relatively minor reason: suspicion, long-held belief or fears, the similarity of the drug name to others which are known to be dangerous. These problems are best dealt with by clear explanation at the initiation of drug therapy.

More difficult to deal with is the patient who conceals her non-compliance. Drugs may be hidden, spat out or hoarded; where failure of treatment occurs, this possibility should be explored. Hoarded drugs are a potential danger; they may be found by other patients and used or distributed by the patient for others, without anyone being aware of the potential hazard.

CASE HISTORY

Mrs N was originally prescribed nembutal as a sedative during a United States Air Force (USAF) alert in Norfolk — the noise of the planes kept her awake. The drug was added to those on her repeat prescription card by the general practitioner's secretary and on all subsequent occasions she was issued with a repeat prescription which included nembutal with her other drugs. When the USAF alert was over she only took the drug on 'bad nights' and accumulated quite a backlog of capsules. One day a friend complained of not sleeping well, so Mrs N kindly gave her a few capsules and then a bottle. Other customers followed and the prescription was subsequently accepted, so that she could supply her friends' needs. All these barbiturate-takers were elderly and fortunately well, and not taking much alcohol or drugs which might interact. Mrs N was amazed when she was told of the problems which could have developed and is now a reformed character.

MEDICATION ERRORS

Studies have shown that the main cause of non-compliance is lack of comprehension of the regime. This includes errors of omission, of addition and of mistiming of the treatment regime. In addition to the problem of a failing memory, poor vision, lack of manual dexterity and overall immobility contribute to non-compliance. Many complaints from elderly patients and their relatives, some of which are resolved only after hospital admission, are due to mistakes or misunderstanding of the treatment by patient and relatives.

CASE HISTORY

Mr W, aged 70 years, came to the outpatients department with his wife, who complained that he kept her awake all night and then went to sleep in the morning when she 'had all her work to do'. Mr W was being treated for cardiac failure and had been discharged from hospital three weeks before on a drug regime of digoxin, thiazide diuretic with potassium supplement, and nitrazepam. He had kept very well but admitted that he did have to get up several times at night to urinate. The pharmacist checked his tablets with him, except for the sleeping tablets which he kept by his bed. He explained that he had 'little white ones' (heart tablets) twice a day and the 'white ones' (water tablets) in the morning, together with the 'oblong ones' which 'were to put back what went out with the water'. Unfortunately all the containers were the same and the print rather small, otherwise he might have noticed that he was in fact taking this sleeping tablets, white round tablets, in the morning instead of his 'water tablets' also white and round, which he had by his bed and took at night. The problem was solved by putting a different coloured label on the sleeping tablets and making sure that they and not the diuretic tablets were by his bed.

Muddling tablets is a common problem. Many patients keep all the day's drugs in one bottle and take them randomly. Some even keep their husband's or wife's tablets together with their own.

MEASURES TO IMPROVE COMPLIANCE
Acceptance

Making treatment acceptable to the patient is the first step to compliance. Many patients have fixed ideas about drugs or may expect strange things to happen to them, such as becoming impotent or 'queer in the head'. Such ideas are often based on old wives' tales or stories they have heard about under completely different conditions. Even so, the worry is real and must be dealt with honestly, with the benefits and possible difficulties encountered by patients starting on the drug explained.

Helping patients to obtain drugs

Patients who leave hospital are supplied with drugs to take with them and subsequent prescriptions when required are normally obtained through the general practitioner. This should be explained to the patient and reassurance given that her doctor will know which drugs she is to take. The patient should be informed that the tablets she receives from the pharmacy may look different from those she receives from the general practitioner and that a repeat prescription should be ordered at least a week before supplies run out. In some cases it may be necessary for a relative or home help to collect prescriptions. For people of retirement age (60 years for women and 65 for men) prescriptions are free of charge if they fill in and sign the reverse of the prescription form and any patient receiving drugs after this age should be reminded of this.

Improving professional practice

It is essential that doctors, nurses and elderly patients learn to discuss drug treatments with one another.

The concept of 'blind compliance' with an apparently useless or unacceptable regime is inappropriate. In fact, non-compliance is more likely, the hoarding of drugs then follows, with the final scenario being the elderly person taking the drugs at random from their 'geriatric confectionary', thus making adverse reactions almost inevitable (Burns & Phillipson 1986 p. 96).

As Burns and Phillipson advocate, therapeutic regimes are required for elderly patients which rely on fewer drugs and which experiment with alternative or complementary medicine. A careful balance is needed between the valuable use of effective drugs and the dangers of their excessive use — especially with old people, whose adverse reactions to drugs increase with age. Non-compliance to a drug regime is likely to be due to misunderstanding by the patient or a wise decision by the patient to stop taking the drug because the

side-effects are worse than the health problem. The likelihood of 'intelligent non-compliance' is greater than stubbornness, awkwardness or forgetfulness on the part of the individual.

ACCURATE ADMINISTRATION

Labelling

In the past, labels on medicine bottles lacked explicit instructions for taking the tablets and did not include dispensing or expiry dates. They were also frequently illegible. Since 1984, the British Pharmaceutical Society has required large, typed labels so that old people, and anyone else, can read them. Now, rather than vague instructions such as 'take as directed', the label should contain clear details for administration as well as the purpose of the drug, e.g. 'two tablets four times a day if necessary for pain'.

Memory aids

The routine for drug administration varies in different hospitals, but for patients starting a new drug it is the hospital routine which is taught. On discharge from hospital, this routine may need to be adapted to fit in with the patient's home life. Remembering when to take drugs is a difficult problem for elderly patients. The problem is increased in proportion to the number of drugs to be taken and the different regimes of administration. Where possible, patients should be taught to administer their drug before discharge, an innovation which has proved a useful aid to compliance (Baxendale et al 1978). Simple measures such as linking drug-taking to events in the daily routine (getting up, washing, mealtimes) or marking a diary when the drug is taken may be all that is needed for some patients. Calendar-packed drugs are also helpful in this respect. For patients with greater difficulties it may be necessary to make use of 'dose boxes'. These are compartmentalized boxes, or collections of tablet containers, which are filled with a supply of drugs, usually weekly (Hatch & Tapley 1982). Each dose is placed in an individual compartment and the patient can check that the drug has been taken by seeing the compartment empty. This method requires the recruitment of a relative, neighbour or friend who can prime the box if the old person cannot do so herself, but it means that the patient remains independent. The final resource for a patient who cannot remember drugs, is to employ another to administer them. This could be difficult, however, because elderly friends and relatives may also have memory problems.

Another memory aid which should improve compliance is to give the old person and her relatives clearly understandable information about her drug regime. A simple treatment card with a sample tablet stuck down with transparent tape against an easily understood description ('water' tablets, pain tablets, breathing tablets) can be prepared for each patient.

Aids for physical disability

Many adults have difficulty in opening child-proof drug containers, and this problem increases with age. Drugs can be dispensed in conventional containers or in containers with winged caps; these are very helpful for stiff hands. Small tablets may be difficult to handle and wide-necked bottles or tablet dispensers can help with this problem. Where these are used, they must be adequately labelled and help may be needed in filling them. Calendar packs may have to be snipped with scissors if the patient cannot tear the foil.

Poor sight should be compensated for with large print or identifiable symbols for tablet container recognition. Braille labels are available, but not all blind people read Braille. Dose boxes are also useful because the patient can feel which compartments are empty. For liquid, a medicine measure cut down or painted clearly to the level of the exact dose, or a fixed volume syringe, may be useful.

All innovations should, however, be tried out with the patient to check that they work for her. As patients get older they may well require more help. For example, a nurse who can give an injection in a now inaccessible site would be welcomed by elderly diabetics. Reappraisal of the situation is important and should be remembered by nurses in outpatients and general practitioners' clinics, as well as by the visiting district nurse (see Chapter 27).

Complete compliance is only possible with obsessional patients. For most drugs the occasional omission has only a minor effect and may at times be useful in reducing side-effects, as with digoxin therapy. Additional doses can, however, be dangerous for the elderly (e.g. sedatives, digoxin, levodopa). The patient should be advised *not* to take an additional tablet to make up for one which she thinks she has forgotten.

CASE HISTORY

Mr J is a very fit, independent 78 year old, successfully treated with Sinemet® (levodopa and carbidopa) for Parkinsonism. One morning he had an important meeting to attend at his local club and in his anxiety not to be late he suddenly wondered, 'Have I taken my morning dose of Sinemet?' Being very conscious of the benefits of the drug, he took another dose before he went out to be sure and drove to the club in his car. On arrival he felt dizzy and had to sit in the car again (postural hypotension), and on entering the club he rushed to the toilet and was sick (gastric irritation). The dizziness remained and a friend telephoned his wife. She suggested phoning the doctor, to which her husband responded by angrily knocking the telephone on the floor (aggression). All these manifestations, postural hypotension, gastric irritation and aggression, are symptoms of levodopa overdose. Mr J had, of course, taken his drug as normal with his breakfast.

SELF-MEDICATION

Self-medication, the prescribing of drugs for one's self, has an important role in self-care and the maintenance of independence. Traditionally, the treatment of common ailments such as colds, coughs, headaches, constipation and symptoms such as aches and pains, together with first aid in the home, has rested on the individual or the family carer (mother). The purchase of medicines 'over the counter' (OTC) also rests with the individual or the one in charge of shopping. Choice of drugs may be traditional, influenced by advertising or by discussion with neighbours or friends. Occasionally, the advice of a nurse at the health clinic, the doctor, or the pharmacist may be sought, generally because the condition is one not encountered previously. The treatment of symptoms related to feeling 'unwell' is common. In 1972 a study made by Dunnel and Cartwright (1972) reported that nine out of every 10 people interviewed said they had felt unwell in the previous two weeks, describing one or more symptoms. Drugs purchased OTC for self-treatment may be obtained from many outlets (slot machine, pharmacy, etc.). The drugs taken most commonly, such as antipyretic analgesics (e.g. aspirin), are obtainable in many shops. The controls placed on them by the Medicines Act of 1968 are related to the number and strength of tablet on sale through the different outlets. Large quantities of most OTC drugs are only allowed to be sold when a pharmacist is present. Many OTC drugs, including cold cures, contain a number of ingredients which may include aspirin, paracetamol, antihistamines, stimulants and alcohol, all possible interactors with prescribed drugs.

The symptoms suffered by elderly people tend to be ascribed to 'old age', and these patients tend therefore to collect drugs in case they need them and to take drugs to maintain 'normality'. This may delay their visit to the doctor or mask the symptoms of disease.

PROBLEMS ASSOCIATED WITH SELF-MEDICATION

Overdose may result from patients' 'doubling up' on drugs already issued on prescription, for example taking a 'cold cure' containing aspirin when prescribed soluble aspirin for rheumatic pain. This may result in frank overdose symptoms such as tinnitus or accentuated side-effects such as gastrointestinal bleeding.

Interactions with prescribed medicines may result if the patient is not advised of the possibility occurring, for example, between cold cures and monamine oxidase inhibitors (MAOIs) or between aspirin and coumarin anticoagulants. Patients tend not to consider that patent medicines are drugs, or that they might cause problems in relation to prescribed drugs.

Masking symptoms, as mentioned above, can be

a problem; the symptoms of illness of elderly patients often present in an unusual fashion. Pain which might be diagnostic of myocardial infarct in younger patients is often mild or absent in old people. Thus the taking (or giving) of an analgesic for mild chest pain or discomfort might rob the doctor of a useful diagnostic pointer.

Abuse of OTC drugs is common, particulary in relation to laxatives, analgesics, and vitamins. In general, OTC drugs are only able to relieve symptoms; they are therefore of no use in prophylaxis. For example, the habitual taking of laxatives by elderly people who believe that only a daily motion is normal, can lead to dependence verging on addiction. The patient feels normal only if she has the laxative, and her bowel is incapable of evacuating without it. This may in time lead to fluid loss, malabsorption, irritation and a loss of normal function.

NON-DRUGS

Few people, other than pharmacologists, consider alcohol, tobacco, coffee, tea or herbs to be drugs. However, they all contain pharmacologically active ingredients with known action in the body. Many, such as alcohol, caffeine and nicotine, are known to have addictive properties as well as personal and social attributes. In moderation they may be useful and advantageous, but in excess can cause physical damage. Alcohol, for example, can be useful in the form of sherry as an appetite stimulant, whisky is a useful night sedative, and beer or stout provide useful energy and nutrients. Excessive use of alcohol may accompany loneliness or depression and can lead to damage of the liver and brain.

Alcohol has been consumed for thousands of years and early historical records refer to the beneficial effects of moderate consumption for medicinal purposes or to 'forget the sorrows of old age' (McKinn & Mishara 1987). Wine was recommended for health and vigour in old age and, as McKinn and Mishara observe, the thirteenth century inventor of brandy, Arnaud de Villeneuve, thought his discovery of 'aqua vitae' (the 'water of life') would increase longevity, maintain youth and relieve depression.

The beneficial effects of moderate alcohol consumption (less than two drinks, or 30 ml of ethanol per day) has been confirmed in more recent times. It is associated with a reduced risk of coronary heart disease compared with the risk for either heavy drinkers or abstainers, and has been found to promote sleep and well-being and lift depression of elderly people (McKinn & Mishara 1987). These effects were found by Mishara and his co-workers with elderly people living in nursing Homes or in their own homes. It was unclear whether the benefits of alcohol were due to the chemical benefits of ethanol or to psychological reactions by the old people to being treated as responsible adults, or to psychosocial benefits of drinking and participating in a social setting. The authors recommended, however, that alcohol should be served in a social setting rather than as a medicine.

In recent years herbalism has become more popular as an alternative to conventional medicine and is considered to be safer. The tests used on, and regulations such as quality control for herbal remedies are less stringent than for drugs in spite of the fact that many contain pharmacologically active ingredients. For example, herbs reputed to act on the heart or as diuretics (Adonis, False Hellebore, Yellow Foxglove) contain cardiac glycosides and will therefore potentiate the effect of prescribed drugs such as digoxin.

WHERE THE NURSE CAN HELP

When patients enter hospital they enter an institution which has organized routines, where many individuals from different disciplines with different levels of knowledge and at different stages in training all have a role in the organization of patient care. The routines of organization are there to ensure that many activities are undertaken in an approved manner, for reasons of efficiency, tradition, safety, and so on. The rules for drug ordering, care and issue are controlled for these reasons, but different activities are undertaken by different professionals. Prescription is usually the doctor's responsibility, issue the pharmacist's and administration the nurse's. At home the patient is responsible for administration and for the prescription and acquisition of non-prescription

drugs. In taking over the role of drug administration the nurse imposes routines, often based on tradition, which suit the hospital setting. For elderly patients who have been managing their drugs at home, these changes may be muddling and lead to non-compliance on discharge from hospital. Removing independence makes the patient incapable of self-care later and imposes physical changes which alter the drug response. Most of these problems can be avoided if the nurse appreciates the situation and the patient takes an active part in the drug routine. The patient should, for example, participate in a supervised self-medication programme before discharge from hospital if at all possible. The value of community psychiatric nurses, dental nurses, health visitors, nurse practitioners and therapists can be most effective in teaching patients and their relatives about their medicines and in encouraging compliance and monitoring adverse reactions. This nursing role is important for residents of old people's Homes as well as those living in their own homes.

ON ADMISSION TO HOSPITAL

The patient is usually asked to hand over the drugs taken at home when entering hospital. This action offers the nurse an ideal opportunity to obtain a drug history in which information on drugs currently taken, past problems with drugs and self-medication preferences can be acquired. Where possible, the hospital routine can be adapted to the patient's and changes in routine explained to the patient. Information on self-medication can be relayed to the doctor so that, where suitable, the patient's favourite laxative, analgesic or indigestion mixture can be prescribed and be available when required. The drug history need not be collected all in one session, particularly if the patient is already exhausted by questioning. Some information may be more easily obtained from relatives or friends.

CHECKLIST FOR A DRUG HISTORY

1. *Prescribed drugs* from the general practitioner or hospital outpatients department will already have been discussed with the medical staff. Information obtained by the nurse may, however,

supplement and check this and some estimate of compliance should be gained. The list of drugs, numbers and times taken should be checked with the medical record. In the confusion of admission the patient may have forgotten about a drug or told the doctor incorrectly that it was taken. These incidents occur particularly where there are many drugs or memory problems.

2. *The drug-taking routine* should be discussed, such as the times drugs are taken, their relationship to meals, sleep and other daily activities. Some patients will develop sleep problems if thyroxid or diuretic drugs are given too late in the day for them. A small alteration in nursing routine may prevent a sedative being given. A change in the routine of taking drugs either before or after meals will often alter the absorption pattern and response. Discussion of the routine will also give an estimate of compliance problems to be encountered on discharge.

3. *Self-prescribed drugs* are often forgotten but for many patients form a part of their everyday life. The discussion should include drugs routinely used, habits of use, any allergies, herbal treatment and dietary products such as bran, vitamins and slimming pills. The current fashion for dietary fads is often taken to extremes by people who do not fully understand what is intended, like the man who ate a pot of yoghurt after every meal because he was told it was good for slimming. The information given may provide clues to symptoms such as diarrhoea when laxatives are used daily, and may ensure that abnormal readings are not obtained in tests. Throat lozenges containing iodine can make the thyroid function test of a myxoedemic patient appear normal.

4. *Non-drug stimulants* (coffee, tea) or *sedatives* (alcohol) should also be discussed and their pattern of use established. Many people routinely use sherry to promote appetite (it activates gastric secretion) or whisky as a sedative, and there is generally no reason why this should not be continued for most people. Where bizarre treatments are established it may be necessary to wean the patient gradually from the drug, otherwise they could be physically upset and lose confidence in medical treatments.

DURING THE HOSPITAL STAY

Through their role in drug administration nurses are in an ideal position to monitor the patient's drug progress, reporting responses and side-effects. They are also the people the patient asks about the drug, what it should do or how it works. Educating the patient about drugs is a very important task. The nurse should, however, be equipped to do so, checking in advance what response should be expected or the side-effects that are possible, so that the information is available when the patient asks questions. This education need not be restricted to current treatment but extended to cover first aid and self-medication. In the course of administration it is often possible to identify problems which may occur on discharge. The patient's physical ability to take drugs (vision, manual dexterity, swallowing) can be assessed and some idea of their ability to remember details obtained. Before discharge from hospital, direct patient involvement in her own drug administration, under supervision, is desirable. Such steps have been used in some institutions (Hatch & Tapley 1982) but problems with rules and traditions are often encountered.

Throughout the patient's hospital stay the nurse should be preparing her for discharge, so that when the day comes the patient is not pushed (in a wheelchair) out of the door with a bagful of drugs, unprepared to take them.

ON DISCHARGE FROM HOSPITAL

Going home might be as big a shock and change as hospital admission. The patient might be unsure about coping with meals at home, shopping, cleaning, as well as with drugs. If instructions and routines have been well established in hospital and are understood, the problems are reduced. Preparation should include liaison with the general practitioner, district nurse, pharmacist and relatives as the need arises. Instructions should be written clearly as well as given verbally. To ensure that they can be read and understood, ask the patient to repeat the instruction. Advice on possible adverse effects and interactions with self-medication drugs should be included where they may occur.

For the patient going home, discharge is often not the last contact with hospital. Nurses in the outpatients department can make use of their contact to help elderly patients with any problems which develop after discharge, to check and adapt their drug routine, or to help with compliance aids as they are required.

It is often the case that patients are unclear about their drug treatment when they are discharged from hospital, and so they continue taking the medicines they had been prescribed before admission as well as those supplied on discharge. After discharge from hospital the drug regime may be altered by the hospital doctor in the outpatients department or by the general practitioner or by the patient herself with very little communication among them, so confounding the problem for the patient still further. It is essential that hospital discharge notes should reach the general practitioner promptly. It is wise to give the patient a copy of the discharge note to take with her when she next visits the GP in case of postal delays.

THE DRUGS INDUSTRY

DRUG MONITORING AND LIMITED DRUG LISTS

There is a great need for an effective drug surveillance system so that adverse reactions to specific drugs are made known to official bodies such as the Committee for Safety of Medicines. The Drugs Surveillance Research Unit at Southampton University invites local doctors to provide information on drug effects and adverse reactions. This enables a data base on drug effects and toxicity to be built up which can be fed back to doctors, so keeping them up-to-date (Burns & Phillipson 1986).

Recommendations for limiting the drugs available under the NHS were published in the Greenfield Report (DHSS 1983). The Report advocated generic prescribing as being safer and cheaper than choosing from the variety of different brands of the same product. An example is

Valium®, which cost £24 per 1000 tablets in 1985 compared with its generic equivalent, diazepam, which cost £1.75 per 1000 tablets in the same year.

The DHSS, however, was not convinced that generic prescribing would save money, and it did not accept Greenfield's recommendations, at least not immediately. Yet, a year later, in 1984, the government introduced, in great haste and with very little consultation, its own limited list 'for minor self-limiting illness', in the expectation that £100 million per year would be saved from the NHS bill. This sudden decision evoked a widespread critical attack from medical bodies, Community Health Councils, the drugs industry and trades unions, with the result that the government revised its list in April 1985. Anxiety concerning the comprehensiveness of the limited list for elderly people's needs is widespread, although the cost saving of generic prescribing, the need for monitoring drug administration, and safer prescribing are welcomed (Burns & Phillipson 1986). The limited list should reduce lucrative gains and unjustifiable claims being made by drug firms for the safety and effectiveness of their products, as was the case with the NSAID, Opren® (benoxaprofen).

THE DRUGS INDUSTRY AND HEALTH EDUCATION

The dramatic imagery and the commercial language of advertising are inappropriate for drug advertising, yet are commonly used. Information given should be precise and factual and should include dosage, side-effects, contraindications and drug interactions as well as the benefits. Burns and Phillipson (1986) recommend that for every glossy advertisement that extols the virtue of a new anti-arthritic drug, for example, the pharmaceutical industry should pay for an equally glossy advertisement that promotes the virtues of other therapies, such as diet, exercise, self-help and counselling. This strategy would ensure that equal weight is given to drug promotion and health education in advertisements published in medical journals and popular magazines.

Health educators find it difficult to compete

with the glossy 'hard sell' approach of drug companies. The problem is partly financial; the budget of the Health Education Council (now the Health Education Authority) for 1983–1984 was £9.5 million, whereas £180 million was spent in the same period by the drug industry on promotion, and £400 million was spent on advertising by the food industry (Burns & Phillipson 1986).

The battle between the health educators and the drugs industry is well illustrated in the case of smoking. Campaigns against smoking have always been weakened by the powerful tobacco industry (Taylor 1984). In the early 1970s, a government working party set up to assess the economic implications of a reduction in smoking concluded that a 40% reduction in smoking over a 30-year period would result in a saving of half a million lives. However, the 'costs' of this saving were regarded as unacceptable for the country's economy in that a reduction in smoking would leave a larger number of retired people, more social security payments and high unemployment with closure of the tobacco factories. The full report of the working party was never published and it only came to light when a copy reached the Guardian newspaper 10 years later.

Research on smoking continues to show that there are benefits for health from giving up smoking, even for lifelong smokers aged over 65 years (Burns & Phillipson 1986). The implications of this research are that, without stronger government action against smoking, many of the chronic illnesses common in old age in this country will continue.

Similarly with food. Throughout the 1970s and early 1980s committees debated diet and nutrition but publication of their reports was obstructed by the vested interests of the government and the food industry (Burns & Phillipson 1986). An example of this is the NACNE Report (National Advisory Committee on Nutrition Education), which was not published until 1983, four years after the Committee was set up, and only after considerable pressure was put on the government by the mass media and after publication of extracts of the report in the Lancet. Burns and Phillipson (1986) highlight the continuing controversies over food policy. For example, they report that pressure from the dairy and meat industries persuaded the government to re-word its guide to healthy eating in their favour. It was only after the head of the team which produced the guide threatened to resign and the chairman of the College of Health declared he would release the truth to the press, that the Department of Health agreed to the guide's publication in its original form.

Thus, the messages conveyed to the public and to health professionals about prevention of ill health — through healthy eating, healthy living, giving up smoking, etc. — are difficult to interpret and open to political manipulation. By contrast, messages about drugs are much clearer, less ambiguous and offer immediate, if only short-term relief. It is easier, too, for doctors to rely on evidence for the effectiveness of drugs in research publications, whereas the benefits of preventive practices and health education are much more difficult to confirm from conventional scientific research.

Burns and Phillipson (1986) argue strongly that the power of the drug companies and the medical establishment are significant factors in maintaining the nation's ill-health. They urge that greater priority be put on prevention rather than treatment, which means that responsibility for health should be much less the sole preserve of the medical profession and should pass to the government, to industry, to health educators and to the individual. For further discussion of self-care in old age, see Bernard's and Phillipson's Chapter 23 in this volume.

The idea of controlling and directing our own ageing is largely foreign to our culture, and partly explains our vulnerability to the short-cuts offered by many drugs . . . [T]he time has come for a massive programme of education about the claims and promises of the drug companies. Older people, as the biggest consumers of drugs, must be a key group in this educative process. If professionals, and other workers and carers, fail to develop campaigns on drug awareness and drug use, then the spiral of suffering from the overzealous use of drugs will continue (Burns & Phillipson 1986, p. 146).

Nurses are in an ideal position to take a major role in health education and in raising the awareness of old people and their families of the benefits and limitations of drugs.

REFERENCES

Baxendale C, Gourlay M, Gibson I I J M 1978 A self-medication retraining programme. British Medical Journal 2: 1278–1279

Bender A D 1965 The effect of increasing age on the distribution of peripheral blood flow in man. Journal of the American Geriatric Society 13: 192

Bergman U, Norlin A, Wiholm B E 1979 Inadequacies in hospital drug handling. Acta Medica Scandinavica 205: 79–84

Burns B, Phillipson C 1986 Drugs, ageing and society: social and pharmacological perspectives. Croom Helm, London

Christopher L J, Ballinger B R, Shepherd A M M, Ramsay A, Crooks G 1979 A survey of hospital prescribing for the elderly. In: Crooks J, Stevenson I H (eds) Drugs and the elderly. Macmillan, London

Cook P J, Huggett A, Graham-Pole R, Savage I T 1983 Hypnotic accumulation and hangover in elderly inpatients: a controlled double-blind study of temazepam and nitrazepam. British Medical Journal 286: 100–102

DHSS 1983 Report to the Secretary of State for social Services of an informal working group on effective prescribing (Chairman P R Greenfield) HMSO, London

Dunnel K, Cartwright A 1972 Medicine takers, prescribers and hoarders. Routledge and Kegan Paul, London

Freeman G K 1979 Drug prescribing patterns in the elderly: a general practice study. In: Crooks J, Stevenson I H Drugs and the elderly. Macmillan, London

Hatch A M, Tapley A 1982 A self-administration system for elderly patients at Highbury Hospital. Nursing Times 78 (42): 1773–1774

McKinn W A, Mishara B L 1987 Drugs and aging. Butterworths, Toronto

Misra D P, Loudon J M, Staddon G E 1975 Albumin metabolism in elderly patients. Journal of Gerontology 30: 304–306

Novak L P 1972 Ageing, total body potassium, free fat mass and cell mass in males and females between 18 and 85 years. Journal of Gerontology 27: 438–443

Norris A H, Lundy T, Sheck N W 1963 Trends in selected indices of body composition in men between the ages of 30 and 80 years. Annals of the New York Academy of Science 110: 623–639

Platzer H 1988 A study into the causes of post-operative confusion in the elderly. Unpublished MSc Thesis, King's College, University of London

Taylor P 1984 The smoke ring: tobacco, money and multinational politics. Sphere Books, London

Wade B E, Sawyer L, Bell J 1983 Dependency with dignity. Occasional Papers on Social Administration, No 68, Bedford Square Press, London

FURTHER READING

Coleman V 1982 The good medicine guide. Thames and Hudson, London

David J A 1983 Drug round companion. Blackwell, Oxford

Heaney C R, Dow R J, MacConnachie A M, Crooks J 1982 Drugs in nursing practice. Churchill Livingstone, Edinburgh

Li Wan Po A 1982 Non-prescription drugs. Blackwell, Oxford

CHAPTER CONTENTS

Causes of death in the elderly 392

Where people die 393
General hospital 393
Hospice 393
Home for incurables 393
Continuing care unit/geriatric ward 393
Nursing Home 394
At home 394

Managing the problems of the dying elderly person 394
Pain 394
Anorexia and mouth care 395
Breathlessness and cough 395
Nausea and vomiting 396
Insomnia 396
Pressure sores 396
Constipation and incontinence 396
Confusion and terminal restlessness 397
Emotional reactions to dying 397
The relatives and carers 398

The hospice movement — could all elderly people benefit? 399

Euthanasia and elderly people 400

22

Death and dying

Jo Hockley

Nothing is more certain than death; nothing less certain than the time of its coming (Translation of the Latin inscription once present on official wills).

Discussion on the care of elderly people would be incomplete without some consideration of dying. Chalmers (1982) says that the best way to come to terms with old age is first to come to terms with death. This holds a great deal of truth, but as La Rochefoucauld (1613–80) wrote: 'Neither the sun nor death can be looked at with a steady eye.' Often there are no straightforward answers; there is only a willingness not to run away.

Each individual should take the opportunity to look at death, and perhaps beyond, before it becomes a threat to his or her own life. A doctor or nurse who has not come to terms with the fact of his or her own death will find it difficult to support the dying (Twycross 1982). In the following few pages we hope that what is so often considered to be a taboo subject might be seen as a positive opportunity to care, so fulfilling the needs not only of elderly dying people but also of the relatives and carers.

Many patients have remarked, 'It is not death that I am afraid of but rather *how* I am going to die that frightens me.' There is no doubt that this fear of the process of dying has not decreased over the years. Advance in medical science has enabled people to live longer, but many fear that it has been at the expense of dignity. However, with the advent of the hospice movement attitudes towards death and dying have started to change from that of a rather hopeless and depressing one into that of growth — growth not only for the patient, family and carers involved, but for society as a whole.

A century or so ago the greatest proportion of deaths occurred between the ages of 0 and 14 years. There has been an enormous change in this distribution over the past century, with 75% of deaths now occurring over the age of 65 years and as much as 55% of deaths taking place in those over the age of 75 (Office of Population Censuses and Surveys (OPCS) 1986). In dividing the elderly age group in two (those 65–74 years and those over 75 years of age) the percentage of male deaths in each category is much the same. However, when comparing female mortality in these two groups those dying at over 75 years of age are nearly three times as many as those dying in the 65–74 year age group (OPCS 1981).

CAUSES OF DEATH IN THE ELDERLY

In looking at the main causes of death in elderly people, heart disease accounts for just over a third of their deaths in England and Wales (OPCS 1981). Respiratory disease, cancer and cerebral vascular disease have consistently been the next most common causes of death. Until recently, deaths from cancer in elderly people were significantly high only in the 65–74 year old group, but statistics for 1986 show cancer overtaking cerebral vascular disease to become the second most common cause of death of people over 75 years of age. This may be because of the increased number of elderly people having more investigations to establish a diagnosis prior to death. All these diseases mentioned tend to cause a relatively *slow death*, often being accompanied by a certain amount of physical and psychological distress. The gradual awareness of deterioration can appear a wearisome burden both for the patient and the carer.

Sudden death

This is occasionally seen among elderly people, and a national survey (Bowling & Cartwright 1983) showed that 4% of elderly deaths were sudden, without any warning of illness. For the partner who is left, this kind of death can be one of the most difficult to cope with as there is no warning or anticipation of loss. Other relatives, however, may say, 'It was a nice way to go . . . she did not suffer,' which the grieving spouse may not find particularly helpful.

Natural death of old people

This kind of death is rarely observed among elderly people, partly because few of this age group die at home. Pneumonia, once known as 'the old man's friend' often continues being treated until it becomes a major decision whether to treat or not to treat. Cardiac resuscitation of old people may prevent natural death. A recent account of the attempted resuscitation of an 85-year-old man with a 10-year history of heart disease supports this. He had mentioned on several occasions that he did not wish to have his life prolonged, and the failed resuscitation only succeeded in producing unnecessary suffering for the patient, little comfort for the relatives and a feeling of failure on the part of the hospital staff. Bernard Levin (1980) reminds us of the macabre and repulsive scenes which accompanied the postponed deaths of General Franco of Spain and President Tito of Yugoslavia. Allowing life to move peacefully towards its close is much more preferable for dying people than endeavouring to keep them alive at all costs.

In many primitive societies where one might expect to see the acceptance of natural death, one sees a different concept — that of the acceleration of death. Hinton (1967) describes how nomadic tribes would leave the frail old person behind at the camp site to die, while the rest of the tribe moved on. In other societies it was traditional for the aged to request to be buried alive once they thought they were dying.

Suicidal death

This occurs especially amongst elderly bereaved people. They may feel that now their lifelong partner has gone there is no incentive to go on living.

Mr Day was a 75-year-old man who was admitted having attempted suicide by taking an overdose of sleeping tablets. His wife had died six months previously and although he went to luncheon clubs and got invited out by his attentive daughter at the weekend, he could not cope with the fact of being in the house alone.

The adjustment many bereaved elderly people have to make especially after a long happy marriage is often an uphill struggle, even with willing family and friends to help. (Suicide is discussed in more detail in Chapter 20.) If an actual suicide is not attempted one commonly hears of a widow or widower dying of a 'broken heart'.

WHERE PEOPLE DIE

In 1973 Cartwright et al estimated that about 60% of deaths occurred in hospital or similar institutions; 10 years later this was estimated at nearer 70%. In America, as many as four out of five elderly people spend their last days in a hospital, nursing home or other type of institution (Lerner 1970). However, Bowling and Cartwright (1983) found that if a patient was aged 80 or over at the time of death these were the ones least likely to die in hospital.

GENERAL HOSPITAL

The 'acute' setting of the general hospital, despite its superior medical facilities, is in many ways not the most ideal place for dying elderly people. The rigid routine and pressing physical needs of other patients easily takes time away from the psychosocial and spiritual care of the dying. The opportunity to just 'be' with dying people is given lower priority than all the things to 'do' for those patients getting better. Bowling and Cartwright (1983) found that patients dying in hospitals were more likely to die alone; even when the spouse had stayed overnight at the hospital they were often absent at the time of death. Nurses, medical students and doctors often lack the teaching and experience to initiate the different care the dying require, and so dying patients may feel isolated.

HOSPICE

A hospice incorporates a homely atmosphere with medical and nursing expertise. Since hospices are small (the largest in England having only 62 beds) patients are able to receive individualized physical, psychosocial and spiritual care. Within these units tests and observations are kept to a minimum so that the patient is not unnecessarily disturbed. The grieving family will be cared for for as long as is necessary even after the death of the patient. Hospices are ideal for caring for dying patients and their families because nurses and doctors are trained and motivated to do this work. Unfortunately, except in a few cases, beds are provided only for those dying from cancer.

HOME FOR INCURABLES

These long-stay units provide excellent care for patients dying from non-malignant disease. There is the time to build relationships between staff and patient in a homely atmosphere. Both this kind of Home and the hospice rely heavily on voluntary help and well-motivated personnel for practical and financial support.

CONTINUING CARE UNIT/GERIATRIC WARD

These units are perhaps the most used to caring for dying elderly people outside the hospice setting. People working in these units are often highly motivated but they can become frustrated because low staffing levels prevent them from giving adequate care. Many of the patients are in this setting because they have no one to care for them at home, and consequently few visitors are available to help with needs such as feeding and sitting with these patients. The great demand on the physical needs in these units again often detracts from the needs of the dying. However, because patients dying on these wards may have been nursed in the unit many months and sometimes years, a close relationship has often been established between patient and nurse and between patient and doctor, which helps to foster an understanding of the patient's specific needs.

The standard of care varies greatly from unit to unit, but unfortunately public and professional opinion is, often mistakenly, rather gloomy. There is still a stigma attached to being a patient in a geriatric ward.

NURSING HOME

These Homes vary in the quality of care they give to dying elderly residents. They rely on the community service of general practitioners and district nurses and although often providing a more homely setting than hospital, they might not be able to provide the expertise required to nurse the dying. The current pilot scheme in England of National Health Service nursing Homes may provide the necessary expertise. These are discussed briefly later in the chapter, and in more detail in Chapter 29.

AT HOME

For old people, dying at home is often preferred. They will suffer tremendous hardships to be able to stay in the familiarity and comfort of their own home where they can feel in control of what happens to them. However, few relatives can stand the pressure of giving 24-hour care over a long period of time without considerable back-up, medical care and support.

With the gradual emergence of domiciliary terminal care support teams attached to both hospitals and hospices, keeping the dying patient at home has been made a possibility in some areas. This would appear to be the ideal sort of care, but unfortunately this limited service is again generally confined to those dying of cancer.

MANAGING THE PROBLEMS OF THE DYING ELDERLY PERSON

Hinton (1967) states that most people will have a terminal period lasting a few days or weeks — not usually exceeding three months. The art of caring for the dying refers mainly to this period of terminal illness and, irrespective of the length of the terminal phase of an illness, control of the problems that may arise is essential in order to achieve a good quality of life. Unfortunately, the terminal phase for the old person dying from a non-malignant disease is not always easy to define.

In Cartwright et al's (1973) study, relatives or friends of the deceased reported several symptoms which either they or the patient had found distressing: pain (66%), sleeplessness (49%), loss of appetite (48%), dyspnoea (45%). As was said earlier, it is often 'how' someone is going to die that frightens them more than the actual concept of death.

PAIN

Most people fear pain more than anything (Saunders & Baines 1983), and many patients associate this fear with dying. It is important to remember that what presents as physical pain in dying people might be due to psychological, social or spiritual factors. 'Total' pain (Saunders 1978) is a phrase used in a deliberate attempt to encourage people to look at various factors of a dying patient's distress. Twycross (1978) states that pain is often not just a physical sensation but an emotional reaction to it. People's pain thresholds vary considerably but can be lowered and raised by certain factors (see Table 22.1).

Table 22.1 Factors modifying pain threshold. From Twycross 1978.

Threshold lowered ↓	Threshold raised ↑
Anger	Diversion
Anxiety	Sympathy
Depression/sadness	Elevation of mood
Discomfort	Relief of symptoms
Fatigue	Rest
Fear	Understanding
Insomnia	Sleep
Introversion	Drugs
Mental isolation	Analgesics
Past experience	Anxiolytics
	Antidepressants

There has been a considerable improvement in the control of pain over the past 10–15 years through the work of hospices and the wider use of opiates, nerve blocks and electrical stimulators, but Parkes and Parkes (1984) showed that pain was still a problem at home causing a 'very great anxiety' for spouses.

To believe the patient when he says he has pain is essential, but one must not stop there. The nurse's duty is not just to report pain but to know its site or sites, duration and description, whether it is most likely the result of the illness or of other factors such as infection, position or constipation, and how long after analgesia it recurs. Both body and pain charts can be helpful in recording and assessing pain on certain patients and allow for a better continuity of care. The assessment of pain has been described in detail in Chapter 17.

For the dying patient adequate relief of 'useless' or 'chronic' pain is paramount — without it, patients will often die sooner. Analgesics must be given regularly in a therapeutic dose before the pain returns. Charles-Edwards (1983) explains in detail the various analgesics available. The use of opiate medication (morphine and diamorphine) for the dying will almost always relieve any discomfort or suffering. The right dose of elixir for each patient (beginning with 2.5 mg) must be given every four hours for the proper control of pain. The 'Brompton cocktail' (a mixture of diamorphine, chlorpromazine and cocaine in an alcoholic base) was for many years the drug of choice, and is still used by some doctors. However, more recently it has been found that just diamorphine or morphine made up in chloroform water gives adequate pain relief without making the patient too sleepy.

An anti-emetic is also given with the opiate but prescribed separately to prevent any nausea. It can be discontinued after 2–3 days if nausea is not a problem. If and when a patient is unable to take oral medication, then suitable alternative measures must be taken, such as giving the analgesia sublingually, by suppository or by subcutaneous injection. Four-hourly subcutaneous injections can be substituted by a battery-operated 'syringe driver' which administers a steady dose of medication, usually diamorphine, over a 24-hour period.

ANOREXIA AND MOUTH CARE

Cartwright et al (1973) and Ward (1974) found that 76% and 61% respectively of their terminally ill patients complained of anorexia — second only to pain. Although a lot of people when they are very ill do not feel like eating, factors which reduce the appetite must be detected.

Dirty mouths, sore gums, constipation, nausea and badly presented food are all factors contributing to anorexia. Alcohol before or with a small, nicely presented meal with the willing offer of assistance can be a great help. Prednisolone 5 mg three times daily or dexamethasone 2 mg daily are both used to stimulate the appetite of the terminally ill person. However, these drugs can cause fungal infection in the mouth, and so strict and regular mouth care is most important.

Cleaning the teeth with toothpaste and brush is the most effective way of keeping the mouth clean, together with a reasonable fluid intake. Alternatively, a gloved hand and swabs can be used. Once the mouth has become dirty, corsodyl mouth-wash (and if infected, nystatin suspension) is effective. A solution of lime cordial on swabs is refreshing for the weak and dying patient whose sucking/swallowing reflex is often present right up until near the end. Small pieces of crushed ice placed in a piece of gauze can also be given to the patient to suck on or even be placed between the gums and the cheek. In this way the ice slowly dissolves without the danger of the patient choking. Relatives will often feel more relaxed and 'useful' if they are shown how to assist with this care.

BREATHLESSNESS AND COUGH

Breathlessness can be one of the most distressing symptoms for the patient and carer (whether relative or nurse). It is most often present in patients dying from chronic bronchitis, fibrosing alveolitis, heart failure and carcinoma of the lung. Breathlessness produces a vicious cycle of anxiety, fear, tension and increased breathlessness. All possible factors causing the breathlessness must be considered and treated appropriately. When these measures are ineffective, small doses of oral morphine or diamorphine with or without a phenothiazine given four-hourly (or just at night for some people) can reduce anxiety without reducing the rate of respirations. The use of oxygen via a humidifier and nasal specula can be continued if this is what the patient is accustomed to. Oxygen masks can act as a barrier to conversation with relatives and staff.

A tiresome cough can be extremely irritating and exhausting for the terminally ill patient. Codeine linctus is often quite adequate but, if the sputum is thick and tenacious, bromhexine (Bisolvon®) tablets or elixir is more effective in making the sputum less thick. Linctus methadone 5–10 ml is especially useful at night. In the last stages, if excessive secretions have accumulated ('death rattle') in the lungs, then hyoscine 0.4–0.6 mg given subcutaneously with an opiate can help to dry up secretions.

NAUSEA AND VOMITING

Nausea and vomiting can be two of the most demoralizing of all symptoms, and adequate control is essential. Hinton (1963) found that these two symptoms as well as breathlessness were the three most difficult to relieve and were particularly common for patients dying from heart and renal failure. Distinguishing between the causes of nausea or vomiting before prescribing the most appropriate antiemetic is the first important step in finding a solution to the problem. Often the cause is one or more of the following:

(a) the use of certain drugs prone to produce nausea, e.g. opiates, gastric irritants
(b) obstruction of the alimentary tract due either to disease or constipation
(c) raised intracranial pressure
(d) metabolic disturbances (e.g. uraemia, hypercalcaemia).

INSOMNIA

Insomnia in the terminally ill is a lot more common than is generally believed. Unfortunately, this problem is often accepted by both patient and nurse as part of being in hospital and is not taken seriously. A good night's sleep is very important if the terminally ill patient is going to be able to cope with the next day. Cartwright et al (1973) showed that sleeplessness in the dying patient is most common for patients suffering from a malignant or respiratory disease. If symptoms such as pain, breathlessness, anxiety, depression or urinary frequency can be relieved, insomnia should improve. However, if not, medication such as Welldorm®, temazepam, or Heminevrin® should

be given. The mistake is often made of omitting night sedation when a patient is receiving opiate medication. The latter is not a sedative.

PRESSURE SORES

Immobility, incontinence and malnutrition are some of the factors contributing to pressure sores in the elderly dying person. Once these patients get pressure sores it is extremely unlikely that they will heal, and so prevention is paramount. Unfortunately, pressure sores often appear to be accepted as a necessary evil in terminal care. With more people dying in hospital, pressure sores will increase (Barton & Barton 1981). Norton et al (1975) found that 54% of elderly dying patients had pressure sores, 24% developing them while in hospital. In a more recent but smaller study (Hockley et al 1988), where the average age of the elderly dying patient was 71 years, 61% of the patients had one or more pressure sores, 38% developing them after admission to hospital.

Nurses often appear to be more alert to the risk of sores developing in patients dying from malignant disease than they are in the case of patients dying from other diseases. We hope this will change now that the approach to nursing is more 'problem oriented' than 'disease oriented'. Good observation and nursing care with the help of 'ripple' mattresses, soft sheepskins and Spenco Silicore® mattresses should prevent sores from developing. Time taken to explain the necessity of relieving pressure to both patient and relatives is time well spent.

CONSTIPATION AND INCONTINENCE

Constipation and urinary incontinence are the two problems likely to make the dying patient feel most undignified. The constipating effect of opiates, weakness, and lack of fluid intake are a few of the factors making the regular prescription of aperients important.

Bulk aperients such as lactulose (Duphalac®) syrup and dioctyl sodium sulphosuccinate (Medo or Forte) are very useful for softening the stool. Stimulant aperients to increase peristalsis such as bisacodyl (Dulcolax®) tablets or sennoside B (Senokot®) tablets can be used. More often than not, however, for the terminally ill patient a combination of a bulk softener and bowel stimulant is preferable.

When the elderly dying patient has had good bladder control, incontinence is often only a problem in the last few hours of life. Continued incontinence is an additional factor in the breakdown of pressure areas, and catheterization should be considered if incontinence persists over a period of 24–36 hours. However, catheterization should not be performed as a matter of routine and patients should be given a clear understanding of what is going to be done whether they are able to respond or not.

CONFUSION AND TERMINAL RESTLESSNESS

Confusion in dying people can be a difficult problem to cope with, especially if the patient is restless at the same time. It can cause a lot of distress to both family and staff. Pain, dyspnoea, a full bladder or rectum may be contributing factors exacerbating confusion, and appropriate treatment of these should be carried out first. For the patient suffering from dementia a move to unfamiliar surroundings is bound to increase the confusion, and isolation may easily make the situation worse.

The use of sedatives and tranquillizers must be selective but the following may be helpful:

- haloperidol (Serenace®) 2–10 mg daily in divided doses
- thioridazine (Melleril®) 25 mg three times daily
- chlorpromazine (Largactil®) 25–50 mg three times daily
- stelazine (Trifluoperazine®) 2–4 mg daily in divided doses.

If muscle twitching is present during the last day or so, diazepam (Valium®) 5–10 mg intramuscularly or by suppository is effective.

When a crisis occurs, such as an acute exacerbation of breathlessness, haematemesis or haemoptysis, an injection of diamorphine 2.5 mg and hyoscine 0.4 mg with or without chlorproma-zine can be effective. This, together with a nurse to sit and hold the patient's hand, will almost always calm the situation.

EMOTIONAL REACTIONS TO DYING

In describing people's emotional reactions to dying, Kubler-Ross (1973) mentions five stages: denial (disbelief), anger, bargaining, depression and acceptance. These are not necessarily everyone's experience but some of these descriptive stages may be present and patients should be allowed to express them and to work through all their feelings.

Hinton (1963) found that depression and anxiety increased for the dying patient with the length of illness and the degree of distressing symptoms. However, intense anxiety is often only really seen when patients are dying with breathing difficulties or where they have continued to deny the imminence of their death. It is very difficult to measure anxiety, although Carr (1982) states that moderate anxiety is experienced by between one quarter and one half of patients, but is less often seen in patients over 60 years of age. Fear of the unknown and the unexplained, of being a burden or becoming helpless can often 'paralyze' dying people into an inability to communicate. If these fears can be identified and discussed it will help decrease anxiety and reassure the patient of the love and care surrounding her.

Hope is a very important ingredient to life and should not be excluded from the care of the dying. To be 'written off' by the doctor with the statement 'There is nothing more we can do for you' is devastating. This need never be said — one can always care. Hope for each day or a realistic event should be encouraged, but there is no place for false hope.

Dying does not usually call for specialized skills in counselling — just a willingness to try to understand and stay near. However, when the question 'Am I going to die, nurse?' is suddenly and unexpectedly thrust upon us it is too easy for the denial 'No, of course not' to be the immediate response. It is important to remember that often a patient does not want an immediate answer and this in itself can be a worthwhile pause. To take time to decide what to say is most valuable and can be found by returning the patient's question with a further question.

THE RELATIVES AND CARERS

Relatives of dying patients are now more often recognized as part of the emotional network from which the patient has come, and they often need as much help to adjust to the situation as the patient does. In trying to help them they must be allowed to express the confusion, fear, anger and grief they feel. The loss of a family member can be the single most feared event in the life of an individual (Kalish 1977). Whatever age one is, this has to be true; but for the elderly spouse there is the heartbreak, loss and loneliness after many years of marriage. To try and encourage the building of links with close friends or family at this time, before the death, can prevent the relative from isolating her or himself and so help in the bereavement process to follow.

Richmond and Waisman (1955) emphasized that the family's involvement in the physical care of the dying person is extremely important — allowing the family to feel they have been able to 'do' something. They should not be made to feel guilty if they cannot help, or do not want to help, in these tasks. Hampe (1975) has identified eight needs of the spouse of a dying patient: visiting at any time; helping with physical care; prompt and competent attention to physical and emotional needs of the patient; awareness of diagnosis and daily progress by the nursing staff; awareness of impending death; expressing anxieties regarding the care given; comfort and support; friendliness by the health professionals to the spouse.

Some relatives feel it is best that the truth be kept from the dying patient. This, unfortunately, causes a conspiracy of silence to be built up, isolating the patient from those around. Relatives often make excuses to go to the toilet in order to see the doctor, and soon further 'lies' have to be told to keep up the façade. Families should be warned beforehand how easy it is to lie to the patient about her condition but how difficult it is to handle the problems and tensions that this creates.

Inevitably there comes the time when the dying

are too weak to 'entertain' their visitors and many relatives feel awkward and helpless. At this point encouraging both relatives and staff to sit by the bed and 'just be there' is often helpful. To the weak and dying patient, the comfort of knowing someone is there is all she needs — knowing that she is not alone. This can, however, be very exhausting for relatives and they may well need to be told to go for a break or go home for a meal with the reassurance that someone will keep a close watch on the patient's condition. One of the dangers of open visiting can be that relatives get overtired, especially if a patient is dying over a number of weeks. In these circumstances, following the idea of many hospices, to make sure the relative has a complete 'day off' is very important.

The anticipation of loss of the loved one should not be discouraged in the case of a terminal illness. Parkes (1972) states that as much as 50% of the grieving should be done beforehand if the person is to cope with the bereavement process. Where anticipatory grief has not taken place, as with sudden loss, it can cause serious physical or mental breakdown of the bereaved person afterwards. The following case illustrates this point. An elderly widow was admitted with an acute attack of asthma, never having had asthma before. She happened to be admitted to the care of the same doctors who had looked after her husband the previous year. Through tears she related how she had been told by the doctors that her husband had chronic bronchitis and when asked if she wanted to nurse him at home, she agreed. After a rapid deterioration he died four days after discharge and on his death certificate the wife noticed the cause of death to be carcinoma of the bronchus. She had not suspected that her husband was going to die and was utterly distraught — 'If I had known I would of done so much more for him, and now he is dead.' With a lot of belated support this lady was slowly able to recover. In being able to give dying people and their relatives the care and respect they deserve enables society once again to recognize a depth of human compassion and understanding.

The following extract describes beautifully how many of us feel when faced with bereaved relatives — but it is our duty in caring to reach out to them.

I did not know what to say to him, I felt awkward and blundering. I did not know how I could reach him, where I could overtake him and go hand in hand with him once more. It is such a secret place the land of tears (Antoine de Saint-Exupéry 1945).

THE HOSPICE MOVEMENT—COULD ALL ELDERLY PEOPLE BENEFIT?

To do all we can to help you, not only to die peacefully, but also to live until you die (Cicely Saunders 1978).

The growth of what has become known as the 'hospice movement' now has an influence reaching far and wide across the world. The United Kingdom alone has over 200 hospices, varying in size from 8–62 bedded units. The advent of the hospice movement has revealed an attitude of care that is relevant not only to the cancer sufferer but to all who are dying, elderly people included. Evidence of the gratitude shown by our needy society must be seen in the amount of financial support and voluntary help people have given to this movement.

The word 'hospice' was first used in the Middle Ages to describe a 'resting place' or inn, where travelling pilgrims throughout Europe could stay, finding food and spiritual comfort to equip them for their journey ahead. This same idea of a resting place for weary travellers — those weary from life's journey — has been adopted by the hospice movement to describe its philosophy of care. The emphasis is still that of a resting place and not a terminus, since death is not seen as the end, but as a passing on.

Within a hospice, basic nursing care is the same as that in hospital but the working environment and philosophy differ greatly. All members of a hospice ward team are motivated to the individualized care of each patient, who in turn receives continual assessment of his or her physical and psychosocial needs as well as sensitive spiritual care. Honesty and openess allow patients to feel secure in the answers to their questions and time is given to talk things through. Families are considered an important part of the patient's emotional well-being and every effort is made to meet all the different needs from the youngest grandchild facing his or her first loss, to the wife, mother, sister or husband of the person dying.

Some hospice units have a few beds for those dying from other diseases, such as motor neurone disease. Others provide a 'holiday relief service that enables relatives caring full-time for someone to go away for a two-week break.

To accommodate within hospices all those who are dying would not be appropriate and certainly was never the idea behind setting them up. If this occurred, death still would run the danger of being hidden away — not in a side-room, as happens now, but in a hospice. Instead, hospices should be seen as providing an opportunity for educating doctors, nurses and the general public in the art of caring for dying people. Cartwright et al (1973) in their nationwide study on 'Life before death' recognized this and recommended that there should be a wide dissemination of these principles into the acute and geriatric hospitals. In this way, they felt, all terminally ill patients, whether old or young, dying from an acute or chronic illness, could benefit from the hospice expertise. To a small degree this has started to emerge with the setting up of symptom control support teams and palliative care units in a few district and specialist hospitals. Unfortunately, the emphasis is often concentrated on patients with malignant disease.

The recent development in this country of state nursing Homes similar to those in Denmark (Dopson 1983, Ch. 29 of this volume) could provide places where the quality of life for elderly dying people is best achieved. The three NHS nursing Homes, accommodating around 20–30 people, plan individualized care for each resident. The Department of Health and Social Security (1983) states that an important requirement of the new nursing Homes is to meet the emotional, psychological and spiritual needs of residents. Although these Homes are not specifically intended to provide terminal care, it is recognized that residents may require support and treatment relating to terminal illness and such care will be provided in the Home. This is a further way in which elderly people may benefit from the dissemination of hospice care principles.

EUTHANASIA AND ELDERLY PEOPLE

Over the last 20 years euthanasia, the literal meaning of the word being 'an easy death' (Gr. *eu*, well, *thanatos*, death), has become one of the moral issues of our day. People have had the power to induce death for many hundreds of years but euthanasia is probably at present more widely discussed, (a) because of the greater ability we now have to prolong life owing to medical advances, and (b) the increasingly secular approach society has towards life. All of us would want an easy death in the sense of it being free from pain and other distressing symptoms, but this is not what is currently meant by the word 'euthanasia'. It has now come to mean 'the deliberate termination of the life of a person who is suffering from a distressing irremediable disease' (British Medical Association 1973).

Euthanasia first became a social issue with the formation of the Voluntary Euthanasia Society (or EXIT, as we now know it) in 1935. Since then, pressure has been put on Parliament to legalize the action of bringing about death when certain criteria are met. Four Bills have been introduced and debated since 1935 but all have been rejected. In 1969 the Representative Body of the British Medical Association passed a resolution that the medical profession had a duty to preserve life and to relieve pain, and they condemned euthanasia.

Carr (1982) states that public support for euthanasia is probably based upon the expectation that death will be unduly lengthy and prolonged because of current medical knowledge and techniques. It is true that for some elderly people dying now produces fears of dependence and pain, as well as physical and psychological indignities. However 'requests' for an 'easy way out' are heard most often from relatives and friends of these patients, rather than from the elderly people themselves. It would appear that one's hold on life is often as strong at 70 or 80 years as it is at 30 or 40 years.

The legalizing of euthanasia poses a very real threat to elderly people, especially the invalid, the demented and the chronically ill. Providing for sick elderly people is not cheap in both economic and social terms; and it will not get any cheaper with nearly half the elderly population of England and Wales now living longer than 75 years. But the question must be, 'What is life about—wealth or people?' The incurable and elderly exist as real people and should be seen as providing an opportunity for our society to express compassion, patience and understanding. What is needed is not a change in the law but a change in people's attitudes towards the dying. If society holds strong ageist attitudes towards the elderly, the atrocities of Germany in 1939 could be repeated. Then, state institutions were required to report on patients who had been ill for five years or more, or who were unable to work. From brief information such as name, race, marital status, next of kin, who visited them and who bore the financial burden, decisions were made on their extermination (Shaeffer & Koop 1980).

Reliance on their families or on the state for help can become an enormous burden for old people. This burden can easily pressurize them into thinking that 'they are a nuisance' or that 'they would be better off dead'. With the legalization of euthanasia this pressure could be even greater, and could run the risk of making elderly people feel obliged to decide when to die. Every tablet or injection prescribed or given would be a threat to the original trust between patients and their carers if doctors and nurses had the right to 'kill'.

Euthanasia, in its current meaning, is also inconsistent with the biblical view that human life should be cherished. In saying this, one is not advocating life being preserved at all costs; this would be as unacceptable as euthanasia. Each person, old or young, should be seen as a unique individual, and loved right up until the end of his or her life.

Over the last 10 years it has become increasingly popular in the United States to sign a 'living will'. Although the legal status of such a document is unclear, its purpose is to record the person's own preference for medical treatment in the event of his or her having a critical illness or injury. This seems to be a reasonably safe compromise which Britain could also adopt. There will always be the distinction between tender, loving and appropriate care for elderly people and that of deliberate killing. The former kind of care has been exemplified in the work of the hospice movement.

Postscript

This poem was written by a woman of 90 years shortly before her death.

Thoughts at ninety

If I could choose the method of my death
Would it be sinking into soundless sleep?
The wild confusion of a storm-swept sea?
Or the sharp mercy of the headsman's sword?

There is no dread in these, no trembling fear
When swept in silent speed to the unknown.

Or with a smile, as did my little son—
Eyes closed as if in sleep, but his small hands
Curling around my hand until he felt
The golden circle of my wedding ring
And stroked that finger as he always had
From smallest babyhood. He found the ring,
Smiled a contented smile . . . and went to
    heaven.

Or as my mother, opening suddenly
Eyes that lit up to see a happy vision
And cried a loving greeting with their names
Of those of us who had gone before.
Any of these so varied deaths I'd die
But with the wistful hope that I might be
Not quite alone to face what waits for me.

Adelaide de Cabsonne, September 1983. (Published with the author's permission.)

REFERENCES

Barton A, Barton M 1981 The management and prevention of pressure sores. Faber, London
Bowling A, Cartwright A 1983 Life after a death — a study of the elderly widowed. Tavistock Publications, London
British Medical Association 1973 The problem of euthanasia. In: Trowell H (ed) The unfinished debate on euthanasia. SCM Press, London
Carr A T 1982 Dying and bereavement. In: Hall J (ed) Psychology for nurses and health visitors. Macmillan, London
Cartwright A, Hockey L, Anderson J L 1973 Life before death. Routledge and Kegan Paul, London
Chalmers G L 1982 Caring for the elderly sick. Pitman, London
Charles-Edwards A 1983 The nursing care of the dying patient. Beaconsfield Publications, London
de Saint-Exupéry A 1945 The Little Prince. Heinemann, London
Department of Health and Social Security 1983 The experimental NHS nursing homes for elderly people — an outline. DHSS, London
Dopson L 1983 Having your own front door. Nursing Times 79 (October 19): 10–12
Hampe S O 1975 Needs of the grieving spouse in a hospital setting. Nursing Research 24(2): 113–119
Hinton J M 1963 The physical and mental distress of the dying. Quarterly Journal of Medicine 32: 1–21
Hinton J 1967 Dying. Penguin, London
Hockley J, Dunlop R J, Davies R J 1988 A survey of distressing symptoms in terminally ill patients and their families and the response to setting up a symptom control team. British Medical Journal 296: 1715–1717
Kalish R A 1977 Dying and preparing for death: a view of families. In: Feifel H (ed) New meanings of death. McGraw-Hill, New York
Kubler-Ross E 1973 On death and dying. Tavistock Publications, London
Lerner M 1970 Why and where people die. In: Brimm, Freeman, Levine and Scotch (eds). Dying patient. Russell Sage Foundation, New York
Levin B 1980 Generalissimos die in bed. The Times April 29: 24–27
Norton D, McLaren R, Exton-Smith A N 1975 A study of factors concerned in the production of pressure sores and their prevention. In: An investigation of geriatric nursing problems in hospital. Churchill Livingstone, Edinburgh
Office of Population Censuses and Surveys 1981 Mortality statistics. HMSO, London
Office of Population Censuses and Surveys 1986 Mortality Statistics. Series DH2 no 13. HMSO, London
Parkes C M 1972 Bereavement studies of grief in adult life. Penguin, London
Parkes C M, Parkes J L N 1984 Hospice versus hospital care: re-evaluation of ten years of prognosis in terminal care. Post-Graduate Medical Journal 60 (February): 120–124
Richmond J B, Waisman H A 1955 Psychological aspects of management of children with malignant disease. American Journal of Diseases of Childhood 89 (January): 42–47
Saunders C 1978 The management of terminal disease. Arnold, London
Saunders C, Baines M 1983 Living with dying. Oxford University Press, Oxford
Shaeffer F, Koop C E 1980 Whatever happened to the human race? Marshall, Morgan and Scott, London
Twycross R G 1978 Relief of pain. In: Saunders C (ed) The management of terminal disease. Arnold, London
Twycross R G 1982 Euthanasia — a physician's viewpoint. Journal of Medical Ethics 8: 86–95
Ward A 1974 Telling the patient. Journal of the Royal College of General Practitioners 24: 465–468

Part 3

The organization of care for elderly people

CHAPTER CONTENTS

The social context 405

Definitions of self-care and self-help in old age 407
Self-help 407
Self-health care in old age 409

Case studies 410
Health information and self-care skills: pensioners' health courses 410
Emotional support, information and advice: peer health counselling 412

Conclusion: problems and prospects for self-care and self-help 413

23

Self-care and health in old age

Miriam Bernard, Chris Phillipson

The theme of this chapter is the concept of older people taking more active control of their own health. The areas to be discussed are that of self-health care in old age and the development of self-help groups. The former refers to actions taken by individuals with regard to health issues; the latter denotes activity by groups of individuals who share similar health and social concerns. In this chapter we shall, first, consider the background to the development of activities in these areas; secondly, review in more detail various definitions of self-health care and self-help; thirdly, describe some examples of initiatives and projects developed with older people; and finally, examine the linkages between broader discussions in the field of old age and self-help and self-health care.

THE SOCIAL CONTEXT

The idea of personal responsibility for health is now well-established (Barker 1985). It is clearly the case, as Porter has observed, that 'a great deal of healing in the past . . . has involved professional practitioners only marginally or not all, and has been primarily a tale of medical self-help or community care'. In medicine's history, Porter writes, 'the initiatives have often come from, and power has frequently rested with the sufferer, or with lay people in general, rather than with the individual physician or the medical profession at large' (Porter 1985, p. 175). Yet this historical truth is open to some variation, depending, in particular, on the extent of professionalization of health care and the accessibility of medical knowledge. There are some periods when medicine (and its practitioners) play a dominant role in influencing ideas about health; other periods where, by contrast, they are much weaker. The post-war period from the 1950s to the early 1970s was probably a case of the former (Burns & Phillipson 1986). Over the past ten years, however, we have seen a growing interest in the idea of individuals taking more control over their own health, with older people being a key group behind this development. What are some of the reasons that can be identified to explain this growing concern with issues relating to self-care in old age?

The emergence of self-care and self-help can be attributed to a number of factors. They reflect, in the first place, a disenchantment with aspects of conventional medicine as experienced by older people (for example, the problems associated with the use of drugs in old age). Concern about the over- and under-prescribing of drugs has stimulated an interest both in non-pharmacological approaches to treatment and to methods which reduce the social dependency implicit in the doctor-patient relationship (Lipton & Lee 1988). At a wider level, the interest in self-care and self-help reflects changes in attitudes towards old age itself. Here we are seeing a questioning of traditional stereotypes of old age, both by older people and by their informal carers (Fennell et al 1988). There is an analogy here, we would suggest, with debates in the women's health movement. In the 1960s and 1970s there was a concern, for example, to replace the medical view of women as inferior and 'sickly' people, with a recognition of their status as normal, healthy human beings — the so-called 'well woman' approach (Doyal 1983). This entailed struggling against sexist beliefs and practices in health care. At the same time, there was growing awareness that certain areas of knowledge, previously monopolized by doctors, were potentially of immense value to women. Systematic efforts were therefore made to demystify medical knowledge and to make it more widely available.

The 'well woman' approach is now being developed in similar ways by groups of older people (Porcino 1983). First, there is the attempt to define growing old as a normal process, and to challenge its presentation as an illness and a deviation from a well-established path. Secondly, there is a concern to restore to older people knowledge and control of the ageing process. The parallels with the women's movement are clear: older people must be brought back into the arena of prevention and care. They have skills and abilities which can be used to ensure that growing old is a positive and affirmative experience (Thornton 1989). Depriving older people of the necessary health and social care skills makes a positive ageing that much harder to achieve.

An additional influence supporting self-care and self-help has come from within the field of health education and health promotion. The justification for such activity in relation to older people has typically rested on a number of arguments, all of which rely on an element of self-care/self-help. In America, the National Research Council (Gilford 1988) has cited the following reasons for adopting a health promotion and disease prevention approach with older people: first, because of the plasticity of the ageing process; secondly, because of the risks associated with normal ageing and the predominance of care rather than cure in terms of the focus of health care work.

As regards the plasticity of ageing, the evidence suggests that some harmful conditions are capable of modification given appropriate interventions in later life. For example, research on osteoporosis indicates that moderate exercise can retard age-related bone loss and even in some cases increase bone density in very elderly women (Smith 1985). Secondly, it is important to recognize the extent to which the various changes associated with normal ageing carry increased risk of conditions such as cardiovascular disease, cerebrovascular disease and mature onset diabetes. Brody (1988) refers to these as age-dependent diseases, i.e. conditions which appear to be closely related to the ageing of the individual. For such conditions, he suggests, specific cures and treatments offer little promise. Instead, 'postponement of morbidity by interventions by research methods intended to delay body ageing, or by modification of health habits and diets, will be our great allies' (Brody 1988, p. 214). In a similar way it has been argued that it may be better to substitute the term *usual* instead of *normative* ageing, to recognize the possibility of adverse effects accompanying the changes associated with advanced age. At the same time, we need to consider the importance of considering techniques to modify these usual but not necessarily harmful, characteristics (Gilford 1988, p. 114). Greater use of self-care/self-help approaches will undoubtedly be an important feature of such techniques and should be seen as a valuable adjunct to conventional therapies (see, for example, Lorig & Fries 1983).

DEFINITIONS OF SELF-CARE AND SELF-HELP IN OLD AGE

As we have argued, the idea and concepts involved in self-care are not new and there is now a growing body of research in Europe and North America addressing the theory, methodology and practice of self-care (Social Science and Medicine 1989). However, because British work in these areas is as yet limited, it is important to map out precisely what is meant by terms such as self-care and self-help. In this section, then, we shall review various definitions of these terms as well as illustrating some practical examples.

SELF-HELP

Self-help is perhaps the key term to begin with in any discussion of developments in the field of self-health care. It is a term which symbolizes the shift during the 1980s towards a much wider acceptance of a social model of health: a model which acknowledges and emphasizes that health and illness are not narrowly defined medical phenomena, but are affected and influenced by social, economic and environmental factors (Kickbusch & Hatch 1982). Such a view is also very much in keeping with the WHO/UNICEF declaration on primary health care, which made clear that health should be considered as 'a state of complete physical, mental and social well-

being, and . . . a fundamental human right' (WHO 1978).

Kickbusch and Hatch identify a self-help continuum for health care 'which ranges from individual involvement in self-care to possibly large scale action on the part of self-help organisations' (Kickbusch & Hatch 1982, p. 66). Self-help implies purposeful organization into groups which have a common aim or purpose and which, in turn, connote mutuality rather than simple self-interest. Knight and Hayes (1981) for example, outline seven key features of self-help groups:

1. They are voluntary
2. Members have shared problems
3. They have meetings for mutual benefit
4. The helper/helped role is shared
5. The group is concerned with constructive action towards shared goals
6. Groups are self-run
7. Groups exist without outside funding.

These characteristics, they argue, serve as a model against which actual groups can be compared, as in their studies of self-help community initiatives in four inner city areas of London (Knight & Hayes 1981), and their review of nine innovatory economic self-help projects (Knight & Hayes 1982). More recently Vincent (1986), in her study of self-help groups in health care in the East Midlands, adopted a broader three-fold 'prescriptive ideal' in which self-help groups are characterized by:

1. Members sharing a problem
2. Reciprocity being the primary mode of exchange
3. Participative democracy informing organizational arrangements.

Groups were then defined as self-help if they had one or more of these features. Whatever definition or categories one adopts, it is important to recognize that the development of self-help activity can take new forms and may in fact render existing definitions outmoded (Posner 1989).

Alternative care services

These have often developed in the context of self-help groups and may in fact be provided by them. In essence, they are services which would otherwise not be available to particular groups or are services which promote forms of treatment or care other than those provided by the formal health care system. One example is the development in some American states of refuges for older people who have been subject to domestic violence. This initiative reflects the significant debate surrounding this issue during the 1980s (Pillemer & Wolf 1986).

Self-help support systems

This refers to organized support systems for self-help groups, such as clearing houses or centres, health shops and health centres. Support is given through networking such groups, and by providing resources such as rooms, telephones and organizational help; speaking on behalf of a network of such groups; initiating groups; publishing directories, news bulletins and so on. In Britain, such self-help support systems are most well developed in respect of support to carers. The Alzheimer's Disease Society and the Carers National Association, for example, take a particular interest in the development of respite care, carers' support groups and other means of assisting carers. They also develop training and information for professionals and carers, as well as guidelines for policy-makers and service providers.

Self-help organizations and pressure groups

These can vary enormously in scope and size and may be organized around general or specific health care issues. They may focus on health care organization, health promotion or disease prevention, and are aimed at bringing about changes in the health system or society at large. This is often the most visible, action-oriented part of self-help. Again, the carers' organizations are particularly active in this field, whilst the national Age Well campaign has been concerned since 1985 with encouraging a positive approach to health in old age. It has concentrated on motivating older people,

professionals and community organizations to develop and expand their work by initiating Age Well shows, study days and workshops, as well as by establishing a variety of health promotion groups around the country.

Kickbusch and Hatch (1982) contend that the women's health movement most adequately reflects the self-help continuum, and that many of its radical ideas 'have now become commonly accepted by the self-help movement in general' (p. 7). These key ideas are particularly pertinent to our current discussion about older people and include:

- the idea that self-reliance is possible
- giving back to people the confidence in their own knowledge and skills
- letting people trust their own experiences
- convincing them that they can help themselves and each other.

Some examples of activity by older people include: widow's support groups; self-help groups for carers of people with Alzheimer's disease; hypertension clubs; and pensioner health groups. An interesting example of a self-help group concerned with the problem of high blood pressure is cited by Lafaille:

There are two parts to the meeting of the group. In the first part, both blood pressure and weight are recorded. This enables the noting of developments and changes, and individuals can find out which factors are influences on blood pressure. In the second part, the influences on blood pressure are discussed. The information for such discussion are recorded by the members themselves. So the members talk to each other about their way of life and try to find the connection between factors causing high blood pressure and the blood pressure of each member of the group (Lafaille 1983, p. 173).

Riessman et al (1984) describe an arthritis clinic in New York which uses self-help techniques. They write:

The Arthritis Clinic at the Downstate Medical Center in Brooklyn, New York, operates a self-help project for its patients. Group members share their experiences and focus on ways to cope with the problems of living and dealing with families, jobs, neighbors, and physical incapacitation. Some of the most important skills discussed are how and when to ask for help (and how to ask people *not* to help when help is not required); how to question doctors and nurses; and how to perform the exercises patients have developed for themselves. A social network has developed outside the meetings, with members calling each other frequently and planning activities together (Riessman et al 1984, p. 20).

Riessman et al highlight a number of criticisms that have been made of the self-help approach: that it involves blaming the victim; that it diverts attention from basic structural change, and that it fragments problems. However, they also find (along with many others, e.g. Macfadyen 1985) many positive features of self-help care. Such activity can raise consciousness about the inadequacy of existing health resources; can increase confidence when dealing with health (and welfare) professionals; can assist in combating iatrogenic disease; and can widen the scope and effectiveness of health education. In addition, self-help can help to demystify the nature of the ageing process, revealing it to be a natural and positive feature of the life-course. This realization may also allow individuals to place the role of drugs and other medical interventions into their proper perspective, seeing them as just one element in a range of strategies for experiencing a healthy old age. Whether such ideas can be translated into reality will be considered in our later discussion of various case studies.

SELF-HEALTH CARE IN OLD AGE

Activities in health-related groups have come to form an important role in the lives of many older people. However, this itself reflects the central role of self-care in old age. This activity has been defined as 'all the actions that an individual takes to prevent, diagnose, and treat personal ill health; all individual behaviours calculated to maintain and improve health, and decisions to access and use both informal support systems and formal medical services' (Coppard et al 1984, p. 3).

Dean (1982) has argued that 'self-care is the individual health behaviour component of self-help' (p. 20). At the individual level, the research

evidence shows that while self-medication is the most extensive form of self-care behaviour, health knowledge and basic treatment skills are poor, especially amongst older people (Dean 1982). That such 'skills are relatively easy to teach and pose few risks for health complications even in the absence of a professional' (Coppard et al 1984, p. 3), would suggest that there is considerable scope for promoting self-care amongst elderly people (Health Education Council 1985).

In their review of self-health care and older people for the World Health Organization, Coppard and his colleagues (1984) outline five skills or components of such care. These are:

- *Simple diagnostic skills* which the individual can use to make an estimate of her health status e.g. checking temperature, taking pulse rate, breast self-examination
- *Skills relevant to simple acute conditions*, e.g. treatment of the common cold and everyday illness, first-aid for non life-threatening injuries
- *Skills needed to treat chronic illness*, e.g. self-monitoring, following prescribed regimens
- *Skills for disease prevention and health promotion*, e.g. exercise, diet, avoiding tobacco and alcohol abuse, good dental hygiene, healthy life styles
- *Health information skills*, e.g. what steps to take prior to seeking professional treatment, how to obtain health information, how to gain access to formal care.

Work in the area of arthritis provides an example of the self-health care approach. Lorig et al (1984) report on an arthritis self-management course given to older people (20% of whom were over the age of 75) in Northern California. The course examined areas such as: nutrition, doctor/patient communication, use of drugs, a relaxation and joint protection programme, and the design of individual exercises. According to Lorig et al:

The course utilized a highly experiential process with emphasis on decision-making. For example, participants were not given specific exercises but instead were taught principles for designing an exercise program. Rather than discuss the evils of arthritis quackery, participants were taught how to evaluate what they read in the popular press and how to make judgements about new treatments. The techniques of group discussion, brainstorming, demonstration, and verbal contracting were used extensively throughout the course (Lorig et al 1984, p. 456).

Coppard et al (1984) describe the 'Growing Younger Program' in Boise, Idaho, which has focused upon doctor-patient communication and practising self-diagnosis skills. Over 1500 neighbourhood groups in Boise have been exposed to the programme over the past three years, and it is beginning to reach more frail elderly as well as fitter senior citizens.

The 'Healthy Lifestyles for Seniors' project, another American development, had a number of goals aimed at improving older people's control over their health. Savo (1984), in her monograph on self-care and self-help, summarizes these goals:

1. To increase participants' knowledge of the normal physiological and psychological processes of ageing and the adaptations required by these normal changes

2. To increase participants' positive feelings and attitudes about the ageing process and their ability to make positive lifestyle changes

3. To increase the incidence of participants' accepting responsibility and taking action to improve and maintain their health, and

4. To improve measurable indicators of health.

Some of the objectives were normalized weight and blood pressure; increased strength, flexibility and feelings of relaxation; and decreased physical pain, stress symptoms and muscle tension.

A final point to be made is that rather than being outside the remit of health professionals, such initiatives should and could be facilitated by medical and nursing staff, given appropriate gerontological training and experience. Indeed, the pioneering Well Elderly Program for medical students, directed by Robert Butler at the Mount Sinai Medical Center in New York, has shown that ageist attitudes amongst health care professionals can be effectively countered through the exposure of students to healthy older adults in mutual learning activities (Aldeman et al 1988). Results from

this experimental programme are still being analysed, but it has already been suggested that it could be extended to include both nursing and social work students (see also Phillipson and Strang 1986).

CASE STUDIES

HEALTH INFORMATION AND SELF-CARE SKILLS: PENSIONERS' HEALTH COURSES

In 1981 the health education unit of the London borough of Barnet was approached by Taskforce (now Pensioners Link) and the Community Health Council to help in initiating a health course for older people. As a result, eight local pensioners joined forces with two health and community workers to plan a 12-week course. The course provided pensioners with information about how their bodies work and the meaning of medical conditions as well as information about rights and services. It included sessions on ageing; bones, backs and joints; blood pressure and heart conditions; bowels and water-works; diet; hospital stays; yoga and relaxation. All of the sessions were aimed at challenging the negative stereotypes surrounding pensioners' health. Information sheets were provided for course participants, and relevant books from the local library could also be borrowed.

As a result of the success of the first health course, a number of other programmes were arranged by professional workers working with local pensioners. No two courses were the same, and the range of topics covered was extensive. Moreover, the courses were not 'ends in themselves' and a variety of follow-up activities have developed, including ongoing social activity clubs with a health education input, health groups, a swimming club, keep-fit classes and a lip-reading class. The implication seems to be that if professional workers actively involve pensioners from the outset in the planning and development of a course, such programmes can act as a trigger for long-term activities.

In February 1985, Barnet Pensioners Link was

awarded funding by the (then) Health Education Council for a two-year project aimed at consolidating and developing this initial work. The initial task was to review the work already undertaken, and to explore what could be learnt from the experiences of people attending and running the health courses. Between May and July 1985, 187 pensioners, 19 speakers and 14 pensioner group co-ordinators completed questionnaires. The main findings from this review highlight a number of important issues in relation to self-health care and the role of professional workers (Meade 1986). For pensioners, the chance to make new friends and to go to something which offers more than the traditional game of bingo is a decided attraction. In addition, over 60% of attendees said that their main reason for coming was an interest in keeping themselves healthy. Many have made use of the information, seeking out practical help from various services or taking positive steps to maintain their own health. Self-confidence and understanding have also been enhanced as the following comments illustrate (see Age Well Ideas Pack):

I've learnt more about my blood pressure. I've had it for seven years. I've found out what the pills are doing for me.

The health club's lovely. It brings us out, gets us mixing with people socially — we're making a lot of friends.

I think these talks help us because doctors have very little time — they prescribe pills. When we come to these meetings, things are explained to us about illnesses. And we know what to do to look after ourselves.

For the professional workers and speakers, the findings relate both to the structure, style and content of courses, and to their own professional role. In particular, there is a need to:

• involve pensioners in planning the course content, both in general terms and in relation to individual topics
• challenge the traditional pattern of pensioner health education whereby one-off talks on broad health topics are given to large groups of older people
• brief speakers about the interests, needs and knowledge of the particular group

• allow time for the sharing of ideas and information, and for 'private chats'
• provide good teaching aids and leaflets.

Moreover, the majority of co-ordinators recognized their role as enablers, although the process of actively involving the 'consumers' in decision-making is often a slower and more complex process than is first anticipated. Thus, workers need to have sufficient time in which to nurture such developments and to respond to any longer-term initiatives. Crucially, too, it was evident that this kind of health education work is frequently 'squeezed in' between other commitments and is often not recognized as a legitimate part of many health professionals' jobs. Thus, it is of critical importance that such preventive work becomes a recognized priority amongst a range of professionals involved in helping to sustain the health and well-being of older people.

Arising out of this work, a 'how to' guide was developed to provide guidelines, activities and resources for people interested in developing health promotion courses with older people (Meade 1987). Five principles have guided the approach taken in the pack, and these clearly echo the self-health care and self-help/mutual aid philosophies outlined earlier:

• a belief that older people want to learn more about maintaining their health
• a recognition that old people themselves have considerable knowledge and valuable experience to share with each other and with health professionals
• the knowledge that older people can take steps both to improve their own health and to prevent illness
• a commitment to involve pensioners at every stage of the planning process
• appreciation that an individual's health is influenced not only by their own attitudes but also by the political, social and economic world in which they live.

The pack is intended for use in a variety of settings in the hope that many more older people will be enabled to gain the information, skills and support which they want in order to promote their own health.

EMOTIONAL SUPPORT, INFORMATION AND ADVICE: PEER HEALTH COUNSELLING

Promoting one's own health is, as we have already noted, but one facet of self-health care. Arising out of the kinds of health courses and discussion groups described above, a Stoke-on-Trent based organization has been developing a Peer Health Counselling Project. In early 1984 the Beth Johnson Foundation, in partnership with the Centre for Health and Retirement Education in London, set up three health issues discussion groups. Participants explored a range of concerns related to health in retirement, and tried out experimental materials being developed for use on pre-retirement courses. Participants in these groups made a number of pertinent comments about the ways and means of promoting health in old age, including these:

What we need is somewhere to go when we're well; somewhere to ask about anything that is worrying you, where you can chat over the little things.

We ourselves have to encourage other people to come and join us.

As a consequence of all these developments, it became increasingly evident that a number of older people were expressing an active interest in becoming leaders or facilitators themselves. By way of response, the Foundation initiated an experimental training programme in 1985 in which older people were offered the opportunity to acquire some basic skills needed to lead groups of their peers in health-related discussions and activities, or to engage in individual counselling and support work (Bernard & Ivers 1986). Subsequent to this training, four avenues of work were identified:

• one-off days, fairs and exhibitions at which Peer Health Counsellors are on hand to pass on information and discuss health-related issues
• individual counselling and support work to help people (re)establish self-health care programmes and self-confidence, by means of diet, exercise, activity-based pursuits and stress-management strategies
• long-term groupwork in residential homes,

sheltered housing complexes etc., leading gentle exercise and relaxation groups and discussing health issues
• short-term groupwork as above, but for an agreed period, after which staff and/or residents and tenants then manage the programme for themselves.

In addition, Peer Health Counsellors received ongoing professional support and training at regular monthly meetings.

In 1986, Peer Health Counselling became integrated into a much wider self-health initiative: The Self Health Care in Old Age Project. This project has been funded jointly for four years, by the European Economic Community under its Second Poverty Programme and by the Beth Johnson Foundation. Three underlying principles have guided its development, namely:

• to raise older people's awareness of the need for health care and maintenance
• to encourage the involvement of more older people in health-care programmes
• to assist older people in identifying the skills and strategies they require to obtain the resources to meet their needs.

In addition to expanding the Peer Health Counselling Scheme, the project comprises three other elements: a Senior Health Shop; Careline — a telephone link scheme; and health-related courses and activities (Bernard 1989). By linking these four innovatory and practical schemes, the aim is to provide an accessible, attractive and popular means of furthering health education and promotion amongst a group who are not generally the target of such initiatives. The Project also highlights the associated issues of powerlessness amongst older people, particularly in relation to their poor knowledge of what constitutes a healthy old age; their poverty of opportunity and access to existing services; and their lack of command over resources (Bernard 1988).

The work of the Peer Health Counsellors addresses all these issues and, since 1985, four training courses have been set up and 41 older people have received training. The work these volunteers currently undertake falls into two categories: group work and individual work. Peer Health Counsellors now work with residents and tenants in six residential homes for elderly people and in two sheltered housing schemes. In addition to the gentle exercise and discussion groups which have proved extremely popular, a recent innovation has been the development of a reminiscence project in which four counsellors, in collaboration with the City Museum and the City Library, using relevant photographs and artefacts, are running four-week programmes at residential homes for elderly people. In the longer term, the intention is to produce a tape/slide pack and/or video presentation on 'Life in the Potteries' which can then be used in a variety of settings.

In terms of individual work, counsellors are on hand to help, advise and support people in the Senior Health Shop, in the Senior Centre and at other venues where groups operating under the auspices of the Foundation meet, e.g. swimming pools, leisure centres, etc. During 1988, the counsellors' weekly logs of the kind of advice and activities in which they engage showed a total of 1018 discussions on 25 topics over the period February to December. These included discussion of the physical, mental, social and emotional aspects of health and well-being, as well as enquiries for various information about services or activities. By far the most discussed topic was aches and pains, including arthritis and rheumatism. This was followed by physical exercise and activity; the use of social services; reduced mobility; and depression and anxiety. The least discussed topics were, interestingly, those relating to specific health issues such as diabetes and osteoporosis, and accommodation issues such as residential care and housing. Where appropriate, the counsellors refer enquiries on to other agencies and professionals.

Peer Health Counsellors receive ongoing training and support and, since late 1987, a part-time (seven hours a week) Support Worker has been in post. She provides a point of contact for the counsellors; organizes training; monitors and reviews the work programmes and helps set up new contacts and initiatives. It is hoped that this might prove a model for other organizations (agencies who might designate one aspect of, for example, a community nurse's or social worker's workload

to provide similar professional support for a group of trained, older volunteers). Thus, peer health counselling, as part of a much wider self-help health initiative, is directed at increasing the use of preventive health measures amongst older people themselves as well as trying to encourage more positive images of old age and ageing amongst professionals and lay people. In the longer term it is hoped that this will enable people to challenge and ask for the type of health and social care they most need and want.

CONCLUSION: PROBLEMS AND PROSPECTS FOR SELF-CARE AND SELF-HELP

The emergence of interest in self-care/self-help issues is part of an important trend within the field of work with older people. This is exemplified by critical perspectives in social gerontology, with important contributions from researchers such as Estes (1979) and Townsend (1986). Estes, for example, in her major study *The Aging Enterprise*, highlighted the inequalities between expert and client and the way that services invariably focused on the deficiencies rather than the strengths of older people. By the early 1980s, Townsend (1986) was referring to the structured dependency of elderly people, a situation fostered both by state policies and by passive forms of institutional and community care. Finally, in a different context, Maggie Kuhn and the American Gray Panthers were raising criticisms of health and social services, arguing that important though all of these services were, their paternalism could often 'demean and diminish older people' (Kuhn 1986).

An important element of this debate is the critique of the biomedical model, with its emphasis on the pathological and decremental aspects of ageing. The argument proposed by critical gerontology is that people can exert more control over the quality of their life in old age, through a combination of statutory support, political empowerment and self-care (Phillipson & Strang 1986). As with the Women's Movement, we are also concerned with demystifying the process of ageing. This involves demonstrating, first, that the problems faced by older people are often created and sustained by social processes; secondly, it requires making the knowledge base of gerontology itself more accessible to older people and their carers (Porcino 1983).

Self-care and self-help are clearly central elements in achieving this new perspective about old age. At the same time, some cautionary points need to be made about these important areas of activity. First, we should be careful about claims for the success of particular self-care initiatives and self-help projects. Many such schemes are poorly evaluated (if evaluated at all) and may be difficult to replicate amongst other individuals and in other geographical areas. Secondly, the very success of self-care/self-help may create barriers and promote distrust amongst professional carers. Attention must therefore be given to changing the attitudes of health and social care staff to enable them to see encouraging self-care and self-help as an essential part of their involvement with older people. This issue should be reflected in the training received by formal carers, both at a qualifying and post-qualifying level.

Finally, it will be a mistake to see self-care/self-help as a means of replacing professional care. The two must be seen as complementary elements in any developed health care system. Indeed, we would argue that an extensive network of self-help groups and self-care activities will itself place fresh demands on professional carers. This should be the case for a number of reasons: older people should have raised expectations about the range of health care facilities they have a right to expect; they should have greater confidence in challenging poor standards of care; and they should demand a sense of greater empowerment through their involvement with formal carers. Above all, intensification of self-care/self-help may well raise the potential and standard of life in old age. This would seem to be an important outcome of this major social movement amongst older people.

REFERENCES

Age Well Ideas Pack (no date) Pensioners' health courses in Barnet. Ideas Sheet 19. Health Education Council and Age Concern, London (first edition)

Aldeman R, Hainer M S W, Butler R N, Chalmers M 1988 A well elderly program: an intergenerational model in medical education. Gerontologist 28(3): 409–413

Barker J 1985 New initiatives in self-health care. In: Glendenning F (ed) New initiatives in self-health care for older people. Beth Johnson Foundation, University of Keele, Stoke-on-Trent

Bernard M, Ivers V 1986 Peer health counselling: a way of countering dependency? In: Phillipson C, Bernard M, Strang P (eds) Dependency and interdependency in old age: theoretical perspectives and policy alternatives. Croom Helm, London

Bernard M 1988 Taking charge: strategies for self-empowered health behaviour amongst older people. Health Education Journal 47 (2/3): 87–90

Bernard M 1989 Research in action: self-health care and older people, Hygie — international journal of health education VIII (2) June: 11–15

Brody J A 1988 Changing health needs of the aging population. In: Evered D, Whelan J (eds) Research and the ageing population. Wiley, Chichester

Burns B, Phillipson C 1986 Drugs, ageing and society. Croom Helm, London

Coppard L C, White-Riley M, Macfadyen D, Dean K 1984 Self health care and older people — a manual for public policy and programme development. WHO, Copenhagen

Dean K 1982 Self-care: what people do for themselves. In: Hatch S, Kickbusch I (eds) Self-help and health in Europe — new approaches in health care. WHO, Copenhagen

Doyal L 1983 Women, health and the sexual division of labour: a case study of the women's health movement in Britain. Critical Social Policy 3: 21–33

Estes C 1979 The aging enterprise. Josey-Bass, San Francisco

Fennell G, Phillipson C, Evers H 1988 The sociology of old age. Open University Press, Milton Keynes

Gilford D 1988 (ed) The aging population in the twenty-first century. National Academy Press, Washington

Health Education Council 1985 Health education and promotion among older people. HEC, London

Kickbusch I, Hatch S 1982 A re-orientation of health care? In: Hatch S, Kickbusch I (eds) Self-help and health in Europe — new approaches in health care. WHO Copenhagen

Knight B, Hayes R 1981 Self help in the inner city. London Voluntary Service Council, London

Knight B, Hayes R 1982 The self help economy. London Voluntary Service Council, London

Kuhn M 1986 Social and political goals for an ageing society. In: Phillipson C, Bernard M, Strang P Dependency and interdependency in later life. Croom Helm, London

Lafaille R 1983 A new perspective for self-health care. In: Hatch S, Kickbusch I (eds) Self-help and health in Europe. WHO, Copenhagen

Lipton H L, Lee P R 1988 Drugs and the elderly. Standford University Press, California

Litman T 1971 Health care and the family: a three generation analysis. Medical Care 9: 6–7

Lorig K, Fries J 1983 The arthritis handbook. Souvenir Press, London

Lorig K, Laurin J, Holman H 1984 Arthritis self-management: a study of the effectiveness of patient education for the elderly. Gerontologist 25: 455–57

Macfadyen D 1985 Self-health care: international

perspectives. In: Glendenning F (ed) New initiatives in self-health care for older people. A Beth Johnson Foundation Publication in Association with the Health Education Council, Stock-on-Trent

Meade K, 1986 Challenging the myths — a review of pensioners health courses and talks. Age Well (joint Health Education Council/Age Concern Campaign), London

Meade K 1987 Helping yourself to health — health courses for older people: a 'how to' guide. Pensioners Link Health Education Project in association with the Health Education Council, London

Phillipson C, Strang P 1986 Training and education for an ageing society. Health Education Council in association with the Department of Adult Education, University of Keele, Stoke-on-Trent

Pillemer K, Wolf R 1986 Elder abuse: conflict in the family. Auburn, Massachusetts

Porcino J 1983 Growing older, getting better. Addison-Wesley, Massachusetts

Porter R 1985 The patient's view: doing medical history from below. Theory and Society 14: 167–174

Posner T 1989 The development of self help organizations: dilemmas and ambiguities. In: Humble S, Unell J (eds) Self help in health and social welfare — England and West Germany. Routledge, London

Reissmann F, Moody H R, Worthy E H 1984 Self-help and the elderly. Social Policy 14: 19–26

Savo C 1984 Self-care and self-help programmes for older adults in the United States. Health Education Council in association with the Department of Adult and Continuing Education, University of Keele, Stoke-on-Trent

Smith R 1985 Exercise and osteoporosis. British Medical Journal 186: 1376–1377

Social Science and Medicine 1989 Special issue on self-care 29(2)

Thornton H 1989 A medical handbook for senior citizens and their families. Auburn, Massachusetts

Townsend P 1986 Ageism and social policy. In: Phillipson C, Walker A (eds) Ageing and social policy. Gower, Aldershot

Vincent J 1986 Constraints on the stability and longevity of self-help groups in the field of health care. Centre for Research in Social Policy, Loughborough

World Health Organization 1978 Primary health care. Report of the International Conference, Alma-Ata, USSR, 6–12 September, WHO, Geneva

CHAPTER CONTENTS

Demographic trends and social circumstances 418
Size of elderly population 418
Women and men 418
Housing and income 418
Dependency 419
Care of dependent or sick elderly people 419
Some implications 420

Division of labour in care provision for elderly people 421

Historical development of services for the elderly 421
Legacy of the Poor Law 421
The beginnings of change 421
Health and social services 422
Government policies on the elderly 422
Some practical implications of service organization and government policy 423

Organization of geriatric medicine and nursing 424
Geriatric medicine: the specialty 424
Geriatric medicine: contemporary organization 427
Geriatric nursing 429
Relationship of geriatric nursing and geriatric medicine 432
Towards organizational solutions? 433

Conclusion 434

24

Care of the elderly sick in the UK

Helen K. Evers

In this chapter some of the topics which seem important in understanding contemporary trends in the organization of care for sick old people are discussed. In the first part of the chapter we outline some of the characteristics of our elderly population and the implications regarding need for and availability of care. Most old people live in private households, and the bulk of the care they need comes not from services but from families and other lay people.

Today's array of services and the division of labour among them is complex and not always logical. This reflects the process of historical development. In the second part of the chapter, we note briefly some of the landmarks in historical development of services for elderly people, together with the implications of government policies for old people and their carers, both lay and professional. The needs of old people seldom fit neatly with the organizational divisions among services.

Although most dependent elderly people are looked after at home by lay carers, the development of geriatric medicine as a specialty has had a profound influence on health care for the elderly. In the third part of the chapter, we give a short summary of its history in the United Kingdom and outline the major ways in which it is organized. As the dominant health care profession, medicine and its organization is a prime influence in setting the parameters for the work of other health professionals, and we go on, in the fourth part of the chapter, to review what we know of the practice and organization of geriatric nursing. We explore some tentative ideas about its relationship with geriatric medicine; and offer some thoughts about approaches to what seem to be perennial problems in care provision.

DEMOGRAPHIC TRENDS AND SOCIAL CIRCUMSTANCES

SIZE OF ELDERLY POPULATION

In 1986 there were 8.5 million people aged 65 years and over living in Britain, constituting just over 15% of the total population (Central Statistical Office 1989). The proportion of the population who are more than 65 years old has risen dramatically during this century. In England and Wales, less than 5% of the population was aged over 65 years in 1901. Of these, a quarter were more than 75 years old. In 1986, 42% of the numerically much larger elderly population were 75 or older (Central Statistical Office 1989). By the end of the century, the proportion of the population aged 65 years or more will not increase dramatically, but within the elderly population, there will be a slight decline in the proportion of 'young' elderly, and an increase in the proportion of 'old' elderly people. These changes in population reflect in part the fact that fewer people die during earlier stages of the life-cycle. This has resulted primarily from environmental improvements: better housing, sanitation, clean water, adequate diet and general improvements in the standard of living.

WOMEN AND MEN

What do we know about these growing numbers of elderly people? Women tend to live longer than men do, thus they outnumber men by 2:1 in the 75 years and over age group. Women also tend to marry men who are older than themselves. For both reasons widowhood is very common. In 1986, 64% of women aged 75 or over were widows and 21% were still married, whereas only 30% of men in the same age group were widowed, and 61% still married. Thus among the elderly population, it is no surprise to find that 50% of women over

60 live alone, but only 5% of men (Office of Population Censuses and Surveys 1985). The death of a spouse often brings social and psychological distress, of course, but in addition, and particularly for women, socioeconomic disadvantage tends to ensue. This derives mainly from societal structures and processes which tend to systematically disadvantage women across the lifespan (see Harrison 1983 for further discussion).

HOUSING AND INCOME

Wheeler (1986) reviews a range of evidence regarding the housing of elderly people. Over 90% of older people live in their own homes, around 5% of these in sheltered housing with a warden. Home ownership is on the increase — just under half of all elderly households live in owner-occupied housing, as compared with just over half of all households. Elderly owner-occupiers are more likely than their younger counterparts to live in older housing that lacks basic amenities and is in a poor state of repair. Older people are also more likely to be private tenants — again, in relatively poorer, older housing stock. On average, then, households containing an elderly person tend to have a lower standard of housing and poorer access to basic amenities (Tinker 1981).

Old people are among the poorest members of society (Townsend 1979) although, as in all age groups, there is a great range in wealth and income level. For example, the 1980s have seen an unprecedented boom in sales of exclusive newly-built retirement housing, which bears witness to a new affluence among a significant minority of the older population.

Although financial circumstances in late life bear a relationship to those at earlier stages of the life-cycle — the retired professional person will be relatively well off compared with the retired manual worker — income is drastically reduced for almost all after retirement. On average, about half the weekly household income in cases where the head of household is aged 65 or over derives from social security benefits, as compared with less than a tenth of the household income where the head of household is under 65 years of age. Households occupied by lone women have the lowest weekly income of all types of household occupied by elderly people; and of households containing one person past retirement age dependent mainly on state pension as a source of income, 78% are those of women (Department of Employment 1987). Extreme old age is the life-stage featuring the greatest material poverty, just at a time when extra expenses — e.g. for heating, transport or special diet — may accrue, particularly for those in poor health or with a disability (Martin & White 1988).

DEPENDENCY

A survey by Hunt (1978) and a special section of the General Household Survey for 1980 (OPCS 1982) provide data on health problems, mobility and capacity for self-care, as reported by old people. Martin et al (1988) show that both the prevalence and severity of disabilities of all types are markedly higher among those aged 60 and over, the rates increasing with advancing age. There are various sex differences worth noting. In all age groups, old women are more likely to report a long-standing illness which limits their activities and more likely to report mobility problems (Hunt 1978, OPCS 1982).

While the majority of the elderly population do not suffer from dementing illnesses, the significant minority who do may well require considerable help and support at some stage in their illness, as work by Levin et al (1983) and Sidell (1986), among others, shows. Estimates of prevalence vary according to methods of assessment (see Badger et al 1989a, for a critical review of methods of assessing dementias, and Ch. 19). But commonly accepted estimates are that up to 10% of the elderly population as a whole, rising to around 20% among those over 85, suffer from some form of dementing illness.

As we have seen, most elderly people live at home. A majority live full lives, are independent and take care of themselves and also, in many cases, other people too. But some of those living at home are dependent on others for many kinds of essential help. Dependency in old age can be increased or even created by low income, poor

housing and other disadvantages arising from the relatively low status which is assigned by society to the elderly population (see Fennell et al 1988, for further discussion of these issues).

What does the demographic picture mean in human terms, and who helps those elderly people who become sick or disabled?

CARE OF DEPENDENT OR SICK ELDERLY PEOPLE

A majority of old men have wives to look after them if they become sick. But their wives, although on average a little younger, are likely, as they age, to have their own health problems, which may limit their activities. In contrast, a minority of women have husbands to take on the care-work should they become unable to do this for themselves. Female spouses are thus a major source of help, after which children — primarily daughters or daughters-in-law — make an essential contribution (Equal Opportunities Commission 1982, Nissel & Bonnerjea 1982, Rossiter & Wicks 1982). Green (1988) found that, nationally, 14% of adults are carers of sick, disabled or dependent people. Where the dependant shares a household with the carer, 12% of carers are unrelated. Where the dependant person lives in a different household from the carer, in 26% of cases the carer is a friend or neighbour and not a relative.

What role, then, do formal services play? Government policy (examples are DHSS 1976, 1981b) has for some time indicated that home-based rather than institution-based care provision is to be preferred on humanitarian grounds, and because it may be cheaper; though this last assumption is now widely challenged. In the state care sector, 'cheap' community care probably means 'inadequate' community care. Policy also explicitly states that services are intended only to supplement what the major care givers, the women of the family, provide by way of support (DHSS 1981a). For the 1990s, the policy emphasis is still on community care as the preferred option (Secretary of State for Health, Social Security, Wales and Scotland 1989). Data on patterns of service provision are scant and suffer from limitations.

They tell us nothing about the circumstances of those who receive no services, yet we cannot assume these non-recipients need no help.

Elderly people are major users of the health and social services. But the available evidence on community services suggests that 'unmet needs' are commonplace (e.g. Chapman 1979) and that allocation of services depends not just on need but also on availability and mix of services in a given geographical area (Levin et al 1983), local professional policies — implicit as well as explicit — and gender-based assumptions. An example of the last is that dependent elderly men with wives as carers are far less likely to receive home help and other support services than are women looked after by their husbands, despite the fact that the dependent men have greater support needs. Women are apparently assumed to be able to cope with far more by way of domestic work and caring than are men (Evers et al 1988).

Since most old people live in private households, health care is in the main provided by the primary care team. People over 60 years of age account for between a quarter and a third of all general practitioner (family doctor) consultations (Age Concern 1977, Wilkin et al 1987). According to Wilkin et al, the average consultation rate for this age group is around 3.1 per annum, irrespective of variations in the proportion of older people in the population served by the doctor.

The community nursing service is extremely important in providing personal care to older people at home. Overall, 74% of district nurses' time with patients is devoted to those aged 65 years or more. Looking just at auxiliaries, the figure is even higher at 89% (Dunnell & Dobbs 1982).

With increasing age, the probability of contact with the hospital services also increases. As with primary health services, elderly people are also major users of hospital services. Around 50% of all hospital beds (excluding maternity and geriatric departments) are occupied by people who are 65 years of age or older.

SOME IMPLICATIONS

The decreasing proportion of 'young elderly' in re-

lation to 'old elderly' means that fewer relatively fit people in the 65–74 age group will be available to look after increasing numbers of frail and much older kin: parents, spouses or siblings. Where carers come from a pre-retirement generation, not only are demands and obligations to look after an older family member more likely to arise, but also the women carers must cope with other pressures. These include the needs of their own families, and the need and often the desire to work outside the home. The increasingly common incidence of divorce, often followed by remarriage, may have profound effects on family structure which will affect availability of younger-generation carers for sick elderly people.

At the same time, government policy endorses community-based care in a general way but without obvious diversion of resources into state community services. In effect, this places greater demands on family and other lay carers. The current picture, in 1990, offers a little encouragement. In response to a bleak prospect on community care offered by the Audit Commission (1986), the Griffiths report (Griffiths 1988) called for provision of earmarked budgets for community care services, designated care managers with responsibility for assembling 'packages' of care services, and a Minister for Community Care, among other proposals. The proposals were greeted by widespread expression of professional and public concern about community care issues. Indeed, anxiety about the well-being of long-term disabled or sick elderly people was increased by the proposals for NHS reorganization contained in the White Paper, *Working for Patients* (DH 1989). Self-governing hospitals and budget-holding general practices, geared to cost-effective performance, may find themselves in a difficult position in relation to such patients. This does not bode well, of course, for the patients themselves, who will often be elderly people.

In late 1989, the government responded to the Griffiths proposals in its White Paper, *Caring for People* (Secretary of State for Health, Social Security, Wales and Scotland 1989). The general framework holds promise for improving community care. It assigns responsibility for deciding priorities, assessing individuals' and carers' needs, and devising packages of care to social services departments, under the supervision of designated care managers. Automatic social security funding of residential care is to cease, with management of budgets for social care, whether provided in a residential or a community setting, carried out by social services departments. This will end the perverse disincentive to community care provision. Better co-ordination of a range of services, provided by statutory bodies, voluntary and private organizations, should result, and lead to improved access by those in need of community support. However, the proposals for community care budgets remain vague. Without clearly designated funds, whether the supposed benefits of the new arrangements will accrue in practice must remain an open question.

DIVISION OF LABOUR IN CARE PROVISION FOR ELDERLY PEOPLE

Although lay people provide the bulk of care received by dependent or sick old people, a formidable array of professional and non-professional paid and voluntary workers is also involved, not to mention complex arrangements for a range of state cash benefits. The paid workers include members of the primary health care team — doctors, nurses, remedial therapists and health visitors — and hospital staff, home helps, social workers, providers of the meals-on-wheels service, day centre and day hospital staff, staff of residential Homes and ambulance drivers, to mention only some. While this proliferation of types of worker and the services they supply may have obvious advantages for their clientèle, our present systems of service delivery feature many anomalies and confusions. It is not unusual to find elderly people or their carers bemused by the distinction between the roles of social worker and health visitor, or health visitor and district nurse, for instance.

Services for the elderly have evolved in a piecemeal fashion. Some understanding of the pattern of care services we have today can be gained through a brief look at how they have developed.

HISTORICAL DEVELOPMENT OF SERVICES FOR THE ELDERLY

Many writers have traced the historical development of government policies and of services vis-à-vis elderly people. Macintyre (1977) and Tinker (1981) are two examples, and Brocklehurst (1975) provides an overview of the development of geriatric services. Mears and Smith (1985) offer a detailed analysis of the development of welfare services, including health services, for elderly people between 1939 and 1971. In this chapter, we have space only for a very brief summary of these complex developments.

LEGACY OF THE POOR LAW

At the turn of the century, the main provision for elderly people in Britain derived from the Elizabethan and the New Poor Law of 1834. Outdoor relief was provided to the destitute and infirm, from Poor Rates collected from all occupants of property in a parish. The workhouse became the repository of the destitute and infirm, and in 1834 the principle of 'less eligibility' was enshrined as a deterrent. Provisions in the workhouse were to be less attractive than the lowest level of subsistence 'enjoyed' by anyone outside, although it was suggested that elderly people of 'good report' might deserve some special arrangements. Workhouse infirmaries provided accommodation for the aged and chronic sick.

THE BEGINNINGS OF CHANGE

The Old Age Pension Act of 1908, which gave people over 70 years a small weekly — but at first means tested — pension, was an important landmark. It began to establish provision for elderly people outside the framework of the Poor Laws. As to institutional provision, in 1929 the Local Government Act made the local authorities responsible for the work of the former Poor Law guardians, including the administration of Poor Law institutions. These now became known as public assistance institutions. The stigma of Poor

Law relief of destitution was probably significantly diminished as a result of this new arrangement. Amulree (1951) considers, however, that this Act had an unexpectedly negative consequence for the elderly sick. Under a permissive clause, local authorities could choose to transfer infirmaries attached to public assistance institutions to the health authorities, the idea being to improve standards. This happened but as standards improved these infirmaries became highly selective of the patients they admitted, and many elderly people could no longer gain access. The statutory right of admission had been lost with the transfer of control of infirmaries to the health authorities.

HEALTH AND SOCIAL SERVICES

The National Health Service Act of 1946 and the National Assistance Act of 1948 were both important in setting the stage for the development of today's pattern of health and social service provision for elderly people. The 1946 Act brought the former public assistance infirmaries, the municipal hospitals, the voluntary hospitals and community-based health services together into the National Health Service. It also empowered local authorities to employ home helps and to make provision for the care and aftercare of the sick. The 1948 Act enabled local authorities to concern themselves with the welfare of those who were deaf, dumb, blind or otherwise substantially handicapped. Under Part III of this Act, local authorities were required to make accommodation available for all who needed care and attention because of age, infirmity or other circumstances. Many large former workhouses were used to this end and are now referred to as 'Part III' accommodation. Section 31 of the 1948 Act empowered local authorities to make a financial contribution in support of the work of voluntary organizations, for example voluntary Homes and meals services.

In 1971, the Local Authority Social Services Act (1970) was implemented. This aimed to provide a co-ordinated approach to the family by bringing together, in social services departments, the former children's and welfare departments. Some writers (e.g. Harris 1979) imply that the generic approach to social work has served to reinforce the pre-eminence of work concerning children — deriving from numerous statutory imperatives — to the detriment of professional social work with elderly people.*

GOVERNMENT POLICIES ON THE ELDERLY

Macintyre (1977) shows how policy concerns about the elderly as a 'social problem' between 1834 and 1976 oscillated between organizational considerations such as the 'burden' on society of the cost of supporting a dependent sector of the population, and humanitarian concerns about responding to the health or welfare problems occasioning hardship to old people. The tensions between organizational and humanitarian perspectives are evident today, for example in policy statements about community care (DHSS 1976, 1978, 1981a, b). The official line is that service provision for old people should be grounded in the assumption that being looked after at home is best, both because old people prefer this and because it is cheaper. If it is in fact cheaper, this may be because types and levels of service provision are inadequate (Opit 1977). This is now implicitly recognized in the present government's policy line for the 1980s and beyond: that family care of old people, supported by community services, is the 'best' model for service development on both organizational and humanitarian grounds. The tension between these two perspectives has been 'resolved' by firmly locating responsibility with the family, thus, among other things, rendering the human plight of some sick old people less publicly visible.

From the late 1980s, important service developments have become more widespread. Two examples are the growth of a range of services for dementia sufferers and carers; and 'intensive' domiciliary care services, organized by social services and district nursing auxiliaries or both in collaboration. The needs of carers particularly are now becoming more visible and attracting some response from health and social service providers.

---

* Others (e.g. Court 1976) have suggested that preventive health services for children have suffered through increasing involvement of health visitors with elderly people.

One issue which has yet to receive the attention it warrants, other than in a few pioneering locales, is the care of old people from ethnic minority groups. In those areas where they are concentrated, their numbers are set to rise dramatically and, in the main, culturally appropriate service delivery is sadly lacking (see, for example Glendenning & Pearson 1988, Cameron et al 1988, Atkin et al 1989, Badger et al 1989b).

Uncertainties regarding future developments in services for older people derive from proposals to reform the organization of the NHS (DH 1989) and of Community Services (Secretary of State for Health, Social Security, Wales and Scotland 1989). By the mid 1990s, the nature of these changes and innovations will be clearer.

SOME PRACTICAL IMPLICATIONS OF SERVICE ORGANIZATION AND GOVERNMENT POLICY

In the post-war period, both the health and personal social services have undergone various changes in their respective organizations. Yet the needs of their elderly clientèle cannot be so neatly divided between health and social services — not to mention housing or financial considerations, which have not been discussed here. Furthermore, needs do not remain static: classification and response is not a once-for-all activity. Thus collaboration among families, health and social services professionals is essential in the care of dependent or sick elderly people. The historical development of separate health and social service organizations — whose territorial boundaries often do not coincide — in some respects militates against easy co-ordination. The mix of institutional and community bases of provision in both services compounds the difficulties. Undoubtedly, there are many examples of effective co-ordination in service delivery, but one may speculate that these occur despite rather than because of service organizational features, and are mediated through the efforts of individual workers and managers to establish mutually harmonious and complementary interrelationships.

Voluntary and private sector provision must be mentioned in this context. Voluntary and chari-table organizations have a long history of providing community and institutional services for the elderly; and old people with the financial means to do so have always had the option in practice of buying the support they deem themselves to need, whether at home or in an institution.

From the early 1980s, private sector provision of residential and nursing home care has risen dramatically. In 1979, private Homes were looking after 17% of the 152 897 occupants of residential facilities; 67% were in local authority Homes and the remainder in the voluntary sector. By 1986, the overall number of residents had risen to 204 382, of whom 38% were in the private sector (House of Commons 1988). This unprecedented growth was prompted by changes in the social security system, which allowed payment for private sector places to be fully met, up to a defined ceiling level, and subject to means test qualification of the potential resident. Such funding is to cease for new residents from 1991 (see Secretary of State for Health, Social Security, Wales and Scotland 1989), thus encouraging a shift away from residential and towards community care.

There is continuing concern about the criteria and process of registration of private residential and nursing Homes, and about monitoring standards, for which statutory authorities are responsible. Another type of concern is the escalating cost to the state of supporting long-term institutional care of older people. Challis (1989) notes that the cost to the state for 'board and lodging' payments rose from £18 m in 1980 to £102 m in 1983, and that costs continue to rise. Further, professionals continue to urge that assessment of people's need for residential care should be mandatory. From 1991, assessment of individual need will be a requirement for admission to care, rather than mere agreement between the home and the old person and/or her relatives. The Wagner Report (1988) calls for more attention to be paid to the consumer's viewpoint, in an effort to make residential care a positive rather than last-resort choice. While it is now widely accepted that collaboration with the private sector is to be encouraged, it is only with the White Paper on community care (Secretary of State for Health, Social Security, Wales and Scotland 1989) that the establishment of organizational systems for doing this is formally called for.

The growth of private sector care has had an impact on the provision of long-term care within both local authorities and health authorities. The number of residential places in the local authority sector fell slightly between 1979 and 1986, and there is evidence that the proportion of beds dedicated to long-term care of elderly people within the NHS is falling. While it is now widely accepted that collaboration with the private sector is to be encouraged, there is at present no means for tackling joint planning of service delivery.

Today's professional carers for elderly people work within a complex pattern of service organization. The territorial and functional boundaries of its components have assumed their present limits after years of development and change, shaped significantly by Acts of Parliament. These boundaries do not necessarily coincide neatly with the presenting problems of real old people and their lay carers.

ORGANIZATION OF GERIATRIC MEDICINE AND NURSING

We have emphasized that care of sick and dependent old people is provided by many different workers, paid and unpaid, and that this work is mainly done outside the hospital. Why, then, is it necessary to pay specific attention to the hospital-based specialty of geriatric medicine, and to geriatric nursing? There are four main reasons.

1. The organization of professional hospital-centred delivery of care for elderly people has received, perhaps, a disproportionate amount of professional and research attention as compared with health care provided in other settings. There are good reasons for this: the prestige of hospital-based medicine; the 'visibility' of the hospital; the managerial challenges and economic costs of today's hospital care. Rightly or wrongly, hospital-centred care of the elderly occupies considerable attention. Thus we need to analyse its implications for nursing and for patients.

2. The geriatric department is important for its contribution to raising expectations and status of health care of the elderly as a legitimate and valuable occupation, whether it is done in primary care, geriatric departments, other hospital departments or settings outside the hospital.

3. Most health professionals receive much of their education and training in the hospital, and, increasingly, the geriatric department features — if fleetingly for some — on the agenda. As such, it has a vital role to play in educating those who will meet elderly people in their professional practice, in whatever setting it may be carried out.

4. Solutions to problems in geriatric nursing care, as we hope to show below, are more likely to be found if nurses have a clear understanding of how medical philosophy, priorities and organization of practice affect their own position and that of their patients.

GERIATRIC MEDICINE: THE SPECIALTY*

Geriatric medicine as a specialty is generally deemed to have begun with the work of Marjory Warren at the West Middlesex Hospital in 1935. The patients of a former Poor Law infirmary became her responsibility, and she carried out assessments of the patients contingent upon which treatment and rehabilitation was started. The effects of this were soon apparent: it became possible to discharge some patients and to challenge the prevailing practice of nursing a majority of elderly and chronic sick patients in bed. The concentration of elderly chronic sick patients in London's peripheral hospitals during the war provided opportunities for development of practice. The

*There is no definitive history, to date, of the development of geriatric medicine in the UK. A number of geriatricians have written about aspects of the specialty's history; and others provide a resumé as a preface to considering contemporary themes. I have drawn on various sources of this kind in my account of the specialty's development; including Amulree 1951, Brocklehurst 1975, Macintyre 1977, Ferguson Anderson 1981, and Clark 1983.
Carboni's (1982) comparative analysis of geriatric medicine in the UK and the US is another important source.

setting up of the National Health Service, more than 10 years after Warren's pioneering work, added impetus to the beginnings of geriatric medicine. When the NHS brought the voluntary and the municipal hospitals together, the largely custodial role of the latter in the care of the elderly and chronic sick was increasingly questioned.

Also there were fears that the acute beds of the former voluntary hospitals could be overwhelmed by elderly people who previously would have had the right of access only to the municipal hospitals. For example, Thomson et al (1951) wrote:

When the National Health Service Act became operative . . . it seemed certain that many of the aged sick, no longer able to obtain admission to overcrowded infirmaries under statutory orders, would either remain at home or find their way into the wards of acute general hospitals and choke their beds with cases it was impossible to move. In either event grave hardship and public scandal would result (p. 1).

Dr Trevor Howell, who established one of the early geriatric units in London, and the first geriatric research unit, was instrumental in establishing the Medical Society for the care of the Elderly in 1947, to become the British Geriatrics Society (BGS) in 1959. The first appointments of physicians in geriatric medicine were made from the 1940s onwards, and since then the specialty has continued to grow. In 1982 there were more than 470 consultants in England and Wales. The first university chair in geriatric medicine was established in 1965, and by 1983 there were 14 chairs in Great Britain.

By 1985, there were 243 consultants with a commitment to old age psychiatry (Royal College of Physicians of London and Royal College of Psychiatrists 1989). As we enter the 1990s, consultant numbers continue to increase, and some further university chairs of geriatric medicine have been established. While geriatrics and psychogeriatrics, and their associated services, continue to grow, developments are patchy. As Hall (1988) points out, services remain woefully inadequate in some parts of the country. More than double the number of consultants is required to bring the total in England and Wales close to the norm of 0.143 consultants per 1000 population over the age of 65

recommended by the British Geriatrics Society (Andrews & Brocklehurst 1987).

Despite its rapid growth, geriatrics faces continuing dilemmas over its relationship with other medical specialties which are involved in care of the elderly sick, and a range of organizational solutions is to be found in practice. These can best be discussed in the context of a description of trends in the organization of the hospital geriatric service.

In the early days, as a legacy from the former workhouse infirmaries, geriatric departments tended to have the image of custodians for long-stay patients who had proved untreatable in other departments of the hospital. Thus almost all admissions came from other wards or hospitals, and the geriatric wards were very often housed in under-resourced buildings remote from the general hospital. It was quickly realized that if geriatric medicine was to establish itself on a par with other medical specialties, and to provide a service for a defined elderly population, it had to do more than serve as custodian for the failures of other branches of medicine. Two things had to be done: geriatricians needed to establish that they had a unique contribution to offer to the care of the elderly sick; and they had to change the practice and organization of their departments, and their relationship with other hospital departments and the community.

The claim to a unique contribution in care of the elderly sick seemed to derive primarily from two arguments. First, that the presentation of illness in old age is often distinctive as compared with illness in younger adults. Not only may the clinical picture present differently, but very often multiple conditions are found, which may also be directly related to social and environmental factors. Geriatricians have special knowledge and skills in understanding the presentation, and thus the management, of illness in old age.

The second argument is that geriatricians have special expertise in rehabilitation, and experience in organizing hospital care so as to meet patients' rehabilitative needs. Thus many of the patients whom the acute wards find hard to discharge and who come to be seen as 'bed blockers' would perhaps never have found themselves in this predicament, it is argued, had they been admitted directly to the geriatric department and received the benefits of its expertise and special organization from the outset. In the acute ward, mobilizing the patient with a fractured femur or stroke illness when the patient is elderly may receive low priority, and the chance of rehabilitation may be completely lost if the management of the early days of the illness does not pay close attention to mobilization.

A vital change in the organization of practice is the acceptance of direct admissions to the geriatric department. Achieving direct rather than second-hand admissions both enables geriatricians to demonstrate their special skills, and requires a different kind of departmental organization from that which featured in the largely custodial long-stay, back wards. Various ways of receiving direct admissions are possible, for example adopting a policy of taking all hospital emergency admissions of medical patients of a particular age; or taking age-defined emergencies of particular diagnostic categories. Direct acceptance of all, or of defined types of, emergency patients above a certain age referred by general practitioners is another strategy, as well as accepting general practitioner requests for home assessments. As a result of this at least some elderly patients may be admitted directly to the geriatric department. Taking direct admissions means that the variety of patients' services will need to increase: besides those needing long-term hospital care, there will be increasing numbers of acutely ill patients for whom active treatment, perhaps followed by a period of rehabilitation, will be needed prior to discharge. Assessment of patients becomes very important, including seeking out factors which the patient may erroneously attribute to 'old age', and positive rather than residual criteria for admission must be identified. Emphasizing treatment in the geriatric department also requires a reorientation of work priorities among existing staff — nurses and doctors — and greater involvement with other professionals having a therapeutic role to play, e.g. physiotherapists, occupational therapists and social workers. A wider repertoire of skills will be needed by all these staff when they are dealing not just with long-term care, but also with acutely ill

patients and rehabilitation. Thus the nature and quality of their training, experience and calibre become crucial.

Successful discharge of an elderly patient who has responded to treatment and rehabilitation requires different strategies, very often, from discharge of 'cured' patients in younger age groups. Remember that the elderly patient may have some limitations of day-to-day activities even when deemed 'cured'; that she is very likely to live alone or with an elderly spouse and in less than ideal housing circumstances. So it is an advantage if staff of the geriatric department know something of the social and environmental circumstances of the elderly patient at home, such that steps can be taken to compensate for inherent problems through initiating provision of aids and adaptations or services. Health education in its broadest sense, including practical ways of making self-care or care of an elderly spouse easier, is also essential to achieving a successful discharge.

'Community orientation' of the medical specialty has for many years been seen by geriatricians as a basic requirement for providing a good service to a defined elderly population. Home assessments originally offered a way of screening patients referred for admission and reducing waiting lists by suggesting alternatives to hospitalization. When a patient is admitted to hospital, first-hand knowledge of her home environment and social and family circumstances may help in planning the treatment strategy and in organizing a well-supported discharge when she recovers. Home assessments also enable geriatricians to constantly review their admissions policies in relation to the range of presenting needs among the elderly population, as well as to maintain working relationships with primary health workers and with agencies involved in providing care for elderly sick people. The development of day hospitals, the increasing importance of outpatient clinics run by geriatricians and the provision of beds for short-term admissions to relieve caring relatives are other features of the specialty's community orientation.

In establishing its unique contribution and evolving new approaches to organizing its practice, geriatric medicine has come to set great store by multidisciplinary team-work. The needs of elderly patients are so varied, and health factors so often inextricably linked with environmental and social factors, that a range of professional skills must be brought to bear on assessment, treatment and rehabilitation and planning a patient's discharge.

Ferguson Anderson (1981) summarizes the features which differentiate geriatric medicine from general medicine as follows:

1. The practice of health education for the elderly.
2. The use of the members of the health care team . . . to seek out unreported illness.
3. The knowledge of the home conditions of the individual patient before admission; of the atypical presentation of disease in older people, often accompanied by multiple pathology; of the frequent combination of physical and mental illness in the elderly, and of problems with medication.
4. The need for comprehensive patient management and for continuity of care (p. 122).

Much of this could, incidentally, be applied to other branches of medicine not organized around specific disease processes, for instance general practice, or paediatrics, which, like geriatrics, is concerned with an age-defined rather than disease- or organ-defined patient category. Isaacs (1981) reflects that geriatric medicine has been mainly concerned with problems of organizing practice in order to provide a quality service to the elderly population. For the future, Isaacs sees increasing emphasis on exploiting the opportunities for the scientific study of human ageing which the specialty of geriatric medicine affords.

GERIATRIC MEDICINE: CONTEMPORARY ORGANIZATION

Like other mainstream medical specialties, geriatric medicine is now firmly committed to active treatment and patient turnover, and it is around this general aim that most geriatric departments are organized. Providing long-term care, which was the most common base from which the early geriatric departments developed, now fits uneasily into a cure-oriented service.

There seems to be an unresolved tension here. The existence of large numbers of chronically sick elderly hospital patients, on whom medicine had

'given up', provided the early impetus to the development of the specialty. The British Geriatrics Society (1983) notes,

The largest number of patients under the geriatrician's care at any one time are those in need of continuing nursing care which cannot be given at home . . . [T]he continuing care wards are very much part of the 'shop window' of the specialty. . . . The medical attention given to such patients is relatively small but the way in which it is given is absolutely vital (p. 3–4).

Yet, at the same time, geriatric departments are striving to establish themselves by the same criterion of 'success' commonly applied to other medical specialties: high rates of patient turnover. The issue of long-term care is one about which many geriatricians are both profoundly concerned and profoundly uncomfortable. The Hull geriatrician Peter Horrocks (1982) is committed to the organization of geriatric medicine as an age-related specialty. In explaining why, he provides an excellent review of the three major approaches to organization, which are a 'residual', an integrated and an age-related service.

A 'residual' service

Horrocks' view is that the quality of service for the elderly population would remain poor if geriatrics were only a rehabilitation and long-term care specialty taking its admissions largely from other hospital departments. This is probably uncontroversial. That policy serves to deny the special contribution of geriatric medicine in care of the elderly sick; to reinforce the second-class status of geriatric medicine, which would in turn ensure that the specialty's claim on scarce resources and on staff would always be secondary, and that training and recruitment in the specialty — lacking any coverage of acute illness, and suffering inadequate resources — would always be a problem.

An integrated service

A model which has been adopted by various departments, and which was favoured by a working party of the Royal College of Physicians (1977), features integration between geriatric and general medicine. This might take the form of appointing general physicians with an interest in geriatric medicine who would divide their attention between general and geriatric beds; or, Horrocks describes, a geriatric physician working alongside general physicians, all of whom would admit patients to the same wards. There might be back-up wards, under the sole control of geriatricians, for slow-stream rehabilitation and long-term care.

An integrated service — a model put into practice in some areas — is said to have the advantages that the special skills of the geriatrician would be available to sick old people; that the access of sick old people to diagnostic and treatment facilities would be secured; that recruitment and training in the specialty would be assured since it would be a part of mainstream medicine; and that the status and resource control of geriatric medicine vis-à-vis other specialties would be improved. But Horrocks has reservations about integration. He questions whether the physician with an interest in geriatric medicine, or even the full-time geriatrician within an integrated service, would in practice be able to accord sufficient priority to work other than with acute patients; and suggests that there are practical difficulties in providing the appropriate equipment and environment for sick old people in a general medical ward. Horrocks cites other medical writers who are worried that the geriatrician's patient in the general ward may be resented and accorded low priority.

The integration model has much to commend it as a strategy for securing higher levels of recruitment into geriatric medicine. Indeed this consideration was a major influence on the deliberations of the Royal College of Physicians' working party, at a time when numerous articles and letters in professional journals were both bemoaning the persistent shortage of geriatricians relative to funded consultant posts, and discussing with alarm the possible effects on medical care generally of the rising numbers of elderly people, in particular the very old.

An age-related service

In this third type of service, which Horrocks reviews, the geriatrician offers comprehensive care — acute, rehabilitation, long-term care, community involvement and continuing responsibility when needed for patients known to the department — for all patients with non-surgical conditions above a particular age: commonly, 75 years old and over. Organizationally, this requires that emergency cases are admitted at the discretion of the patient's general practitioner or via the casualty department, along with patients who have been assessed at home by the geriatrician. A department set up along these lines would feature relatively high turnover rates (Horrocks provides some data on the age-related service he manages) and would deal with a wide variety of medical conditions. As such, the department would offer valuable experience, and would be in a good position to attract doctors and other staff of the necessary calibre to work in this broad-based and challenging arena. For patients, continuity of care by specialists in geriatric medicine has obvious advantages. It improves their chances of recovering former well-being. The need for long-term care is said to be minimized where appropriate diagnostic, treatment and rehabilitation skills, along with advance planning of appropriately supported discharge, are brought to bear from the moment of first presentation of the sick old person at the hospital. Thus the turnover rate can be maintained, and beds be kept available to meet the needs as they arise from the geriatric department's catchment area. Horrocks notes his experience that actual numbers of beds are less important than the quality and range of services associated with available beds. That is, a good proportion of the patients need to have full access to all the facilities of the district general hospital.

In comparing the resources and performance of several geriatric services run along differing lines, Grimley Evans (1983) endorses this point. He also observes that various modes of service organization can achieve the desired objective of ensuring access of elderly patients both to the facilities of the district general hospital and to appropriate — i.e. geriatric — expertise (Grimley Evans 1981).

Horrocks quotes data from a 1980 survey carried out by the British Geriatrics Society of 49 geriatric departments. This showed that consultants having dual responsibilities for general and geriatric medicine were very much in a minority. Twenty-nine of the 49 departments took emergency admissions, and 20 of these only admitted patients above a certain age. When asked about 'ideal' policies, four out of five respondents favoured age-related admissions, the majority opting for a rule-of-thumb age limit somewhere above the minimum pensionable age.

Isaacs (1981) remarks that the age-related model can be criticized 'on grounds of illogicality, segregation, ageism, duplication — but it succeeds' (p. 228). He also notes that most departments of geriatric medicine embody some characteristics of an age-related service. Grimley Evans (1983) uses data on the operation of an 'integrated' service compared with data from three other services including Horrocks' service in Hull, to argue that an 'integrated service' is the most viable option where access to district general hospital beds for elderly patients is very restricted.

A 'best buy'?

Having set out the basic elements of three general approaches to organizing geriatric departments, it is not our intention to attempt to identify a consumer's 'best buy'. Expediency and professional interests may have a great influence on chosen strategies of organization, and we have already mentioned that the stark realities of unfilled consultant posts in geriatric medicine may have influenced the Royal College of Physicians' hearty endorsement of an integration model.

An age-related model, if it succeeds in achieving a healthy turnover level and minimizing its devotion of resources to long-term care, has clear advantages in raising the prestige of geriatric medicine as a specialty on a par with mainstream acute hospital specialties. This may in turn have real advantages for patients: the prestigious geriatric department is likely to be able to muster stronger claims to resources and staff than its less prestigious counterpart, and to gain support from other specialties, if it is seen to be taking care of its share of the older age groups, from among whom the 'bed blockers' of the acute wards would otherwise emerge.

Local contingencies may reinforce or preclude particular possibilities; valuable accounts of the practicalities of developing effective psychogeriatric and geriatric services in two different locales are provided by Jolley et al (1982) and Harrison (1984).

GERIATRIC NURSING

Having discussed the medical context, we now turn to the implications for geriatric nursing. The discussion is divided into four sections: origins; research-based analyses of practice and problems; the relationship with geriatric medicine; organizational solutions.

Origins

Baker (1978) draws parallels between the development of geriatric medicine and geriatric nursing. She refers to White's (1978) study of the development of nursing, and argues that the voluntary hospital nurses shared the prestige accorded to the medical élite who serviced the voluntary hospitals and developed their mainly curative work with acutely ill patients. The Poor Law nurses of the workhouse infirmaries, which became the municipal hospitals, worked with chronically sick, bedridden patients who embodied all the stigma of the workhouse, providing routine bedside care. This was in stark contrast to the nursing work of the voluntary hospitals, and it was this low status group, the Poor Law nurses, who became the first geriatric nurses.

Research-based analysis of practice and problems

The British literature on geriatric nursing does not seem to have begun to emerge until well after the founding fathers had become established in medicine. The work of Doreen Norton and her colleagues (1962) is perhaps the pioneering research-based text in the field. Their *Investigation of Geriatric Nursing Problems in Hospital* reported detailed studies of patients and of nursing work, aimed towards the practical ends of improving patient care and easing the workload of nurses. Specific areas included individual patient care studies; assessment of patients; furniture and equipment; design of suitable clothing; and, perhaps best-known, a study of the identification of patients liable to develop pressure sores, and nursing care strategies for their prevention and treatment.

Two of the most important British studies which illuminate the nature of geriatric nursing are those of Baker (1978) and Wells (1980). Wells' research began in 1972, before Baker's, and her aim was to describe current nursing practice in order to develop a potential model for geriatric nursing. She felt that the specialty lacked a distinctive body of nursing knowledge and skill. Her three starting assumptions were: that nurses' behaviour was influenced first by their physical work environment; second, by their attitude towards geriatric ward patients; and third, by their knowledge of the causes and treatment of patients' needs. The findings of Wells' research were on the whole depressing. She concluded that the environment posed many problems and, on top of that, most nurses lacked the understanding and knowledge necessary to cope with the nursing care problems of their patients, never mind to promote change. This was true of both trained and untrained staff. But trained staff had positive attitudes towards old people, and saw the answer to all their problems as resting in the provision of more staff. Wells shows that life is not so simple: she found that nursing problems often featured lack of awareness about current practices; unclear aims; lack of planning; and lack of communication and co-ordination of routine and of innovative work practices. Commonly, there was no monitoring of work progress either. In observing how geriatric nurses spent their time, Wells found:

The nursing work on the geriatric wards was not focused on the patients' needs but on ward routines which might or might not be appropriate for each patient. The work routines were based on minimal, universal needs such as meals, commoding/changing wet pads, 'getting up', and 'going to bed'. Work was not organised in the sense that it was assigned in any manner. Routines were determined by the time of day, and the work progressed in bursts of frantic activity by nurses working in pairs or a group of three to complete the routine from one end of the ward to another.

Further, not only was work not assigned or even focused on individual patients but there was no nursing record of individual patient preferences and such information was not regularly transmitted verbally in nurse communication. Moreover, individual patient preference or even necessary variation in care appeared to be obstructive to the work goal, which was completion of the routine. Thus, the problem of nursing work in geriatric wards was not so much shortage of staff as the fact that such work was neither sensibly organised nor provided the likelihood of helpful care for patients.

Patients' physical care problems were not the central issue. Nursing staff were not concerned about any specific patient problem; their prime concern was the completion of ward routines (Wells 1980, p. 127–128).

Baker (1978) was interested in the relationship between nurses' perceptions of their work and their actual work behaviour. In a participant observation study, she found that patients in geriatric wards were on the whole perceived as enjoying less than adult status, and that the prevailing style of nursing was what she called 'routine geriatric' — the application of broad-based routines to whole groups of patients, irrespective of considerations of individual need or preference. She accounts for this in terms of medical priorities and expectations first of all. Little medical attention is accorded to those patients deemed unlikely to make a speedy recovery to a point at which they can be discharged. The low status accorded to patients who do not fit this category is mirrored, on the whole, in nurses' perceptions of such patients. This arises through the traditional primacy of the doctor's role and the pervasiveness of the idea of and desirability of cure and discharge — a widespread emphasis in most departments of geriatic medicine. The 'routine geriatric' style of nursing is reinforced by various organizational factors. Wards which attract low levels of medical attention tend to have poorer levels of staff and other resources; administrative priorities of nursing managers and some doctors — tidy wards, a quiet life, for example — are best met by following the 'routine geriatric' style. A patient-centred style might mean, for example, that beds remained unmade for long periods while patients' needs were attended to; or that doctors might have to wait for the completion of essential personal care of patients by nurses before beginning a ward round.

There were some exceptions to the 'routine geriatric' style, for which it was only possible to speculate as to the explanation. Overall, Baker's findings, suggesting as they do a lack of humanitarian concern for patients in the delivery of care, lead her to consider some radical changes. She calls for a complete reorientation of the nursing profession such that nursing care is provided to individual patients *as* individuals: remember that Baker's research pre-dates the nursing process 'revolution' in the United Kingdom. She also states that raising the status of geriatric nursing is a prerequisite to improving things: the caring along with the curing role of nursing care deserves and indeed demands proper recognition. Baker is an advocate of organizing long-stay institutional care outside the hospital system, under the clinical management of the nursing profession (see Ch. 29 of this volume for further discussion of long-stay care).

By the 1980s, we saw the emergence of optimistic literature from geriatricians concerning the successes of their departments judged by medical criteria — e.g. increased turnover. It has often been implied that a better service for a larger slice of the elderly population of a catchment area results (Harrison 1984).

What evidence do we have from other sources that things are in fact better from the nursing and the patients' angle? There are some instances where improved practices have been described — e.g. Cullen (1983), Storrs (1982), and Stevens (1983), and by finalists in the West Midlands Institute of Geriatric Medicine and Gerontology's Ward of the Year Competition (1982).

The initiatives taken at the Nursing Development Unit at Burford Cottage Hospital (Pearson 1983) are particularly impressive. These led to the setting up of nurse-controlled beds for patients who are past the acute stage of their illness. 'Primary nursing' is practised, by which each nurse has responsibility for a group of patients, and care is individualized, planned and evaluated (see Ch. 33). The nurses receive continuing education and support in introducing change. Other Nursing Development Units have been and are being set up in different parts of the UK, but their vulnerability when in competition with a hostile and powerful medical establishment for scarce resources has been demonstrated with the closure of the highly acclaimed Nursing Development Unit at Oxford's Radcliffe Infirmary (Salvage 1989). This unit was closed in spite of its demonstrated higher-quality and cheaper care when compared with conventional hospital treatment; and in spite of support from some physicians (McCarthy & Kendall 1989). As Salvage emphasizes, clinical excellence alone will not guarantee success; nurses need political acumen too in order to implement enduring change in the face of hostility from the medical profession. One suspects, therefore, that the problems described by Wells (1980) and Baker (1978), and in my own work (Evers 1981), will remain part of the scene in many geriatric departments. Further discussion of Nursing Development Units can be found in Chapter 29.

Godlove et al (1981) found that apathy and inactivity were major features in long-term care wards. In my own research, I found that in eight unremarkable geriatric wards in different hospitals, housing predominantly long-stay patients, a 'warehousing' approach to geriatric care, similar to that described by Miller and Gwynne (1972) in residential homes for the physically handicapped, predominated. There was some evidence of personalized care in five of the eight wards (Evers 1981, 1984). But there remained considerable evidence of inhumane treatment of patients, and patterns of care in many respects failed to match the various professional and policy statements about appropriate standards of care, e.g. the joint statement by the British Geriatrics Society and the Royal College of Nursing (1975). Wards providing some personalized care were distinguished from those which did not in the stance adopted by the consultants towards the work of slow-stream rehabilitation and long-term care. They expressed the belief that such work was valuable and important, no less so than cure-work. In different ways, they provided positive support in practice of the nurses' primacy in this area of patient care. In the other wards, the consultants saw care-work as necessary but less attractive and interesting than cure-work. They had in effect handed the responsibility to the nursing staff and withdrawn from the arena. Not surprisingly, these nursing staff felt discouraged and disaffected in their work because patients were implicitly labelled by the doctor as 'second class', or 'less eligible'.

The medical argument that a modern, high turnover geriatric department is offering a quality service to the elderly population of the catchment area rests not only on what happens to its patients for whom rapid cure and discharge is the aim, but also — less explicitly — on the presumption of quality non-medical care for its 'backstage' patients (those for 'slow-stream' rehabilitation and possibly eventual discharge; patients needing long-term care; and some dying patients). They occupy the majority of geriatric beds, so what goes on in these beds is crucially important. Writing about their services, many geriatricians devote little explicit attention to the organization of care for patients other than 'fast stream' treatment and rehabilitation patients. Could this be because they believe that if their practice and organization succeeds in relation to discharging patients, then appropriate practice and organization of care for the other patient categories will automatically follow?

From my own research findings — in line with common sense — it seems that the opposite may be true, unless active measures are taken to identify and institute positive care strategies for *all* categories of patient. That is, where high turnover is a chief criterion of success, work with patients who do not fit this category is in danger of becoming devalued medically and therefore in nursing and remedial therapy terms too. In some of the wards I studied there was a mixture of patient types. There were three common trends in the provision of care, which sometimes occasioned much suffering — albeit unintentionally — to patients. First, efforts were sometimes made to define patients as candidates for rapid cure and discharge and treat them accordingly, when from the patient's perspective this was not necessarily appropriate. Second, there was often an avoidance of explicitly defining care goals for manifestly 'non-cure' patients, who then suffered from aimless residual care. A third trend was to reject or ignore patients who did not fit a ward's preferred repertoire of care and treatment strategies and its

established routines; or even — more rarely — to eject them, by redefining them as psychiatric cases, for example (Evers 1984). Multidisciplinary teamwork, commonly assumed to be beneficial for patients, seemed not to be successfully applied in practice to any patients other than those for whom rapid cure and discharge was the agreed goal (Evers 1982). Fairhurst's work (1977) also suggests that teamwork fails to fulfil its promise for patients, but serves instead as a medium for professionals to try to resolve conflicts over status and resources.

Nursing and social research, then, continues to paint a picture of geriatric care and attendant quality of life for patients which is not altogether cheerful. What, if any, are the implications of research evidence for the nature of care provision within the differing medical strategies for organizing geriatric departments?

RELATIONSHIP OF GERIATRIC NURSING AND GERIATRIC MEDICINE

For the future, the main viable alternatives seem to be age-related and integrated types of service; thus just these two will be considered. We do not know of any research analysis of the relationship between overall medical policy and organization of geriatric departments and the nature and organization of non-medical care. But on the basis of the studies discussed above, some tentative speculations can be made. Perhaps these might form the basis for a future research study. In both the age-related and integrated geriatric department, acute-type nursing care aimed towards cure or amelioration and rapid discharge is likely to be done satisfactorily if we assume minimal levels of competence and resources. This is what all nurses learn to do during their training, and is directly and obviously linked with the miracles of modern medicine. In our 'ageist' society, however, people who have chosen to work with elderly people in a geriatric department may not have to confront the same dilemmas regarding priorities which could arise for those working with acutely ill patients of all ages. Where pressure of work is extreme, elderly acutely ill patients may be accorded less priority than younger ones in an integrated service.

The research studies described above show that work with types of patients who command little medical attention and regard tends to feature depersonalization, routinization and unintended suffering for at least some patients. Thus, so long as patient care is carried out within a medicalized arena, the age-related type of service, whose staff have largely chosen to work there, is perhaps best placed to confront these perennial problems.

TOWARDS ORGANIZATIONAL SOLUTIONS?

Organizational strategies for continuing to improve the status and quality of work with sick elderly people are needed. The medical emphasis on turnover serves a vital purpose in this regard, and has succeeded in mobilizing improved resources to offer a service to larger numbers of elderly people. However, there may be room for improvement in the extent to which the needs and problems of patients who cannot be rapidly 'turned over' are met. A case can be made for removing what is primarily care-work outside the medicalized arena of the hospital. A nursing-based care facility could, in the British context, enhance the status of nursing care-work, and at the same time create the conditions in which the practice of nursing *care* could be expected to flourish. The feasibility of this has been studied by Bond and Bond for the Department of Health (see, for example, Bond 1984). This research is described in Chapter 29. This approach perhaps offers fresh promise; but it certainly embodies familiar problems. Such an arrangement could serve simply to aggravate existing fragmentation of care of the elderly sick. It could also create a new kind of institutional ghetto for nurses and patients. To avoid this, access to material and professional resources would need to be assured, and 'openness' of organizational boundaries actively maintained. It might appear unlikely that the Department of Health would take on board further development of Nursing Home facilities, given trends in the late 1980s to a decline in long-term care in the NHS, and the increase in

private sector residential and nursing Home provision.

But, so long as care of the elderly sick continues along established lines in this country, it is vital for the medical profession to articulate and practise explicit and positive strategies in relation to *all* categories of elderly patient. The medical strategy, rightly or wrongly, sets many of the parameters within which patient-care work done by others is practised.

Education and training are important in spreading the word throughout the caring professions that care-work as well as cure-work is important and valuable, even when performed with the very old. As Norton (1965) pointed out, geriatric nursing well done epitomizes good nursing care. Yet care-work is often described as 'basic', and by implication seen as boring, low status and less important. I sometimes heard, during my research, newly qualified nurses remarking sadly that geriatric nursing was 'a waste of all that training'. But on the educational front there are promising developments. Geriatric experience is now compulsory for all nursing pupils and students — and the quality of that experience is, we hope, improving along with developments in nursing practice and education more generally, as well as in geriatric care and its organization.

A more obviously patient-centred and flexible service should in our view incorporate ways of bridging the Great Divide between the hospital and the rest of the world. We have already noted that hospital-centred care commands a disproportionate level of attention. Although geriatricians see themselves as fostering a community orientation and indeed may spend much of their time working outside the hospital, geriatric nurses commonly have no community involvement. Firsthand knowledge of the patient and her home, family and social environment might result in numerous benefits for patients and nurses; most obviously, the enhanced opportunity for planning, together with the patient, a personalized care regime. Conversely, community-based health professionals might usefully cross the boundary into the hospital more often than is currently the case. The importance of a 'community orientation' cannot be overstressed, given that is where 95% of the elderly population live — and cope — and are likely to continue to do so.

CONCLUSION

Services for care of the elderly sick in the United Kingdom are, like other health care services, currently feeling the effects of austere economic policies. Even greater responsibility for care will, as a result, be vested in families and other lay carers, given the facts of demography.

Innovative responses to the needs of elderly sick people and their lay carers are called for on the part of service providers. Despite problems of the cost, and of putting new ideas into practice, our formal and voluntary services have a strong tradition of developing innovative responses to unmet needs, and we hope this tradition will continue (Isaacs & Evers 1984).

Health care professionals who work with elderly people can do a great deal, individually and collectively, to capitalize on the strengths and combat the problems of our current patterns of service provision. Nurses, being the largest group, perhaps have the greatest responsibility here. We have suggested that the conventional relationship with geriatricians might be challenged and revised in the interests of improved long-term care. Further, there is a strong argument for an extension of nurse-controlled patient-centred care environments — with some caveats. Interchangeability of hospital and community staff is urgently needed, and nurses are well placed to take a major initiative here. Breaking down some of the barriers between hospital-centred and other bases of care provision would facilitate continuity of care in the endeavour to understand and respond to the needs of old people and their lay carers in their own social environment. The hospital is a small but disproportionately visible part of the care network. The family and other lay carers contribute the greatest part, and are the least visible. The nursing profession does much, but could do more, in support of the latter.

REFERENCES

Age Concern 1977 Profiles of the elderly 4: their health and the health services. Age Concern, Mitcham

Amulree 1951 Adding life to years. National Council of Social Service, London

Andrews K, Brocklehurst J 1987 British geriatric medicine in the 1980s. King Edward's Hospital Fund for London, London

Atkin K, Cameron E, Badger F, Evers H 1989 Asian elders' knowledge and future use of community social and health services. New Community 15: 439–445

Audit Commission 1986 Making a reality of community care. HMSO, London

Badger F, Cameron E, Evers H 1989a Cognitive and psychological testing in the elderly: a brief overview. Working Paper No 30, Community Care Project Working Papers, Department of Social Medicine, University of Birmingham

Badger F, Cameron E, Evers H, Atkin K, Griffiths R 1989b Why don't GPs refer their black patients to the district nurses? Health Trends 21: 31–32

Baker D 1978 Attitudes of nurses to the care of the elderly. Unpublished PhD thesis, University of Manchester

British Geriatrics Society 1983 Geriatric medicine: a career guide. Geriatric Medicine 13 (Mimeo): 3–4

British Geriatrics Society and Royal College of Nursing 1975 Improving geriatric care in hospital. *RCN*, London

Bond J 1984 Evaluation of long-stay accommodation for elderly people. In: Bromley D (ed) Gerontology: social and behavioural perspectives. Croom Helm, London

Brocklehurst J(ed) 1975 Geriatric care in advanced societies. MTP, Lancaster

Cameron E, Badger F, Evers H 1988 Old, needy — and black. Nursing Times 84(32): 38–40

Carboni D 1982 Geriatric medicine in the United States and Great Britain. Greenwood Press, London

Central Statistical Office 1989 Social Trends No 19. HMSO, London

Challis L 1989 A system to suit the customer. Community Care January 12: 28–30

Chapman P 1979 Unmet need and the delivery of care. Occasional papers on social administration No 61, Bedford Square Press, London

Clark A 1983 The historical perspective: development of geriatrics in the United Kingdom. In: Graham J, Hodkinson M (eds) Effective geriatric medicine. Department of Health and Social Security, London

Court S 1976 Fit for the future. Report of the Committee on Child Health Services. HMSO, London

Cullen M 1983 Nursing care. In: Denham M (ed) Care of the long-stay elderly patient. Croom Helm, London

Department of Employment 1987 Family expenditure survey 1986. HMSO, London

Department of Health 1989 Working for patients. HMSO, London

Department of Health and Social Security 1976 Priorities for health and social services in England and Wales. HMSO, London

Department of Health and Social Security 1978 A happier old age. HMSO, London

Department of Health and Social Security 1981a Growing older. HMSO, London

Department of Health and Social Security 1981b Care in the community. HMSO, London

Dunnell K, Dobbs J 1982 Nurses working in the community. HMSO, London

Equal Opportunities Commission 1982 Caring for the elderly and handicapped: community care policies and women's lives. EOC, Manchester

Evers H 1981 The creation of patient careers in geriatric wards: aspects of policy and practice. Social Science and Medicine 15A: 581–588

Evers H 1982 Professional practice and patient care: multi-disciplinary teamwork in geriatric wards. Ageing and Society 2: 57–75

Evers H 1984 Patients' experiences and the social relations of patient care in geriatric wards. Unpublished PhD thesis, University of Warwick

Evers H, Cameron E, Badger F 1988 Community Care Project: Overview of findings and issues. Working Paper No 28, Community Care Project Working Papers, Department of Social Medicine, University of Birmingham

Fairhurst E 1977 Teamwork as panacea: some underlying assumptions. Unpublished paper read at Annual Conference of the Medical Sociology Group of the British Sociological Association, University of Warwick

Fennell G, Phillipson C, Evers H 1988 The sociology of old age. Open University Press, Milton Keynes

Ferguson Anderson W 1981 The evolution of services in the United Kingdom. In: Kinnaird J, Brotherston J, Williamson J (eds) The provision of care for the elderly. Churchill Livingstone, Edinburgh

Glendenning F, Pearson M 1988 The black and ethnic minority elders in Britain: health needs and access to services. Working Papers on the health of older people No 6, Health Education Authority in association with the Centre for Social Gerontology, University of Keele. Health Education Authority, London

Godlove C, Richard L, Rodwell G 1981 Time for action. Joint Unit for Social Services Research, University of Sheffield

Green H 1988 Informal carers. OPCS Social Survey Division, Series GH5 No 15 Supplement A HMSO, London

Griffiths R 1988 Community care: agenda for action. A report to the Secretary of State for Social Services. HMSO, London

Grimley Evans J 1981 Institutional care. In: Arie T (ed) Health care of the elderly. Croom Helm, London

Grimley Evans J 1983 The appraisal of hospital geriatric services. Community Medicine 5: 242–250

Hall M 1988 Geriatric medicine today. In: Wells F, Freer C (eds) The ageing population: burden or challenge? Macmillan, Basingstoke

Harris J 1979 More than going grey: a preliminary examination of gerontological theory and social work practice with old people. Unpublished MA thesis, University of Warwick

Harrison J 1983 Women and ageing: experience and implications. Ageing and Society 3: 209–235

Harrison J 1984 Making a geriatric department effective. In: Isaacs B, Evers H (eds) Innovations in the care of the elderly. Croom Helm, London

Horrocks P 1982 The case for geriatric medicine as an age-related specialty. In: Isaacs B (ed) Recent advances in

House of Commons 1988 Public expenditure on the social services. Memorandum from the DHSS to the Social Services Committee. HMSO, London

Hunt A 1978 The elderly at home. HMSO, London

Isaacs B 1981 Is geriatrics a specialty? In: Arie T (ed) Health care of the elderly. Croom Helm, London

Isaacs B, Evers H (eds) 1984 Innovations in the care of the elderly. Croom Helm, London

Johnson M 1983 A sharper eye on private homes. Health and Social Services Journal August 4: 930–932

Jolley A, Smith P, Billington L, Ainsworth D, Ring D 1982 Developing a psychogeriatric service. In: Coakley D (ed) Establishing a geriatric service. Croom Helm, London

Levin E, Sinclair I, Gorbach P 1983 The supporters of confused elderly persons at home. Extract from the main report. National Institute for Social Work Research Unit, London

McCarthy S T, Kendall G 1989 Letters. Nursing Times 85(19): 15

Macintyre S 1977 Old age as a social problem. In: Dingwall R, Heath C, Reid M, Stacey M (eds) Health care and health knowledge. Croom Helm, London

Martin J, White A 1988 The financial circumstances of disabled adults living in private households. OPCS surveys of disability in Great Britain, Report 2. HMSO, London

Martin J, Meltzer H, Elliot D 1988 The prevalence of disability among adults. OPCS surveys of disability in Great Britain, Report 1. HMSO, London

Mears R, Smith R 1985 The development of welfare services for elderly people. Croom Helm, London

Miller E, Gwynne G 1972 A life apart. Tavistock, London

Nissel M, Bonnerjea L 1982 Family care of the handicapped elderly: who pays? Policy Studies Institute, London

Norton D 1965 Nursing in geriatrics. Gerontologia Clinica 7: 51–60

Norton D, McLaren R, Exton-Smith A N 1962 An investigation of geriatric nursing problems in hospital. Reprinted 1975, Churchill Livingstone, Edinburgh

Office of Population Censuses and Surveys 1982 General household survey for 1980. HMSO, London

Office of Population Censuses and Surveys 1985 General Household Survey. HMSO, London

Opit L 1977 Domiciliary care for the elderly sick — economy or neglect? British Medical Journal 1: 30–33

Pearson A 1983 The clinical nursing unit. Heinemann, London

Royal College of Physicians 1977 Report of the working party on medical care of the elderly. The Lancet 1: 1092–1095

Royal College of Physicians of London and Royal College of Psychiatrists 1989 Specialist services and medical training. Royal college of Physicians of London and Royal College of Psychiatrists, London

Rossiter C, Wicks M 1982 Crisis or challenge? Family care, elderly people and social policy. Study Commission on the Family, London

Salvage J 1989 Setback for nursing. Nursing Times 85(11): 19

Secretary of State for Health, Social Security, Wales and Scotland 1989 Caring for people: community care in the next decade and beyond. (White Paper) Cmnd 849. HMSO, London

Sidell M 1986 Coping with confusion. The experience of 60 elderly people and their formal and informal carers. Unpublished PhD thesis, University of East Anglia, Norwich

Stevens P 1983 It's not the tidiest ward in the hospital. British Journal of Geriatric Nursing 3: 6–8

Storrs A 1982 What is care? British Journal of Geriatric Nursing 1: 12–14

Thomson A P, Lowe C R, McKeown T 1951 The care of the ageing and chronic sick. E and S Livingstone, Edinburgh

Tinker A 1981 The elderly in modern society. Longman, Harlow

Townsend P 1979 Poverty in the United Kingdom. Penguin, Harmondsworth

Wagner G 1988 Residential care — a positive choice. Report of the Independent Review of Residential Care. HMSO, London

Wells T 1980 Problems in geriatric nursing care. Churchill Livingstone, Edinburgh

Wheeler R 1986 Housing policy for elderly people. In: Phillipson C, Walker A (eds) Ageing and social policy: a critical assessment. Gower, Aldershot

White R 1978 Social change and the development of the nursing profession: a study of the Poor Law Nursing Service 1848–1948. Kimpton, London

Wilkin D, Hallam L, Leavey R, Metcalfe E 1987 Anatomy of urban general practice. Tavistock, London

CHAPTER CONTENTS

Introduction 437
A note on terminology 438

Black and ethnic minority elders in Britain 439

Social and material circumstances 440
Financial resources 440
Housing 440
Family networks 441

Health and well-being 441
Mobility and independence 442
Specific diseases 442
Mental health 443

Contact with health and welfare services 443
Domiciliary service and day centres 444
Health services 444

Community responses 444

The response of the statutory sectors 445

A way forward 445

25

Care of black and ethnic minority elders

Maggie Pearson

INTRODUCTION

Although black people have a long history in Britain, dating back at least to Roman times when black African soldiers defended Hadrian's Wall (Fryer 1984), they and their experiences have been largely 'invisible' to the rest of the population. Only very recently have the needs and experiences of black people and ethnic minorities in Britain been addressed within organizations providing services, including the health service.

If black and ethnic minority communities have been 'invisible' in Britain, their elders have been all the more so. 26 400 elderly black and ethnic minority people were recorded in the 1971 Census, but one London borough with a large Afro-Caribbean community claimed in 1973 that such elders could not exist, because they had no files on them (Sevedin and Gorosch-Tomlinson 1984). There are now almost half a million elderly people living in the United Kingdom who were born abroad (OPCS 1983), but many nurses may never have looked after a black or ethnic minority elder, and fewer still will have had any training with regard to the issues which underpin the delivery of care in a multiracial society.

An increasing number of health professionals are now becoming aware of their inability to deliver effective and sensitive care to their minority patients. Unfamiliar with, and ignorant of, everyday life in black and ethnic minority British communities, they cannot plan appropriate patient-centred care. Nurses, who may first come into contact with black and ethnic minority elders in distressing circumstances (e.g. after an emergency admission) may be so worried about offending their patients by doing something inappropriate or unacceptable, that they unintentionally avoid them, delivering the minimum of care for fear of offending. The policy of care in the community sharpens these issues still further; support and maintenance of patients at home demands an even greater knowledge and understanding of their social and material world, and of their access to resources which would maximize their independence.

Often it has been assumed that cultural information will be enough to enable professional carers to provide appropriate and sensitive care for their minority patients. 'Cultural packages' are often sought in the form of training days, packs or booklets, but all too often an emphasis on culture alone has involved simplistic, ill-founded stereotypes of minorities' lifestyles, just as 'the elderly' are often treated and stereotyped as a single, homogeneous group. Much damage has been done by reproducing cultural information without first considering and challenging the ways in which black people's lifestyles are often stereotyped and defined as deviant and inherently problematic (CCCS 1981).* Although it is important to understand patients' and clients' social and cultural frames of reference, these are only a *part* of black people's experience. Their choices are constrained, and their prerequisites for health denied, by the impact of racism and discrimination on their lives.

This chapter aims to reverse both the invisibility and the misplaced emphasis on culture, drawing together the findings of several surveys of black and ethnic minority elders in Britain today to set out the context within which their health problems arise, and in which nurses will be giving care. It describes their family circumstances, living conditions, health and well-being and the failure of established services to meet their needs; it also briefly discusses community projects which have emerged in response to this legacy of neglect. There are, therefore, no potted guides to minority cultures in this chapter. Nor are there any recipes for instant solutions to which nurse managers and practitioners can turn. Instead, there are examples of the achievements and resources of local black and ethnic minority communities, to whom nurses can refer elders needing help, and with whom they can consult and work to ensure that their care responds to the everyday experiences of all elderly people.

A NOTE ON TERMINOLOGY

First, however, it is important to clarify some terms, and to identify the potential patients about whose care this chapter is written. Writing about racial and ethnic groups, racism, and racial discrimination is always difficult and controversial, not least because 'race' is a *social* category or construct, not a distinct biological entity (Husband 1982).* There is no one word which embraces all people who experience discrimination, hostility or oppression because of the colour of their skin and/or their ethnic origins.

The word increasingly used by people of Afro-Caribbean origin and Asian origin is 'black', underlining their united experience of discrimination because their skin is not 'white'. At the same time, there are 'ethnic minorities' who do not identify themselves as black, but who nevertheless share a common experience of discrimination and inequality because of their country of birth, ethnic origins, language, culture or religion. The government's Office of Population Censuses and Surveys uses the term 'ethnic minority' to refer to people who are not white. Their definition therefore excludes Irish people, or people from Eastern Europe, who may have different traditions, languages or life chances from those of the majority of white people in Britain.

No single term is completely acceptable to everyone, but throughout this chapter the phrase *black people and ethnic minorities* is used to refer to the wide group of people whose language, culture and religion are different from the white British norm, and those whose skin colour is not white.

---

* See Pearson (1986) for a fuller discussion.

* See Pearson (1985a) for a brief review.

Terms referring to national or ethnic origin, such as 'Afro-Caribbean', 'Asian' or 'Polish' are used to refer to specific groups of people. *None* of these terms implies, or is meant to imply, that the people discussed are not British citizens.

Writing about 'elderly' people is similarly sensitive. People of the same chronological age often have very different abilities, attitudes and lifestyles. In many ethnic minority communities, however, people are 'elders' from their mid-fifties, a reflection of the respect which older people are often accorded, and of the reality that from their mid-fifties onwards they may be some of the oldest people in their communities. The term *elders* is therefore used throughout this chapter to refer to older people aged 55 and over who are often, in reality, retired from work. The term is also used to project a more positive image of older people, implying wisdom and experience, as opposed to the more commonly used 'elderly', which all too often has pejorative connotations.

BLACK AND ETHNIC MINORITY ELDERS IN BRITAIN

Almost 400 000 elderly people living in the United Kingdom were born abroad, constituting just less than 4% of the total population of 10.5 million aged 60 and over (OPCS 1983). This figure includes all migrants from Ireland and other EEC countries (50 000); Poland (93 000) and other Eastern European countries (80 000); China and East Asia, including Vietnam (4 000). Almost 90 000 are from the New Commonwealth and Pakistan; of these almost 20 000 were born in the Caribbean and approximately 55 000 are of Asian origin from the Indian subcontinent and East Africa.

Many of the migrants from Poland and Eastern Europe were adults when they came during and after the Second World War. In future years, the number of their elders will not therefore increase differentially, since their communities' age structures already approximate that of the total British population, of whom 20% are aged 60 and over. Amongst the black and ethnic minority communi-

ties with origins in the New Commonwealth and Pakistan, however, the picture is different. Whilst their elders currently comprise less than 5% of the population, this proportion will increase sharply over the next twenty years, as the cohorts currently between the ages of 45 and 65, who comprise over 15% of the population, age. The current number of 16 000 Afro-Caribbeans of pensionable age will increase to over 100 000. Similarly, the number of elderly Asians from the Indian subcontinent and East Africa will increase from under 55 000 to more than 160 000.

The black and ethnic minority elders have a wide variety of histories and backgrounds. Some were born in Britain, but because ethnic origin is not recorded in the Census with country of birth, we do not know how many. Those who migrated from the Caribbean and the Indian subcontinent came principally in the post-war years of acute labour shortage in Britain. They were actively recruited and invited here to fill the low-paid jobs and shift work which the British population would not do, and to staff the rapidly expanding public services such as transport and the health service. Others, from Poland and other East European countries, from Vietnam, and people of Asian origin from East Africa came as refugees, arriving here after years of horrendous persecution and harassment in many cases. Many Chinese people who came to Britain for work stayed here as refugees after the Chinese Revolution of 1948.

The majority of black and ethnic minority communities are established in inner city areas: in Greater London, the West Midlands and Manchester; in textile towns such as Leicester, Derby, Nottingham; the West Yorkshire woollen towns such as Bradford and Leeds; and the Lancashire cotton mill towns such as Rochdale and Oldham. Few currently live in rural areas.

Nearly 2000 elders in black and ethnic minority communities have been interviewed over the last decade in six studies in Birmingham (Bhalla & Blakemore 1981), Nottingham (Berry et al 1981), Manchester and London (Barker 1984), Bristol (Fenton 1986), Derby (Lambert & Dolan 1986) and Leicester (Farrah 1986). These studies give a detailed picture of their personal, social and material circumstances, and of their health and welfare needs; they are drawn on heavily here, to describe the circumstances in which black and ethnic minority elders live, and the context in which their hospital and community care is given.*

SOCIAL AND MATERIAL CIRCUMSTANCES

FINANCIAL RESOURCES

Almost half of our black and ethnic minority elders approach retirement age redundant, unemployed, or permanently sick. The older manufacturing industries, in which they were employed, declined drastically during the 1970s. Many of these elders have poor health associated with the semi-skilled and unskilled manual occupations in which they were concentrated (Brown 1984). With few personal or financial resources, including pensions, their new-found leisure may be bleak, with very few real choices. Their employment history in precarious and poorly paid occupations, often with frequent job changes, has left many elders with no entitlement to a full state or occupational pension and little opportunity to accumulate savings. Between one third and one half of the elders in studies in Birmingham (Bhalla & Blakemore 1981), Manchester (Barker 1984) and Derby (Lambert & Dolan 1986) did not receive a full state pension.

Despite the prevalence of poverty and the lack of pension rights, low take-up of social security benefits is a consistent feature of the six local studies. In Leicestershire, for example, 35% of the Afro-Caribbean elders entitled to Supplementary Benefit (now Income Support) and 88% of those entitled to a single payment for household goods had not made a claim. Similarly, 34% of those entitled to reduced bus fares were not claiming them (Farrah 1986).

Asian elders in Birmingham (Bhalla & Blakemore 1981) and Derby (Lambert & Dolan

---

* For a fuller review of this and other material, see Glendenning and Pearson (1987).

1986) were less likely to have a pension or state benefits than were Afro-Caribbeans, possibly because information on social security is not easily available in languages other than English. Because most Asian migrants worked in declining manufacturing industries, rather than in the public sector, many have had interrupted work histories, and may not have a complete national insurance record. Polish elders, for example, and those from the Indian subcontinent whose first language is not English may have minimal access to language lessons and little chance to speak much English, often working with fellow mother-tongue speakers and on the night-shifts in textile mills and other factories (Jagucki 1983). In both Birmingham (Bhalla & Blakemore 1981) and Derby (Lambert & Dolan 1986), almost three quarters of the Asian elders interviewed said they needed an interpreting service when dealing with the health and welfare services.

Language is not the only factor affecting take-up of benefits. People may not be aware of their entitlement when little information is readily available and may be reluctant to ask, particularly if previous enquiries or claims have met with hostility and suspicion from social security staff. There is evidence from several localities that black people have been asked to produce passports to certify their entitlement when claiming benefits (Lalljie 1983).

HOUSING

The majority of black and minority elders live, like the younger generations, in inner-city areas, often the victims of subtle or blatant discrimination in the housing market (CRE 1984a, 1984b). Owner-occupiers are often in older terraced property, and those who are council or private tenants are consistently allocated lower-quality accommodation. Whether owners or tenants, black and ethnic minority elders are likely to have poor household amenities. They are very unlikely to have a downstairs toilet inside the house (Brown 1984, Lambert & Dolan 1986, Farrah 1986). Almost a quarter of Asian elders in the Birmingham study had no piped hot water, compared with 15% of white elders in the same neighbourhood (Bhalla

& Blakemore 1981). For some families, the size of the accommodation available and regulations about overcrowding mean that large families or several generations cannot be properly housed together.

FAMILY NETWORKS

It is perhaps in their family circumstances that the situation of black and ethnic minority elders is most varied. Whilst a significant number of elders have no family in Britain at all, others may have children and grandchildren living with them.

Women comprise almost 60% of the national population over the age of 60 (CSO 1989), but whilst they comprised a similar proportion of the various samples of Afro-Caribbean elders interviewed (Berry et al 1981, Farrah 1986), less than 40% of the Asian elders were women (Bhalla & Blakemore 1981, Barker 1984, Lambert & Dolan 1986). Many elderly Asian men have no immediate family in Britain, and have faced protracted problems in trying to secure the immigration rights of their wives and families.

Thirty six per cent of elderly people in Britain live alone, but in Derby (Lambert & Dolan 1986), Nottingham (Berry et al 1981) and Leicester (Farrah 1986) less than 30% of Afro-Caribbean elders were on their own, whilst in Bristol the proportion was a third (Fenton 1986). Almost a tenth of Afro-Caribbean elders in Birmingham had no relatives in Britain, and almost a half had no family in the neighbourhood (Bhalla & Blakemore 1981). In Leicestershire, 8% of Afro-Caribbean elders had no family contact at all (Farrah 1986). In Nottingham, 18% of Afro-Caribbean elders had no living children (Berry et al 1981).

In both Derby (Lambert & Dolan 1986) and Birmingham (Bhalla & Blakemore 1981), over 95% of Asian elders lived with others, but these statistics mask the potential for deep-rooted loneliness, since over a quarter of the Asian elders in Birmingham had no family in Britain, and a further 31% had no family living locally (ibid).

This evidence of isolation and solitary living is particularly important, since it has often been assumed that minority elders have not, in the past, taken up the available benefits and services because their extended family meets all their needs.

In Bristol, many elders felt that although materially easier than their parents', their life was blighted socially and psychologically by the absence of their children (Fenton 1986).

The potential isolation of living alone may be avoided if other family members live nearby, but again the situation is very varied. In Leicestershire, nearly two thirds of the Afro-Carribbean elders interviewed had 'frequent' contact with relatives, and a fifth had children living locally (Farrah 1986). Over half of the Afro-Caribbean elders interviewed in Nottingham had children living locally, including 37% who had one or more child living with them (Berry et al 1981). Even where families live in close proximity, relationships between the generations may, however, have changed in Britain:

[C]are of grandchildren or other children is mentioned only by one per cent of the Afro-Caribbean, five per cent of the Asian and none of the European sample as something they would like to do. . . . [W]hatever the cause of the low proportion of elders who mention care of grandchildren [emphasis added], it means that we have to revise the view that grandparent-grandchild relationships are always a strong feature of minority group family life. (Bhalla & Blakemore 1981, p. 24).

Feelings of isolation from the younger generation are often attributed to problems of 'culture' or 'generation' clash between the minority elders and their children. But the poverty and poor housing which are more likely to be the lot of black elders may exacerbate disputes and differences which commonly arise between generations in all communities. In the case of Liverpool, it has been suggested that elderly Chinese prefer to stay in familiar surroundings in central Liverpool rather than move into their children's homes in suburbia (Chan & Leung 1987).

HEALTH AND WELL-BEING

The potential distress of ageing and retirement in the social and material circumstances outlined above is particularly complex for black and ethnic minority elders. In the societies with which many of them identify, they would have assumed an important role within the family and within the community. At no point would they have been dismissed as useless or roleless (SCEMSC 1986). In Britain, however, the situation is less happy. Later life may bring reflections of sadness, disappointment and dashed hopes on their years here (Fenton 1986). Many feel very lonely and trapped in a country which wanted only their labour (Fenton 1986, Farrah 1986).

MOBILITY AND INDEPENDENCE

The ability to maximize economic, social and family resources, and to maintain the dignity of independent living is profoundly affected by physical mobility and mental well-being. For the elders with no family in Britain, physical mobility is crucial to their social interaction in their community's place of worship and other meeting centres.

In Birmingham the Afro-Caribbean sample reported more health and mobility problems than their Asian or European counterparts, despite being younger overall (Bhalla & Blakemore 1981). Sixty one per cent had visual impairment, which varied in severity from almost total blindness to inconveniently restricted vision, compared with just over half the Asian and white elders. Walking posed a problem for over half the Afro-Caribbean sample, who did not get out of the home each day. By contrast, 66% of Asian elders and 60% of white elders went out of the home daily (Bhalla & Blakemore 1981).

The elders in Derby were 'reasonably fit and mobile people' (Lambert & Dolan 1986). In contrast to the Birmingham sample, Afro-Caribbean elders in Derby reported the least illness and had the fewest problems with eyesight and hearing. The Pakistani elders, on the other hand, had the most health problems: 75% had problems with their eyes and 30% had hearing problems.

A fifth of the Afro-Caribbean pensioners in Nottingham had difficulty getting about at home and in getting out of the house on their own (Berry et al 1981). Almost a quarter of those aged over 65 had problems with at least one of the everyday personal tasks such as having a bath, dressing, getting in and out of bed, and cutting toenails. Cutting toenails was the most problematic: an awkward but not onerous task which could improve mobility and could be undertaken by community nursing staff if necessary. The major source of help with these personal and domestic tasks was the respondent's spouse but, as we have seen, almost a third of elders live alone.

The ability to undertake domestic tasks such as housework, cooking and shopping are also vital for many elders' pride and independence, but a deterioration of physical or mental function may render household chores impossible. Approximately 15% of the Nottingham respondents needed help with one or more of these tasks, and spouses (where available) were again the major source of help.

SPECIFIC DISEASES

These disabilities may have several causes. The only national data on the prevalence of disease are mortality statistics, so we know relatively little about ethnic differences in the incidence of non-fatal disease, because data on 'race' or ethnic origin are not routinely recorded by health authorities.*

The Immigrant Mortality Study identified causes of death during the period 1970–78 by country of birth (Marmot et al 1984), and indicates the major diseases which affect black and ethnic minority communities, some of which have an undoubted impact on later life. The principal causes of death are not, as some would believe, 'special' diseases, but the common health problems of hypertensive disease, cerebrovascular disease, heart disease and diabetes. These diseases are, however, significantly more prevalent in black and ethnic minority communities.

Death rates from diabetes were high in migrants born in the Caribbean and in the Indian subcontinent. In Afro-Caribbean migrants, mortality from hypertensive disease was four to six times as

---

* But see Beevers and Cruickshank (1981), Tunstall Pedoe et al (1975), Cruickshank and Beevers (1989).

high as the average rate for England and Wales, and twice as high for cerebrovascular disease. Deaths from ischaemic heart disease were 19% higher than average in men born in the Indian subcontinent, and 28% higher than average in women. Gastrointestinal and breast cancer mortality was low amongst Indian subcontinent migrants.

These major causes of death amongst black and ethnic minority people are potentially very disabling. Poor eyesight, peripheral neuropathy and gangrene may be the degenerative results of diabetes. The poor housing in which many black and ethnic minority elders have to live may exacerbate their mobility problems. Renal problems associated with hypertension and diabetes are also more common causes of death amongst Afro-Caribbean and Indian subcontinent immigrants.

The Coronary Prevention Group points to the high incidence of diabetes, and the stress and deprivation generated by racial discrimination, as possible explanatory factors of the high incidence of ischaemic heart disease among Asian-born men (CPG 1986).

The epidemiology of disease amongst migrants becomes very similar to that of the rest of the population in the country to which they move after a few generations of settlement. At present, it is too early to say whether this will be the experience of black and ethnic minority people who have migrated to Britain.

MENTAL HEALTH

Black and ethnic minority elders' mental health is an issue of great and increasing concern. Older people who came to Britain as refugees from Eastern Europe during the Second World War, or more recently from East Africa and Vietnam, may have endured horrendous experiences. Painful and harrowing memories dulled and buried with the passage of time may return during the long days and solitude of a lonely retirement. There is considerable evidence that East European elders in particular experience mental health problems in later life (Hitch & Clegg 1980, Rack 1983, Littlewood & Lipsedge 1982).

The Leicestershire study was one of the first to include questions about mental health and found that just over a quarter said they felt very depressed (Farrah 1986). Only 4% were depressed and receiving treatment. This iceberg of undetected mental ill health highlights the need for relatives, neighbours and professionals to be alert to the signs of depression and to see them as such, rather than as inevitable consequences of growing old.

Depression is, of course, commonly experienced among older white people, but it is more likely to be misdiagnosed or not diagnosed at all in the black population (Burke 1984). If the ill person attributes her illness to the stress and alienation of being black in Britain, this may be misconstrued by professionals as 'paranoia'. Moreover, a misunderstanding and ignorance of the desperate isolation, powerlessness and poverty in which some black and ethnic minority elders live can result in misdiagnosis. We are warned of the pitfalls of such professional ignorance:

In France surveys have shown that the ratio of mental illness among immigrants [sic] is two or three times higher than among French citizens, but the category of mental illness is suspect. It would be more, not less, scientific to say that immigrants [sic] suffer twice or three times as much from insecurity and unhappiness. (Berger & Mohr 1975).

If health professionals are unable to communicate with clients and patients effectively, whether because they do not speak their client's language, or because they do not have a real understanding of their plight, culture or health beliefs, then serious misdiagnoses can be made, with far-reaching and long-lasting consequences for the patient and his/her family.

CONTACT WITH HEALTH AND WELFARE SERVICES

Elders' experience and use of health and social services are discussed briefly here, since both are important resources which may enable elders to maximize their independence and maintain their autonomy.

DOMICILIARY SERVICE AND DAY CENTRES

The problems of lack of information about benefits are mirrored for domiciliary and day services. In Birmingham (Bhalla & Blakemore 1981), Nottingham (Berry et al 1981) and Derby (Lambert & Dolan 1986), between a half and three quarters of elders in several minority communities had not heard of home help services, meals-on-wheels, or day centres. Just as worrying, however, are those who know of the range of services available, but would not use them. Almost a fifth of Afro-Caribbean elders interviewed in Nottingham said they would reject a home help and three-quarters would refuse meals-on-wheels (Berry et al 1981). In Birmingham, while a fifth of white respondents interviewed received a home help, only 6% of Afro-Caribbeans and no Asians did so. Six per cent of Europeans and 2% of Afro-Caribbeans received meals-on-wheels. The Asians did not use the service (Bhalla & Blakemore 1981).

A similar picture emerges regarding use of day centres. Those who know of them may decline to use them because they anticipate hostility from staff and other clients, particularly if they are only one or two among a large number of white visitors. After years of hostility from white people in Britain, such pessimism is, sadly, wholly understandable, and poses a real challenge for nursing and other care staff, who may find themselves required to mediate in such situations. Many black elders who attended day centres in Nottingham rejected them, and those who remained were isolated and ignored, or found themselves the butt of all the jokes (Lalljie 1983). Others simply feel they do not fit in to facilities designed for white clients. In Derby, Afro-Caribbean elders who attended a local day centre would have preferred somewhere of their own, where they could talk, understand and help each other (Lambert & Dolan 1986).

HEALTH SERVICES

We know very little about black and ethnic minority elders' contact with the NHS. Sixty-eight per cent of Afro-Caribbeans, 70% of Asians and 53% of Europeans interviewed in Birmingham had visited their general practitioner during the previous month (Blakemore 1982), compared with between 25% and 30% of elders in Derby (Lambert & Dolan 1986), where the GP consultation rate was similar to the national average of 33% for people over the age of 65 (OPCS 1987). There is not always confidence in the GP. In Nottingham, more than half the Afro-Caribbean elders had sought and paid for a second opinion in order to get 'better treatment' (Berry et al 1981). When one considers that many black elders are living on the minimum state pension, or on supplementary benefits, paying for a private consultation may be an expense which they can ill afford.

In Birmingham (Bhalla & Blakemore 1981) and Leicester (Farrah 1986), a considerable number of elders were receiving no treatment for their common health problems. If elders are unable to communicate effectively with their general practitioner, they may ignore a problem until it becomes an emergency or an accident occurs (Chan & Leung 1987). Although this pattern of referral for the elderly has been generally recognized — particularly for those who live alone (Dove & Dave 1986) — when an elder whose first language is not English presents as an emergency, communication becomes a major problem, not least for the nurse. Interpreters are rarely available at short notice, and elders' competence in their acquired English may well be reduced by their illness or the stress of the moment.

COMMUNITY RESPONSES

If it had not been for self-help groups which have emerged in many local minority communities, often without any formal resources, many black and ethnic minority elders would be in dire straits indeed. Moreover, it has often been the community's action which has prompted statutory authorities to take action to make their own services more accessible and relevant.

Various projects have been established throughout Britain by black and ethnic minority organizations, sometimes in collaboration with other voluntary bodies, providing day care and domiciliary services for their elders (see Glendenning & Pearson 1987 for fuller discussion). At luncheon clubs, which often provide transport to enable immobile elders to attend, elders can meet without being the odd one out. The entertainment and food are to their liking, and they can reminiscence with people who have had a similar history. Some of these projects also supply a meals-on-wheels service to elders who are housebound. Unlike in local authority facilities, however, participants usually have to make a financial contribution, because budgets are very tight.

Housing associations and other non-statutory organizations have set up sheltered housing or 'group homes' so that elders in specific communities can be housed together, with support and warden services provided by their own people. Unlike the day care schemes, for which statutory funding is rarely available, these community-based residential schemes have made imaginative use of social security residential care payments so that there is no extra cost to their clients (Finn 1986).

Like most community projects in the voluntary sector, however, the luncheon clubs, home-help schemes and group homes are precariously financed on short-term, 'soft' money outside the mainstream budget; run on a shoe-string from year to year, often in borrowed premises and vulnerable to changing financial priorities. If there are paid staff, they are usually preoccupied with the pursuit of funds for subsequent years. With such an immediate agenda, there is little scope for development. This, too, is a form of indirect discrimination, that the only services truly accessible to black and ethnic minority elders are so marginalized and vulnerable.

THE RESPONSE OF THE STATUTORY SECTORS

Against the backcloth of disability, poor health and isolation which many black and ethnic minority elders endure, the low uptake of, and lack of faith in, health and other welfare services is worrying. Campaigns to promote the use of existing services are not necessarily the answer. Any sense of alienation engendered by the nature of the service may be reinforced if there are no other elders from the same community. Even if there are other minority elders and a genuinely warm reception from staff and white clients, the services offered might be inappropriate. For example, if the food provided is 'standard British fare', then it will be unacceptable to many groups, including vegetarians, or orthodox Jewish and Muslim elders who require their meat to be ritually slaughtered. Many elderly refugees will not have any 'good old days' about which to reminisce or romanticize. For them, therapies or activities which involve recall of memories may be overwhelmingly painful, and one which they have devised various strategies to avoid. As Bhalla and Blakemore (1981) conclude:

[A]ll the services looked at are to some extent culturally if not racially exclusive. Thus 'integration' of Asian and Afro-Caribbean elders in the use of services and institutions as they are now structured would in fact mean integration on the terms of the dominant white culture — that is, a form of cultural domination (p. 38).

A WAY FORWARD

The problem of low uptake of services by black and ethnic minority elders stems from their image of the statutory services being provided *by* white people *for* white people. As long as black people and ethnic minorities are under-represented in the higher echelons of the services, being concentrated in positions, occupations and sectors seen as inferior, then this image and reality will persist. No progress can be made, therefore, without an active equal opportunities policy which aims to encourage the recruitment and promotion of under-represented groups.*

If black and ethnic minority elders' needs cannot be met within the mainstream services, then specific provision within the statutory sector, or in

---

* Strategies for achieving equal opportunities in the NHS are discussed more fully in Pearson 1985b.

the voluntary sector supported by mainstream funding may be required. However, grounded in the fundamental principle that people should be treated the same, no matter who they are, many health professionals find such demands for specific or separate provision unacceptable, incredulous that the service they provide excludes black people and ethnic minorities by failing to meet their needs. Often, the cost of initiatives such as providing appropriate food is cited by statutory authorities as being the prohibitive factor. Yet with some imagination and creative management, relevant and appropriate food could be cooked for use in residential care, hospital services, day centres and for distribution to people at home, to ensure that black and ethnic minority elders, like their white counterparts, have real access to domiciliary support and appropriate food. Similarly, interpreters could be employed in a consortium of services.

Some authorities have made considerable changes to their services in response to community pressure. For example, a few local authorities have allocated a certain number of places in residential Homes for elders from specific communities. Others have set up working parties and employed specialist race equality or ethnic minorities officers to review services and implement changes. The statutory services in many of the relevant districts, however, have yet to respond or to implement a process of real consultation with their local communities.

It is all too easy to reproduce initiatives taken elsewhere, or to consult through established channels, seeking recipes for quick and acceptable change. However, sound knowledge and dialogue with the local community is vital, both when planning services and in responding to specific problems or issues. The voluntary sector representatives on local authority and health authority joint planning committees, who are often assumed to speak on behalf of the consumer, are rarely aware of the concerns of black and ethnic minority elders. The Standing Committee for Ethnic Minority Senior Citizens (SCEMSC) was established in 1981 to raise the profile of black and ethnic minority elders, and argues that:

The black voluntary sector is no longer prepared to have their needs articulated for them by the established white voluntary sector who have little or no concept of what these needs really are (SCEMSC, 1986).

Professional bodies and statutory authorities should make contact with local community organizations and Community Relations or Racial Equality Offices, so that pre-emptive action can be taken before crises arise. If nurse training schools and employers implement a training programme so that all those delivering care understand why black and ethnic minority elders have so little faith in the established services, they will be able to recognize how their services should change.

As they become more frail, an increasing number of black and ethnic minority elders who are currently fully or partially independent will be in need of intensive support. Domiciliary services may suffice, but some will need sheltered or residential accommodation or nursing care. Plans must be made now, before the numbers of minority elderly people increase significantly, to ensure that the existing services take account of the needs and experiences of black and ethnic minority elders. If action is taken now, within a firm commitment to equality for all service users, then a golden opportunity could be grasped to prevent the distress and serious mistakes that have sometimes arisen in other sectors, because the service was unable to respond adequately to a patient's needs.

REFERENCES

Barker J 1984 Black and Asian old people in Britain. Age Concern England, Mitcham

Berger J, Mohr J 1975 Seventh man. Penguin, Harmondsworth

Beevers D G, Cruickshank J K 1981 Age, sex, ethnic origin and hospital admission rate for heart attack and stroke. Postgraduate Medical Journal 57: 763

Berry S, Lee M, Griffiths S 1981 Report on a survey of West Indian pensioners in Nottingham. Nottinghamshire Social Services Department, Nottingham (mimeo)

Bhalla A, Blakemore K 1981 Elders of ethnic minority groups. All Faiths for One Race (AFFOR), Birmingham

Blakemore K 1982 Health and illness among the elderly of minority groups living in Birmingham: some new findings. Health Trends 14: 69

Brown C 1984 Black and white Britain. The third PSI survey. Gower, Aldershot

Burke A W 1984 Is racism a causatory factor in mental illness? International Journal of Social Psychiatry. 30: 1

Central Statistical Office (CSO) 1989 Social Trends 19. HMSO, London

Centre for Contemporary Cultural Studies (CCCS) 1981 The empire strikes back. Hutchinson, London

Chan M C K, Leung T 1987 The elderly in the Chinese community in Liverpool (unpublished paper)

Commission for Racial Equality (CRE) 1984a Race and council housing in Hackney. Report of a formal investigation. CRE, London

Commission for Racial Equality (CRE) 1984b Race and housing in Liverpool: a research report. CRE, London

Coronary Prevention Groups (CPG) 1986 Coronary heart disease and Asians in Britain. CPG, London

Cruickshank J K, Beevers D G 1989 Ethnic factors in health and disease. Butterworths, London

Dove A F, Dave S H 1986 Elderly patients in the accident and emergency departments and their problems. British Medical Journal 292: 807

Farrah M 1986 Black elders in Leicester: an action research report on the needs of black elderly people of African descent from the Caribbean. Leicestershire County Council (mimeo)

Fenton C S 1986 Race, health and welfare. Afro-Caribbeans and South Asian people in central Bristol — health and social services. Department of Sociology, University of Bristol, Bristol

Finn J 1986 Supported living scheme for ethnic elders. Liverpool Personal Service Society. Liverpool (mimeo)

Fryer P 1984 Staying power: the history of black people in Britain. Pluto Press, London

Glendenning F (ed) 1979 The elders in ethnic minorities. Beth Johnson Foundation in association with the Department of Adult Education, University of Keele and the Commission for Racial Equality. Stoke-on-Trent

Glendenning F, Pearson M 1987 The health needs of black and ethnic minority elders. Working papers on the health of older people No 8. Health Education Authority in association with the Department of Adult Education, University of Keele, Keele.

Hitch P J, Clegg P 1980 Modes of referral of overseas immigrant and native-born first admissions to psychiatric hospital. Social Science and Medicine. 14A: 369

Husband C 1982 'Race' in Britain: continuity of a concept. Hutchinson, London

Jagucki W 1983 The Polish experience: 40 years on. In: Baker R (ed) The psychosocial problems of refugees. British Refugee Council. London

Lalljie R 1983 Black elders: a discussion paper. Nottinghamshire County Council Social Services Department. Nottingham

Lambert P, Dolan J 1986 Ethnic elderly of Derby. Derby CRE, Derbyshire Social Services and Derbyshire College of Higher Education, Derby

Littlewood R, Lipsedge M 1982 Aliens and alienists. Penguin, Harmondsworth

Marmot M G, Adelstein A M, Bulusu L 1984 Immigrant mortality in England and Wales, 1970–78. Studies on medical and population subjects No 47. HMSO, London

Office of Population Censuses and Surveys (OPCS) 1983 Census 1981: country of birth, Great Britain. HMSO, London

Office of Population Censuses and Surveys (OPCS) 1987 General household survey 1985. HMSO, London

Pearson M 1985a The politics of ethnic minorities health studies. In: Rathwell T, Phillips D (eds) Health, race and ethnicity. Croom Helm, Beckenham

Pearson M 1985b Equal opportunities in the NHS: a handbook. National Extension College for Training in Health and Race and the Health Education Council, Cambridge

Pearson M 1986 Racist notions of ethnicity and culture in health education. In: Rodmell S, Watt A (eds) The politics of health education. Routledge and Kegan Paul, London

Rack P 1983 Race, culture and mental disorder. Tavistock, London

Standing Conference on Ethnic Minority Senior Citizens (SCEMSC) 1986 Ethnic minority senior citizens: the question of policy. SCEMSC, London

Sevedin A M, Gorosch-Tomlinson D 1984 They said we didn't exist. Social Work Today April 2: 14

Tunstall Pedoe H, Clayton D, Morris J N, Brigden W, McDonald L 1975 Coronary heart attacks in East London. Lancet ii: 833

CHAPTER CONTENTS

The case for preventive care 449

Health visitors and elderly people 450

Health surveillance 451

Health promotion and preventive care 453

Alternative approaches to health visiting 456

Growing old in inner cities · 457

Violence against elderly people 458

Violence outside the home 458
Violence inside the home 459

**The value of health visiting for elderly people —
conclusion** 460

26

Health visiting and elderly people

Alison E. While

Seedhouse (1986) has argued that issues of 'health' cannot be separated from issues of life, and indeed it is generally agreed that health is a matter of universal concern. For elderly people, health is of particular importance because it is in staying reasonably well that they will be able to remain independent. In order to enable elderly people to remain healthy, attention should be given to the prevention of ill health, the detection of deviation from the healthy state and to rehabilitation. It is this positive approach upon which the health visitor's contribution is based.

THE CASE FOR PREVENTIVE CARE

The health of elderly people is one of the major concerns of the National Health Service, since large financial resources must be devoted to their care. Since 1900 the population of England and Wales has grown from about 32.5 million to just over 49 million. This growth in population has been accompanied by the steady improvement in the life expectancy of both males and females, although the rates for females exceed those for males (Alderson 1986). The Census data have also revealed that the distribution of persons of pensionable age across the country is not uniform, with many coastal areas — especially those in the South and South-West, together with an area in mid-Wales — supporting particularly high proportion of older people (20.99% or over of their constituent population) (OPCS 1984). This change in the age structure has necessitated a review in health care provision — especially in the present economic climate, in which issues of efficiency and cost effectiveness are primary considerations.

In 1976, the DHSS (1976a) suggested that early detection of disability among the elderly would be of great benefit not only to elderly people themselves but also in terms of cost-effectiveness. Detection of early signs of ill health is achieved by a variety of methods, including prophylactic visiting and screening clinics. The case for this work is based upon the following evidence: a. elderly people are frequently admitted to hospital (Alderson 1983); b. these admissions are often because of a crisis; c. the events leading up to the crisis usually have a long history (Williamson et al 1964, Hendriksen et al 1984, Vetter et al 1986). The need for health surveillance of older people is particularly acute because not all old people readily report their medical problems, seemingly because they do not know that many symptoms constitute ill health rather than the assumed natural process of ageing (Williams et al 1972, Currie et al 1974, Brocklehurst 1975, Hay 1976, Williams 1979, Barber & Wallis 1982). This failure to acknowledge ill health can lead not only to serious illness being unnoticed in their early stages, but also to failure to treat minor conditions which later have a cumulative effect.

HEALTH VISITORS AND ELDERLY PEOPLE

Health visitors are unique in the field of health care in that they determine their own clientele by selection from the population. Indeed, it seems that health visitors initiate most of their care (HVA 1970, 1980), although they also accept referrals. This means that health visitors are able to offer support on their own initiative, based upon their own assessment of health visiting needs, without waiting for a specific request for help. This professional judgement is of course reflective of professional competence, attitudes and values for which all practitioners are held accountable (RCN 1984). This is not to say that client views may be

overlooked — elderly people have the right to refuse ministrations and indeed a minority find health visitor contact intrusive and suggestive of frailty and dependency (Luker 1981a). Like district nurses, health visitors have no statutory right of entry into people's homes and therefore enter homes as guests. Midwinter (1988) draws to our attention the professional's tendency to arrange services to suit her or his convenience rather than respond to the views of the consumer, which would acknowledge an individual's dignity and autonomy. Good health visiting should of course be consumer sensitive.

However, despite demographic changes it seems that health visitors, as in the past, continue to draw their clientele from families with young children (DH, 1989a) whom they have a statutory responsibility to visit. This apparent concern for the welfare of young children and their families may be a reflection of the early history of the health visiting service (MacQueen 1962). However, the health visitor's ability to determine her clientele according to need and her professional responsibility should enable her to exercise her function in the prevention of ill health, in surveillance and in rehabilitation among the elderly population. Luker (1979) found evidence of much variation in the number of elderly people receiving visits from a health visitor; more recently Phillipson (1985) has noted a decline from 15% in 1979 to 13% in the proportion of elderly people in health visitor caseloads. Luker (1979) asserted that the variation in elderly-centred health visitor practice reflected four factors:

1. Age structure of the population served
2. Health visitor organization, that is, attachment to general practice or geographical location
3. Local health authority policies
4. Personal preference of the health visitor.

Phillipson (1985) has argued that current health visitor practice has many limitations not only in terms of its extent and coverage but also because concern with older people appears to be centred upon deficiencies caused by health and social problems rather than upon positive approaches to growing old. He is particularly critical of basic and continuing health visitor education, which he perceives as failing to address demographic needs and the changing attitudes of older people themselves. In the wake of his criticism of lack of leadership in the health visitor profession, the Health Visitors' Association has facilitated the continued development of a group specifically concerned with health visitor work with the elderly. The Health Visitors' Association together with the British Geriatrics Society have issued a joint policy statement (BGS and HVA 1986), in which they call for health visitor contact with all people over 75 years of age and argue that health visitors should promote the health of elderly people no less than that of other groups. It is noteworthy that health visitor education is also responding to the challenge with changes in curricula and with the publication of professional texts devoted exclusively to health visitor activity with the elderly (McClymont et al 1986).

As long ago as 1955, Anderson and Cowan suggested extending the role of the health visitor to include health promotion and health maintenance among the elderly. Anderson and Cowan identified the health visitor's role in terms of offering support during family crises and potentially improving the elderly person's morale. This is an interesting perspective in view of Hodkinson's (1975) research which suggested that a successful outcome owes more to mental factors such as personal motivation than to the degree or nature of the physical disability. Health visitors can, therefore, make a significant contribution to the rehabilitation of elderly people after episodes of ill health, assisting them in the achievement of their optimum level of independence.

Dingwall (1977) has argued that health visitors have a role to play as the case-finding agency of the welfare state. Health visitors are qualified for this in view of their post-registration training in health and social work skills and their knowledge of the individuals and services in their practice area. They are therefore able to refer clients appropriately or apply for aids on their behalf. This is an important point, since it identifies the health visitor as a facilitator in the community and perhaps also as a 'stop gap' in a large bureaucratic health care system. Indeed, primary health care

provisions in the inner cities undoubtedly require a health worker with a flexible role. Possible role overlap between health visitors and district nurses has been of concern in some quarters, but the demands of the acutely sick or those requiring fundamental physical care must and will always take precedence in the district nurse's caseload. Health visitors have no such conflict, since they make no curative or physical contribution to care, which leaves all their time for case finding, health teaching and surveillance (While 1986).

A decade ago the Royal Commission on the National Health Service (1979) suggested that there was considerable scope for expanding the role and responsibilities of health visitors and district nurses:

We consider that there are increasingly important roles for community nurses, not just in the treatment room, but in health surveillance for vulnerable groups and in screening procedures, health education and prevention programmes, and as a point of first contact, particularly for the young and elderly (p. 79).

This statement reiterated that of the DHSS (1976b), which specifically suggested that health visitors should increase their involvement with elderly people. Indeed, the Cumberledge Report (DHSS 1986a) advocated that health visitors should reduce their work with young children and increase their work with the elderly. More recently, Government initiatives (DH 1989b) have proposed changes in health care provision. The exact nature of future community provision was made at the time of going to press.

HEALTH SURVEILLANCE

A reappraisal of health visiting principles outlined one of the functions of health visiting as:

identifying and fulfilling self-declared and recognised, as well as unacknowledged and unrecognised, health needs of individuals and social groups. (CETHV 1976 p. 8).

Surveillance is therefore an important activity, since it permits the identification of those with unmet health needs. It is now a feature included in all future general practitioner service contracts.

A number of studies have been carried out in which the health visitor was involved in screening for problems among elderly people. Barber and Wallis (1976) describe a system in which the health visitor made assessments of elderly patients (65 years and over) who were already in contact with a general practitioner or health visitor. Apparently no extra staff were required to carry out the comprehensive assessments, but the newly identified problems generated more work for the primary health care team. Interestingly, the health visitors felt that their visits based upon the assessment schedule were more useful than their previous visits had been. Barber and Wallis (1978) discuss the benefits to the elderly of a surveillance programme based upon a comprehensive assessment using their schedule. The schedule requests demographic data about the elderly person, together with details of her acceptance of the interview. The second section includes questions on such topics as mobility, vision and hearing, which are all socially as well as physically important. Another section of the schedule notes the domiciliary services and support currently being provided. The final section includes questions of a specifically medical nature. Barber and Wallis conclude that such a continuing programme of geriatric assessment is valuable. The greatest improvements for clients were found in such areas as clothing, bedding, heating, dentition, diet, vision and hearing, and the least improvement in level of dependency, home hazards and problems with a caring relative.

Do you live on your own?
Are you without a relative you could call on for help?
Are there any days when you are unable to have a hot meal?
Are you confined to your home through ill health?
Is there anything about your health causing you concern or difficulty?
Do you have difficulty with vision?
Do you have difficulty with hearing?
Have you been in hospital during the past year?

Fig. 26.1 Questions in the screening letter of a geriatric assessment programme for the elderly. *Source: Barber, Wallis and McKeating 1980. Reproduced by kind permission of the journal of the Royal College of General Practitioners.*

Subsequently, Barber et al (1980) developed and tested a postal questionnaire (Fig. 26.1) as a screening procedure in a comprehensive geriatric assessment programme for all elderly people over 70 years of age. The authors concluded that the questionnaire was acceptable to elderly people and that it safely identified all those who could benefit from further assessment by a health visitor. This successfully reduced the enormous workload that would be generated in routine assessment visiting of all elderly people.

Where no screening procedures exist, it seems that the subsequent implementation of screening substantially increases the workload for all health workers during the 'intervention' phase. However, after this phase the general practitioner's workload decreases considerably, whereas although the district nurse's and health visitor's workload with elderly people decreases it is still higher than before the 'intervention' (Barber & Wallis 1982). Once a surveillance scheme is established, Barber and Wallis (1982) have estimated, the time required to continue a full screening and assessment programme for those aged 75 years and over is 11–18 hours per week throughout the year. Jones (1976) attempted to extend Tudor Hart's Inverse Care Law to geriatric screening. This states that the quantity of unmet need discovered at geriatric screening reflects the lack of care that elderly people usually receive from their general practitioner. Thus, Barber and Wallis's estimate may need to be considered with caution, and further, Barley (1987) has argued that unless health visitors change their practice to accomodate this time demand, between 3000 and 6000 more health visitors would be required nationally!

Drennan (1986a) adapted the postal questionnaire of Barber and Wallis (1978) for use in an inner London health district and concluded that it was one way of contacting elderly people which was perceived as worthwhile by the people themselves. She, however, admits to the need for the revision of some of her questions to reduce their ambiguity and improve the sensivity of the questionnaire in identifying those at risk. Stanton (1987) has described how successful a shortened version of the Barber and Wallis questionnaire was as a friendly and unintrusive method of screening the well elderly. The shortened questionnaire is included in birthday cards which are sent to those aged 65, 70, 75, 80, 85 and over.

An alternative model has been developed by Williams (1986). He argues that his 'social performance model' is useful for estimating the type of 'social' help needed in planning anticipatory care. The model is based upon three levels of function — social, that is, activities outside the home; domestic, that is, activities inside the home; and, personal, that is, tasks specific to the individual. However, Williams has not described rigorous testing of the model.

Munday's research (1979) revealed that between 9% and 21% of those aged 75 years or over registered at four general practices in Devon were seen by neither a doctor nor a health visitor during the course of a year. This research developed and tested an Elderly At Risk record card (Fig 26.2) to facilitate the care offered to elderly people in the community. The record card is similar to Williams' (1974) schedule and was considered not only a useful assessment tool but also a means of co-ordinating the support available to elderly people.

The shortage of manpower resources is likely to be a constraint upon the development of surveillance and screening programmes. In an attempt to reduce the manpower implications, Barber (1988) has described a system of self-screening of the elderly using a newly developed personal health record which old people are asked to complete at three- or six-month intervals. Barber acknowledges that such a system is only an adjunct to more formal systems of screening and assessment.

An alternative to home visiting and the use of questionnaires is the establishment of clinics. Such a clinic has been successfully established in central London and particularly focuses on 'younger' elderly people, aged between 60 and 75, with the aim of promoting positive attitudes to health by offering information and health education as well as appropriate referral (Phillips 1988). Screening clinics for 'well-adults', that is, people of working age, have also been successfully established elsewhere (Diment 1988, Hutchinson 1988) and these also provide the opportunity for promoting healthy habits as well as identifying health problems which require treatment in order to prepare people for a healthy old age.

A more resource-intensive approach to surveillance is home visiting. Carpenter (1987) has argued that the home assessment of an elderly person is a crucial element of any surveillance process; indeed, he has suggested that a change in the appearance of the house can be as significant as a change in an individual's demeanour. Within this context, it is important to acknowledge the generally inferior household amenities of those over 75 years of age (OPCS 1984); care prescriptions must clearly acknowledge the circumstances under which individuals live. Shultz and Magilvy (1988) have found that different strategies yield different health-needs data — thus, census data provide demographic data; a survey can elicit rates of illness, use of and need for health care; while informal interviews provide insight into lifestyle and more detailed information pertaining to individual experience.

Despite the wealth of literature describing how one might identify the elderly at risk, Bowling's (1985a) survey of the four Thames regional health authorities was disappointing. It appeared that just under one fifth of the district health authorities surveyed had attempted to identify elderly people within their boundaries or to develop 'at risk' registers. Bowling (1985b) rightly argued that without fairly accurate computerized registers of the elderly, there can be little hope of developing and maintaining comprehensive, district-based 'at risk' registers, and that fragmented preventive care is all that is possible through the activities of individual health visitors and district nurses. She advocated the employment of clinical medical officers for the elderly and the establishment of elderly people's health clinics with provision of home assessment for the housebound. Indeed, Bowling suggested that well-organized, well-advertised and well-placed clinics with a positive image (which therefore attract a good attendance) could play an important part in meeting the needs of the 'ageing' population.

HEALTH PROMOTION AND PREVENTIVE CARE

Fundamental to health promotion is the belief that

Front

NAME

ADDRESS

Date of birth

Special disability

Social worker

Telephone

GP

HV

Address 2

Address 3 (or next of kin)

ASSESSMENT/SERVICES: Requestd (R) Provided (✓)

YEAR & AGE	ASSESSMENT DATE	CATE-GORY OF RISK	OTHER RISK FACTORS	G.P.	Health visitor	District nurse	Chiro-pody	Day care	Social worker or O.T	Home help	Meals on wheels	Warden scheme	Resi-dential Home	OTHER	MARITAL STATE (M S W D SEP)	HOUSING

ELDERLY AT RISK REGISTER

Back

Back

CATEGORY OF RISK

Codes for use overleaf

Minimal or no risk (0) (✓)

- Adequate mobility
- Can shop, clean & cook unaided
- No incapacitating illness

Some risk (1) (✓)

- Mobility restricted/Housebound
- Unable to shop
- Mental deterioration (a) Mood / (b) Memory present but coping
- Risk of physical illness

Severe risk (2) (✓)

- Movement restricted to 1 or 2 rooms
- Unable to cook
- Severe mental deterioration (a) self / (b) others with danger to
- Debilitating illness

HOUSING

- A – Lives will spouse
- B – Lives alone
- C – With friends/relatives
- H – Own home
- J – Rented accomodation
- K – Sheltered accomodation
- L – Lodgings

OTHER RISK FACTORS

- X – Social isolation
- Y – Financial need
- Z – Family under strain
- ZZ – Family cannot cope
- V – Inadequate housing
- W – Inadequate heating

DATE	NOTES

Fig. 26.2 'Elderly At Risk' record card — modified version. *Source: Munday 1979. Reproduced by permission of the King's Fund Centre.*

people should be able to increase their control over their health and well-being. This control requires full and continuing access to information about all aspects of health. The prominence of health promotion in current literature lies in the belief that it has the potential to change the worrying trend in which the United Kingdom is falling behind other countries in the life expectancy league table (London School of Hygiene and Tropical Medicine et al 1988). Health visiting is the only profession wholly dedicated to health promotion and preventive care.

Preventive care may be considered to fall into three distinct levels derived from the work of Caplan (1964) in the field of mental health. Primary prevention involves education, information-giving, persuasion and continual comparison against the norm which, with appropriate prophylaxis, can prevent the development of the disease process or the delay of a disease process. Examples of work in this field include health education and advice regarding healthy eating (Gray 1987, Holmes 1987) and accident prevention (Cave 1988, Livesley 1988) and the involvement of health visitors in pre-retirement education (McClymont et al 1986). Encouraging acceptance of the influenza vaccine by vulnerable older people is also an important contribution at the primary prevention level (Shukla 1981).

Secondary prevention is the detection, through screening and other means, of health problems in their early stages. The involvement of health visitors in this work has already been described, in the section entitled Health Surveillance. Tertiary prevention is undertaken when illness or disability have already occurred and prevention is concerned with the maximization of health potential and the avoidance of complications and relapse. Examples of health visitor work in this field are the education of elderly people regarding medication and encouraging compliance (Denham 1988) and the provision of aids and adaptations at home. A recent survey (George et al 1988) of 140 people aged over 75 revealed that many disabled people required aids for the bath and toilet; up to half the aids already provided were not in use and many (47%) of the walking aids were faulty. The needs of carers are also of fundamental importance to the well-being of the older disabled dependent person, for if the pressures on carers are ignored, the family situation may deteriorate and result in abuse of the old person. The health visitor clearly has a role in supporting carers and while Crossroads Care Attendant Schemes have pioneered a successful service in this field, they do not exist in every area and are usually overstretched and plagued by the vagaries of voluntary sector funding (Brotchie 1988). Arber et al (1988) found in their research that carers who are married women under 65 obtained least domestic (home help, meals-on-wheels) and personal health (district nurse, chiropodist) support when compared with other carers of similarly disabled elderly. They also found that old people living alone and elderly men received somewhat more domestic and personal health services than elderly women. The unremitting nature of caring for elderly dependents was also borne out by Jones and Vetter (1985).

Two schemes outside the Crossroads Care Attendant Schemes which support carers are the Share the Care Scheme in Lincoln (Morley 1988) and a neighbourhood care scheme set up by a health visitor in the Chilterns (Enticknap 1987). This latter scheme, like the caring-sharing scheme established in the Isle of Wight (MacHardy 1988) also provides physical support such as gardening or handiwork and emotional support through befriending.

ALTERNATIVE APPROACHES TO HEALTH VISITING

Drennan's (1986b) survey revealed that health visitors are no longer constrained to work with their clients only through home visiting and clinic attendance. The survey revealed that health visitors were involved in community-orientated iniatives in 83 of the 130 district health authorities which completed questionnaires. The health visitors were involved in a wide variety of projects, which included community aid for the elderly and active elderly groups as well as involvement in running groups within the clinic setting, such as groups for elderly people. Drennan (1988) has described her contribution to one such group and how this culminated in a health festival and the subsequent production of a health handbook for pensioners. An alternative approach to group work through an Age Well Forum is described by Enderby (1989). While Kewley's (1984) health visitor work involved campaigning for a community centre to serve an estate; from this effort, an autonomous self-help group for the elderly residents developed.

Health visitor skills have been used in several experimental schemes to give special attention to the needs of elderly people. A health visitor was seconded to a social services department under a joint finance scheme and given responsibility for preventive care, health education and liaison (between health and social services staff). She also had a particular responsibility to foster the welfare of elderly and handicapped people in that district (Day & Magridge 1981). This scheme is currently under evaluation but it demonstrates that the training and skills of health visitors can be utilized in the community and not just within the primary health care team. Indeed, health visitors may have a role in community action to improve the care of local elderly residents.

In a pilot scheme in Manchester funded by inner city money, a geriatric team is led by a health visitor who acts as the liaison between hospitals, community health services and social services (Halladay 1981). Geriatric liaison health visitors increasingly are being appointed throughout the country in an attempt to ensure continuity of care of patients on discharge from hospital. Thursfield (1979) reports on such a scheme, which aims to give support to elderly patients and to assess their progress while also avoiding the duplication of visits by different care workers. Griffiths and Eastwood (1974) describe the work of a psychogeriatric liaison health visitor and, increasingly, other health visitor liaison schemes are being documented. For instance, Gordon (1983) has described geriatric liaison health visitor work in Barnet and claimed that it resulted in an efficient use of available resources, a point developed by Marshall and Levett-Williams (1987), who stated that a new method of liaison work was evaluated and found to be an effective use of time and that as a consequence a full-time liaison post

was established. Indeed, lack of an efficient hospital–health visitor referral system in the absence of a liaison post prevented good follow-up of discharged elderly patients in one study (Victor & Vetter 1985).

GROWING OLD IN INNER CITIES

Enough is known about the decay, poverty and socially unstable nature of our inner cities for the conclusion to be reached that such environments can exert strong negative influences upon many of the people who live there. Elderly people are a vulnerable group who feel particularly threatened by their apparent demise in our youth-oriented society.

Housing is often substandard and some areas are poorly maintained or polluted and are clearly a hazard to health. The deprived inner city frequently lacks the kind of social institutions in which elderly people can participate and, in view of the indisputable evidence of higher crime rates (Smith 1981), many perceive the environment as physically threatening. The environment is further disadvantaged by its often poor aesthetic appearance — uncollected litter, pavements covered with broken glass, graffiti-covered walls and deserted buildings. Despite this catalogue of negative features, residents in inner city areas frequently display tolerance. Lawton (1980) points out that it is possible to ignore disturbing or irritating elements of the environment. Indeed, one must be wary of imposing outsiders' judgements of what it is like to live in inner city neighbourhoods upon individuals who have spent much of their life in them. Sometimes it is possible to overstate the degree of change to which the physical appearance of inner city areas has been subjected. For example, rebuilding does not necessarily mean a new layout of the facilities because in many instances the shops are rebuilt on their original sites. Thus the basic geography of the shops and other facilities continue to be familiar, although inner urban development has tended to be associated with the demise of the cheap corner shop and its replacement by chain stores and superstores which are aimed at a higher income consumer and frequently located for the shopper who has a car (While 1989).

Recent years have seen changes in the area of transport provision. The 1985 Transport Act introduced competitive tender to bus provision. While the Government believes this will improve services at the same time as reducing costs and subsidies, others have argued that it will increase the cost of local transport. The particular problem of rural transport appears to have been largely ignored and the assumption that elderly people have their own means of transport is not borne out by the statistics; further, local village shops are an increasing rarity, so forcing the elderly people to be dependent upon the charity of their neighbours in meeting their shopping needs. Indeed, elderly folk may well become captive in their village and may experience a different kind of social isolation as they are deprived of contact with the world outside their small community.

There is also increasing evidence that different groups have different experiences in the inner cities. The ageing experience of ethnic minorities is addressed elsewhere in this text (Ch. 25). Norman (1987) has argued that the particular needs of elderly Irish people are rarely met. She points out how their working lives do not provide the opportunities for the acquisition of stable homes or the learning of domestic or budgeting skills, or, in many instances, for the accumulation of money or possessions and a complete National Insurance record upon which a pension may be based. It is estimated that elderly Irish people represent about a quarter of inner city hostel residents, providing a lifestyle well known for its poverty, social isolation and instability. It is no wonder that this same group has double the national rate of suicide and mental health admissions to hospital.

While generally accepting that the inner city environment may be less healthy than others, inner city life has some advantages. Lawton (1980) cites American data to show that elderly people living in inner city areas are significantly more mobile and less hampered by chronic illness than those living in rural areas. There is also the positive advantage of the relative ease of access to health service facilities in densely populated areas. In general, however, the disadvantages for inner city elderly people are greater than those experienced by their suburban counterparts, affecting health and other aspects of daily life.

VIOLENCE AGAINST ELDERLY PEOPLE

VIOLENCE OUTSIDE THE HOME

Prominent press coverage of violence against elderly people may lead one to suppose that they are under continuous threat from the mugger and vandal. However, there seems to be a discrepancy between fears of such crimes and the actual risk of them (Mawby 1983). The 1975 Sheffield victim survey (Bottoms et al 1981) found that old people were statistically less likely to have been victims of crimes than younger respondents, and this finding was supported in a London victim survey (Sparks et al 1977). Thus, contrary to popular opinion old people are relatively safe from crime.

The research indicates, however, that elderly men are more at risk than elderly women, and those living in 'problem' areas are not more at risk than those living in any working-class area. It seems also that those previously employed in unskilled work are less likely to be victims. The research indicates that household size is unimportant, while those with few local friends are at more risk. Although criminal assault is a very traumatic experience and should attract intensive care for the old person wherever it occurs, the research findings do not support the impression that elderly people are a particularly vulnerable group in comparison to others. For example, burglary rates are lower for elderly people than for the population as a whole (OPCS 1982) and elderly people are least likely to be victims of violent crime (Home Office 1983).

Mawby (1983) suggests that violence against elderly people is relatively low because they venture out of doors less frequently than younger people and so expose themselves less to the possibility of attack. Indeed, where crime is rationally planned it would seem that elderly people offer little reward since old age is associated with poverty (Townsend 1979). The fact remains that much crime is unplanned. Mawby (1983) points out that certain locations are especially vulnerable to crime such as city centres, near empty streets, and the vicinity of public houses. These are places not often frequented by elderly people since they are more likely to be at home. It is also worth noting that crimes against property are more likely if the property is empty, so that those remaining at home are doubly protected. Unfortunately, if policies are pursued which encourage more participation by elderly people in activities outside the home, the risk of crime against them may be expected to rise. The Sparks et al (1977) survey demonstrates clear relationships between age, crime and activities. They found that more activity outside the home increased the risk of being a victim of crime.

Health visitors can assist in the prevention of crime against elderly people. They can influence the various vulnerability factors by mounting crime prevention campaigns, encouraging neighbour support and minimizing the isolation of elderly people. They may affect the 'visible target attractiveness' by encouraging old people to refrain from displaying obvious signs of possessions which may attract offenders. They can inform old people of dangerous locations, and can sponsor the rehousing of those who feel trapped or endangered by their environment, especially those who have been victimized. They can also contribute to the care of victims and perhaps help in setting up schemes similar to Victims-Aid, to which the police are asked to refer elderly victims of crime so that they may be counselled or referred to others. Victims of Violence is an example of one such scheme (Melville 1987).

VIOLENCE INSIDE THE HOME

It is difficult enough to find valid statistics of violence against the elderly outside the home. It is even more difficult to assess the extent to which 'granny-battering' inside the home occurs. As with crime against elderly people outside the home, abuse in the domestic setting is a popular subject for the press. However, as Cloke (1983) points out there is no unanimous view among researchers as

to what constitutes 'old age abuse'. A working definition has been provided by Cloke: 'the systematic and continuous abuse of an elderly person *by the carer*, often, although not always, a relative, on whom the elderly person is dependent for care' (para 2.2, emphasis added).

Eastman argues that abuse includes physical assault, threats of physical assault, neglect, exploitation and abandonment, sexual abuse and psychological abuse (Eastman & Sutton 1982, Eastman 1982, 1988). Eastman contends that this is not an exhaustive list but a useful framework within which to view granny-battering, and that abuse by people other than caring relatives constitutes something quite different.

Eastman and Sutton (1982) estimate that 500 000 elderly people in the United Kingdom are at risk from old age abuse. This is based upon their report that 42% of those over 65 years of age in the United Kingdom are supported by care-giving relatives. They use American research which suggests that 10% of such people are at risk from abuse. However, the application of American research findings to a different society is dubious. America does not have a comprehensive welfare system for the elderly, which forces most elderly people to be wholly dependent upon their younger relatives. The suggestion that 42% of those over 65 years in the UK are supported by care-giving relatives is not confirmed by the Office of Population, Censuses and Surveys study (1978), which found only 12% of elderly people living with their children. In summary, although it has been established that old age abuse occurs in the United Kingdom there is insufficient research evidence to establish its prevalence.

Similarly, knowledge about the predisposing factors of old age abuse is scanty. The only data for analysis have been gleaned from a limited number of reported incidents and adequately detailed case history information is seldom available. A number of factors individually or jointly may contribute to old age abuse: lack of support to carers; low income; poor and overcrowded housing; poor family relationships and poor communication within the family; the carer's responsibility for another person such as a spouse or child; a history of psychological problems in the carer; an alcoholic carer; changes in the carer's lifestyle; and a lack of understanding by the carer of the ageing process and the capabilities of elderly people (Cloke 1983). The lack of research findings in this field means that health visitors must be mindful of the possibility of abuse in all settings and should be particularly supportive to caring relatives. Warr (1980) gives a moving account of her personal experience as a carer of an elderly relative, clearly outlining some of the problems involved; and case studies recounted by Seabrook (1988) further question society's commitment to supporting elderly people and their relatives.

Despite the lack of good research to reveal reliable predisposing factors behind abuse, the abused person invariably has the following profile: over 75; female; functionally disabled and dependent for fulfilment for at least some basic survival needs; lonely and tearful; living at home either with or near adult children; and roleless within the family (Eastman 1988). Health and social services differ in their procedures upon the discovery of abuse, but professionals clearly have a responsibility to maintain the safety of an elderly person in the domestic setting; increasingly, case conferences are being used to identify which agencies should be involved and what they can do to meet the needs of the elderly person and her carer.

THE VALUE OF HEALTH VISITING FOR ELDERLY PEOPLE — CONCLUSION

Clearly, health visitors have a role to play in the care of elderly people. In the future they should perhaps become the principal case-finding agency at work in the community, exercising their training and skills to the full so that every elderly person may be aware of their entitlements to welfare benefits as well as knowing the facilities and services to which they could have access in their locality. The use of age-sex registers in general practices is one means of locating elderly people, which is an extremely difficult task if no such register exists. Alternatively, active case searching by health visitors may prove more rewarding, making use of

registers concerning those in receipt of meals-on-wheels or the home help service, or attendance registers at luncheon clubs or self-help groups.

Health visitors have a major role to play in the maintenance of well-being among elderly people. Uninvited visits allow the health visitor to carry out regular surveillance, anticipating future needs while advising old people about diet, hypothermia, financial entitlements and so on. Health visitors can make an enormous contribution to health teaching among elderly people.

The counselling skills of health visitors are particularly important with regard to the care of the bereaved. Elderly people are more likely than any other age group to lose the companionship of someone close to them, and the loss of a partner or friend may cause grief, shock, anger and bitterness. By 1991 over 3 million elderly people are expected to be living on their own (CSO 1979). The importance of understanding mourning and the need for skilled professional help is underlined by Parkes (1975) and Pincus (1976). Williams (1974) suggests that there is a need for this work to be accorded higher priority and that perhaps health visitors should allocate more of their time to it.

The application of an analytical approach to health visiting may become a helpful innovation in the care of the elderly and overcome Luker's (1983) criticism that health visitors do not focus their interactions with elderly clients. Rogers (1982) describes the successful introduction of the 'health visiting process' and the development of a new record card in a health district in southern England. The use of such an approach offers a systematic method of record keeping in which client needs and problems and health visiting plans can easily be identified. It also enables health visitors to audit the effectiveness of their care and intervention. This is important because the needs and problems of an elderly person constantly change, and so the health visitor must continually assess whether her or his actions are effective. If they are not, she (or he) must make alternative plans, and these in turn should be evaluated. As Hedley et al (1982) point out, given the limited working time available in which the health visitor must address unlimited health needs there is much to be gained from using an improved method of record keeping. They suggest that the use of the health visiting process records has promoted logical thought which enables the visitor to formulate the needs of their clients. They also suggest that it has helped the visitor's assessment of priorities and their planning on a daily and weekly basis. Furthermore, they argue that the use of the health visiting process has improved their practice with the formulation of short- and long-term plans for clients, so helping to focus the health visitor intervention and to evaluate the effectiveness of the advice or subsequent action.

The health visitor is an ideal link between the individual in need and available help. The adoption of focused health visitor intervention should offer much for the future welfare of elderly people. The use of one of the described assessment tools together with the health visitor process may provide a helpful starting point for improved health visitor care of the elderly. Robertson (1988) describes the use of different assessment tools, giving examples of health visitor work with the elderly.

Two studies have attempted to evaluate the effect of health visitor intervention upon the well-being of elderly people. Luker (1981b) used two groups of elderly women in a 'cross-over' study (that is, both groups alternately acted as the 'experimental' and 'control' groups). She found that their health problems improved with 'intervention' although there was no clear improvement in 'life satisfaction'. Ninety-five per cent of her sample (n = 100) reported that they had enjoyed the health visitor visits. Luker attributes this to the benefits accruing from 'therapeutic anticipation' before the next expected visit; the well-being generated by the fact of another person taking an interest in one's welfare is described by Luker as the 'worthy of interest syndrome'. Sixty-two per cent of the sample reported that they had been helped by the visits if only through the social contact, while others felt that they had been helped directly with health-related matters such as the maintenance of a reducing diet or identifying possible household hazards. The overseeing or surveillance function of the health visitor was also acknowledged with 92% of the sample agreeing

that it was a good idea for health visitors to visit elderly people. Luker's study also demonstrated the long-term effect of health visitor intervention with the benefits of 'intervention' continuing to accrue at the follow-up visit after six months.

Vetter et al (1986) examined the practice of two health visitors making an annual unsolicited visit and related follow-up visits to the over-70 age groups. Interestingly, the two study health visitors adopted quite different approaches to the elderly. The one who used a more generally orientated approach as compared to the other's medically orientated approach was more effective and was found to reduce mortality, although such an approach did not affect disability. Of particular note was the marked increase in the provision of services to the elderly people visited by the 'generally orientated' health visitor and this was associated with some improvement in the general quality of life of the clients. Indeed, Vetter et al have claimed that a good health visitor is better at obtaining a complete understanding of an elderly person's home circumstances than are general practitioners (family doctors). They argue, therefore, that health visitors have a role complementary to that of general practitioners.

Taylor and Ford (1983) suggest a hierarchy of 'at risk' elderly people which provides health visitors with a potential priority scale from which to organize their work. They suggest, contrary to popular opinion, that the isolated, childless and never married are the least disadvantaged, whereas the recently widowed, those living alone, the poor and those from social class V (Registrar General's classification) form an intermediate group. The most 'at risk' elderly are those who have recently moved, those recently discharged from hospital, the divorced or separated and the very old.

A common theme of recent government publications (DHSS 1986b, 1987) is the promotion of health and the prevention of illness. In the light of this, the functions of the health visitors as outlined by the Council for the Education and Training of Health Visitors (CETHV 1976) are as applicable to elderly people as to any other age group:

1. Prevention of mental, physical and emotional

ill health or alleviation of its consequences

2. Early detection of ill health and the surveillance of high risk groups
3. Recognition and identification of need, and mobilization of resources where necessary
4. Provision of care; this will include support during periods of stress, and advice and guidance in case of illness.

Health visitors should use their skills to assist in the care of elderly people so that the wish of most to remain in their own homes may be a reality. This should enable old people to enjoy the maximum quality of life.

REFERENCES

Alderson M R 1983 An introduction to epidemiology, 2nd edn. London, Macmillan

Alderson M 1986 An aging population — some demographic and health trends. Public Health 100: 263–277

Anderson W F, Cowan N 1955 A consultative health centre for old people. Lancet 1: 239–240

Arber S, Gilbert G N, Evandrou M 1988 Gender, household composition and receipt of domiciliary services by elderly disabled people. Journal of Social Policy 17(2): 153–175

Barber H 1988 Self screening by the elderly using a new personal health record. Health Visitor 61(3): 73–74

Barber J H & Wallis J B 1976 Assessment of the elderly in general practice. Journal of Royal College of General Practitioners 26: 106–114

Barber J H, Wallis J B 1978 The benefits to an elderly population of continuing geriatric assessment. Journal of Royal College of General Practitioners. 28: 428–433.

Barber J H, Wallis J B 1982 The effect of a system of geriatric screening and assessment on general practice workload. Health Bulletin 40(3): 125–132

Barber J H, Wallis J B, McKeating I 1980 A postal screening questionnaire in preventive geriatric care. Journal of Royal College of General Practitioners 30: 39–51.

Barley S 1987 An uncompromising report on health visiting for the elderly. British Medical Journal. 294: 595–596

Bottoms A E, Mawby R I, Xanthos P D 1981 Sheffield study on urban social structure and crime, Part 3. Unpublished Report to the Home Office.

Bowling A 1985a Tracking down the elderly risk. Health and Social Service Journal Feb 28: 254–255

Bowling A 1985b 'At Risk' registers for the elderly. Health Visitor 58(12): 354–356

British Geriatrics Society, Health Visitors' Association 1986 Health visiting for the health of the aged. BGS & HVA, London

Brocklehurst J C 1975 Geriatric care in advanced societies. Blackburn Times Press, Blackburn

Brotchie J 1988 Caring is not a commodity. Social Work Today 1 Dec 14–15

Caplan G 1964 An approach to community mental health. Tavistock, London

Carpenter I 1987 The home assessment. General Practitioner Oct 30: 34

Cartwright A, Hockey L, Anderson J 1973 Life before death. Routledge & Kegan Paul, London

Cave J 1988 Growing old dangerously. Nursing Times, Community Outlook Oct: 18–19

Central Statistical Office 1979 Social trends 9, HMSO, London

Cloke C 1983 Old age abuse in the domestic setting. Age Concern, London

Council for Education and Training of Health Visitors 1976 An investigation into the principles of health visiting. London, CETHV

Currie G, MacNeill R M, Walker J G, Bernie E & Mindie E W 1974 Medical and social screening of patients aged 70 to 72 by an urban general practice health team. British Medical Journal 2: 108–111

Day L, Magridge J 1981 Health visitor who stayed. Health and Social Services Journal 91: 1114–1115

Denham M 1988 Medication and the elderly. Health Visitor 61(4): 112–113

Department of Health and Social Security 1976a Prevention and health: everybody's business. HMSO, London

Department of Health and Social Security 1976b Priorities for health and social services in England. HMSO, London

Department of Health and Social Security 1986a Neighbourhood nursing — a focus for care. Report of the Community Nursing Review. Chairman: Mrs J Cumberlege. HMSO, London

Department of Health and Social Security 1986b Primary health care: an agenda for discussion. Cmnd 9771, HMSO, London

Department of Health and Social Security 1987 Promoting better health. Cmnd 249, HMSO, London

Department of Health 1989 Statistics and research form LHS 27/3 DH, London

Department of Health 1989b Working for patients : caring for the 1990s. HMSO, London

Diment Y 1988 Evaluation of a health screening clinic for those in their mid-fifties. Unpublished MSc Thesis, Department of Nursing Studies, King's College, London

Dingwall R 1977 What future for health visiting? Nursing Times 73: 77–79

Drennan V 1986a A feasibility study into the screening of elderly people in an inner city area. In: While A (ed) Research in preventive community nursing care. Chichester, John Wiley

Drennan V 1986b Developments in health visiting. Health Visitor 59(4): 108–110

Drennan V 1988 Celebrating age. Nursing Times. Community Outlook June: 4–6

Eastman M 1982 Granny battering: a hidden problem. Community Care May 27: 12-13

Eastman M, Sutton M 1982 Granny battering. Geriatric Medicine 12(11): 11–15

Eastman M 1988 Granny abuse. Nursing Times Community Outlook Oct 15–16

Enderby V 1989 Ageing well in Thetford. Health Visitor 62(2): 61

Enticknap B 1987 Village volunteers. Nursing Times. Community Outlook Sept 19–22

George J, Binns V E, Clayden A D, Mulley G P 1988. Aids

and adaptations for the elderly at home: underprovided, underused, and undermaintained. British Medical Journal 296: 1365–1366

Gordon H 1983 Liaison: the vital link. Nursing Mirror, Community Forum 3 Aug i–iv

Gray J 1987 Nutrition in the elderly. Midwife, Health Visitor and Community Nurse 23(11): 488–489, 492, 496

Griffiths A, Eastwood H 1974 Psychogeriatric liaison health visitor. Nursing Times 70: 152–153

Halladay H 1981 A geriatric team within the health visiting visiting service. Nursing Times 77(38): 1039–1040

Hay E H 1976 A geriatric survey in general practice. Practitioner 206: 443–447

Health Visitors' Association 1970 Health visiting manifesto. London, HVA

Health Visitors' Association 1980 Health visiting in the 80s. London, HVA

Hedley C, Grieve L, Hood J, Leyshon Y 1982 Health visiting and the nursing process III. Health Visitor 55: 211–215

Hendricksen G, Lund E, Stramgard E 1984 Consequences of assessment and intervention among elderly people: a three year randomised controlled trial. British Medical Journal 289: 1522–1524

Hodkinson H M 1975 An outline of geriatrics. Academic Press, London

Holmes S 1987 An acquired taste. Nursing Times. Community Outlook Dec: 16–17, 19

Home Office 1983 The British crime survey. HMSO, London

Hutchinson B 1988 Establishment of a screening clinic for well-adults. Midwife, Health Visitor and Community Nurse 24(9): 368, 370, 374

Jones D A and Vetter N J 1985 Formal and informal support received by carers of elderly dependents. British Medical Journal 291: 643–645

Jones R V H 1976 Recognition of geriatric problems in general practice. Update 13: 643

Kewley J 1984 Self-help for the elderly. Community View April: 9

Lawton M P 1980 Environment and ageing. Brooks/Cole, New York

Livesley B 1988 Safety in the home in old age. Health Visitor 61(9): 284–286

London School of Hygiene and Tropical Medicine, Institute of Gerontology King's College London and King's Fund Institute 1988 Promoting health among elderly people. King Edward's Hospital Fund, London

Luker K A 1981a Elderly women's opinions about the benefits of health visitor visits. Occasional Paper Nursing Times 77(9): 33–35

Luker K 1981b Health visiting and the elderly. Occasional Paper Nursing Times 77(51): 137–140

Luker K A 1983 An evaluation of health visitors' visits to elderly women. In: Wilson-Barnett J (ed) Nursing research — ten studies in patient care. John Wiley, Chichester

McClymont M, Thomas S, Denham M J 1986 Health visiting and the elderly. Churchill Livingstone, Edinburgh.

MacHardy L 1988 Your caring sharing friends and helpers. Community Care. Jan 7: 24–25

MacQueen I 1962 From carbolic powder to social counsel. Nursing Times 58: 886–888

Marshall B, Levett-Williams S A 1987 Liaison between the community and an acute hospital for the elderly. Health Visitor 60(10): 328–329

Mawby R I 1983 Crime and the elderly: experience and perceptions. In: Jerome D (ed) Ageing in Modern Society. Croom Helm, London

Melville J 1987 Helping victims survive. New Society Nov 6: 18–19

Midwinter E 1988 Our masters' voice. Community Care March 10: 30-31

Morley S 1988 How can we help you? Nursing Times Community Outlook October: 32, 34, 37

Munday M 1979 Care of the elderly in Devon. King's Fund Centre, London

Norman A 1987 Down and out in Britain. Community Care 12 Nov: 20–21

Office of Population Censuses and Surveys 1978 The elderly at home. Audrey Hunt. HMSO, London

Office of Population Censuses and Surveys 1982 Nurses working in the community. Dunnell K, Dobbs J. HMSO, London

Office of Population Censuses and Surveys 1984 Dicenial report of censuses for England and Wales 1951–1981. London, HMSO

Parkes C M 1975 Bereavement: studies of grief in adult life. Pelican, London

Phillips S 1988 Growing old gracefully. Nursing Times Community Outlook June: 15–18

Phillipson C 1985 Health visiting and older people: a review of current trends. Health Visitor 58(12): 357–358

Pincus L 1976 Death and the family. Faber and Faber, London

Robertson C 1988 Health visiting in practice. Churchill Livingstone, Edinburgh

Rogers J M 1982 Health visiting and the nursing process I. Health Visitor 55: 204–208

Royal Commission on the National Health Service 1979 Report Cmnd 7615 Chairman: Sir A Merrison HMSO, London

Royal College of Nursing 1984 Further thinking about health visiting. London, RCN

Schultz P R, Magilvy J K 1988 Assessing community health needs of elderly populations: comparison of three strategies. Journal of Advanced Nursing 13(2): 193–202

Seabrook J 1988 Old in a cold season. New Society Jan 8: 8–9

Seedhouse D 1986 A universal concern. Nursing Times Jan 22: 36–38

Shukla R B 1981 The role of the primary care team in the care of the elderly. The Practitioner 225: 791–797

Smith S J 1981 Negative interaction: crime in the inner city. In: Jackson P, Smith S J (eds) Social interaction and ethnic segregation. Academic Press, New York

Sparks R, Genn H, Dodd D 1977 Survey victims. Wiley, Chichester

Stanton A 1987 Happy birthday. Nursing Times Community Outlook March 20, 21, 24

Taylor R C, Ford E G 1983 The elderly at risk: a critical examination of commonly identified risk groups. Journal of Royal College of General Practitioners 33: 699–705

Thursfield P J 1979 The hospital that doesn't say goodbye. Nursing Mirror. 150(6): 50–52

Townsend P 1979 Poverty in the United Kingdom. Penguin, Harmondsworth

Victor C R, Vetter N J 1985 The use of the health

visiting service by the elderly after discharge from hospital. Health Visitor 58(4) :95–96

Vetter N, Jones D, Victor C R 1986 Health visiting with the elderly in general practice. In: While A (ed) Research in preventive community nursing care. Chichester, John Wiley

Warr J 1980 Caring for an elderly relative: a personal experience. Health Visitor 53: 525–529

While A E 1986 The value of health visitors. Health Visitor 59(6): 171–173

While A E 1989 Health in the inner city. London, Heinemann Medical

Williams E I, Bennett F M, Nixon J V, Nicholson M R, Garbert J 1972 Sociomedical study of patients over 75 in general practice. British Medical Journal 2: 445–448

Williams E I 1986 A model to describe social performance levels in elderly people. Journal of Royal College of General Practitioners 36: 422–423

Williams I 1979 The care of the elderly in the community. Croom Helm, London

Williams J C 1974 Death and bereavement. Age Concern, London

Williamson J, Stokoeo I H, Gray S et al 1964 Old people at home: their unreported needs. Lancet 1: 1117–1120

CHAPTER CONTENTS

Primary health care 465
Attachment 466
The primary health care team
Neighbourhood nursing 466

The role of the district nurse 467
Functions of the district nurse 467
Drugs and old people in the community 471
Community nursing aids and equipment 472
The day hospital 473
The community hospital 473
Aftercare for the elderly 473
Ethnic minority elders 474
Elderly mentally frail people 474

Personal social services 475
Services in the home 475
Social day care 476

Housing 477

Social security benefits 477

The role of the voluntary sector 478
Voluntary organizations 478
Neighbourhood care groups 478
Mutual aid groups 479
Informal carers 479

Current policy on community care — the implications 480

Current developments in district nursing practice for elderly people 480
Hospital-at-home scheme 481
Out-of-hours nursing care 481
Innovations in care 481

27

Nursing old people in the community

Fiona M. Ross

Nursing old people at home is complex, challenging and rewarding. The patient is seen as part of a family, in her own home with memories, rights and dignity; community nursing functions in this context. Nursing care is patient-oriented and family-centred and aims to support old people in living independently.

PRIMARY HEALTH CARE

Primary care in the United Kingdom is the first level of health care provided outside institutions. It is characterized by patient-initiated consultations for health or social problems or by a case-finding approach. The patient's encounter with a health professional triggers a sequence of events that results in the patient becoming part of the health care system.

The members of the primary health care team with key roles in the care of old people are the general practitioner, district nurse, nursing auxiliary, and the health visitor with support from specialists such as stoma nurses and continence advisors. The focus of this chapter is on the district nurse.

Old people make frequent use of the general practitioner's services. On average a general practitioner has five consultations per annum with each patient aged 65–74, as opposed to 3.8 for patients aged 5–64. For patients aged 75 and over the number rises to 6.3, which is reflected in higher prescribing rates (DHSS 1987).

Although district nurses spend the majority of their time with old people (DHSS 1982), the evidence suggests that the district nursing service only reaches a small proportion of the elderly population. Figures vary from 8% in a national survey (Hunt 1978), rising with age to 20% of those aged 85 and over (Bond & Carstairs 1982). Within this there are inequalities in the provision of care in terms of gender and ethnicity (Cameron et al 1989), and region (Bowling 1987).

The district nurse has an important actual and potential contribution to make to the care of old people, including the well elderly. As well as analysing need and providing care and support for old people in their own homes, residential care and sheltered accommodation, she is, ideally, involved in health promotion, the mobilization of professional and voluntary resources, and the support of carers. These key issues are addressed in this chapter.

There is no one standard model of district nurse organization in primary health care. Many and various interpretations of attachment, primary health care team, and neighbourhood nursing exist.

ATTACHMENT

A district nurse may be 'attached' to one or a group of general practitioners. She is responsible for the nursing care needs of all patients registered with these general practitioners. Doctors and nurses are formally based in the same location, health centre or general practice surgery. In reality there are several interpretations of this system. Some attached nurses pay only fleeting daily visits to the practice, others may genuinely use it as a working base. This is not always related to the availability of premises. Although attachment provides a structure for improved communication it does not necessarily imply effective teamwork; success probably depends on attitudes and facilities available for the key workers.

THE PRIMARY HEALTH CARE TEAM

The primary care team has been defined as:

an interdependent group of general medical practitioners, secretaries, receptionists, health

visitors, district nurses and midwives who share a common purpose and responsibility, each member clearly understanding his or her own function and those of other members, so that they can all pool skills and knowledge to provide an effective primary care service (Standing Medical Advisory Committee 1981, p. 2).

Fundamental to the concept of teamwork is the division of labour, co-ordination, and task sharing, each member making a different contribution, but one of equal value towards the common goal of patient care. During the late seventies and early eighties mainstream policy advocated multidisciplinary approaches as essential for the care of elderly people because of their complex psychological and physical health care needs (DHSS 1978, 1981). However, the gap between the rhetoric and reality reveals that teamwork is not only a problematic, inadequately defined concept but that there are difficulties experienced by professionals in practice (Bond et al 1985).

NEIGHBOURHOOD NURSING

The Cumberlege review (DHSS 1986) recommended that community nursing services be organized for a population of between 10 000 and 25 000. The rationale for the proposals was to develop a locally based, decentralized service to facilitate the definition of consumer need within the social and political context of the community. The emphasis was upon broadening the scope of the service from the individual to the community and upon exploiting the expertise of community nurses in collaborative and collective strategies. Cumberlege was at pains to point out that there was room for many local interpretations of an appropriate model, and that on no account should neighbourhood nursing replace existing good primary care teams.

Health centres

Primary care teams may work either in health centres or in a general practice setting with office space, clerical support, and facilities for professional activities. Health centres are units where family doctor services, child health and health education services are carried out. Accessible to the community, they provide a non-institutional setting for the integration of specialist skills. The special needs of old people may be catered for by chiropody, audiology, dentistry, optical, medical and nursing services. In addition, the health centre may serve as a setting for welfare advice or an outlet for publicity such as the Age Concern prevention of hypothermia campaign.

Health centres have several advantages. First, they provide a base for different professionals which facilitates interdisciplinary communication and the exchange of information. Secondly, they enable experiments such as a shared, centralized patient record system to be accessible to all members of the team. This kind of innovation clearly has important implications for the delivery of informed care to the elderly. Finally, health centres may be the focus of primary care developments such as computerization of records, or multidisciplinary screening of the elderly using an age–sex register.

THE ROLE OF THE DISTRICT NURSE

The district nursing sister is employed by the Health Authority to give skilled nursing care to all persons living in the community at home, in health centres and in residential accommodation. She (or he) is the leader of a nursing team which includes registered nurses, enrolled nurses and nursing auxiliaries to whom she delegates work as appropriate. She is professionally accountable for assessing and reassessing the needs of the patient and the family and for monitoring the quality of care. To this list of professional responsibilities, Mackenzie (1989) has added: leadership, referral to other agencies, recognition of the importance of research and analysis of caseload.

FUNCTIONS OF THE DISTRICT NURSE

1. Identification of physical, emotional and social needs of patients in their own homes, as well as the wider needs of the community.

2. Planning and provision of appropriate programmes of nursing care particularly for the following groups: the chronically sick, disabled, frail elderly, terminally ill and post-operative patients
3. Mobilizing community resources, both professional and voluntary
4. Identification of the special needs of the carer and family
5. Ensuring continuity of care between home and hospital in both directions
6. Promotion of health education and self-care with individuals and groups
7. Rehabilitation
8. Counselling

Other activities may include nursing care in the health centre and participation in multidisciplinary screening.

The district nurse spends 75% of her time with old people, the majority of whom are female (DHSS 1982). The following discussion will use a nursing process framework to focus on the key issues of the district nurse's role, referred to above, that are particularly relevant to the care of the elderly.

Assessment

The aim of the assessment is to obtain sufficient information to identify the old person's health and nursing needs. The assessment includes information gathered during the patient interview, observation of the patient, family and environment, and information from the medical records, referral agency and other health workers.

The use and application of nursing models as a means of shaping the assessment and critically evaluating practice are in their infancy in district nursing. The value of using models has been described by Damant (1988). The Roper framework (Roper et al 1980) is probably the most commonly used, perhaps because its focus is upon individual behaviour and abilities rather than upon disabilities. However, adapting models for the community which were originally designed for an acute setting is problematic.

The principles of the assessment of elderly people in the community should include:

- a continuous cycle of assessment and reassessment
- assessment of the carer's needs alongside the patient's
- assessment starting from the patient or carer's concerns
- access to information from other agencies/professionals
- multidisciplinary assessment
- acknowledgement of intuitive and subjective assessment.

It is the conceptualization of assessment in terms of nursing and health needs rather than an emphasis on medical problems that is important. Instead of a series of predetermined questions, the district nurse's approach should be the exploration of needs and feelings which are common to everyone, but may have assumed troublesome significance for the patient.

The first visit is of enormous importance in establishing a relationship with the patient and determining a baseline of information which can be built on over a period of nursing intervention. Handling information in an accepting, non-judgemental way is essential. The ability to do this in some circumstances is a challenge to and a measure of the district nurse's professional skills. The nurse is a guest in the patient's home, with no right of entry. The patient therefore has ultimate authority and can play a major part in negotiation for change.

Important information is obtained on the doorstep at the first visit. The appearance, access to the property and state of the garden give useful clues. The response when the doorbell rings — whether there is the noise of boisterous children, a dog barking or a long silence followed by the shuffle of bedroom slippers — should also be noted. This, combined with observation of the person's expression of anxiety, relief, fatigue or despair contribute to the nurse's assessment.

There may only be a single problem contained in the referral, but others may emerge during the interview and through discussion with neighbours, family, etc. A referral for the assessment of a patient with a leg ulcer may reveal an isolated old man, cut off from his remaining family, with grossly oedematous legs, sleeping in an armchair because the bed evokes the pain of his wife's terminal illness.

Care planning

Information obtained during the assessment is used to define the patient's needs. Both patient and carer should be involved in setting realistic goals in order of priority, preferably using their own words. The reason for this is twofold. It involves the patient directly in goal-setting and self-care and, secondly, since the care plan is left in the home and is accessible, it may avoid anxiety and misunderstanding if the language is that of the patient rather than the jargon of the nurse.

Identifying to what extent the problem is that of the patient and not the nurse is central; for example, persuading the old man to sleep in his bed to allow passive drainage of the leg and therefore promote healing of the ulcer is pointless if the real problem is unresolved grief for his wife. This raises several key issues. The patient must determine the pace of the nursing intervention. There would be no value in setting up a comprehensive rehabilitation programme if the patient were unprepared to cope with change. Secondly, there may be a conflict between the patient's and the nurse's values and priorities. For instance, an old lady may be preoccupied with unbearable loneliness and not with a weekly bath. Finally, there may be a conflict of the nurse's aims with the resources, services and staff available. For example, the nurse may agree that the problem with the chairfast patient is stress incontinence and that the long-term aim should be the promotion of continence with the short-term goal strengthening the muscles of the pelvic floor by exercise and regular toileting. However, staff shortages may make this kind of labour-intensive rehabilitation programme difficult to implement.

Implementation

The implementation of the care plan combines clinical skills with those of health education and counselling. This approach will be illustrated by the nursing management of venous leg ulcers.

It has been estimated that about 400 000 people have leg ulcers (Callum et al 1985). It is commonly a problem for elderly people and is on the increase. In a recent survey, district nurses indicated that it was the most common condition they treated (Journal of District Nursing 1987). Treatment of leg ulcers is based on two principles: adequate compression, and treatment of the ulcer itself (Gilchrist 1989). But it is also important that nursing care embrace the psychological and educational needs of the patient and avoid focusing entirely on the ulcer (Ross 1989a). Many patients have strongly held beliefs about their ulcers based on folklore that the ulcer was the outlet for bad humours from the body (Loudon 1981). Because of the chronic, intractable nature of many ulcers, patients may be anxious, protective and even obsessive about their treatment. In order to treat the underlying condition the nurse should adopt a strategy to teach the importance of good nutrition, losing excess weight, exercise and rest with leg elevation. Furthermore, it has been found that the majority of ulcers are a recurrence, and so the nurse has an important role in prevention and in teaching maintenance care, such as the use of support stockings.

The home circumstances may pose constraints and limitations on the implementation of nursing care. If the only table is littered with papers and cigarettes then it may be better to use a chair or the end of the bed to do the dressing. The kingsize double bed which the 74-year-old overweight amputee shares with her husband may make nursing very difficult. The patient, with justification, may resist advice for a hospital bed because of the symbolic importance it has for their relationship.

Adaptation and improvisation in the home depends on the patient's condition, the environment and the available equipment. Circumstances may be such that, for example, in the final stage of a terminal disease a decision not to carry out an insensitive and probably unnecessary dressing using a meticulous aseptic technique would be wise, because it would cause anxiety to the patient and additional stress for the family. Improvisation and the imaginative use of available equipment and resources are important — for example, using a wire coathanger to make a catheter stand.

Suggesting or making too many changes at once, particularly in a new, complex and personal situation, may be stressful for the patient. It may also be interpreted as interference or a painful reminder of the loss of independence and deterioration in health, or it may threaten the balance of a relationship where the carer's role is sustained by looking after a dependent member of the family.

Evaluation

Assessing the effectiveness of nursing care for elderly people is central and should be done regularly. Evaluation completes the cycle, making the process continuous. Sometimes changes take place almost inconspicuously in the patient, carer, or care given. Care must therefore be adjusted gradually to meet changing needs.

The community nursing record is a legal statement of care given in the home. Conventionally, records are kept in the home as well as the health centre or nurse's working base (with the inevitable problems of duplication). Problem-oriented recording is developing alongside the nursing process. These allow the clear definition of nursing goals and interventions and facilitates audit and the evaluation of care.

Future developmental strategies in the community should recognize the importance of the record as a vehicle for multidisciplinary communication not only among members of the primary care team, but also between primary and secondary care.

1. A shared professional record kept in the home at the point of delivery of care would promote co-ordination and prevent fragmentation of professional resources, especially for the housebound elderly.
2. Communication between hospital and community through the transfer of nursing care plans in both directions would enhance the exchange of information.

Prevention and health education

Prevention has been classified by Caplan (1961) as primary, secondary and tertiary. District nurses are involved to a varying degree in all three. The following discussion will focus on the district nurse's role in prevention of ill health in the elderly.

Primary prevention entails intervention to prevent the incidence of disease, for example by immunization. An old person with an abrasion following a fall may alert the district nurse at an encounter either in the home or health centre to organize tetanus toxoid through the general practitioner.

Secondary prevention involves the early detection of illness using tested screening techniques, for instance measuring blood pressure or testing the urine for glucose. This may take place routinely at a first visit or if a clinical problem is suspected. District nurses increasingly participate in multidisciplinary screening programmes. In addition to undertaking some technical procedures such as venepuncture for haemoglobin levels, sight testing and electrocardiographs, they may be involved in promoting health advice on diet, exercise and leisure activities.

Tertiary prevention is defined as the measures taken to alleviate an existing condition, prevent complications and modulate the effects of illness. The district nurse uses this preventive approach in many ways:

1. Implementing a rehabilitation programme for the aftercare of a stroke patient at home, helping with adjustment to disability and preventing complications.
2. Teaching patient safety such as measures to prevent accidents and falls caused by unsuitable footwear, torn floor coverings and unlit passages.
3. Teaching old people about environmental problems that may cause ill health, such as the risks of hypothermia, the problems of muscle wastage caused by immobility, apathy and withdrawal and constipation owing to a low-roughage diet and insufficient exercise.
4. Teaching relatives how to prevent pressure sores, and demonstrating the principles of safe lifting to ensure comfort to the carer and prevent damage to the patient's delicate skin tissues. Preparing relatives to come to terms

with imminent death in order to avoid abnormal grieving behaviour.

Health education may take place in the home at an individual level with the patient or carer, or in a group in a health centre, community centre, day centre or residential Home. The district nurse is in a unique position to promote health education as an accepted visitor in the home. She may become a well-known and trusted figure over time and therefore will be in a position to influence and change existing behaviour. Group work may take several forms and is usually a response to a community health need or a personal interest in a particular area; examples are obesity groups exercise sessions for maintaining mobility of the well elderly or leg ulcer groups associated with clinics. The move towards neighbourhood nursing means that health needs of a community can be identified and a strategy developed to meet them.

It is clear from the above that the district nurse has a crucial role to play in prevention and health education. This is in line with government policy that district nurses should be committed to advising about prevention and health maintenance (DHSS 1986, 1987). In a national survey, it was shown that only 17% of the district nurse's time is spent on 'advice, counselling, reassurance and health education' (DHSS 1982). It may be that this figure conceals the fact that many nurses are engaged in these activities implicitly in the course of practice.

Counselling

As well as providing health advice, district nurses are often able to listen and offer support, because of their continuous, regular, often long-term contact with patients in their own homes. The process of giving practical, personal help often elicits trust:

1. The nurse's interest and sensitive directed concern for the old person may help to promote change and allow discovery of new methods of coping.
2. Insight into the feelings of an old person may be explored by looking at the barriers to communication and defensiveness about illness and disability.

3. The traumatic life event of rehousing can be very stressful for old people. There may be intense ambivalence: e.g., a longing to move out of the damp, cold flat with the peeling wallpaper and conflicting sadness at leaving the familiar and the known.
4. The relatives' involvement in care should be continuously valued, supported and regenerated. Attentive listening may help carers come to terms with role changes and the effects of illness in the family and share some of the burden of the caring task.

Decision making and the district nurse

District nursing involves making complex decisions. The isolation of district nursing practice increases the responsibility for making decisions alone with few opportunities for sharing with peers. Several studies have reported that district nurses have difficulty with decisions, especially those affecting elderly people. McIntosh (1979) found that decisions were frequently ritualized, task-oriented and unsystematic.

Kratz (1978) looked at nursing care given to patients recovering from a stroke at home. She developed a continuum of care theory that identified appropriate valued and focused care for the acutely ill and inappropriate and diffuse care for those patients who were getting better but still suffered from a residual disability. The conclusion reached from this study was that district nurses have difficulty defining goals for the long-term and chronically sick and fail to value their care as highly as that of the acutely ill. It was confirmed by White (1979) that district nurses found it easier to discharge patients following a clearly defined programme of treatment such as postoperative dressings than the elderly chronic sick requiring 'supervisory' visits.

These findings highlight a real dilemma faced by district nurses today. On the one hand, a goal of community care is to promote self-care. However, to an elderly person, independence may mean loneliness and isolation (Gray & McKenzie 1980). How much anxiety is generated when finally the venous ulcer has healed? The nurse may

feel a sense of achievement but the old lady may only feel the loss.

District nurses are often criticized on the grounds that their long-term nursing intervention fosters patient dependency. The real problem is more complex. The district nurse may fill the gap between the termination of professional care and the absence of community support because the alternative is making a complete statement of withdrawal.

DRUGS AND OLD PEOPLE IN THE COMMUNITY

The district nurse gives parenteral, rectal, and oral medication to elderly people and drugs by inhalation. She has a responsibility for monitoring compliance, observing for adverse reactions, and ensuring safe storage. The reader is referred to Chapter 21 for a detailed discussion of drugs and the elderly. In this section, the problems experienced by patients at home, which are encountered by the district nurse, are highlighted.

Drugs are the property of the patient for whom they are prescribed. The administration of drugs in the community therefore involves adapting principles of safe practice to the particular needs of the patient at home. The rules governing controlled drugs may seem more relaxed in the home, but the nurse must be vigilant to make sure that written prescriptions are available, meticulous records are kept, storage is safe and the patient's or family's permission is obtained for disposal of the drugs when no longer required.

The district nurse should be aware of the factors associated with poor compliance, such as multiple pathology, polypharmacy, complex drug regimes and isolation from medical advice (Parish et al 1983). It has been found also that complex drug regimes cause considerable anxiety to the elderly patient (MacDonald et al 1977) and reduce comprehension and compliance (Parkin et al 1976).

One of the most serious problems in the community is the breakdown of communication which often occurs at the interface between primary and secondary care. The separate systems of hospital and community often lead to failure or delay in the communication of a patient's drug information in both directions (Bliss 1981). For example, the patient often does not understand that the drugs given on discharge have replaced the old ones she was taking before admission. It has also been found that general practitioners and district nurses looking after the same patients, and in principle having access to medical and nursing records, were in some disagreement over the prescribed drugs in the majority of cases (Ross 1989b).

There are several strategies that the district nurse can follow to help the patient understand and follow drug regimes. First, the problem-oriented approach of the nursing process enables individual assessment and encourages active participation and understanding of drug regimes. In practical terms drug regimes can be tailored to the patient's own routine and requirements. Secondly, the district nurse has an important role in prevention. Because of her continuous regular contact with elderly people she is in an excellent position to notice early signs of adverse reactions, and to anticipate and prevent drug misuse. This is a sensitive area because some old people may feel checked up on, or criticized, if too intrusively supervised. Therefore, it is important to adopt tactful, imaginative, innovative strategies with the aim of preventing hazards and at the same time to protect the patient's independence. These measures may include ensuring that labels are clearly typed in large print, including name, strength of drug, date of dispensing and expiry (Kiernan & Isaacs 1981). Directions for use should be simple, but specific, using words patients understand. Old people find child-resistant containers notoriously difficult to open and often transfer tablets to alternative bottles with inappropriate labels, which is an obvious potential source of error.

Simple systems to aid memory can be devised, for example counting tablets into an egg-box to be taken at specified times of the day, or devising charts with instructions on time and dosage. Written instructions for drug use have been found to be an inexpensive method of improving compliance amongst hypertensive patients (Laher et al 1981), and effective when used in conjunction with counselling (Macdonald et al 1977). A drug guide given to elderly patients on the district nurses caseloads in one primary health care team was found to contribute to increased knowledge of the drug regime and improved agreement of the patient, nurse and doctor (Ross 1988).

Prescribing by nurses, recommended by the Cumberlege report (DHSS 1986) and now on the political agenda (DHSS 1987) will have important implications for the care of old people.

COMMUNITY NURSING AIDS AND EQUIPMENT

Aids and equipment supply is a confused area of service provision, affecting the disabled, the elderly and the terminally ill. Different agencies are involved, including district health authorities, local authority social service departments, artificial limb appliance centres, voluntary organizations and the private sector. In theory, health authorities provide nursing aids (sick room equipment), while social service departments are responsible for 'aids to daily living'. In practice this distinction is often arbitrary, and probably meaningless to the client. It is not surprising that the result is a poorly co-ordinated and confusing system of patchwork provision; getting necessary equipment is a complex, time consuming and often frustrating business (Beardshaw 1988), and there is a lack of accessible information for consumers (Tester & Meredith 1987).

In the absence of an appropriate aid, the district nurse often needs to be imaginative and adaptive, for instance using a cardboard box as a bed cradle. Realistic and careful planning is important. Often the solution is a compromise between the ideal piece of equipment and that preferred by the patient. Some old people find it hard to accept the use of aids, which may be a reminder of their deteriorating health, loss of independence and represent a threat to an accustomed way of life. For example, the 90-year-old lady living alone in a neglected basement flat with restricted mobility, spending all sleeping and waking hours in her armchair, refused to contemplate reorganization of her room to accommodate the single bed because of the disruption it would cause to the work on her autobiography. The personal space of this lady was intensely private, and no reassurance would change her mind. In this situation the nurse must recognize that her patient's priorities are different from her own and that the nursing environment is far from ideal.

THE DAY HOSPITAL

Day hospitals provide a bridge between hospital and the community. They are often located within the geriatric department of a general hospital. The aim is to provide a therapeutic environment during office hours, with multidisciplinary specialities including occupational therapy, physiotherapy, speech therapy and chiropody. The reasons for referral to a day hospital include continuity of care on discharge, rehabilitation, treatment to maintain the progress of an intensive hospital programme, medical and nursing procedures that cannot be carried out at home, and social care.

Day hospitals have been criticized for low patient turnover, and an emphasis on social care other than rehabilitation.

THE COMMUNITY HOSPITAL

The concept of the community or general practice hospital is an exciting new development in primary care. The aim of the community hospital is to provide a service for rehabilitation, respite care, terminal care, and for patients with acute medical problems not requiring intensive treatment.

An innovative example of this in London's inner city is the Lambeth Community Care Centre. There, general practitioners provide the medical care and work with a multidisciplinary team of nurses, physiotherapists and occupational therapists. The philosophy of self-care and empowerment gives patients their own records and the right to be involved in decision-making (Wilce 1988). The Community Care Centre is discussed further in Chapter 29 of this volume.

AFTERCARE FOR THE ELDERLY

There is considerable evidence to suggest that the co-ordination of aftercare is unsatisfactory (Skeet 1974, Roberts 1974, Turton & Wilson-Barnett 1981). Skeet's study (1974) identified the dis-

charge of old people as a matter of particular professional concern.

There are three major problems in the provision of follow-up care: communication between hospital and community, absence of discharge planning by hospital staff and family expectations.

1. Communication. The exchange of information between hospital and community in both directions has been found to be unsatisfactory. There is often a delay of up to three weeks before the general practitioner is notified of a patient's discharge (Continuing Care Project 1979). Parnell (1982) found that in 93% of cases the district nurse received information, but in only 48% of these was it 'reasonable' enough to facilitate the planning of appropriate care. There are three methods of communication that take place: direct contact between professionals, which in practice happens rarely; referral forms, which vary in quality; liaison nursing staff who function as co-ordinators. Communication from the community to hospital has also found to be lacking. Forty-six per cent of hospital nurses 'rarely' or 'never' receive information (Parnell 1982). This communication failure in both directions has implications for elderly people. Reliable information should be transferred with the patient in order to prevent this major change being traumatic and unsettling. Future developments of the nursing process could adopt a problem-oriented care plan to promote the exchange of information.

2. Discharge planning. The urgent need of a hospital bed often results in a precipitate and ill-conceived decision to discharge a patient. Lack of time to co-ordinate services, an unprepared home and uninformed relatives mean confusion and insecurity for the old person.

3. Family expectations. Relatives are the main carers for recently discharged dependent patients (Roberts 1974, Age Concern 1980). Poor communication among the services places additional strain on the family. Whereas the old person may minimize her health and social problems because of an overriding desire to return home, families may have different expectations. They may undervalue their own role, feel guilt for previous failure which led to hospital admission, or resent renew-

ing the inevitable exhausting and continuous caring tasks.

Where an old person lives alone many relatives find it hard to accept the element of risk. This raises the question of how much support to give. Too much can lead to over-dependence and too little may expose undesirable risk. Coping with the anxiety of risk is as hard for relatives as it is for involved professionals.

Awareness of the 'care gap' has led to attempts to improve the continuity of care, notably through the development of hospital/community liaison posts. These posts are held by health visitors or district nurses and have evolved in various ways. A study describing the structure and process of liaison comments that the role should be developed from an 'intermediary' to an 'advisory' one through educational and organizational change (Jowett & Armitage 1988).

Planned early discharge is the practice of discharging selected surgical patients to the follow-up care of community nurses and family doctors after a minimum stay in hospital. Candidates may in the past have been excluded because of age, but this is likely to change, because of demand for beds (Ruckley et al 1980, Plant & Brendan Devlin 1978).

ETHNIC MINORITY ELDERS

The needs of ethnic elders have been ignored for a number of reasons, which include the assumption that this group of old people are cared for by the extended family. However, Barker (1984) found in his study of ethnic elders in Manchester and London that the majority reported loneliness, loss of role and dignity. Common problems identified were poor housing, low income, difficult access to health and social services, and feelings of powerlessness.

Most new initiatives for ethnic minority elders have come from the voluntary sector, for example AFFOR (All Faiths For One Race), a multiracial resource based in Birmingham, which has made a number of innovations including Asian meals-on-wheels, home helps and housing schemes and which promotes community action and self-help groups. There are some housing schemes that pro-

mote sheltered accommodation, for example the Carib Housing Association in Kensington and Chelsea, London, for elderly West Indians, and Aram House for old Asian men in Newham, London. In addition, special day clubs and resource/advice centres have been set up, for example the Black Elderly Project in Wandsworth, London, which has Local Authority funding. The special housing needs of ethnic elders has been studied by Age Concern (1984) whose researchers identified a lack of awareness amongst service providers of housing needs and recommended ethnic monitoring and closer collaboration among agencies.

The health services have also been slow to recognize ethnic needs. There is evidence that black elders tend to be unrepresented among health service users. Many of the factors that contribute to low uptake stem from service ethnocentrism, stereotypical views of black people, and inflexibility in the organization and delivery of care. This has been highlighted in the district nursing service by Cameron et al (1989). Clearly, there is a need for improvements in training, as well as management support and professional development. These issues are discussed in detail in Chapter 25 of this volume.

ELDERLY MENTALLY FRAIL PEOPLE

At the end of the 1960s in the UK, a small group of psychiatrists with a special interest in old people began to develop local services for elderly people with mental disorders. These services are extremely patchy across the country today, but where they exist they concentrate on supporting patients (and their families) in their own homes whenever possible and on improving the quality of long-stay care (RCP and RCPsych 1989). These initiatives include home assessments and joint assessments by medical, psychiatric and social services teams in units for old people with physical and mental frailty. Unfortunately, the administrative and financial separation between health and social services, which could be compounded further by the health–social care distinction advocated in the Griffiths Report (Griffiths 1988), coupled with the uneven growth of private sector provision, have resulted in incoherent service planning and major cutbacks in both health and social service provision.

The health professionals most closely involved in caring for elderly mentally frail people (particularly dementia sufferers) in the community are community psychiatric nurses (CPNs). These specialist nurses help families with practical, financial and emotional difficulties, and act as counsellers and advocates for old people and their carers. They can mobilize extra support when family carers are unable to cope and predict the time when admission to a long-stay institution will become necessary. Quite often, short-term hospital admission is recommended for medical assessment or respite care, and the CPN is able to work actively with occupational therapists, social workers and medical staff to ease the transition home. Day hospitals, day centres and 'sitter' services are particularly appropriate for the elderly mentally frail and their families, but are often woefully inadequate. The psychogeriatric care team that can cope with emergencies, admit old people to hospital when required with no waiting list, prevent breakdown in family support and offer a flexible system of planned relief is the most successful (RCP and RCPsych 1989). The CPN has a crucial role in enabling the carer at home to cope and in providing someone to turn to whenever this is required. It is essential that the CPN, the psychogeriatric unit social worker and the general practitioner work closely together to meet the needs of the elderly person and family carers, and this support is likely to be required for the remainder of the old person's life.

Sheltered housing wardens and home helps provide a valuable service in helping old people with mental frailty to remain at home. In addition, the voluntary sector is increasingly active through local self-help groups, neighbourhood support groups and organizations such as Age Concern, MIND and the Alzheimer's Disease Society (RCP and RCPsych 1989). These activities help to plug some of the gaps in statutory provision.

PERSONAL SOCIAL SERVICES

The local authority personal social services are re-sponsible for important supportive care of old people in the community, including services in the home, day centres and residential accommodation. The elderly and particularly the very elderly represent one of the largest care groups for social services. A study by the National Institute of Social Work found that over 20% of referrals to the social work department were from the 75+ years age group (Phillipson 1982).

Social service provision includes:

1. Social workers employed by and based in the social work department of the local authority. Occasionally, they may work in a health centre, which clearly facilitates communication with the primary care team. Social workers have been criticized for giving old people a low priority. Rethinking a new approach is urgent, in view of the implementation of the Griffiths (1988) proposals on community care.

2. Domiciliary occupational therapists based in social work departments. They assess old people's needs for aids to daily living. The Chronically Sick and Disabled Person's Act 1970 obliges local authorities to make necessary adaptations to the home, such as installing ramps, handrails, hoists, stair lifts, etc. Other services provided under this Act include help in obtaining radios and televisions, the allocation of telephones and enabling elderly people to have holidays.

3. Social services are also responsible for specialists (such as social workers for the blind), laundry for the incontinent, and welfare benefit advice.

4. Respite care is organized by social services to give relatives a rest from the continuous and exhausting demands of caring. This may entail organizing a bed in residential accommodation or perhaps arranging board with the growing number of families willing to look after an elderly person for payment.

SERVICES IN THE HOME

Home help

Traditionally, the home help service has provided regular help with domestic and household tasks, including shopping, collecting prescriptions, cleaning and the preparation of meals. Provision is patchy; typically, the London boroughs and metropolitan districts provide greater cover and intensity of service compared to that of the shire counties (DHSS 1988).

Innovations in home care

Demographic, economic and policy pressures on local authority social service departments have resulted in a recent shift away from the more traditional home help service to more comprehensive personal and domestic care (Davis & Ferlie 1982). The Social Services Inspectorate has noted that most social service departments are at various stages of planning and implementing change in this direction (DHSS 1988).

'Domiciliary care assistant', 'home care assistant' and 'domiciliary aide' are various terms to describe a worker engaged in personal care and homemaking tasks to enable elderly people to stay in their own homes. 'Community carer', a term coined by the Audit Commission (1986) and used in the Griffiths report (1988), describes a key worker who, given adequate training, could undertake a wide range of basic nursing and occupational therapy tasks, as well as providing personal and domestic help.

It is the role of the domiciliary care assistant that, so far, is at the heart of the change in service provision, and the types of scheme vary. Some provide short-term assistance for those discharged from hospital, in an attempt to ease the transition and prevent readmission (Townsend et al 1988). However, a review by Salvage (1984) of over 40 schemes showed that the majority provide long-term support to frail old people in an attempt to maintain them at home.

An essential feature of these new schemes is flexibility, in terms of hours, frequency of visiting, and work undertaken. Thus it is a service of high intensity and low cover. The second important characteristic is the emphasis on personal care, for example washing and dressing. Undoubtedly this is a valuable service and a lifeline for many dependent people, but it raises some interesting issues. For example, it is likely that, because of resource constraints, targeting services for a smaller group

of dependent people will reduce the cleaning-only service, which some would argue has an important preventive function. Secondly, there are the professional questions of training, assessment, management, support, and interface with other agencies such as the district nursing service and occupational therapy (Ross 1989c).

Meals-on-wheels

This is a domiciliary service to provide a subsidized, hot two-course meal for frail elderly or disabled people. More than 50% of the 26 million meals in 1978/79 were provided by the local authority, and the remainder by the Women's Royal Voluntary Service (WRVS) (DHSS 1981). The availability of the service is variable. In some areas elderly people are restricted to weekly visits, and in others clients may receive meals seven days a week according to need. Most receive three meals or fewer a week, although this may be an overestimate, given current cuts in spending. Special diabetic or low-roughage diets can be arranged on request. The meals service also often fulfils a surveillance function. If an old person fails to answer the door or suddenly deteriorates, then the appropriate agency can be informed.

SOCIAL DAY CARE

Day care is provided by the local authority or a voluntary organization. Day centres offer a hot lunch, entertainment, diversionary activities, adult education, bathing, chiropody service and facilities for self-help or health education groups.

The majority of elderly people do not go to any social centres (Abrams 1978, Hunt 1978). One of the reasons for low uptake may be the problem of access and transport. It is for the housebound, isolated old person that day centre provision is important and it is for precisely this group that places are restricted, because of the shortage and unpredictability of transport. Many old people are frustrated by long circuitous journeys, the uncertainty of picking-up times and uncomfortable seating. This illustrates the frequent absence of collaboration among services when planning new programmes.

HOUSING

The majority of elderly people live at home, often in inappropriate accommodation. Just over half of elderly couples, and 38% of older people living alone are home owners. Forty-two per cent of single elderly households, and just over half of old couples live in local authority housing. Although only 8% of the population live in private rented accommodation, this includes a disproportionate number of old people (Wheeler 1986), and only 6% of the elderly population live in sheltered accommodation (Tinker 1982). Housing Associations have a developing role in service provision for old people, including specialist housing, peripatetic wardens, specialist housing for ethnic minorities, high-care schemes or 'very sheltered' housing, and care and repair services.

It is now more widely recognized that there is a high proportion of owner-occupiers in unsatisfactory housing. There are a number of reasons for this, including the older nature of properties, low incomes and failure to apply for statutory improvement grants. Dowling and Enevoldson (1988), in a study of housing needs of elderly people, suggest that the extent to which elderly householders consider their dwelling to be in a good state of repair may influence their well-being. Although the Black report (Townsend & Davidson 1982) describes a link between housing status and mortality, this is an area which needs further research.

The main focus of housing policy over the last 20 years has been to promote sheltered accommodation, funded in the main by local authorities, sometimes by housing associations and, increasingly, by the private sector (the latter mostly in the south-east of England, where the market exists). Sheltered housing consists of grouped accommodation (flats or bungalows) with some communal facilities, an alarm system and a warden on site. The resident warden provides a regular and continuous 'friendly neighbour' support, making daily visits, providing emergency domiciliary care and liaising with other community workers and members of the primary care team (Heumann 1981). Sheltered accommodation pro-

vides a vital part of assisted housing stock for the old.

While it undoubtedly meets a need, there are various problems with sheltered accommodation in that it creates age-segregated housing, with little consideration for the views, and the increasing frailty, of old people. One of the main conclusions from the research on sheltered accommodation is that for some people it is resorted to for want of a better alternative. There is little doubt that many old people move to escape loneliness, only to find a greater alienation in unfamiliar surroundings.

Housing policy is beginning to shift from 'moving on' to 'staying put'. This involves various strategies initiated by local authorities and housing associations, including 'care and repair' and advice on alterations, insulation and modernization. However, progress in this area is often limited by the lack of co-ordination between housing and social service departments in the local authority, and by the structural separation between the public and private sectors.

SOCIAL SECURITY BENEFITS

The evidence suggests that the old in Britain are poor. While just under one in five (18%) of all persons in Great Britain are over retirement age, this group accounts for two in every five of those living on incomes on or below the supplementary benefit level, i.e. the official social standard of poverty (Walker 1986).

The system of state financial support for old people is complex and the following section will outline the main groups of benefits available. The government department responsible for administering social security benefits is the Department of Social Security.

The benefit level is adjusted annually, and current information and further details can be obtained from:

- local Social Security offices
- freephone Social Security 0800 666555
- local Citizens' Advice Bureaux
- Child Poverty Action Group.

The **Retirement Pension** is payable to men at 65 years and women at 60 years. In 1988/1989 the pension was set at £41.65 for a single person and £65.90 for a married couple. There is a non-contributory age addition for those over 80 years.

Attendance Allowance is tax free and is not means-tested. It is payable at two rates. The higher rate is for a dependant requiring continual supervision both day and night, and the lower rate for a person requiring frequent attention by day.

Invalid Care Allowance is a weekly cash allowance. It is payable to those under pension age unable to enter employment because of responsibilities to care regularly and substantially at least 35 hours a week for a dependant.

Income Support is a means-tested benefit that aims to top up income to the level the government defines is necessary to live on. It was designed to simplify the old system of separate benefits, for example, heating, laundry, diet etc. These have now been incorporated into an average amount, which is payable at two levels, one for those over 60 years, the other for those over 80 years or who are receiving disability benefit. In spite of the fact that pensioners form the bulk of claimants for supplementary benefit, there is a low take-up rate.

Housing Benefit is a scheme run by local authorities to help with rent and rates for those on a low income. The rules for calculating benefit changed in 1988 so that everyone must pay 20% of rates, and savings of more than £6000 rule out entitlement. Old people on income support would normally get the maximum housing benefit.

The **Social Fund** was introduced in 1988 to replace the legal framework of urgent need and single payments. It is a cash-limited and discretionary scheme to help people with exceptional expenses which are difficult to meet from regular income. The payment is in the form of a recoverable loan and may be provided in the following circumstances:

- budgeting loans for items such as furniture or repairs
- crisis loans; for example, if an elderly person was burgled or had a fire
- community care grant to help meet the needs of people moving out of long-term care.

In addition to these discretionary loans, funeral payments are made from the Social Fund. People have a legal right to them if they qualify.

The **Independent Living Fund** was set up in 1988 with the objective of helping severely disabled people on low incomes to live independently in their own homes by providing money to employ a personal care assistant or domestic help. Claimants should be receiving attendance allowance and income support. If they do not get income support it is still possible to claim if their income is less than the cost of the care needed, and their capital is less than £6000.

THE ROLE OF THE VOLUNTARY SECTOR

The activity of the voluntary sector in the United Kingdom is dynamic and changing according to local need and individual initiatives. It includes the work of the formally constituted voluntary organizations, neighbourhood care groups, mutual support groups and informal carers.

VOLUNTARY ORGANIZATIONS

These provide support for old people in the community and include groups such as Age Concern, Red Cross and WRVS (Women's Royal Voluntary Service). They offer services such as transport, help with gardening, shopping, visiting the isolated elderly, offering respite for carers, bereavement counselling, aids for nursing old people at home, supplementary linen and hypothermia packs.

NEIGHBOURHOOD CARE GROUPS

These are organized attempts to mobilize local resources to increase the amount and range of help and care they give to one another, such as offering support to someone during an acute phase of illness and skill swapping — for instance, exchanging plumbing expertise for knitting a pullover.

MUTUAL AID GROUPS

These offer mutual support and a focus for social contact for people with similar problems or a common concern; examples include stroke clubs, carers' organizations and pensioners' self-help groups (see Ch. 23). There is often an intrinsic element of pressure group activity, which has meant that many professionals regard their existence with suspicion.

In recent years there has been a growth in radical mutual aid groups such as pensioners' action groups. Often achieving a strong community identity, they fight local campaigns to improve services for old people, for example by providing evidence on the association between number of falls by the elderly with disrepair of pavements.

INFORMAL CARERS

The consequences of community care policies, and the current vogue for efficiency savings means that old people tend to be cared for longer at home, and are discharged at an earlier stage of recovery. Policies over the last ten years have emphasized the caring role of the family. An informal carer is anyone whose life is in some way restricted because of the need to take responsibility for the care of a person who is mentally ill, mentally handicapped, physically disabled or whose health is impaired by sickness or old age.

It has been estimated that Britain's informal carers number 7 million; the majority of carers are women — daughters, wives, mothers, friends and neighbours (General Household Survey 1985). While 35% of carers are male it has been noted that daughters tend to care for the more highly disabled elderly people and they often receive the lowest level of community-based services e.g. home helps and meals-on-wheels (Evandrou et al 1986).

Most research on carers has been consumer-led, taking one of two main approaches, which to some extent overlap. The policy lobby, for example, has criticized the inadequate funding of community care (Parker 1985), and feminist researchers have focused on the way in which society makes assumptions about women and caring, which may restrict their opportunities. Nissel and Bonnerjea's (1982) case study of 22 families revealed that husbands rarely gave direct help to their wives with the care of a dependent relative, even when the wife was employed outside the home.

From both perspectives the majority of this descriptive research discusses caring in terms of 'burden', that is, the physical, psychological, social and financial costs. This separation is somewhat artificial because, for example, the physical demands of the caring tasks, the duration of the caring episode, and the time spent are likely to take their emotional toll. Further, the ageing of the population means that carers will increasingly be frail spouses and elderly children.

In summary, the nature of the task is often continuous, exhausting, and frustrating, The tendency to emphasize the burden of caring overlooks what for some is a positive experience. The concept of 'mutuality', or reciprocity, suggests that the caring relationship may be meaningful and satisfying as well as frustrating. Hirschfield (1978) concludes from a study of confused elderly people and their carers that mutuality was a crucial factor in determining a carer's ability to cope. More recently, in a collection of case studies, Lewis and Meredith (1988) have described the ambivalence and confused feelings coming from 'love and labour' that characterize many caring relationships.

The carer's lobby criticizes the erratic and ad hoc nature of service provision, and it is often noted that the presence of a carer will mean reduced service input. Exceptions are made to this if the carer is male or if there is a crisis. This has been studied in relation to district nursing and there is a growing consensus that unspoken criteria are used to ration visits in terms of who the carer is (Luker & Perkins 1988, Badger et al 1988).

Twigg (1989) has developed a framework for explaining the relationship between professionals and carers. Her discussion focuses on social services, but parallels can be drawn with health services. Carers are described as 'resources', 'co-workers' or 'co-clients'. If the carer is viewed as a 'resource' her needs are subordinated to the dependent person's. In contrast, a 'co-client's' needs (often when the carer is elderly) are acknowledged and met, albeit at a secondary level. The third description, 'co-worker', suggests the carer works in parallel with the professional. These models could be used as a useful frame of reference for clarifying and understanding the carer/nurse relationship.

There is little doubt that the district nurse has an important role in providing carer support. Some interesting initiatives have been taken by district nurses in setting up and facilitating carer support groups. The Kings Fund informal caring unit has developed teaching packages to alert professionals to the needs of lay carers, and is in the process of preparing a carer's charter (Richardson et al 1989).

CURRENT POLICY ON COMMUNITY CARE — THE IMPLICATIONS

The last thirty years have seen a remarkable political consensus with regard to community care. Elderly people have been identified as a priority group for community care initiatives in a number of statements (DHSS 1976, 1978, 1981, 1987). The failure of community care has been attributed to inadequately defined objectives, and to the gap between policy rhetoric and practical reality (Walker 1982). The Audit Commission (1986) highlighted the funding problems and the complex network of relationships and responsibilities at local level that lie at the root of poor communication. It recommended a thorough review, which resulted in the Griffiths report (1988). Griffiths recommendations were based on the keystones of responsibility, accountability and, inevitably, quality assurance, and proposed that community care should be the responsibility of local authorities with clear policy and management direction from central government. However, the implications for old people must be considered within the context of the White Paper on the NHS (DH 1989). The main thrust of the government's plans are to increase the competitiveness and efficiency of the acute sector and to promote consumer choice. These themes are reflected in the proposals to change the general practitioner contract, giving GPs purchasing and provider rights; to introduce targets for some preventive functions; and to implement peer audit.

In general, these proposals are likely to increase the vulnerability of elderly people for the following reasons:

● the pressure to make services more competitive will mean that priority will be given to acute, short, sharp treatments rather than to elderly care which is often lengthy, expensive and uncertain

● buying services outside the district may be cheaper, but it would increase travelling time for patients and their carers

● early discharge and more day care as a measure of efficiency may not necessarily be matched by appropriate community support

● contracted-out hospitals empowered to set independent salaries, terms and conditions may mean that the negative stereotypes of the chronic care groups will be reinforced with the further drift of good calibre staff away from hospitals for elderly people and the community

● the proposal to link general practitioner salaries more closely with 'capitation' may mean a tendency to increase patient list size, with consequences for reduced quality of care

● the emphasis on medical care will marginalize the contribution of other health workers.

Interestingly, Griffiths emphasizes in his report the distinction between health and social care and that these branches of service are to be dealt with by separate agencies. It is accepted by many that health needs are best understood in a social context, which makes this an arbitrary separation, with the inherent risk that clients such as elderly people, will fall through the caring net.

CURRENT DEVELOPMENTS IN DISTRICT NURSING PRACTICE FOR ELDERLY PEOPLE

The district nurse is usually described as a generalist. In recent years there has been an adaptation of her role in specialist areas, which include stroke rehabilitation, coronary, terminal, stoma and diabetic care, promotion of continence, hospital/community liaison, care of children and the treatment of venous leg ulcers.

The argument put forward in favour of specialization is that it provides greater nursing expertise and support to patients and other practitioners. There are also misgivings and anxieties that specialization not only devalues the role of the district nurse but also fragments care.

HOSPITAL-AT-HOME SCHEME

This experimental scheme which started in Peterborough, England, using the district nursing service aims to provide intensive nursing care for patients during an acute phase of illness at home (Mowatt & Morgan 1982). Evaluation of the project shows that the average age was 71 years, 33% were aged 80 years and over and 31% lived alone. The specific events that precipitated referral to the scheme included 14% who rejected hospital admission and 25% of families no longer able to cope. It is interesting that in 4% of cases district nurses identified the inseparability of the patient and spouse as a clear personal problem affecting treatment choices. The advantages of the scheme were that it allowed families to stay together and avoided expensive social service support for the frail or disabled partner left behind at home. Families, patients and nurses were positive about the programme. Relatives were able to take a more active role in care and the district nurse found the work gave her more job satisfaction.

OUT-OF-HOURS NURSING CARE

An out-of-hours service is defined as functioning between 17.00 h and 08.00 h. There are two sorts of provision: the evening service which covers the 'twilight hours' between 17.00 h and 21.30/22.00 h, and the night service which provides cover throughout the rest of the night.

The evening service provides mostly long-term nursing care for the elderly, disabled and chronic sick. Patients are often highly dependent, living alone or with frail relatives. Nursing care may be the administration of drugs by injection such as insulin, antibiotics or opiates, help with activities in preparation for bed such as washing, toileting, pressure area care, or contributing to a rehabilitation programme such as the promotion of continence. Occasionally, help is needed during a crisis, for instance helping relatives to nurse a patient

through the early stages of a stroke. For many, the evening nurse is often the last visitor of the day before the long and probably lonely night.

The night service covers 20.00 h to 08.00 h. It overlaps with the evening service, and the functions are twofold. First, crisis or short-term care may take place during an episode of acute illness or an acute phase of a terminal disease. Referrals may be made to unblock a catheter, give an enema or sort out a patient who has been discharged from hospital with a leaking wound and no dressing supplies. The second type of care is long-term and may involve providing a night sitter to give exhausted relatives a good night's sleep.

Unfortunately, provision of out-of-hours service is patchy. Some districts are carrying out experimental programmes. Where schemes have been implemented and monitored they have been found to be valued highly by patients and their relatives (Martin & Ishino 1981).

INNOVATIONS IN CARE

There are many ways in which district nurses are making innovatory contributions to the care of elderly people through the development of clinical, teaching and management skills. Such innovations include:

1. Combined programmes with social services for district nurses to work in day centres and residential accommodation to provide health advice to residents and staff.
2. Collaboration with social services in domiciliary aide programmes.
3. Liaison between housing departments and health districts to promote closer working relationships between district nurses and wardens of sheltered housing.
4. Participation in training and support programmes for home care aides for elderly people.
5. Utilization of day care facilities to provide night nursing care for the elderly.
6. Offering increased availability to consumers through open access clinics.

In summary, there are several issues central to the provision of community nursing services for the elderly. Research should be carried out into the nursing needs of old people. Future developments of housing schemes, social service provision and primary care programmes should recognize the professional implications for other relevant departments and adopt joint planning strategies. The primary care team should be aware of the implications of cuts in spending on social and health services in a system already constrained by regulations in health care. In particular, the district nurse, practising at the sharp end of policy implementation, should recognize her professional responsibilities to oppose social and economic policies that militate against the well-being of the community.

The district nurse's work with the elderly raises many questions such as her own attitude to ageing, dependency, old peoples' rights, uncertainty and the stress of coping with the complex problems culminating from many years of neglect. Sharing, listening and finding support from her peer group, opportunities for professional development and close working relationships with other members of the primary care team are of central importance for the delivery of effective community nursing care to old people.

REFERENCES

Abrams M 1978 Beyond three score and ten. Age Concern, London
Age Concern 1980 Discharge from hospital — the social worker's view. Age Concern, London
Age Concern 1984 Housing for ethnic elders. Age Concern/Help the Aged Trust
Audit Commission 1986 Making a reality of community care. HMSO, London
Badger F, Cameron E, Evers H 1988 Facing cares unequal shares. Health Service Journal 98 (5128) 1392–1393
Barker J 1984 Black and Asian old people in Britain. Age Concern, London
Beardshaw V 1988 Last on the list. Community service for people with physical disabilities. Kings Fund, London
Bliss M R 1981 Prescribing for the elderly, including problems of instructions, supervision and liaison between hospital and general practice. British Medical Journal 283: 203–206
Bond J, Carstairs V 1982 Services for the elderly. Scottish Health Service Studies no 42. Scottish Home and Health Department, Edinburgh
Bond J, Cartlidge A, Gregson B, Phillips P, Bolan F, Gill K 1985 A study of interprofessional collaboration in primary health care organisation. University of Newcastle, Health Care Research Unit, Newcastle-upon-Tyne

Bowling A 1987 Community health services. In: Harrison A, Gretton J (eds) Health care UK. Public Money, London
Callam M, Ruckley C, Harper D, Dale S 1985 Chronic ulceration of the leg: extent of the problem and provision of care. British Medical Journal 290: 1855–1856
Caplan G 1961 An approach to community mental health. Tavistock, London
Cameron E, Badger F, Evers H 1989 District nursing the disabled and elderly: who are the black patients? Journal of Advanced Nursing 14: 376–382
Continuing Care Project 1979 Organizing aftercare. National Corporation for the Care of Old People, London
Damant M 1988 Innovations in assessment. Journal of District Nursing 6(9): 9–12
Davis B, Ferlie E 1982 Efficiency and promoting innovations in social care: social services department and the elderly. Policy & Politics 10: 181–203
Department of Health 1989 Working for patients. Review of the NHS. HMSO, London
Department of Health and Social Security 1976 Priorities for health and personal social services in England. A consultative document. HMSO, London
Department of Health and Social Security 1978 A happier old age. HMSO, London
Department of Health and Social Security 1981 Report of a study on community care. HMSO, London
Department of Health and Social Security 1982 Nurses working in the community. Office of Population Censuses & Surveys, London
Department of Health and Social Security 1986 Neighbouring nursing — a focus for care. Report of the community nursing review (Chairman: Julia Cumberlege) HMSO, London
Department of Health and Social Security 1987 Promoting better health. Cmnd 247, HMSO, London
Department of Health and Social Security 1988 Managing policy change in home help services. Social Services Inspectorate, London
Dowling M, Enevoldson H 1988 The elderly at home project. Liverpool Housing Trust, Liverpool
Evandrou M, Arber S, Dale A, Gilbert G 1986 Who cares for the elderly? In: Phillipson C, Bernard M, Strang P (eds) Dependency and independence in old age: theoretical perspectives and policy alternatives. British Society of Gerontology, London
General Household Survey 1985 Informal carers Office of Population Censuses and Surveys, London
Gilchrist B 1989 Treating leg ulcers. Nursing Times Community Outlook, February 25–26
Gray M, McKenzie H 1980 Take care of your elderly relative. Allen and Unwin, London
Griffiths R 1988 Community care: agenda for action. HMSO, London
Heumann L F 1981 The function of different sheltered housing categories for the semi-independent elderly. Social Policy and Administration 15(2): 164–180
Hirschfield M 1978 Home care versus institutionalisation: family care giving and senile brain dementia. International Journal of Nursing Studies 20: 23–32
Hunt A 1978 The elderly at home. HMSO, London
Jowett S, Armitage S 1988 Hospital and community liaison. Journal of Advanced Nursing 13: 579–587

Journal of District Nursing 1987 Your data on leg ulcers. Journal of District Nursing 5(9): 4–6

Kiernan P J, Isaacs J B 1981 Use of drugs by the elderly. Journal of the Royal Society of Medicine 74: 196–200

Kratz C 1978 Care of the long term sick in the community. Churchill Livingstone, Edinburgh

Laher M, O'Malley K, O'Brien E, O'Hanrahan M, O'Boyle C 1981 Educational value of printed information for patients with hypertension. British Medical Journal 282: 1360–1361

Lewis J, Meredith B 1988 Daughters caring for mothers: the experience of caring and its implications for professional helpers. Ageing and Society 8(1): 1–21

Loudon I S L 1981 Leg ulcers in the eighteenth and early nineteenth centuries. Journal of the Royal College of General Practitioners 21: 263–269

Luker K, Perkins E 1988 Lay carers views on the district nursing service. Midwife, Health Visitor and Community Nurse 24(4): 132–134

MacDonald E T, MacDonald J B, Phoenix M 1977 Improving drug compliance after hospital discharge. British Medical Journal 2: 618–621

Mackenzie A 1989 Key issues in district nursing. District Nursing Association, London

Martin M H, Ishino M 1981 Domiciliary night nursing service, luxury or necessity? British Medical Journal 282: 883–885

McIntosh J B 1979 Decision making on the district. Occasional paper. Nursing Times 75(29): 77–80

Mowatt I, Morgan R 1982 Peterborough Hospital at home scheme. British Medical Journal 284: 641–643

Nissel M, Bonnerjea L 1982 Family care of the handicapped elderly. Policy Studies Institute, London

Parker G 1985 With due care and attention: a review of research on informal care. Family Policy Studies Centre, London

Parkin D M, Henny C R, Quirk J, Crooks J 1976 Deviation from prescribed drug treatment after discharge from hospital. British Medical Journal 18: 686–688

Parish P, Doggett M A, Colleypriest P 1983 The elderly and their use of medicines. Kings Fund, London

Parnell J 1982 Continuity and communication. Occasional paper. Nursing Times 78(9): 33–40

Phillipson C 1982 Capitalism and the construction of old age. Macmillan, London

Plant J A, Brendan Devlin H 1978 Planned early discharge of surgical patients. Occasional paper. Nursing Times 74(7): 25–28

Richardson A, Umrell J, Aston B 1989 A new deal for carers. Kings Fund, London

Roberts I 1974 Discharged from hospital. Royal College of Nursing Series 2, no 6, Royal College of Nursing, London

Roper N, Logan W, Tierney A 1980 the elements of nursing. Churchill Livingstone, Edinburgh

Ross F 1988 Information sharing between patients, nurses and doctors. Evaluation of a drug guide for old people in primary health care. In: Johnson R (ed) Excellence in nursing: recent advances in nursing. Churchill Livingstone, Edinburgh

Ross F 1989a Leg ulcers are people too. Nursing Times, Nursing Times 85(6): Community Outlook 23–25

Ross F 1989b Doctor, nurse and patient knowledge of prescribed medication in primary care. Public Health 103: 131–137

Ross F 1989c The new community carer. Nursing Times 85(24): Community Outlook 14–16

Royal College of Physicians and Royal College of Psychiatrists 1989 Care of elderly people with mental illness: specialist services and medical training. A joint report of the RCP and RCPsych, London

Ruckley C V, Garraway W Cuthbertson C, Fenwick N, Prescott R J 1980 The community nurse and day surgery. Nursing Times 76(6): 255–256

Salvage A 1984 Developments in domiciliary care for the elderly. Kings Fund, London

Skeet M 1974 Home from hospital. Macmillan, London

Standing Medical Advisory Committee and the Standing Nursing and Midwifery Advisory Committee 1981 Report of a joint working group on the primary health care team. (The Harding Report.) Department of Health and Social Security, London

Tester S, Meredith B 1987 Ill informed? A study of information and support for elderly people in the inner city. Policy Studies Institute, London

Tinker A 1982 Housing elderly people: some theories of current research. Public Health 97: 290–295

Townsend P, Davidson N 1982 Inequalities in health. Penguin, Harmondsworth, Middlesex

Townsend J, Piper M, Frank O, Dyer S, North W, Meade T 1988 Reduction in hospital readmission of elderly patients by a community based hospital discharge scheme: a randomised controlled trial. British Medical Journal 297: 544–547

Turton P, Wilson-Barnett J 1981 Two aspects of nursing care. In: Simpson J E, Levitt R (eds). Going home. Churchill Livingstone, Edinburgh

Twigg J 1989 Models of carers: how do social care agencies conceptualise their relationship with informal carers? Journal of Social Policy 18(1): 53–66

Walker A 1982 Community care. Martin Robertson

Walker A 1986 Pensions and the production of poverty in old age. In: Phillipson C, Walker A (eds) Ageing and social policy. Gower, Aldershot

Wheeler R 1986 Housing policy and elderly people. In: Phillipson C, Walker A (eds) Ageing and social policy. Gower, Aldershot

White C 1979 A study of some of the factors influencing the district nurse's decision to discharge patients from her care. Unpublished MSc thesis. University of Manchester

Wilce G 1988 A place like home: a radical experiment in health care. Bedford Square Press, London

CHAPTER CONTENTS

Patterns of care   486
Admissions policy   486
Multipurpose wards   486
Single-purpose wards   486

Basic requirements   487
Bed areas   487
Day space   488
Dining areas   488
Toilet facilities   489
Lighting   489
Furniture   490
Equipment   490

Assessing the elderly person in hospital   491
Function versus pathology   491
Advantages of functional assessment   491
Reliability and validity   492

Rehabilitation   492

Multidisciplinary working   493

Discharge/transfer from hospital   493
Standard checklist   494

Conclusion   494
Ethos of the geriatric unit   494

28

Nursing old people in hospital

Pauline Fielding

The idea that nursing old people in hospital is a specialized activity has been growing since the 1930s, when Marjorie Warren established the first department of geriatric medicine. But it is not a nursing speciality which any nurse can afford to ignore — ill people aged over 65 years are not only to be found in geriatric beds but are major users of all other hospital beds, with the obvious exceptions of paediatric and maternity beds. In 1973, elderly people occupied 49% of general medical beds, 38% of orthopaedic beds and 47% of psychiatric beds (Owen 1976). More recent figures for the North East Thames Region of England show that the over-75s occupy 29% of general medical beds, 37% of orthopaedic beds and 16% of psychiatric beds. These figures show that the National Health Service resources are directed towards old people more than towards any other age group. In 1984/85, the estimated UK NHS spending per head on hospital and community health services for people over 75 years of age was over nine times greater than that for a person of working age (Office of Health Economics 1987). It is important, then, that nurses working in hospital settings, particularly in medical, orthopaedic and psychiatric wards, should have a working knowledge of the special needs of elderly people and should demonstrate a willingness to cater for those needs.

PATTERNS OF CARE

Many of the issues which confront the care of the elderly ward nurse stem from the historical development of geriatric medicine which has emphasized early diagnosis and the assessment and treatment of reversible conditions in the fashion of acute medicine. This is reflected in the report of the Royal College of Physicians' Working Party on Medical Care of the Elderly (1977), which in turn reflects the attempt to rationalize priorities in health and personal social services in a consultative document (DHSS 1976). This document stated that a primary objective must be to enable old people to remain in the community for as long as possible. To this end, emphasis should be placed on the development of domiciliary services and the provision of adequate facilities in general hospitals with easy access to diagnostic, therapeutic and rehabilitation resources. The aim is that eventually 50% of geriatric beds would be located in general hospitals. However, because of local hospital and community resources, geographical considerations and the influence of the interest of a particular physician, geriatric hospital services throughout the United Kingdom take many different forms (see Chapter 24 for further discussion on the historical development of services for elderly people).

ADMISSIONS POLICY

Central to this diversity is the admissions policy of the geriatric unit. On the one hand, the unit may accept any new medical patient over a certain age and provide an extensive range of diagnostic and therapeutic resources. On the other hand, the unit may accept referrals from other specialties once the acute phase of an illness has passed and rehabilitation or social problems hinder resettlement in the community. Often linked to the admissions policy or consequent upon local hospital resources is the placement of geriatric beds. These may be 'scattered' throughout the general hospital, a policy which has serious implications for the provision of appropriate resources and a therapeutic environment. However, even if beds are provided in a single unit there are two main patterns of organization which have differing strengths and weaknesses.

MULTIPURPOSE WARDS

First, multipurpose wards cater for patients who may require short-term diagnostic and therapeutic facilities, rehabilitation and continuing or extended care services, or a mixture of these (Bagnell et al 1977). Amongst the benefits claimed for this type of service are: higher staff and patient morale; continuity of care; and the need for relatively few long-stay beds. However, Pathy (1982) points out that to provide extended care in a district general hospital is unduly expensive and suggests that the use of smaller local hospitals would be better for this purpose and may also maintain patients near to relatives and friends. Pathy also indicates that, in multipurpose wards, relatives are often reluctant to agree to discharge when it is apparent that other patients receive extended care.

The effects of multipurpose wards on nursing and on patient outcomes are unresearched. One might suppose that some of the problems identified in long-stay care such as depersonalization and institutionalization would be ameliorated if long-stay patients shared facilities with the more acutely ill elderly, but such evidence as exists suggests that 'long-stay' patients on general medical wards fare badly when in competition with patients in more urgent need of attention (Fielding 1986).

SINGLE-PURPOSE WARDS

Secondly, a unit may be divided into wards with separate facilities for assessment, rehabilitation or continuing care. This functional separation allows resources to be applied discriminately where they are most needed and permits an appropriate 'homely' environment to be provided for those patients needing extended care. Pathy (1982) argues that, with efficient organization, this system of functional separation is compatible with a high turnover and a minimal number of long-stay beds provided that the active treatment beds are sited in the general hospital.

In addition to such 'straightforward' geriatric beds, some hospitals have established units for particular areas of need, e.g. joint orthopaedic–geriatric units (Devas & Irvine 1963, 1969) and stroke units (Garraway et al 1980).

BASIC REQUIREMENTS

Wherever geriatric beds are sited, there are certain basic requirements in terms of space and facilities which must be considered. The nurse involved in commissioning a new unit must be aware of these, but the nurse working in a well-established environment can often recommend improvements in existing facilities at little cost, providing she has a good grasp of the issues involved.

BED AREAS

The DHSS (now Department of Health) outlined minimum standard requirements with regard to bed areas for geriatric wards (DHSS 1972). These prescribe a minimum of 60 square feet per person. This should be the floor space available after suitable arrangements have been made for privacy, e.g. bed curtaining or cubicles. Once the minimum standard for space has been met, there are a variety of bed arrangements which can be used, e.g. long and open 'nightingale' wards, four to six beds grouped in bays, or individual rooms. Proponents of the traditional nightingale ward maintain that patients prefer them because nurses are always in view and there is plenty of activity to watch. Opponents of this style of ward cite the lack of privacy such an arrangement affords. These two issues, the need for social stimulation and the need for privacy are the prime factors to be considered when planning bed areas.

Privacy is a basic human need and the difficulties associated with its provision in institutions are well documented. Townsend (1962) writes.

In the institution, people live communally with a minimum of privacy, and yet their relationships with each other are slender. Many subsist in a kind of defensive shell or isolation. (p. 379).

Being admitted to hospital is, for most people, a stressful event. The lack of privacy which follows hospitalization often compounds such stress. Davies and Peters (1983) have shown that nurses are somewhat insensitive to stressful items such as noise, privacy and toileting procedures, so it is important that the structured environment affords the maximum amount of privacy for the patient.

Tate (1980) suggests that the functions of privacy are fourfold. First, personal autonomy — the ability of the individual to exercise control over her life. In a hospital ward this would include her ability to have privacy when she wished. In an acute assessment ward this provision may not be possible at all times because of the competing need for surveillance and monitoring of health by staff, but in less acute settings, professional workers of all kinds should recognize the need for the elderly person to exercise control in her dealings with others. Secondly, privacy affords the opportunity for emotional release. The demands on an elderly person who is also a patient, in terms of pleasantness, compliance and availability, are considerable. Periods of 'time-off' are an important feature in any role and are essential in order to alleviate concomitant tensions. Thirdly, privacy affords the opportunity for self-evaluation. This is particularly important for elderly people whose hospitalization may mark a significant life crisis and herald a major change in lifestyle. Tate (1980) suggests that everyone needs time for reflection, creative imagination and integration of life experiences and that most institutions for old people are not conducive to such activity. Fourthly, privacy provides a base from which the individual can have limited and protected communication. One can share confidences with chosen and trusted individuals and, with the knowledge that privacy is available, one can seek social contact with others. This latter function of privacy has implications for nurses and other health workers who need to give information to, or obtain information from, elderly patients. Personal matters which may be causing great distress may not be dealt with adequately or satisfactorily for either party if the only privacy provided is a thin curtain.

Delong (1970) has shown that single rooms served to decrease aggression amongst institutionalized old people and suggests that this is because there is less need to establish personal territory in public spaces such as corridors and lounges. Furthermore, Lawton (1970) found that younger psychiatric patients in single rooms engaged in more social interactions than patients in multiple occupancy rooms.

From the evidence available, it would seem that single rooms in long-stay facilities have much to commend them and may indeed be valuable in the more acute areas if the need for surveillance can be met.

DAY SPACE

Again, the DHSS specified minimum standards for geriatric wards (DHSS 1972). These state that at least 10 square feet per person should be provided. This specification is usually interpreted to mean a dayroom for the recreational use of patients. However, in some units space is at a premium and dayrooms may double as rest-rooms for staff, interviewing rooms, case conference rooms and physiotherapy or occupational therapy rooms. Multiple use of dayroom facilities often means that the furniture is less homely and the room less comfortable than is desirable. Ideally, no such duplication of use would occur and patients would be free to use the dayroom for a variety of activities at any time.

It is generally considered appropriate that dayrooms in geriatric units should be carpeted. Recent advances in the design of floor coverings and in the management of incontinence have rendered the arguments against carpeting dayrooms null and void. Indeed, there is much to be said for carpeting fostering a positive expectation of continence in patients. A carpeted area is also valuable for the patient who is learning to walk with a frame or for the wheelchair user, as many difficulties associated with floor coverings often come to light only when the patient is at home. Useful information on floor coverings and other items of design can be found in Goldsmith (1976).

Décor in the dayroom is a matter of personal taste but wallpaper rather than painted walls may be appropriate for elderly people; several blending colours may be easier to maintain than one rigid colour scheme when new items of furniture are added; pictures will help to lessen the institutional impact, and lighting should provide both general and local illumination. Even in acute units it is appropriate to provide television and radio in the dayroom for selective use, whilst in rehabilitation or extended care facilities one might expect record and cassette players or perhaps a piano. Thought should also be given to the provision of facilities for patients and relatives to make drinks or snacks as appropriate. This may be provided in the dayroom area or in a separate kitchen.

The arrangement of furniture in dayrooms is a vexed issue. Most nurses are familiar with the chairs-against-the-wall arrangement which does not appear to facilitate social interaction between patients. However, attempts to manipulate seating arrangements have shown that patients feel more secure and comfortable with their backs against either a wall or other physical barrier (Sommer & Ross 1958). In a large dayroom the need for a secure vantage point and for close face-to-face interaction can be provided by the careful use of room dividers. Whatever the seating arrangement, however, staff should always try to respect the individual's claim on a particular chair or a particular space.

DINING AREAS

The importance of mealtimes in the day of any patient of any age cannot be overemphasized. In the case of hospitalized elderly people, the dining experience can influence recovery and rehabilitation to a great extent and can affect the maintenance of dignity and independence. For most adults, social life is linked to a great extent to the pleasures of eating and drinking. Social and psychological significance is attached to eating at certain times and for certain purposes. Beck (1981) points out that mealtimes still assume importance even in institutions, as shown by the fact that in some long-stay units residents will resort to queueing for an hour or more waiting for the dining room to open.

It is essential, therefore, that mealtimes are not merely a physiological event for the purpose of supplying nutrition but that they are a social and satisfying experience. Indeed, it could be argued that if they are not the latter, then there may be a failure to meet nutritional needs. Beck (1981) cites the increased dependency of the elderly patient, staff attitudes and sensory loss as vital factors to consider. Old people may be confronted by strange food at unusual times. Clarke and Wakefield (1975) showed that nutritional scores were lowered when elderly nursing Home residents changed the nutritional habits of a lifetime. Whenever possible, mealtimes should provide continuity with the patient's pre-morbid state. Disabilities and sensory losses should be properly assessed by an occupational therapist, who will recommend appropriate aids. Staff attitudes are crucial in promoting and maintaining independence in eating. The change to plated meals service in many hospitals has taken the provision of food away from nursing staff and encouraged the easy serving of food on trays to individual patients. This should not be allowed to detract from the social experience of mealtimes. Even with a plated meals service it is still possible to provide dining areas where patients can dine in groups of four to six to encourage socializing. Dining tables attractively laid with tablecloth, cutlery, crockery and condiments suitable for the meal will create an environment where independence becomes a real possibility. Nursing staff should be encouraged to circulate at mealtimes not only to assess nutritional intake but to facilitate conversation which will in turn increase interest in eating (Clancy 1975).

TOILET FACILITIES

Continence promotion is an essential part of the work of any elderly care ward and the location of lavatories is crucial. It is generally acknowledged that lavatories should be within 40 feet of bed and day areas. Greater distances will inevitably lead to a high level of incontinence in a disabled population. The amount of space required within the lavatory is debatable. In a rehabilitation unit, too much space may give an unrealistic picture of the patient's level of independence, if her home circumstances are cramped and less than perfect. But

in an assessment or long-stay unit it will be essential to have sufficient space to enable a patient to be assisted by one person or to use a wheelchair. A patient with a walking frame needs up to 30 square feet in order to turn around. Ideally, all wards should have a variety of facilities and standard aids such as grab-rails should be provided. These and raised toilet seats can easily be supplied when the patient returns home. Bailey (1982) suggests that lavatory paper should be provided on a roll and in sheets to facilitate independence for hemiplegic patients.

It should be remembered that outward-opening doors leave more room on the inside and increase the likelihood of doors being closed for privacy.

A range of washing facilities is also desirable. For those patients who will be returning to their own homes, bathrooms with standard aids such as bath seats should be provided. For the more disabled person, hoists or cabinet baths may be necessary, but many elderly people can use showers successfully if seating is provided. Mirrors over wash-basins are essential in order to encourage patients to take pride in their appearance, and some should be fitted at the right height for wheelchair-bound patients. Where wash-basins are located in a communal area, nurses should remember that their elderly clients are probably quite unused to sharing such facilities. It is only in recent years that shops and swimming baths have provided communal fitting and changing rooms. The nurse should endeavour to provide privacy for the often laborious and painstaking procedures of washing and dressing.

LIGHTING

Good lighting is greatly enhanced by natural sunlight and if the building is well positioned, then this can be used to good effect. Low-level windows will enable patients to look outside even when seated. Blinds or curtains can be used to protect from direct sunlight and to darken the ward at night. If the ward is not naturally well lit, fluorescent lighting may be necessary, provided it is shaded to eliminate glare. In dayrooms, local lighting can be used for specific areas. Bailey

(1982) suggests that lighting at floor level can be particularly useful at night — patients who are getting out of bed can see where they are going but the light does not shine in the eyes of those who are in bed.

FURNITURE
Beds

It is desirable that a good range is available to take account of the varied needs of patients. However, in most UK units it is the 'Kings Fund' general purpose bedstead which is supplied and the need for diversity is often overlooked. There are certain general points, however, which should be borne in mind when considering any bed (Andrews & Atkinson 1982).

1. Every bed should be adjustable in height. This enables the patient to transfer from bed to chair or commode with the minimum of difficulty.

2. There should be a safe, simple and effective braking system.

3. All beds should have the possibility of having safety sides attached to them which can be stored when not in use.

4. All beds should be designed to accommodate poles for intravenous infusions and overhead handles, and a few should have facilities for traction in combined orthopaedic/geriatric wards. More specialized beds should be available if they are needed, e.g. turning and tilting beds, flotation beds, low air loss beds and some of the many others now marketed.

Chairs

A wide range of chairs is essential. Nurses should resist uniformity for the sake of appearances in favour of being able to provide a specific chair for a particular patient's need. This will mean chairs with a range of seat heights and angles. General points to be considered are:

1. A stable base is essential to avoid over-balancing for patients who may be able to push themselves up with only one arm.

2. Handgrips should be positioned so that patients can use them when attempting to stand.

3. There should be no crossbar at the front which would prevent correct positioning of feet under the chair for standing.

4. Padded armrests and wings may be comfortable but wings can discourage social interaction if the chair is badly positioned.

The maintenance of chairs, as of all equipment, is extremely important. Vinyl seat covers, which are favoured because of their easy-to-clean feature, can become very hard and brittle with repeated washing. Splits may occur, particularly if the underlying foam collapses. This is not an uncommon sight and it is a potential fire hazard. Wells (1980) in a study of 749 chairs in one geriatric unit found that approximately one third were unsuitable for use because of very low seat heights, low backs, instability and grossly uncomfortable seats. A further 8% were severely damaged and had extensive seat welling and tears in the upholstery. In total, 48% of the chairs in the unit needed immediate replacement.

Lockers

All patients should be provided with a locker which has hanging space as well as drawer space for clothes. Doors and drawers should be easily opened with large handles to accommodate arthritic hands. It should be possible to use the locker on either side of the bed either for patient preference or for some therapeutic purpose such as encouraging a stroke patient to pay attention to her affected side. A mirror should be provided on the outside of the locker and the whole thing should be easily movable on casters.

Over-bed tables

These should be easily adjustable and easily movable and be suitable for use from chairs also.

EQUIPMENT

There are three areas of work in which the nurse

caring for elderly people in hospital should be an expert and which require the use of special equipment. These are pressure sore prevention, the management of incontinence, and the lifting and handling of patients. Pressure sore prevention and the management of incontinence are discussed in detail in Chapters 14 and 12 respectively.

Lifting and handling patients

There are many occasions when the nurse, quite appropriately, lifts or handles the patient without any recourse to special equipment. She or he should, therefore, be familiar with the various techniques recognized for safe handling and lifting. Some of these are discussed in Chapter 8. Where special equipment is necessary, there are many aids available which cater for patients with varying degrees of independence. Lloyd et al (1981) group these under three headings.

1. Aids for the independent patient with a residual disability. Included here are sliding boards which enable a patient to transfer from bed to chair; overhead handles or trapeze lifts which may be attached to the ceiling above the toilet, for example to facilitate transfers; and bath seats which encourage independence in getting into and out of the bath.

2. Aids for the dependent patient who can offer some assistance. In this group are turntables for transfers through 90° for patients who can take some weight through their legs; transit seats or slings which enable the nurse to move a patient from one sitting area to another without having to grasp painful joints. A makeshift sling of this kind can be made by rolling up a drawsheet to either side of the patient, then turning the four corners into 'handles' for the lifters.

3. Aids for the dependent patient for whom hoists may be necessary. Hoists may, of course, be used to facilitate bathing for less dependent patients. They may be fixed to the floor, to the ceiling, or they may be mobile. Hoists are described in more detail by Tarling (1980) and it is essential that the nurse knows how to use them to their best advantage. Information on their use can always be obtained from the Disabled Living Foundation.

ASSESSING THE ELDERLY PERSON IN HOSPITAL

The importance of adequate assessment of the patient cannot be overemphasized. Consideration should be given to a general assessment of the patient's level of independence. This is particularly important if the nurse is to have any indication of the type of nursing intervention needed and is also important in terms of evaluating the effect of interventions on the patient's progress.

FUNCTION VERSUS PATHOLOGY

During the past 20 years or so, there has been a shift of emphasis away from the 'pathology' of the patient to a functional assessment of the patient's ability to carry out the 'activities of daily living'. Hall (1976) illustrates this well by pointing out that many disabilities commonly seen in a population, such as anaemia, cardiac failure, urinary symptoms, deafness and defective vision, could possibly coexist in a single individual and yet that person might lead quite a satisfying life with no functional problems in terms of her activities of daily living. It is important, therefore, that assessment of the elderly person in hospital should focus not simply on a medical diagnosis but on functional disability. For the nurse, the latter is paramount.

ADVANTAGES OF FUNCTIONAL ASSESSMENT

The advantages of functional assessment are at least threefold.

1. It can be used and understood by all members of the multidisciplinary team and provides a tool whereby patient and carers can converse in the same language about common goals. The patient's problem, in this functional sense, will not be her rheumatoid arthritis but will be her inability to perform the fine finger movements necessary for dressing herself.

2. It can be used to assess the degree of independence before, during and after treatment and, if used in conjunction with some visual display, such as a wall chart, gives essential feedback to the patient so that she can monitor her own progress.

3. It provides a means of identifying specific functional deficiencies when the total score is broken down into individual items. Crucial items can also be weighted numerically in order to reflect their importance for certain levels of independence.

A fourth possible use may be in the prediction

of recovery. Work by Stewart (1980) suggests that functional scoring can be used in order to select those patients who will benefit most from rehabilitation, but his findings were not replicated in later work by Fielding (1987).

Perhaps the best-known functional assessment tool is the Barthel index (Mahoney & Barthel 1965) but there are several which the nurse might consider for a variety of purposes — the Kenny rehabilitation index (Schoening et al 1965), the nursing dependency index (Walton et al 1978) and the ADL score used by Stewart (1980). See Table 28.1.

Table 28.1 An activities of daily living (ADL) score. *Based on Stewart (1980).*

Function	Level of independence	Score
Bowel	Faecal incontinence (complete loss of bowel control and/or occasional soiling)	0
	Complete control	15
Bladder/catheter	Urinary incontinence	0
	Dry by day or catheter dry	10
	Complete control and/or manages own catheter	15
Walking	Requires at least two nurses	0
	Walks with one person or an aid	5
	Complete independence safely	10
Dressing/undressing	Requires complete help	0
	Requires limited help, e.g. fastenings	5
	Dresses independently	10
On/off toilet	Requires help at some stage	0
	Independent safely	10
Feeding	Requires feeding	0
	Independent but may need help with food preparation	10
Wheelchair (only for those unable to walk)	Unable to control safely	0
	Complete control	15
Stairs	Unable or unsafe	0
	Able to climb five stairs safely	5

RELIABILITY AND VALIDITY

There are certain issues of reliability and validity, however, which should be addressed when using a functional assessment scale. First, do two observers testing the same patient arrive at the same result? Before any index is used, the inter-rater reliability should be established. Secondly, do the tests in hospital correlate sufficiently well with the tasks facing the patient in her own home? If they do not, then the test's usefulness for information relevant to discharge will be limited. A third question has to do with the likelihood that the patient will perform at home to a similar standard as when in hospital. Many more factors may be involved here, including responses to a different environment or a deterioration in physical or mental status. Assessment in the home will usually be standard practice before discharge from hospital.

REHABILITATION

Rehabilitation has a special place in the nursing care of old people in hospital. Even if the elderly person was fit and independent before her admission to hospital, an acute episode may have reduced her functional ability and it will not be sufficient merely to treat the acute illness. Those old people suffering from more chronic disabilities such as congestive heart failure or stroke will also need varying periods of rehabilitation nursing in addition to the treatment of their underlying pathology.

Boyer et al (1986) demonstrated that early intervention with active rehabilitation resulted in significantly improved functional status of ill, elderly people, when compared with a control group. A key feature of this study is that nurses determined the need for activity, diet and remedial therapy. Acute medical conditions had usually subsided after 48 hours and it was then an early nursing assessment that determined subsequent treatment.

Rehabilitation nursing of elderly people is not only relevant in specialist geriatric units. The principles of rehabilitation, which are founded upon accurate functional assessment, and which aim always to promote the person's independence, can be applied in any setting. There is, for example, particular value to be gained by such an approach with elderly orthopaedic patients. Dubrovkis and Wells (1988) describe the benefits achieved for elderly patients with hip fracture when nurses began to focus on maximizing the functional level and discharge potential of the patient.

This aspect of caring for old people has often been overlooked. There has been a tendency to focus either on the acute medical-led intervention stage or on the (primarily nursing-led) continuing care stage. Insufficient attention has been given to the skills, not easily defined, of rehabilitation care, where the links and interrelationships with other members of the multidisciplinary team are most evident. Waters (1986) discusses the role of the nurse in this area and gives a useful overview of the nurse's range of responsibilities. She suggests that the continuous presence of nursing and the intimate care-giving functions are powerful tools for the process of rehabilitation and, as yet, are poorly understood.

MULTIDISCIPLINARY WORKING (OR TEAMS)

The notion of teamwork is central to modern practice in geriatric medicine (RCN & BGS 1987). The social and psychological needs of the elderly person, together with a combination of pathological processes, require the expertise of many different kinds of staff. Teamwork, which includes the patient and her family, is essential in order to ensure the most appropriate outcome. The composition of the team for any particular patient will obviously vary according to individual need but there is likely to be a 'core' of members, comprising doctors, nurses, physiotherapists, occupational therapists, dieticians and social workers. This 'core' team will call on the services of a wider group from time to time, e.g. on speech therapists, chiropodists, chaplains.

Team members will have well defined, but, in some cases, overlapping skills. It is important, for example, that nurses can carry out therapeutic regimes instigated by physiotherapists as part of their nursing care. Well co-ordinated 'seam-free' care is obviously in the patient's best interest, but for this to be assured there must be clear channels of communication and decision making among the team. A common multidisciplinary care plan, or some other source document where plans and decisions are recorded will help to co-ordinate the work of the team. The nurse is ideally placed to undertake this co-ordinating role and if this responsibility is actively pursued, the efforts of other team members have the best chance of success.

There may, of course, occasionally be conflict among team members. This most often arises out of the need to plan the patient's discharge from hospital. Team members may place different emphases on safety issues and doctors in particular will be conscious of the demand on hospital beds of acutely ill people. The differing viewpoints of team members should be expressed in regular team meetings and the eventual decision taken in the patient's best interest. Resolution of team conflict will be aided by good communication and a flexible and innovative approach to problem-solving.

DISCHARGE/TRANSFER FROM HOSPITAL

Planning for discharge should begin early in hospital treatment. The nurse is in a good position when establishing goals with the patient to find out her wishes vis-à-vis returning to the community, and she or he must try to judge, along with other members of the team, whether or not the patient is realistic in her plans for the future. Many people will be involved in returning the patient to her own home or to some other residential accommodation, but it is vital that all arrangements are co-ordinated and that one person has an overall view; the nurse may be the best person to fulfil that role, because of her extended contact with the patient.

STANDARD CHECKLIST

In planning for discharge, it may be useful to follow a standard checklist. McFarlane and Castledine (1982) discuss the use of standard care plans and point out that it goes against the philosophy of individualized care planning. However, they also argue that it helps to establish safe and helpful routines of nursing care. The value of a standard discharge checklist is that it provides a visible record of arrangements made or to be made and reduces the risk of patients being sent home from hospital with inadequate preparation. It can be particularly useful for those wards that are not used to making the complicated arrangements for discharge normally associated with dedicated geriatric ward patients.

Any checklist should include the following items, with room for indicating special arrangements, names of contact persons and the signature of the nurse responsible:

1. The patient's family/friends to be informed.
2. The home is to be prepared, i.e. clean and warm, food and drink available.
3. Access to the home to be confirmed, i.e. key available or someone already present.
4. Transport to be arranged.
5. All clothes and property to be given back to patient.
6. Occupational therapy assessment carried out in hospital.
7. Occupational therapy assessment carried out at home or in simulated environment.
8. All aids or home adaptations to be provided or completed.
9. All medicines or dressings to be provided.
10. The patient or carer to be instructed (with some check for understanding) in:
    a. the taking of medicine
    b. treatment
    c. exercises
    d. prosthesis/appliance functioning.
11. Community services to be arranged:
    a. home help
    b. meals-on-wheels
    c. community nurse
    d. other.
12. Follow-up appointment to be made with or without transport.
13. General practitioner (family doctor) to be informed of discharge.

This checklist is not exhaustive and the nurse will need to liaise closely with social workers, health visitors and various other professionals, depending on local arrangements and the level of service provision available. It is also useful if the patient is provided with the name, address and telephone number of someone to contact should services not begin as arranged. Service provision may also be precarious at weekends and on public holidays and the nurse should bear this in mind when arranging the patient's transfer to community care.

CONCLUSION

ETHOS OF THE GERIATRIC UNIT

The overall ethos of the geriatric unit should not be ignored. For many elderly people whose hold on independent living is tenuous, a sudden crisis resulting in hospitalization can be a major life event of enormous proportions. In the acute phase of their illness they should receive all the necessary diagnostic and therapeutic treatments which are available for younger patients. However, the elderly patient's resistance to the negative effects of institutionalization should not be overestimated and the nurse is in a key position to protect the patient. Depersonalization can occur in several ways. The mode of addressing patients for example, can reveal something of the nurse's attitude towards them and can also convey something of their perceived social worth. Consider the relative merits of 'Hello, Granny' and 'Hello, Miss Frankland'. The use of first names by nurses and patients should be a matter for individual negotiation.

Depersonalization can also occur by material means. One often sees in institutional environments a misuse of articles for other than their original purpose, e.g. saucers used as ashtrays or cups used as sugar basins. This can convey the message to the patients that they are not worth the provision of the proper item. Routinization also encourages depersonalization. Whilst in any institution certain routines are essential, such as the provision of meals at specific times, other routines, e.g. bathing, getting up, going to bed, going to the toilet, are often instituted for staff convenience rather than for the patients' benefit.

The wearing of hospital garments is another means whereby the person is stripped of personal identity. Unless the patient is acutely ill and confined to bed, there is no justification for wearing nightclothes during the day. Indeed, valuable dressing skills may be lost by such a practice.

However, if elderly patients are to wear their own clothes, then some suitable means of laundering will have to be provided for those patients without relatives, and a personal clothing service would need to be installed for a long-stay unit.

The absence of personal possessions may also have a deleterious effect on the elderly patient. Holzapfel (1982) suggests that being able to surround oneself with familiar items such as pets, albums and heirlooms not only provides a sense of continuity with the past in a new environment, but also serves as a means whereby one can review one's life constructively. In an acute hospital setting, it may not be possible to accommodate large items of furniture but patients could be encouraged to keep photographs and small keepsakes by their beds. In a continuing care establishment every effort should be made to provide as homely an atmosphere as possible.

REFERENCES

Andrews J, Atkinson L 1982 Ward furniture equipment and patient clothing. In: Coakley D (ed) Establishing a geriatric service. Croom Helm, London

Bagnell W E, Datta S R, Knox J, Horrocks P 1977 Geriatric medicine in Hull: a comprehensive service. British Medical Journal 3: 102

Bailey R 1982 The hospital unit. In: Coakley D (ed) Establishing a geriatric service. Croom Helm, London

Beck C 1981 Dining experiences of the institutionalised aged. Journal of Gerontological Nursing 7: 104–113

Boyer N, Christy Chuang J, Gipner D 1986 An acute care geriatric unit. Nursing Management 17(5): 22–25

Clancy K 1975 Preliminary observations of media use and food habits of the elderly. Gerontologist 13: 329–532

Clarke M, Wakefield L M 1975 Food choices of institutionalised vs independent living elderly. Journal of American Dietetic Association 66: 600–604

Davies A D M, Peters M 1983 Stresses of hospitalisation in the elderly: nurses' and patients' perceptions. Journal of Advanced Nursing 8: 99–105

Delong A J 1970 The micro-spatial structures of the older person: some implications of planning the social and spatial environment. In: Pastalan L A, Carson D H (eds) Spatial behaviour of older people. University of Michigan, Ann Arbor

Devas M B, Irvine R E 1963 The geriatric orthopaedic unit. Journal of Bone and Joint Surgery 418: 630

Devas M B, Irvine R E 1969 The geriatric orthopaedic unit. British Journal of Geriatric Medicine 6: 19

Department of Health and Social Security 1972 Minimum standards in geriatric hospitals. DHSS, London

Department of Health and Social Security 1976 Priorities for health and personal social services in England. HMSO, London

Department of Health and Social Security 1978 A happier old age. HMSO, London

Dubrovkis V, Wells D 1988 Hip fracture in the elderly. Canadian Nurse (May): 20–22

Fielding P 1986 Attitudes revisited: an examination of student nurses' attitudes towards old people in hospital. Royal College of Nursing, London

Fielding P (ed) 1987 Research in the nursing care of elderly people. Wiley, Chichester

Garraway W M, Akhtar A J, Prescott R J, Hockey L 1980 Management of acute stroke in the elderly: follow-up of a controlled trial. British Medical Journal 281: 827

Goldsmith S 1976 Designing for the disabled. Royal Institute of British Architects, London

Hall M R P 1976 The assessment of disability in the geriatric patient. Rheumatology and Rehabilitation 15: 59–63

Holzapfel S K 1982 The importance of personal possessions in the lives of institutionalised elderly. Journal of Gerontological Nursing 8: 156–158

Jay P 1983 Choosing the best wheelchair cushion. Royal Association for Disability and Rehabilitation, London

Lawton M P 1970 Ecology and ageing. In: Pastalan L A, Carson D H (eds) Spatial behaviour of older people. University of Michigan, Ann Arbor

Lloyd P, Osborne C, Tarling C, Troup D 1981 The handling of patients: a guide for nurse managers. Back Pain Association and the Royal College of Nursing, London

Mahoney F I, Barthel D W 1965 Functional evaluation of the Barthel index. Maryland State Medical Journal 14: 61–65

McFarlane J, Castledine G 1982 A guide to the practice of using the nursing process. Mosby, London

Office of Health Economics 1987 Compendium of health statistics. OHE, London

Owen D 1976 In sickness and in health. Quartet Books, London

Pathy J 1982 Operational policies. In: Coakley D (ed) Establishing a geriatric service. Croom Helm, London

Royal College of Nursing and British Geriatics Society 1987 Improving care of elderly people in hospital. RCN Publications, London

Royal College of Physicians 1977 Report of the working party on medical care of the elderly. RCP, London

Schoening H A, Anderegg L, Beighstrom D, Fonda M,

Steinke N, Ulrich P 1965 Numerical scoring of self-care status of patients. Archives of Physical Medicine and Rehabilitation 46: 689–697

Sommer R, Ross H 1958 Social interaction on a geriatric ward. International Journal of Social Psychiatry 4: 128–133

Stewart C P U 1980 A prediction score for geriatric rehabilitation prospects. Rheumatology and Rehabilitation 19: 239–245

Tarling C 1980 Hoists and their use. Heinemann, London

Tate J W 1980 The need for personal space in institutions for the elderly. Journal of Gerontological Nursing 6: 439–449

Townsend P 1962 The purpose of institutions. In: Tibbets C, Donahue W (eds) Social and psychological aspects of ageing. Columbia University Press, New York, p 379

Walton M, Hockey L, Garraway W M 1978 How independent are stroke patients? Nursing Mirror 147: 56–58

Waters K 1986 Role recognition. Senior Nurse 5(5/6): 15–16

Wells T J 1980 Problems in geriatric nursing care. Churchill Livingstone, Edinburgh

CHAPTER CONTENTS

The importance for elderly people of living at home 497

Residential provision 498

Characteristics of institutions 500

The quality of long-term residential care 502
What residents want 504
What residents experience 505
Continuing care in hospital 507

Alternative care provision 509
Long-stay hospital or nursing home? 511

Nurse education in long-stay care 515

Conclusion 516

29

Continuing care in long-stay settings

Sally J. Redfern

This chapter looks at care of elderly people in long-term care institutional settings in the UK. It provides companion material to Chapter 30, which discusses choice and flexibility in long-stay settings from the residents' and their relatives' point of view. In this chapter we examine residential and nursing Homes in the state and private sectors and long-stay hospital provision. The improvements made over the last 40 years in geriatric medicine, and the rehabilitation of elderly people suffering from diseases originally thought to be the result of age alone and therefore not treatable, have not been mirrored in long-stay care. Departments of geriatric medicine in British general hospitals can claim great success in acute geriatrics, but we must look to other countries in Europe, such as Denmark, for models of good practice in long-stay care.

THE IMPORTANCE FOR ELDERLY PEOPLE OF LIVING AT HOME

Most old people live in ordinary housing in the community and, in spite of inadequate facilities, they want to stay there (Sinclair 1988). They do not want to be 'put away' in a Home and lose their own home, which would mean loss of identity, privacy and control. Living at home, perhaps alone and lonely, is regarded by many old people as preferable to a Home where one has to live with 'strangers' and surrender one's personal privacy

(Peace 1988). Peace encapsulates the importance and complexity of living in one's own home:

Home is essentially a private place — the centre of domesticity but also a place for intimacy, for solitude, a place from which to gain strength to engage in the public sphere . . . a place where we are in control, where we can permit or deny access. It is a defensible space. . . . [H]ome means people and their relationships. . . . [H]ome has associations with family and related memories, particularly true for older women, for whom home is very much their domain; they feel competent in a familiar environment where disability may appear unremarkable; . . . [home] gives them a sense of control in a world which devalues them, and they find they can trade-off some of the costs of remaining at home by recognising some of the comforts (p. 219).

Only about 6% of the elderly population (over-65 year olds) live in residential or nursing Homes or in hospitals, but with advancing age the likelihood of living in such settings increases, and reaches some 13% of those aged over 85 years (Peace 1988). The numbers of old people over 75 years living in different forms of long-stay care in 1984 are shown in Table 29.1.

Table 29.1 Number of elderly people aged over 75 years in different institutional settings, England and Wales. *From Sinclair (1988).*

	1984 number per 1000 aged over 75
Hospital: geriatric beds	17.1
Local authority Homes	34.5
Nursing Homes	7.6
Voluntary Homes	8.5
Private Homes	17.4

Over the last 10 years there has been a decline in this country in long-stay public-funded hospital beds and in local authority residential care provision, and a very steep rise in residential and nursing Home places in the private sector.

RESIDENTIAL PROVISION

Even though most old people will live out their lives in their own homes, many others find themselves moving into a long-stay setting. Early research into the effects of relocation on the lives of elderly people concluded that relocation was hazardous since mortality was shown to increase during the initial months following admission to residential and nursing Homes (Lekan-Rutledge 1988). Later, however, more methodologically rigorous research has shown that the effect of relocation on mortality is minimal and other factors can mediate the negative consequences of environmental change. Important amongst these other factors are the extent to which the old person was prepared for the change and whether the move was voluntary or involuntary (Lekan-Rutledge 1988). If the elderly person felt she had no choice or control over the relocation decision, then anxiety, depression and apathy may result; but if involved and thoroughly prepared for the change, then the effects of relocation may be altogether more positive.

Until recently in this country, if an old person was unable to remain in her own home (even with social and nursing services), then her options were limited. She might enter a local authority residential Home (Part III Home) or a long-stay geriatric or psychogeriatric bed in hospital, unless she could afford a place in a private sector Home or had access to a Home run for retired employees and their wives enjoyed by some occupational groups. Recently, the growth of residential and nursing Homes in the private sector has mushroomed, and a proportion of old people without private means are living in private Homes but with financial support from the state.

The original purpose of Part III accommodation, as developed under the National Assistance Act of 1948, was to provide Homes along the lines of hotels in which residents were guests who had chosen to live there (Sinclair 1988). However, the hotel concept soon dissappeared as hospital doctors increasingly took control over admissions to Part III Homes in order to cope with the problem of old people 'blocking' hospital beds needed for acute medical cases. Sinclair (1988) refers to Townsend's (1962) survey which reported physical and organizational shortcomings of Part III Homes and which questioned whether they should exist at all because most of the residents wanted to and could be maintained in their own homes with the support of state domiciliary services. Unfortunately, state domiciliary services have not increased sufficiently to achieve Townsend's recommendation, and instead residential provision in the private sector has expanded. Yet the provision of residential and nursing Home care is lower in England and Wales (28.5 per 1000 over-65s in 1984) compared with West Germany (43.0) and the Netherlands (112.5), with the USA and Denmark falling between the German and Dutch figures (Sinclair 1988).

Even though most old people would prefer to remain at home, the increasing numbers of very old and very frail survivors in our population and the falling number of family members to look after them means that the 'need' for residential care is increasing. Sinclair identifies the trends that have contributed to this need:

- The growth in the elderly population — particularly the very elderly (those aged 85 or more).
- The consequent growth in the number of people who are very disabled or suffer from dementia
- The increase in the numbers of elderly people living alone (a group . . . particularly likely to apply for residential care)
- The falling pool of potential care givers (particularly women aged 40 to 49) relative to the numbers of elderly people (a marked trend since 1901, but recently reversing)
- The increasing proportion of women in this age group who work (in 1961, 44% of women aged 45–54 were according to official figures in work, a proportion which rose to 68% in 1981). (Sinclair 1988, p. 245)

Generally speaking, state provision for residential care for elderly people is higher in poorer parts of the country, and private provision is higher in richer areas and in the popular retirement areas of the south (Sinclair 1988). A coherent policy of community and residential care provision is extremely difficult to achieve because liaison and co-operation are required among the health authorities, housing authorities and social services, and also with the private sector, the voluntary sector and the official income support system. As places in long-stay hospital wards and local authority residential Homes decrease, community care provision (day care places, home helps, community nurses) must increase and must do so

before residential care can be reduced by an equivalent amount. Given the public expenditure cutbacks imposed on health and local authorities, it is not surprising that a major shift from residential to domiciliary services has failed to occur (Sinclair 1988).

Two government-initiated reports emerged at the same time which have major implications for the residential and continuing care services in England. The Wagner Report (1988) on residential care is heavily quoted in this chapter, together with its companion volume (Sinclair 1988), which reviewed the research literature as background to the recommendations made. The second paper is the Griffiths report on community care (Griffiths 1988), which did not receive a response from the government for some 16 months (Nursing Times 1989). Both reports recommend a leading role for local authority social service departments in the management of residential and community services.

The Wagner Report emphasizes consumer choice over whether to accept residential Home care and it recommends a trial period for newly admitted residents during which time their previous accommodation would remain available to them. It recommends that social workers should have prime responsibility for creating and co-ordinating packages of care suited to individuals. The report favours social work qualifications over nursing ones and recommends that all senior staff in residential Homes should have a social work qualification or undertake conversion training to acquire this. Not much mention is made of nursing Homes except with reference to elderly mentally infirm people. The recommendation is that nursing Home type facilities should be developed in association with residential Homes.

Another recommendation is that the registration and inspection system should be unified for residential and nursing Homes under the guidance of the then Department of Health and Social Security; with the subsequent separation of Health from Social Security this would now presumably be the responsibility of the Social Security Department.

The recommendations in the Griffiths report that have been endorsed by the government include the proposal that local authority social services departments should organize an assessment of need and individual packages of care in collaboration with family doctors and community nurses as required. The aim is to provide an efficient and co-ordinated service that allows old people to remain at home whenever possible. Funds will be allocated from local authority budgets, but will not be specifically earmarked for the purpose. This means that provision of care will vary markedly across the country according to local authorities' priorities and ability to pay. The Griffiths proposals will separate the social from the health and medical aspects of community care. Thus health workers (community nurses) employed by the health authorities will provide the 'health' and 'medical' components of the care, with social workers and the auxiliary force, based in the local authorities, providing the 'social' care.

Distinguishing in practice between 'health' and 'social' care is not easy in nursing generally but it becomes a nonsense when applied to continuing care. It is difficult to envisage how the co-ordination of health and social services will occur and how community nurses will retain their responsibility for the nursing care of old people at home. The Griffiths report has made an attempt to sort out the existing fragmented community care arrangements, but, as Helen Evers observes in Chapter 24, the demands on lay carers is likely to increase with consequent deterioration in the carer's, and possibly the elderly person's, health and quality of life. A government White Paper with details of the new proposals was published in autumn 1989, and the changes are scheduled to come into effect in 1991 (Secretary of State for Health, Social Security, Wales & Scotland 1989). Further discussion of these proposals can be found in Chapter 18 and 27 of this volume.

So far in this discussion, we have tended to lump residential Homes and nursing Homes in the state and private sectors together under the general rubric of residential care. Although elderly people who require continuing nursing care live in residential or nursing Homes, the proportion of those with severe disabilities in each does vary. The evidence suggests that there is greater disability amongst residents in local authority residential Homes than in private residential Homes, and al-though the severest disabilities are to be found in institutional rather than home settings, the greatest proportion of the very disabled live in long-stay hospitals and the few National Health Service nursing Homes that exist in Britain. Conversely, there is a small but significant number of old people living in hospital wards who do not require continuous nursing care and who are considered by the staff to be 'misplaced' (Wade et al 1983, Atkinson et al 1986, Wilkin & Hughes 1987, Sinclair 1988).

CHARACTERISTICS OF INSTITUTIONS

A considerable amount of research has been undertaken in Britain on life for old people in residential and nursing Homes in both the public and private sectors, but most of the attempts to develop a theoretical understanding of the residential process and its outcomes for elderly people have come from the USA (Willcocks et al 1987). In their review of residential life in local authority old people's Homes, Willcocks and her colleagues identified three research themes which they described as following interactionist, transactional and ecological perspectives. The first theme develops the 'total institutions' thesis of Goffman (1961), the second focuses on person–environment congruence (Kleemeier 1961, Pincus 1968, Kahana 1974), and the third on social ecology (Moos 1974, Lawton 1980).

Goffman (1961) identified characteristics of the total institution as:

- All aspects of life occur in the same place
- Each daily living activity occurs with a large number of people
- All daily activities are tightly scheduled and occur in orderly sequence
- All enforced activities are designed to meet the aims of the institution.

The total institution results in varying degrees of 'psychological extinction' where the emphasis is on discipline, rules, custodial care, and lack of choice.

One proposition is that a whole range of different institutions, set up with different objectives, have common features or can easily regress towards a common type where the differences in *aim* of, say, a long-stay prison, a monastery, psychiatric hospital or old people's home, become less significant than the fact that these are 'people processing organizations' which — sometimes as an accidental by-product of their organization, and sometimes deliberately — make an assault on individuality in order to create compliance to the institutional regime. (Fennell et al 1988, p. 140)

Since Goffman, researchers have looked for aspects of the 'total institution' in various settings (psychiatric hospitals, children's Homes, old people's Homes). One such study is King and Raynes' work in children's Homes (King et al 1971). They identified four institutional dimensions which varied in different settings:

• Depersonalization, providing few personal possessions and limited privacy
• Social distance between residents and staff
• Block treatment, characterized by queueing and batch processing of activities in orderly sequence
• Lack of variation in the daily routine.

These dimensions enabled the authors to describe the Homes they studied as 'institution oriented' or 'child oriented'.

Willcocks et al (1987) observe that the work of Kleemeier (1961) occurred at the same time as Goffman's and focused on psychological characteristics of residential settings for old people. Kleemeier identified three institutional dimensions in which different settings varied:

• Segregation/non-segregation, or the extent to which differentiation occurs between members and non-members
• Institutional control/non-institutional control, or the extent to which control is imposed on the resident
• Congregation/non-congregation, or the extent of batch activity and lack of privacy.

These dimensions formed the basis of Pincus' (1968) institutional dimensions in old people's Homes, described as public/private, structured/unstructured, resource sparse/resource rich and isolated/integrated. Pincus found discrepancies be-

tween the perceptions of staff and residents, and that different residents perceived the environment differently and wanted different things from it. It is important to appreciate that individual perceptions and wishes will vary but that a good match between individual needs and the environment is a significant determinant of morale (Kahana 1974).

The 'environmental docility hypothesis' developed by Lawton (1980) suggests that 'competent' individuals are less influenced by environmental factors than less competent people. This suggests that increasingly frail old people will require a more supportive environment, although it may also mean that an over-supportive environment might exert too few demands on the person, resulting in apathy, submissiveness and boredom.

The work described here on characteristics of institutions provided the basis to the model developed by Willcocks et al (1987) on differences between residential Homes and their effects on elderly residents. In their study of 100 residential Homes, Willcocks and her colleagues identified four dimensions that varied from Home to Home:

• Choice/freedom in residents' lifestyle and daily routine
• Privacy, both personal and in interaction with others
• Involvement in the organization of the Home
• Engagement/stimulation, i.e. staff encouragement of autonomy and independence of residents.

High scores on all these dimensions indicated a relatively progressive style of organization in the Home. The authors found that in the 100 Homes, the degree of choice was on average quite high; privacy and engagement received medium ratings; and involvement was very low.

A Norwegian study of nine nursing Homes revealed a variation in social climate and care provision according to the size of the Home and the leadership priorities of the head of the Home (Slagsvold 1987). The Homes were classified into four types — 'the geriatric hospital', 'the rehabilitation institution', 'the extended family' and 'the guest home' — which corresponded to the degree of medical care, rehabilitation, social contact and personal freedom encouraged by the head of the Home. Slagsvold observed that none of the Homes fulfilled the official guidelines for nursing Homes in Norway and a synthesis of these four types of care in each Home was recommended.

Much of the research evidence suggests that the residential environment itself promotes negative consequences for residents (Booth 1985). It is not unusual to hear staff of Homes or relatives of newly admitted residents comment on how rapidly the old person 'went downhill'. As indicated with the relocation research, it seems that loss of independence, personal autonomy, control and self-help can cause rapid deterioration in previously alert and active old people. There is no doubt that nearly everyone experiences decline in some aspects of physical and psychological functioning as they grow old, and although the impact of any single deficit may be small, the combined effects of many losses may induce feelings of lack of control and helplessness. Seligman (1975) first described the syndrome of 'learned helplessness' from his research with animals. Later, Schulz and his colleagues demonstrated the syndrome in different groups of people, including old people who moved into nursing Homes (Schulz & Brenner 1977, Schulz 1980). Learned helplessness arises when people lose control over events that happen to them. They lose motivation, becoming passive, intellectually slow and socially impoverished. They develop cognitive problems, experiencing difficulty in realizing that their own actions can control outcomes; and they show a flattened emotion which is characterized by depression and a feeling of hopelessness (Robertson 1986).

The suggestion that the residential environment is responsible for over-dependence prompted the 'induced-dependency hypothesis':

[T]he more institutional regimes deny residents control over their own lives the more they tend to foster their dependency. (Booth 1985, p. 129).

Booth made a detailed test of the induced dependency hypothesis in residential Homes, using more rigorous research methods than had been applied to earlier studies. He classified 175 residential Homes into those with 'progressive', client-oriented regimes, those with 'restrictive', institu-tion-oriented regimes, and those with 'mixed' regimes in which some aspects were progressive and others restrictive. He found no support for the induced dependency hypothesis, in that the dependency level of residents in the restrictive regimes was not significantly higher than that of the progressive regimes. The same finding occurred even when he compared the 'very progressive' with the 'very restrictive' regimes.

Although restrictive regimes in residential Homes cannot be claimed to induce dependency, it is likely that the quality of the residents' lives will be enhanced in Homes which have progressive and individualized styles of care, even though the ideal institution may not equal living at home. For example, the ideal Home would allow residents genuine choice, freedom and privacy, would have a minimum of rules and regulations, would be rich in facilities and resources, and would have open access to the world outside. The negative features characteristic of institutionalization, as described in the literature reviewed above, would be avoided, and the likelihood of residents sinking into a state of learned helplessness as a consequence would be minimized. In theory, residents should be able in such conditions to retain and develop, if desired, their capacity for 'learned resourcefulness' (Rosenbaum 1983) or they might win back some lost autonomy. Some residents, paradoxically, may *choose* a state of seeming 'helplessness' rather than 'resourcefulness', a choice that may be a disguised way for them to retain autonomy. There is scope here for more probing research of the 'dependency hypothesis'.

THE QUALITY OF LONG-TERM RESIDENTIAL CARE

Old people's homes are wells of loneliness. For the most part, relationships between residents are about the same as those found in a bus queue. (Booth & Bilson 1988, p. 45)

This conclusion came from a survey of residential Homes for elderly people in Fife, Scotland, which found that loneliness, isolation and depression, frequently intensified by bereavement or loss, were the main reasons for admission to a residential Home (Booth & Bilson 1988).

It is important to elicit the views of residents when trying to establish their quality of life, but much research has ignored interviewing residents because of the inappropriateness for elderly people of standardized interview-based questionnaire schedules and their reluctance to convey their true feelings, especially if they feel negative towards their carers. Wilkin and Hughes (1987) argue strongly for small-scale qualitative studies, which are successful in exploring residents' feelings through in-depth interviews. They succeeded in doing this with residents in six local authority residential Homes. They found a complex mixture of somewhat contradictory feelings — 'gratitude, resentment, resignation, powerlessness, acceptance and dependence'. Most of the residents were bored and lonely, which reflects a poor quality of life, but most accepted this as an inevitable consequence of the forced choice between the battle for survival and independence in their own homes, and equally unpleasant dependence in the institution. It seems unlikely that such an overwhelming sense of resigned acceptance of one's lot will be tolerated by future generations of residents, whose memories will not reach back to the Victorian workhouse.

Horrifying stories of maltreatment of vulnerable elderly residents of old people's Homes have been prominent in the national press over recent years in Britain, and confirmed by the Wagner Report (1988). Some of the reports refer to the unprecedented boom in private residential Homes as a result of the Government's policy of 'community care' for the elderly within the framework of its wider 'privatization' policy. This encouraged unqualified and frankly uncaring people, who anticipated the profits to be made, to set up as proprietors of private residential Homes (see e.g. Halliley 1987). Although admitting that there are many well-run Homes, Halliley's journalistic survey of private Homes in Kent, in south-east England, revealed many instances of verbal abuse, filthy conditions, physical restraint, unheated bedrooms, forceful sedative consumption and harmful

treatment of gangrenous sores (with talcum powder). At best, he found the level of care to be limited and unimaginative:

The typical scene in such homes is of a sparsely furnished lounge fringed with institutional armchairs in which residents pass the day in unattended torpor, unenlivened by the television blaring relentlessly from one corner. (Halliley 1987, p. 4).

It would be wrong to single out the private residential sector as the only setting in which abuse occurs. It has also been found in this country in local authority residential Homes, even where nursing staff are qualified, caring and hardworking. The widely reported scandal of Nye Bevan Lodge, a local authority residential Home in the London borough of Southwark, demonstrates that high stress levels for staff may lead to a situation in which 'elderly, often confused residents are made to eat their own faeces, left unattended, physically manhandled, forced to pay money to care staff and even helped to die' (Vousden 1987, p. 18).

In this case, stress was generated by inadequate training for staff in managing and running a Home. Difficulties for staff are identified by Martin (1984) as important factors in the breakdown of effectiveness in social institutions. His analysis of public enquiry reports into abuses, particularly in long-stay hospitals, showed that the arduous, underpaid and undervalued nature of the work tended to cut staff off from society so that they became as 'institutionalized' as the residents, resulting in self-protection, dishonesty and victimization. In these circumstances not all nurses are able to reconcile the conflict they must experience between being an agent of the institution and acting successfully as the resident's advocate.

There is no doubt that the burgeoning private sector in residential care provision has caused growing concern in Britain about standards of care for elderly and disabled people. In 1984, the Registered Homes Act was passed as a result of this growing concern, which empowers local councils and district health authorities to inspect residential and nursing Homes. The Act enables authorities to refuse or cancel registration or to impose conditions designed to improve standards (e.g. concerning staff, accommodation and resident numbers). The Act also set up a Registered Homes Tribunal which hears appeals by proprietors of Homes against a decision made by the authorities. At the same time, a code of practice for residential care, 'Home Life', was published by the Centre for Policy on Ageing (1985), and was endorsed by the Secretaries of State for England and Wales but which was not given the force of law.

The first 96 decisions made by the Registered Homes Tribunal have been published (Harman & Harman 1989). The authors conclude that the Act is not sufficiently detailed or clear to ensure consistent decisions and unambiguous standards in all Homes. There was particular concern that where there was doubt about the suitability of a proprietor to run a Home, it was the proprietor who was given the benefit of the doubt, not the residents.

The Wagner Report (1988) recommends that local authority, voluntary and private residential and nursing Homes should be subject to the same system of registration and inspection. Further, the Report recommends that national guidelines for inspection should be set up by the Government concerning standards of accommodation, qualifications of management and staff and quality of life of residents.

Tarbox's (1983) research in nursing Homes in Texas may help us to recognize where abuse can occur and that simple environmental changes can enrich the quality of life for residents. He identified neglect concerning the physical environment, nutrition and diet, physical appearance of residents, infantilization, environmental and social deprivation, and what he termed 'abuse by benign neglect', in that the care was impersonal and mechanistic rather than blatantly malicious. Tarbox attempted to enrich the environment and to minimize infantilization by introducing simple activities for residents — games, cards, a record player, a bulletin board, personalized clothing, and beer with biscuits and cheese at 14.00 h. Within a month he had observed significant changes: drug dependency was reduced, incontinence and agitated behaviour had decreased significantly and social responsiveness had mark-

edly increased. Tarbox attributed these improvements to the residents being treated with dignity and as responsible individuals. He also identified the importance of improving the education of nursing Home staff.

WHAT RESIDENTS WANT

We should not underestimate the difficulties facing staff of residential and nursing Homes in providing the environment that residents want; that is, one that offers security and freedom from worry yet also the autonomy, choice and control that is enjoyed when living in one's own home. It is not easy, in fact, to be certain of what residents really do want. As Sinclair (1988) observes, it is difficult to get an accurate picture of residents' views because they tend to express satisfaction with their Home, either through a reluctance to complain because of fear of reprisal, or because they cannot envisage any alternative. Also, residents do not all want the same thing and what they say they want may be different from what caring and sensitive staff feel may give them the greatest comfort.

Notwithstanding the difficulties, the research that Sinclair reviewed gives the following general picture of residents' preferences. They appreciate being looked after, the physical security provided and being free of the worries experienced previously when struggling to cope at home. However, they want a certain amount of independence and control over important aspects of their lives. Fear of losing this control is the principal reason for being reluctant to move into a Home. They want control over choosing their companions, having privacy when they want it, having a room of their own that can be used during the day, and being able to control their own immediate environment (such as opening or closing the window and turning the heating on or off). A finding that emerged from the large-scale critique of residential life in local authority old people's Homes (Willcocks et al 1987) was that most of the residents who expressed a preference said they actually *liked* their chairs to line the walls of communal sitting rooms rather than to be placed in small, sociable groups, a finding that was at odds with the preference of Clark and Bowling's

(1989) residents for small groups. The residents in the Willcocks study may not have wanted to be sociable with other occupants of the small group in which they found themselves. Being a reluctant member of a small group that they did not choose is perhaps less attractive than the anonymity generated by a large group of 'strangers'. Other concerns, such as choosing the wallpaper and paint in their bedrooms and having a resident's committee were desired by only a minority of the residents in the Willcocks study. They valued company and activities of their own choice, especially receiving their own visitors. Yet they were often lonely and bored, feelings that were not relieved by activities arranged for them. Their loneliness often reflected the loss of people close to them and they tended to have no solutions for overcoming this.

WHAT RESIDENTS EXPERIENCE

To the outsider, the daily routine of the residents' lives conveys the impression of inactivity, apathy, lack of stimulation and a low quality of life (Wilkin & Hughes 1987, Sinclair 1988). Most of the time that is not occupied in necessary daily living activities is spent in doing nothing or in sedentary pursuits, like knitting, reading, writing letters or watching television. The daily routine consists of getting up, probably too early and in too much of a rush, eating, sitting, going to the toilet, dozing and going back to bed. Residents who help others, occupy themselves with chores or go out to the shops, the park or the pub are exceptions. In some Homes, residents are not allowed to return to their rooms during the day and so virtually the whole day is spent in public. In contrast, Homes with inadequate communal space are criticized for leaving residents isolated in their rooms.

Nursing and medical care has been criticized not only in the newsworthy scandals reported earlier but also in research studies. Sinclair (1988) refers to horrifying examples of inhumane nursing practice with respect to bathing, toileting and dressing. Few residents receive necessary physiotherapy, specialist services, (such as those for the blind or deaf) or occupational therapy.

Criticism of medical care is largely confined to drug mismanagement: polypharmacy with result-

ant side-effects and overprescribing, particularly of psychotropic drugs. Wade and her colleagues (1983) found that 13% of old people living at home received four or more drugs, compared with about 22% in local authority and private residential Homes, 35% in hospitals and voluntary residential Homes, and 47% in private nursing Homes. Psychotropic drugs were received by 18% of elderly people living at home, compared with 37% in local authority residential Homes, about 45% in voluntary and private residential Homes and hospitals, and an alarming 78% in private nursing Homes. It seems that current concerns about over-medication and iatrogenic disease have not reached the private nursing Home sector to any great extent.

The observer's view of residents' lives as being unacceptably routinized, unstimulating and unnatural is not necessarily shared by the residents. Sinclair's (1988) review of the literature did not reveal that lack of choice, for example, is necesssarily associated with resident dissatisfaction, and, as we have seen, the restrictiveness of the regime is not always associated with functional dependence (Booth 1985). Some residents may want to be waited on for the first time in their lives, and not have to make decisions or choices.

An increase in resident satisfaction was claimed by enthusiastic staff and researchers who together set up small group living units in which residents were encouraged as far as possible to fend for themselves. But more recent research has suggested that residents in these units are less satisfied with their lives than those in conventional Homes, and that their functional abilities do not increase (Sinclair 1988). The provision of small group living units is an effort to reduce loneliness and to encourage friendships among residents. However, the small units do not seem to have been successful in removing the hotel lounge atmosphere of the public spaces in residential Homes, except in the rare instances when close friendships are made. Mostly, relationships are formed at the level of acquaintance only, and residents identify the staff as being more important to them than other residents. Having their own visitors who are members of their family or are friends from the past are more important to them and cannot be replaced by other residents, staff, or volunteer visitors (Sinclair 1988). As Sinclair observes, the turnover of residents through death or hospital admission is fairly high (20–30% of residents die within a year of admission to residential Homes) and so residents may avoid developing a close friendship and be spared the grief of loss should the friend die first.

The mix of residents will affect the atmosphere of the Home and the attitudes of the residents and staff within it. One major concern has been the extent to which confused residents should be mixed with the more lucid. In an early study, Meacher (1972) argued strongly against segregation because it promoted antisocial and aggressive behaviour by the confused residents, and encouraged inhumane practices by staff, such as restraint by sedation and infantilizing procedures. Notwithstanding Meacher's views, confused people are cared for in mixed and segregated settings, with psychiatric and geriatric hospitals providing most of the segregated care. Even so, most residential and nursing Homes contain some confused residents (Sinclair 1988). Sinclair refers to research by Evans et al (1981) which recommended that the proportion of confused residents in a Home should not exceed 30% because then the staff would have to resort to poor practices (such as toileting residents in batches or encouraging incontinence by not toileting them at all). However, Sinclair does not altogether agree with this 30% criterion. He feels that a low staff ratio relative to high resident dependency is the critical factor leading to poor care, rather than the proportion of confused residents. Although confused residents are more likely to present difficulties in their management, staff often prefer caring for them, possibly because they are more malleable and childlike and respond to the staff's parenting approach to caring.

The number of staff in residential Homes and their approach to the work are generally regarded as crucial to the quality of the residents' lives (Sinclair 1988). Local authority Homes have an officer in charge, who usually has a nursing or social work qualification, and supervisors, care assistants and domestic staff. The supervisors are occupied mainly with drug administration, paperwork and residents' social activities, and have little time to

help with the bathing, dressing and toileting duties that form the bulk of the care assistants' work. Preparing food, washing up and cleaning are carried out by the domestic staff. It is the care assistants who tend to be extremely busy with a workload that is often heavy, dirty and exhausting. They are expected to encourage residents to do things for themselves, but this takes longer than doing everything for them, and residents do not always want to look after themselves. There is no doubt that some Homes have insufficient staff to give adequate care to residents; and care assistants have neither the training nor the experience to introduce rehabilitation programmes which might reduce resident dependence. Sinclair (1988) feels strongly that resident dependency is essential to the calculation of staffing requirements if a satisfactory standard of care is to be provided. Although we do not disagree with this, it would nonetheless be unfortunate if the converse were accepted, that is, if necessary staffing requirements were deemed to be lower for residents assessed as less dependent because they can do some things for themselves. Encouraging self-care is a slow, time-consuming business which takes much more effort and patience than doing everything for the resident — which, though exhausting, can at least be done quickly. The standard scales which are often used to assess dependency do not identify which residents require more rather than less time from staff in order to retain their level of independence.

Residential Homes in the voluntary and private sector are likely to have worse staffing ratios than local authority Homes (Sinclair 1988). Often these Homes have a small number of residents, and the proprietor is directly involved, providing night as well as day cover in order to reduce costs. This overtime may be extensive and result in proprietor 'burn out' (Sinclair 1988).

A dilemma facing heads of both state and private Homes is whether they should continue to look after residents whose health deteriorates, or whether they should be transferred to hospital care. Another option is for the residential Home to acquire dual registration as a nursing Home; this would make it subject to much more stringent staffing requirements and regulations. Many residential Homes continue to care for deteriorating residents even though they cannot provide adequate care, because the resident does not want to be moved. A solution would be to call in community nurses to provide additional support and specialist care, but the evidence suggests that community nurses do not give priority to old people in residential Homes. Nursing care should be available as and when it is needed, whether the old person is living at home or in a residential Home (Nisbet 1987).

Summarizing the provision of residential care, the review of the evidence collected for the Wagner Report (Sinclair 1988) drew the following conclusions:

- Most elderly people would prefer sheltered housing to residential care if they cannot look after themselves at home.
- Even so, the provision of residential care places does not meet demand and this imbalance will increase given demographic trends. England and Wales have fewer residential places compared with other European countries.
- There has not been a shift of resources to community care and so widespread implementation of the policy to reduce the number and proportion of old people in residential care has not occurred. The reasons for this have been to do with difficulties of joint planning between the health and social services, restrictions on the funds necessary to expand domiciliary services, and incentives given to private residential provision.
- Private residential care has partly filled the gap left by the reduction in resources for public provision but has not concentrated on areas of greatest need.
- Most old people entering residential care are more able than many remaining in the community who receive comprehensive packages of care. Efforts to prevent admission to residential care should take account of strain on relatives at home and the urgent need for alternative accommodation for the frail old person who is homeless, or in a hospital ward or living in a relative's home.
- The quality of residential life can be assessed according to whether the care meets basic physical and medical needs; allows residents control over key aspects such as security of tenure, finance, privacy and physical environment; and prevents boredom and loneliness without imposing uncongenial company or activities. The extent to which these aspects are met is unknown but problems do occur with respect to:

    a. Physical care when the ratio of staff to very dependent residents is inadequate

    b. Medical care, e.g. management of drugs, incontinence, deafness

    c. Lack of security, privacy, choice

    d. Lack of interesting activities or failure to enable residents to pursue their own interests

    e. Provision of day care or relief care within a Home causing difficulties for staff and a poor standard of care for outside users.

- Methods of regulating Homes have only recently been developed and are hesitantly applied, at least to some Homes. There has been insufficient research into or trial of methods to improve the quality of Homes, such as providing greater professional support, or giving residents greater influence in Home affairs (e.g. advice services, codes of residents' rights, tenure, complaints procedures).

In conclusion, residential Homes for elderly people have a chequered history, and although some provide high standards of care and an environment in which we would be happy to end our days, there is no doubt that all is not well with many others. The rapid growth of Homes in the private sector means that regular inspection and quality control are difficult to achieve. Urgent attention should be given to raising the quality and training of staff so that an optimum balance can be found between the provision of safety and security and allowing the level of independence, choice and control which residents seek. Further discussion of choice and flexibility in long-stay settings can be found in Chapter 30 of this volume.

CONTINUING CARE IN HOSPITAL

In Britain, some enlightened health authorities have recognized the advantages of nursing Homes over hospital wards and are replacing their crumbling backwater wards with purpose-built Homes.

But, by and large, old people who require continuous nursing care from the state face the prospect of living out their lives in hospital.

As discussed by Helen Evers in Chapter 24, the organization of nursing elderly people in hospital is inextricably linked with that of geriatric medicine. Nursing has followed the lead of geriatric medicine and accords higher status to the high turnover acute geriatric service than to the very different skills required and the rewards of continuing care. Nursing, as reflected in the policies of the statutory bodies (e.g. the English National Board for Nursing, Midwifery and Health Visiting), does not seem to consider continuing care as an important part of the nurse's repertoire, since experience in long-stay wards is not a requirement in registered nurse training and, as a consequence, few registered nurses choose to work in continuing care. Like nurses in acute medical wards, nurses in elderly care wards support the energetic diagnosis–treatment–cure–discharge approach of medicine and so accord much higher priority to the 'successful' acute-career patient than the long-stay resident.

The published research on nursing care in geriatric wards presents a dismal picture, particularly for long-stay residents (Clarke 1978, Wells 1980, Evers 1981a, 1981b, Baker 1983 and see Chapter 24). Although nurses were observed to be caring and positively disposed towards the elderly patients, they tended to be over-protective and patronizing, and gave higher priority to getting the tasks done in a 'routine geriatric' (Baker 1983) or 'warehousing' (Evers 1981b) style than to planning and delivering individualized care. Fitting the care into the ward routine of mealtimes, medicine rounds, doctors' rounds, toileting or changing wet pads, getting up and going to bed was the nursing aim implicit in the research studies referred to here. Little was done for the patients outside physical tasks and the primacy of cure-work over care-work left the psychosocial needs of long-stay residents unfulfilled. Thus, the demeaning characteristics of institutions, as discussed earlier in this chapter, often predominated for the long-stay resident.

Helen Evers' research in geriatric wards demonstrates the importance of the consultant geriatrician and, following his or her lead, the ward sister, in determining the standard of care and well-being of long-stay patients:

For long-stay patients, the perceived legitimacy of the caring task in its own right, within the curative ethos of the hospital, was related to the type of care patients received. Unintended suffering and inhuman treatment was markedly less in wards where the consultants subscribed to the importance of care-work, carried this belief through into their own work with long-stay patients, as well as acknowledging and actively supporting the primacy of the nursing role in care-work. The nurses — most importantly, the ward sisters — working with these consultants carried out their work in a distinctive style. They were more likely to make concerted efforts to care for patients as individuals than as work objects and sets of tasks to be accomplished. Despite similar staffing levels, in wards where 'batch processing' and a view of care-work as low status and second-rate prevailed, patients' sufferings as a consequence were observed to be more common. (Fennell et al 1988, p. 157).

Being nursed in traditional task-oriented wards, in comparison to wards where the care is individualized, is positively unhealthy for old people whose hospital stay exceeds one month (Miller 1984, 1985a, 1985b). Although this is not the case for short-stay elderly patients, Miller found that the longer-stay patients in traditional wards were more dependent, more incontinent (urine and faeces), had slower discharge rates and higher death rates than those in the individualized care wards. Nursing priorities in the traditional wards focused on speed and convenience for the staff, so that nurses discouraged slow self-care, slow eaters were often spoon-fed, and catheters were the solution to urinary incontinence.

The style of nursing in Miller's individualized care wards was quite different in that it followed a supportive–educative approach which encouraged self-care and the promotion of independence. The nurses in these wards spent more time talking with the patients, although the amount of physical care given did not exceed that in the traditional wards. In one ward, which changed from task-oriented to individualized care, Miller found that the patients became more independent even though medical policy, admissions and staffing levels remained much the same.

Evidence of iatrogenic disease has also been found in hospitals in the USA. Gillick et al (1982) examined 502 patients in general medical wards for side-effects of hospitalization that were unrelated to the diagnosis or treatment of acute illness. They found evidence of confusion, falling, not eating· and incontinence unrelated to the acute diagnosis in 9% of patients aged under 70 years, compared with 41% of patients over 70 years, a difference that was highly significant statistically. The rate of medical intervention in response to these symptoms (psychotropic drugs, restraints, nasogastric tubes, urinary catheters) was 38% for the younger patients and 47% for the older, a difference that was not statistically significant. The authors noted that these interventions carry a complication rate of 25–30%, which suggests that acute hospital care might not be the best alternative for these elderly people.

ALTERNATIVE CARE PROVISION

Given that the residential Home will continue to exist even if increasing numbers of old people are supported in their own homes, it follows that making the institutional setting as 'like home' as possible would be appreciated by residents. 'Normalizing' the Home could be helped by integrating it into its community as an open system and allowing residents control over their activities and choice of companions. They should be given the opportunity to go out shopping, to the park, pub, theatre, club, visit relatives and friends and have holidays as they wish. Achieving the 'normal' means accepting the risks of everyday life that we all face, which requires the staff of Homes to lessen their concern for too high a degree of security and protection. A Home where accidents never happen is probably too close to the 'total institution' for resident well-being.

Residential Homes have many untapped resources that could be used for the benefit of the surrounding community. Sinclair (1988) sees the Home as a potential resource centre which could: provide the base for the meals-on-wheels service; be the communal centre for sheltered housing complexes; provide short-term assessment apartments with vacancies for emergencies; and provide day care and short-term residential care as well as the conventional long-stay care. More staff are needed in sheltered housing and closer liaison is necessary with community nurses.

Tenants' rights should be explicit, with contracts drawn up and agreed on admission, signed by the tenant, her lawyer and the manager of the Home, which specify exactly what the resident can expect from the Home (Nisbet 1987). Annual reviews should be standard practice so that the resident's changing needs can be considered.

Short-stay residential care is often arranged primarily to give the carer at home a rest rather than to meet any needs the old person may have. Some old people appreciate the change but others do not, and the attitudes of the Home staff and the permanent residents towards the short-stay resident are not always favourable. Important though the short-stay is in terms of the respite it gives the carer at home and the preservation of the carer's mental health (Sinclair 1988), it could also do much more for the elderly person. For example, the opportunity could be taken to make a comprehensive nursing and medical assessment and review the management of any problems; dental, chiropody, sight and hearing check-ups could be arranged; physiotherapy and occupational therapy could be given to meet rehabilitation needs; and the person's home could be assessed for needed improvements, which could be carried out while the old person was away. For the elderly person who is admitted to short-stay residential care on a regular basis (every six weeks or so), an energetic assessment and management programme of rehabilitation could be a continuing process both inside and outside the Home, during which evaluation and updating of the programme would be carried out regularly.

Given the necessary resources and motivation of the staff, all day centres could be raised to the standards of the most successful. These provide care, education and craft activities under the same roof, and bring in teachers from outside as required. The sessions arranged for exercise, music, art, crafts, reminiscence activities, etc. are stimulating, productive and therapeutic rather than organized merely as time-fillers. The successful centres do not engage the clients in mindless, purposeless activity, nor leave most of the old people in 'isolated inactivity' for most of the time (Godlove et al 1982). Combining day centres and day hospitals within the same complex would ensure simultaneous social and health care provision. This could be most successful as long as the complex avoided the temptation of becoming clinical. Further discussion of day centres and day hospitals can be found in Chapter 27 of this volume.

Some researchers have argued for the residential flatlet rather than expanding conventional residential Home provision (Willcocks et al 1987). The residential flatlet would offer private, personal territory, lockable from the inside and under firm control of the resident. It would provide a 'normal, unexceptional, non-institutional' home within the supportive environment of the institution. The accommodation would consist of a bed-sitting room with ample wheelchair and storage space, and a personal shower and toilet cubicle. Personal items of furniture could be installed and tea-making facilities provided. Meals would be taken in the communal dining room, although a nearby kitchenette should be available for residents and their visitors to prepare snacks. A public lounge would be available for communal activities and to encourage residents to meet each other. The value of the lockable flatlet rather than the conventional single room in a Home would give the resident a private as well as a public life. Furthermore, moving into a residential flatlet would be much more like moving house in the conventional sense than like the last move into a Home made so reluctantly by many old people.

An approach designed to maintain elderly frail people in their own homes — even if they are extremely dependent — is augmented home care. Enterprising home care support schemes have been designed for dependent elderly people in general (Challis & Davies 1988, Dant et al 1989) and dementia sufferers in particular (Askham & Thompson 1989). The Kent Community Care Project (Challis & Davies 1988) was set up as an attempt to provide alternative support to residential and long-stay hospital care. It was a complex project in which the Community Care Scheme was compared with standard service provision for matched groups of frail old people who were at the point of needing institutional care. Central to the Community Care Scheme was the appointment of social workers who acted as case-managers and were responsible for developing and maintaining individual packages of care for each old person, thus co-ordinating the necessary social and health services. This idea is similar to the key worker concept discussed by Ian Norman in Chapter 18, and also adheres closely to the recommendations of the Wagner Report (1988) and the Griffiths community care report (1988). The Gloucester project (Dant et al 1989) also identified key-workers as central to the success of the scheme. They demonstrated, too, the value of the biographical approach in assessing individual needs of old people (see Chs 1 and 18 for discussion of the biographical approach).

In the Kent project, individual field workers were drawn from the local community and were 'contracted' to provide the care required. These field workers had manageable caseloads and defined budgets that enabled them to find flexible and imaginative solutions to individual problems which would have been impossible for a centralized service to solve. Close links were made with the local health services, particularly with community nurses and the hospital geriatric unit. The scheme has been introduced in the south-east and north-east of England.

The results of the Kent project show clear advantages for the clients and their carers in receipt of the Community Care Scheme, compared with those who received standard care. Fewer problems remained intractable and unsolved; more old people remained in their own homes (about two thirds compared with one third in the control group); many more (39%) in the control group moved into residential Homes (compared with 1% of the Community Care group). However, the number admitted to long-stay hospitals was much the same. Indicators of quality of life and quality of care of the old people and their carers showed significant advantages for the Community Care group. It is interesting that the option involving receipt of standard services and remaining at home was the least effective in meeting individual needs (compared with receiving Community Care and remaining at home, or Community Care and entering institutional care, or standard services and entering institutional care). This confirms the failure of existing arrangements in the community to provide adequate care. The costs of the Community Care Scheme were not significantly different from those of the standard services.

The success of the Community Care Scheme suggests it could be an effective innovation for the care of old people with very different problems (physical, psychiatric, social and emotional) and who are living in different areas of the country. Askham and Thompson (1987) found, however, that only certain dementia sufferers could manage with augmented home support on a long-term basis. The demented person who is doubly incontinent, aggressive towards others or a constant wanderer is unlikely to be managed successfully at home. Challis and Davies (1988) underline the value of augmented home care which emphasizes decentralized control of resources and effective case-management at the individual level. They are convinced that their 'bottom-up' solution to the fragmentation of care rather than a 'top-down' approach is the key to the success of the scheme.

LONG-STAY HOSPITAL OR NURSING HOME?

There will always be a minority of elderly people who require continuing nursing care which cannot realistically be provided in their own homes or in residential Homes. The case for nurse-managed NHS nursing Homes is strongly advocated by nurses (e.g. Wade et al 1983, Baker 1983) and some doctors (Batchelor 1984), but other doctors are reluctant to lose control of long-stay beds (Millard 1988). The DHSS-sponsored research into the provision of care for old people in long-stay geriatric wards, residential Homes and private nursing Homes (Wade et al 1983) confirmed the inappropriateness of providing continuing care in geriatric wards, and recommended that most long-stay geriatric beds should be phased out. A few should be kept for medical and psychogeriatric assessment and short-term treatment, and for respite care to give families a rest. The authors recommended

that alternative provision should be in state-run nursing Homes in which care is organized along 'supportive model' lines as distinct from 'protective', 'controlled' or 'restrained' models. The supportive model follows closely the open system advocated earlier for residential Homes, and removes the organizational control, lack of resident choice and subordination to the care regime characteristic of the more restrictive models (see Ch. 30 for further discussion of these models).

The DHSS followed the Wade study by funding another major piece of research at the Health Care Research Unit, University of Newcastle (Bond 1984, Atkinson et al 1986, Bond & Bond 1987, Bond et al 1989a, 1989b). Three NHS nursing Homes headed by nurses were established in different areas of England to cater for the same kind of old person normally found in long-stay geriatric wards. The research compared the provision, effectiveness and costs of care and the experiences of the old people in these nursing Homes with those provided in the wards.

The methods of evaluation in the Newcastle research included:

- A randomized controlled trial in which residents in the three experimental NHS nursing Homes were compared with patients receiving continuing care in geriatric wards. The number of residents and patients who participated was 463.
- A multiple-case study of the provision of care in the three NHS nursing Homes and six geriatric wards. In all, 236 residents and patients were observed.
- Two surveys, carried out in 1984 and 1987, of all the continuing care institutions for elderly people within the catchment areas of the three NHS nursing Homes and within three adjoining health authorities. Some 246 Homes and wards were surveyed, which included 2313 residents and patients.
- A cost comparison of the three NHS nursing Homes, the six geriatric wards and other locations included in the randomized controlled trial.
- A survey of all qualified and unqualified nurses working in 15 Homes or wards. 296 nurses were interviewed.
- A survey of 114 relatives who visited residents

and patients in the NHS nursing Homes and the wards.

• An interview survey of 19 volunteers who worked in the NHS nursing Homes and the wards.

The results of the randomized controlled trial on the whole favoured the NHS nursing Homes. Personal well-being was greater for residents of two of the nursing Homes compared with their counterparts in the geriatric wards, although the results were inconclusive in the third Home. Consumer satisfaction was higher in all three Homes. The multiple-case study showed that, although there were differences between the NHS nursing Homes, they provided a more positive environment than that of the geriatric wards. The physical environment of the Homes was of higher quality, especially in the provision of single rooms for most residents. The Homes had more staff than the wards, particularly unqualified staff.

The surveys revealed considerable variation among health authorities in the provision of long-stay accommodation for elderly people. The NHS nursing Homes and the geriatric wards contained the highest proportion of very frail old people compared with residential and nursing Homes in the private sector and with local authority residential Homes. The NHS nursing Home residents were far more occupied in activities than were geriatric ward patients, and the relatives and volunteers favoured nursing Home care rather than hospital care.

The cost comparison showed that NHS nursing Homes were no more costly than NHS hospital accommodation, and were in fact likely to be cheaper:

In revenue terms alone, according to the various assumptions, a 30-bedded NHS nursing home at 100 per cent occupancy would cost a health authority between £72 000 less and £33 000 more per annum than its hospital equivalent (Bond et al 1989, p. 44).

The average cost per resident per week in the NHS nursing Home was £260, which was higher than the average of £215 in private nursing Homes. As the researchers make clear, however, judgement about the relative efficiency of private and NHS nursing Homes cannot be made without knowledge of the type of resident, the quality of care and the provision of care in each setting.

The recommendations that emerged from the Newcastle research are that NHS nursing Homes should be developed as continuing care accommodation and that physicians who are specialists in the care of old people should be responsible for identifying appropriate clients for all long-stay settings. Another recommendation is that research should be undertaken to evaluate the provision of care in the expanding private and voluntary sector.

The study confirmed previous research that old people prefer to live in their own homes. In view of this, the authors recommend further evaluation of non-institutional continuing care facilities, such as 'very sheltered housing' and augmented home care. The Kent Community Care Project (Challis & Davies 1988), described earlier in this chapter, is an example of the latter.

Some health authorities in England went ahead in establishing nursing Homes for the residents of their long-stay geriatric wards without waiting for the results of the Newcastle study. Clark and Bowling (1989) compared the quality of life of elderly residents in two NHS nursing Homes and a long-stay hospital ward. Their observations revealed more evidence of the 'total institution' in the ward than in the Homes, although the hospital's patients' Club, run by an occupational therapy aide, showed that total institution characteristics need not be an inevitable part of hospital life. The quality of life was more positive in the Homes than in the ward, and more positive in one Home than in the other, although there was room for improvement in the better Home too. Routines with respect to getting-up times, going-to-bed times and mealtimes existed in all three settings, although there was more flexibility in the Homes than in the ward.

Patients' requests were ignored and responses to them delayed to the greatest extent in the ward, although not in the Club. The quality of interaction among residents and between residents and staff or visitors was recorded as positive, neutral or negative. The greatest number of positive interactions observed was in the Club, but at only 36% of interactions even this was not high. There was no significant difference between the number of positive interactions across the settings, but the number of negative interactions was significantly higher in the ward and one Home than in the other Home and the Club.

Clark and Bowling (1989) emphasize the importance of encouraging nursing and care staff to take responsibility for organizing programmes of daily activity rather than relying on occupational therapy staff to do this. By taking this responsibility, nurses will increase their communication skills, which they cannot be expected to do successfully by being told merely to talk to the residents. There must be a focus for the conversation based on involvement in an activity chosen by the resident, which would allow communication skills to develop spontaneously. Clark and Bowling maintain that standards of care will continue at an inadequate 'warehousing' level until there is a change in attitude towards the medical and nursing care of old people. This change could occur irrespective of setting, although the less clinical environment of the nursing Home is more conducive to change than is the hospital ward.

Some geriatricians (e.g. Millard 1988) are critical of any move to replace long-stay hospital care with nurse-led units. The pioneering and admirable work done by progressive geriatricians to demonstrate that diseases of old people are treatable and not direct effects of ageing understandably makes them cautious of handing over the responsibility of any patient group to others. Millard (1988, p. 172–173) makes the following recommendations with respect to long-term care; his comments are annotated with our own views:

- Medical responsibility for local authority residential homes should be transferred to the hospital service.

At present, medical care of residents is the concern of the general practitioner (family doctor), who is often not a specialist in the medical care of old people. This may change in the future, now that all doctors receive postgraduate training before going into general practice.

- No one should be admitted to a local authority home or to a government-funded place in a private or voluntary home without prior in-patient assessment in the beds of the Department of Geriatric Medicine, in the District General Hospital.

We would agree with this as long as the assessment is truly multidisciplinary rather than medical alone.

- In those 42 health districts where there are no beds allocated to the Department of Geriatric Medicine in the District General Hospital, those beds should be provided as a matter of urgency.

This is important so that medical assessment, investigation and treatment facilities available for younger patients are equally available for the old. The District General Hospital is not, however, the place for the long-stay resident.

- All who are permanently accommodated in a long-term institution should have the right to be tended in single rooms with en suite washing and toilet facilities. All long-term residents should be able to keep personal belongings in their rooms.

We would go further than this and advocate that long-term residents should not live in hospitals, even if provided with a single room. The residential flatlet in a supportive environment advocated by Willcocks et al (1987) and discussed earlier, is preferable.

- Named (medical) consultants should have contractual responsibility for the standard of medicine *and care* in long-term care wards and residential homes. (parenthesis and emphasis added)

We would agree that physicians who are specialists in the medicine of old age (be they geriatricians or general practitioners) should be responsible for the medical care of residents. They should not, however, be responsible for nursing care which, for long-term residents, should emphasize all aspects of psychosocial and rehabilitative care, drawing on other therapist skills as necessary, rather than focusing on the diagnosis–treatment–cure approach of clinical medicine. Millard also advocates multidisciplinary teamwork but he sees the physician as the necessary leader of the 'team', to which the other members (nurses, physiotherapists, occupational therapists, dieticians, social workers, etc.) would report. This doctor-led approach is appropriate for the acutely ill elderly patient whose medical problems are treatable and who can be rehabilitated sufficiently to return home. Whilst the physician should be involved in the decision to move a patient to long-term care, the responsibility for that care in nursing Home settings should, we believe, be a nursing one.

If NHS nursing Homes are successful and the leadership responsibility for long-term nursing care becomes the nurse's, then geriatricians might be loathe to admit the elderly patient who may fail in the rehabilitation effort to reach a level which enables her to be discharged home. Loss of total control over long-stay beds might encourage the geriatrician to resort to a conservative admissions policy which guarantees no 'bed blockers' (Andrews & Brocklehurst 1987). Geriatrician control of long-stay beds has allowed an admissions policy which could afford the risk of a few 'failures'. Loss of control over long-stay beds might make elderly care wards indistinguishable from acute medical wards in terms of the treatment and care given. However, ensuring that geriatricians are closely involved in decisions to admit to nursing Homes should solve this dilemma. It would be a tragedy if geriatricians became specialists in acute medicine and abandoned their unique expertise in managing the multiple medical problems of old age. The trend in some geriatric units to adopt an age-related policy, in which the *sole* criterion for non-surgical admission is age (over, say, 75 years) is cause for concern. Inevitably the acutely ill, easily diagnosed and rapidly cured patient will take precedence over the slow-speed patient with multiple medical and social problems, who needs the time and skills of the specialist rehabilitation team to make a full or maximum recovery. Yet this is just the patient who has been the geriatric unit's success. We believe the criteria for admission to elderly care wards should include multiple health problems as well as age.

Some unique experimental schemes have been introduced which have questioned the need for a medically dominated, general hospital setting for patients who have progressed beyond the acute stage of their illness. The Clinical Nursing Unit at Burford Community Hospital near Oxford, England is one such scheme (Pearson 1983), and was extended to a second Unit in Oxford (Pearson 1988). The Clinical Nursing Unit (CNU) is based on the principles of the Loeb Center for Nursing and Rehabilitation in The Bronx, New York (Hall 1969). The CNU caters for the patient who is over the acute stage of illness and whose primary need is for 24-hour nursing care supported by medical treatment and paramedical therapy. The CNU therefore comes somewhere between the acute hospital ward and the nursing Home. Its aim is to provide the care necessary to enable the patient to return home or, failing that, to enter a nursing or residential Home.

The proposed clinical nursing unit serves to promote high quality nursing and, in doing so, the development of clinical nursing as a discipline through its practice, education and research. Its activities focus on nursing as a therapeutic agent — an assumption which fundamentally affirms the uniqueness of the unit. (Pearson 1983, p. 31).

As well as providing professional nursing care to people who do not require expensive medical and ancillary services, the CNU provides an opportunity for a professional career structure within clinical nursing. The nurses take full responsibility for the planning and management of the patients' care, and are fully accountable for the care they give. The unit is seen as a centre of excellence in which the quality of care is evaluated, educational programmes are installed, clinical nursing research is carried out and opportunities for career development within clinical nursing are promoted. Rather than bringing about the cessation of research into the clinical problems of the aged (which Millard (1988) fears will occur if medicine gives up responsibility for long-term care) the establishment of CNUs naturally fosters such research activity. The clinical problems of old age which are not amenable to rapid treatment or cure are just those that are the business of the CNU (e.g. immobility, falling, incontinence, pressure sores, leg ulcers, chronic depression, dementia).

The staff of the CNU consists of primary nurses who are independent nurse practitioners, registered associate nurses, care assistants and ward co-ordinators. The services of doctors, physiotherapists, occupational therapists, social workers and community nurses are available. The medical attachment to the unit can be hospital doctors or general practitioners (family doctors) who provide surveillance and treatment as necessary and act as medical consultants to the nurses. The other therapists act largely as advisers to the nurses and become involved in direct patient care only when specialist skills beyond the competence of the nurse are required. The organization of nursing follows a primary nursing approach (Pearson 1988). Primary nursing is described in Chapter 33 of this volume.

Another scheme introduced to provide care at a point intermediate between hospital and home is the Lambeth Community Care Centre in London (Wilce 1988). The initiative for the Centre was taken by the West Lambeth Community Health Council, whose members looked for an alternative to small community hospitals following the closure of Lambeth Hospital. They sought the opinions of local residents and primary health care workers, and the result was a creative architect-designed community care centre for inpatient and day-patient care, and a focal point for health care and educational activities for the local community. The Centre's management team is multidisciplinary, consisting of a senior nurse, an administrator, a therapist (who rotates six-monthly), a general practitioner (rotates six-monthly) and the chairperson of the Centre Advisory Group (CAG). The CAG consists of seven staff members and seven representatives of local people and patients. The chairperson is elected from the non-staff members. The work of the Centre is monitored and evaluated through regular audit meetings; education is a continuous process with student placements, interdisciplinary lectures and seminars, Look After Yourself Courses and a leaflet library.

The staff consists of general practitioners, nurses, therapists, local volunteers and health groups who together provide a comprehensive local primary health service. The patients are those who need skilled nursing and rehabilitation and whose medical care is within the competence of the family doctor. Some patients are in the terminal stages of illness and can be nursed close to their home and family. Others, who are chronically handicapped, can be admitted on a rotating basis to give the family carers a rest. Many, but not all of the patients are elderly people.

The nurses in the Centre act as key workers to the inpatients and practise primary nursing. It has

taken time for the nurses to shed their role as doctors' assistants and to develop the assertiveness necessary for equal team membership; but their self-confidence has grown and with it the confidence to encourage patient choice and autonomy, for example, in the self-administration of drugs. The central role that the nurse takes as the key worker puts her (or him) in an ideal position as the patient's advocate.

New schemes, such as NHS nursing Homes, the Clinical Nursing Units at Burford, Oxford and at Tameside in Manchester, England (Wright 1989), and the Lambeth Community Care Centre will, we hope, expand throughout the country. Nursing Development Units have been encouraged through the competitive funding initiative taken by Jane Salvage, Director of the nursing developments programme at the Kings Fund Centre in London (Nursing Times 1988). That initiative provided the pump-priming funds for four Nursing Development Units in England. These are in different specialties although all four involve elderly people (Heenan 1989). Pearson (1988) dreams of the development of clinical nursing units in all inpatient settings and in every hospital or health service neighbourhood in the country. Unfortunately, the motivation to change by nurses and like-minded pioneers from other professions will not succeed without the co-operation and commitment of the powerful controllers of scarce health service funds. The tragic closure of the Oxford Nursing Development Unit (Salvage 1989), mentioned also in Chapter 24, bears witness to this.

NURSE EDUCATION IN LONG-STAY CARE

We are convinced that the quality of nursing in long-stay hospital wards would be raised if these wards were included as a compulsory part of nursing students' training. At present in British nurse training, the long-stay setting is often considered unsuitable for students, even though the nurse has such a prominent, key worker role in long-term nursing care. The poor standards of care and the unsuitability of the staff to cater for the learning needs of the students are the reasons usually given for keeping students away from these wards. True though these reasons are, the background to the decision has a longer history and may be traced to the position and status of hospital medicine. Until Marjorie Warren's (1943) case that the chronically sick should be the concern of the general hospital, the medical profession did not see treatment of the elderly infirm as its responsibility. Even today, geriatric medicine makes only a minor contribution to the education of medical students and does not include the long-stay wards. Nurse training has followed the lead of medicine and has not recognized the teaching potential of long-stay wards.

We believe this state of affairs should change. Settings which provide long-term and continuing care should become teaching centres. The Teaching Nursing Home, modelled on the university teaching hospital, has developed in several States in the USA (Lekan-Rutledge 1988). The objectives of the Teaching Nursing Home are, among other things, to improve the quality of life and the quality of care for residents, to advance clinical research, to improve the educational preparation of nurses specializing in care of elderly people, to implement successful programmes of assessment and care in the management of health problems commonly found in old people, and to enhance recruitment of nurses into long-stay care. Raising the status of all long-term settings (hospital wards, community health centres and nursing and residential Homes) by installing teaching responsibilities and rotating students through them, will help to increase the quality of care, encourage improvements and increase the likelihood that nurses will choose to work in long-stay care.

CONCLUSION

This chapter has focused on long-stay settings ranging from residential Homes to nursing Homes and hospital wards. Both the public and the private sector have been included, although more emphasis has been given to state provision.

There is no doubt that most old people want to remain for the rest of their lives in their own homes. Those who choose to move into a Home do so with reluctance when they accept that they can no longer cope alone at home and do not wish to burden their families. It remains the case, however, that only a small proportion move into a Home, and the family is the main provider of care in the community. Too often old people who do move into residential care feel that they have no choice, but the move can be a positive one if the elderly person has made the final decision herself.

The quality of residential provision in this country is fragmentary and variable and often not what we would choose for ourselves. Concern is expressed about the current trend of supplementing state provision with private sector Homes. These have increased at such a rate that the procedures for registration and regulation are unable to identify and penalize unscrupulous proprietors who seek to profit from frail old people. It is important that the characteristics of those long-stay institutions that succeed in promoting a high quality of life and quality of care filter through to those that do not achieve adequate quality. The successful institutions avoid restrictive 'people-processing' and offer choice, autonomy and freedom for those who want it.

It is an anomaly that Britain has few NHS nursing Homes, so that hospital provision is often the only alternative for residents requiring continuous nursing care, unless they can afford to buy care in the private or voluntary sector. Concern about the quality of care and quality of life in geriatric wards has increased, as is reflected in government-sponsored research into alternative provision. There is a small but growing trend toward the development of NHS nursing Homes, but such Homes have their critics in parts of the powerful medical lobby. We hope, if only out of enlightened self-interest, that this nursing Home trend continues. It can only succeed, however, if the nurses appointed to run the Homes have shed their medical cloaks and promote the psychosocial as well as the physical well-being of the residents. We recommend that the training of nurses who specialize in continuing care should focus on the psychosocial and physical needs of elderly people. This requires comprehensive education in the health and social sciences and would give nurses the confidence to practise care which transcends that limited by the traditional medical treatment model. The ability of nurses to give up the medical prop would be increased if nurse training included long-stay settings in hospital and the community as compulsory experience for all students.

The integration of health and social science education and health and social care for elderly people runs counter to the proposals of the Griffiths (1988) report on community care. The Griffiths proposals explicitly separate health care from social care, which we have argued to be fundamentally inappropriate for effective continuing care of old people. The idea of a generic key worker for elderly people is our vision for the future. This generic worker will have an integrated education in the health and social sciences and be accorded credibility in what is at present a highly dichotomized health and social care service. Some courses exist in the UK which should produce a generic worker of this kind, such as the Master of Science degree in Gerontology at King's College London. This course is open to suitably qualified nurses, doctors, social workers and others who work with elderly people. Our vision of the future also includes integrated courses at a lower academic level.

Several positive examples of alternative provision in long-stay care have been discussed. These range from augmented home care, residential Homes expanded and opened up to become true community centres, and residential flatlets within a supportive residential Home environment, to community health care centres, nurse-led nursing Homes and nursing development units in hospitals. These developments are exciting and show what can be done by committed and motivated professionals. Integration and collaboration among the various professional groups and among the health, social and housing services is essential in order to achieve the right balance between control over one's own life and the necessary care required to continue to live. Changes are occurring, but change is slow and it will be a long time before the quality of care and the quality of life achieved by the exceptional centres described here reach every old person who faces life in a long-stay institution.

REFERENCES

Andrews K, Brocklehurst J 1987 British geriatric medicine in the 1980s. King Edward's Hospital Fund for London, London

Askham J, Thompson C 1987 Enhanced home support for dementia sufferers. Age Concern Institute of Gerontology, King's College, University of London

Atkinson D A, Bond J, Gregson B A 1986 The dependency characteristics of older people in long-term institutional care. In: Phillipson C, Bernard M, Strang P (eds) Dependency and interdependency in old age. Croom Helm, London

Baker D E 1983 'Care' in the geriatric ward: an account of two styles of nursing. In: Wilson-Barnett J (ed) Nursing research: ten studies in patient care. Wiley, Chichester

Batchelor I 1984 Policies for crisis? Some aspects of DHSS policies for care of the elderly. Occasional Paper No 1, Nuffield Provincial Hospitals Trust, Oxford

Bond J 1984 Evaluation of long-stay accommodation for elderly people. In: Bromley D B (ed) Gerontology: social and behavioural perspectives. Croom Helm, London

Bond J, Bond S 1987 Developments in the provision and evaluation of long-term care for dependent old people. In: Fielding P (ed) Research in the nursing care of elderly people. Wiley, Chichester

Bond J, Bond S, Donaldson C, Gregson B, Atkinson A 1989a Evaluation of continuing-care accommodation for elderly people. Report No 38, Vol 7, Health Care Research Unit, School of Health Care Sciences, University of Newcastle-upon-Tyne, Newcastle

Bond J, Bond S, Donaldson C, Gregson B, Atkinson A 1989b Evaluation of an innovation in the continuing care of very frail elderly people. Ageing and Society 9: 347–381

Booth T 1985 Home truths: old peoples' homes and the outcome of care. Gower, Aldershot

Booth T, Bilson A 1988 Fit for care? Nursing Times 84(29): 42–45

Centre for Policy on Ageing 1985 Home life: a code of practice for residential care. Working Party Report, CPA, London

Challis D, Davies B 1988 The community care approach: an innovation in home care by social services departments. In: Wells N, Freer C (eds) The ageing population: burden or challenge? Macmillan, Basingstoke

Clark P, Bowling A 1989 Observational study of quality of life in NHS nursing homes and a long-stay ward for the elderly. Ageing and Society 9: 123–148

Clarke M 1978 Getting through the work. In: Dingwall R, McIntosh J (eds) Readings in the sociology of nursing. Churchill Livingstone, Edinburgh

Dant T, Carley M, Gearing B, Johnson M 1989 Co-ordinating care: short report. A shortened version of the final report of the Care for Elderly People at Home (CEPH) Project, Gloucester, Open University and Policy Studies Institute, Milton Keynes

Evers H 1981a Tender loving care. In: Copp L A (ed) Care of the aging. Churchill Livingstone, Edinburgh

Evers H 1981b The creation of patient careers in geriatric wards: aspects of policy and practice. Social Science and Medicine 15A 581–588

Fennell G, Phillipson C, Evers H 1988 The sociology of old age. Open University Press, Milton Keynes

Gillick M R, Serrell N A, Gillick L S 1982 Adverse consequences of hospitalization in the elderly. Social Science and Medicine 16: 1033–1038

Goffman E 1961 Asylums. Doubleday Anchor Books, New York

Godlove C, Richard L, Rodwell G 1982 Time for action: an observation study of elderly people in four different care environments. Joint Unit for Social Services Research, University of Sheffield, Sheffield

Griffiths R 1988 Community care: agenda for action. A report to the Secretary of State for Social Services. HMSO, London

Hall L E 1969 The Loeb Center for nursing and rehabilitation, Montefiori Hospital and Medical Center, Bronx, New York. International Journal of Nursing Studies 6: 81

Halliley M 1987 A licence to profit from abuse of the elderly. The Listener 8 October: 4–5

Harman H, Harman S 1989 No place like home: a report of the first ninety six cases of the Registered Homes Tribunal. NALGO, London

Hearnden D 1983 Continuing care communities: a viable option in Britain? Centre for Policy on Ageing Report No 3, CPA, London

Heenan A 1989 Bright spots: Andrew Heenan describes four new nursing development units. Nursing Times 85(33): 19

Kahana E 1974 Matching environments to the needs of the aged: a conceptual scheme. In: Gubrium J F (ed) Late life: communities and environmental policy. Thomas, Springfield, Illinois

Kleemeier R 1961 The use and meaning of time in special settings. In: Kleemeier R (ed) Ageing and leisure. Oxford University Press, New York

King R D, Raynes N V, Tizard J 1971 Patterns of residential care. Routledge and Kegan Paul, London

Lawton M P 1980 Environment and aging. Brooks/Cole, Monterey, California

Lekan-Rutledge D 1988 Gerontological nursing in long-term care facilities. In: Matteson M A, McConnell E S Gerontological nursing: concepts and practice. W B Saunders, Philadelphia

Martin J P 1984 Hospitals in trouble. Basil Blackwell, Oxford

Meacher M 1972 Taken for a ride. Longman, Essex

Millard P H 1983 Long-term care in Europe: a review. In: Denham M J (ed) Care of the long-stay elderly patient. Croom Helm, London

Millard P H 1988 New horizons in hospital-based care. In: Wells N, Freer C (eds) The ageing population: burden or challenge? Macmillan, Basingstoke

Miller A F 1984 Nursing process and patient care. Nursing Times Occasional Papers 80(13): 56–58

Miller A F 1985a Does the process help the patient? Nursing Times 81(26): 24–27

Miller A F 1985b A study of the dependency of elderly patients in wards using different methods of nursing care. Age and Ageing 14: 132–138

Moos R H 1974 Evaluating treatment environments: a social ecological approach. Wiley, New York

Nisbet F 1987 The quality of residential care. Paper presented at the Ageing Well Conference, Brighton, England, September 1987

Nursing Times 1988 The nurses' advocate. Nursing Times 84(29): 20

Nursing Times 1989 Community care: the new mix. Nursing Times 85(29): 16–18

Peace S 1988 Living environments for the elderly 2: Promoting the 'right' institutional environment. In: Wells N, Freer C (eds) The ageing population: burden or challenge? Macmillan, Basingstoke

Pearson A 1983 The clinical nursing unit. Heinemann, London

Pearson A (ed) 1988 Primary nursing: nursing in the Burford and Oxford nursing development units. Croom Helm, London

Pincus A 1968 The definition and measurement of the institutional environment in institutions for the aged and its impact on residents. International Journal of Ageing and Human Development 1: 117–126

Robertson I 1986 Learned helplessness. Nursing Times 17–24 December: 28–30

Rosenbaum M 1983 Learned resourcefulness as a behavioural repertoire for the self-regulation of internal events: issues and speculations. In: Rosenbaum M, Franks C M, Jaffe T (eds) Perspectives on behaviour therapy in the eighties. Springer, New York.

Salvage J 1989 Setback for nursing. Nursing Times 85(11): 19

Schulz R 1980 Ageing and control. In: Garber J, Seligman M E P (eds) Human helplessness: theory and applications. Academic Press, London

Schulz R, Brenner G 1977 Relocation of the aged: a review and theoretical analysis. Journal of Gerontology 32: 323–333

Secretary of State for Health, Social Security, Wales & Scotland 1989 Caring for people: community care in the next decade and beyond. (White Paper) HMSO, London

Seligman M E P 1975 Helplessness: on depression, development and death. Freeman, San Francisco

Sinclair I 1988 Residential care for elderly people. In: Sinclair I (ed) Residential care: the research reviewed. (The Wagner Report), HMSO, London

Slagsvold B 1987 Nursing home quality and role theory. Paper presented at the Ageing Well Conference, Brighton, England, September 1987

Tarbox A R 1983 The elderly in nursing homes: psychological aspects of neglect. Clinical Gerontologist 1(4): 39–52

Vousden M 1987 Nye Bevan would turn in his grave. Nursing Times 83(32): 18–19

Wade B, Sawyer L, Bell J 1983 Dependency with dignity: different care provision for the elderly. Occasional Papers on Social Administration, No 68, Bedford Square Press, London

Wagner G 1988 Residential care: a positive choice. Report of the Independent Review of Residential Care. HMSO, London

Warren M W 1943 Care of the chronic sick: a case for treating chronic sick in blocks in a general hospital. British Medical Journal ii: 822

Wells T 1980 Problems in geriatric care. Churchill Livingstone, Edinburgh

Wilce G 1988 A place like home: a radical experiment in health care. Bedford Square Press, London

Wilkin D, Hughes B 1987 Residential care of elderly people: the consumers' views. Ageing and Society 7: 175–201

Willcocks D, Peace S, Kellaher L 1987 Private lives in public places. Tavistock, London

Wright S 1989 Defining the nursing development unit. Nursing Standard 4(7): 29–31

CHAPTER CONTENTS

Introduction 519

The organization of care 521
The supportive model 521
The protective model 521
The controlled model 522
The restrained model 522

The views of relatives 522
Hospital long-term care 522
Part III Homes 523
Private nursing Homes 525

Loss 526
Coping and confusion 526
Sensory impairment 527
Depression and loneliness 527
Freedom and purpose 527

30

Choice and flexibility in long-term care settings

Barbara E. Wade

INTRODUCTION

The upsurge in research activity in the field of gerontology described by Malcolm Johnson (Ch. 1) reflects an expectation that research, by creating new knowledge, can help in the solution of problems (Illsley, 1983). This chapter draws on some of this research, especially where it is relevant to the long-term care of the elderly in institutional settings.

Approximately 5% of older people are currently receiving long-term care in institutions but the pattern of provision has changed quite markedly over the last few years. For example, between 1976 and 1986 there was a slight decrease in the number of available geriatric beds but the average length of stay was almost halved over the same period. Whereas between 1982 and 1986 local authority residential care provision for those aged 65 and over remained constant, the number of residents in private Homes, a large proportion of whom receive social security support, has increased at an average rate of more than 21% per annum. On the other hand, local authority sponsorship of people in private and voluntary Homes has decreased over the same period (DH 1988).

The wide range of care provision might lead one to suppose that there is a degree of choice available to that minority of elderly people who require long-term care. Indeed, we are told that 'maintaining choice and flexibility in care provision should be a guiding principle underpinning all policy decisions' (Fennell et al 1983, p. 28). Weaver et al (1985) maintain that the concept of choice is relative and that there is only marginally more choice in the private than the public sector, for example, in a large study of private residential Homes, they found that only 38% of old people had visited their present Home before being admitted. Moreover, choice and flexibility do not just depend on the provision of a range of services. The levels of provision, the pressure exerted on that provision and the degree of collaboration and co-operation between professionals, as for example between health and social workers, are also important. Choice and flexibility will be possible only if we have a fully functioning co-ordinated care system with ease of transfer between the different parts.

In 1978 Plank criticized the care system, commenting that 'the major forms of service provision are developing, like Topsy, in an unco-ordinated and isolated manner without benefit of a considered framework of policy and professional practice' (p. 17). The evidence to support these allegations is not hard to find. Elderly people waiting to transfer to other accommodation are seen as 'blocking' beds; admissions to care are mainly crisis-based; there is a high degree of overlap in self-care ability between the elderly in hospital, residential Homes and sheltered housing; there is unmet need in the community and there is evidence of considerable strain upon relatives who undertake the caring role (Wade et al 1983).

The overall picture of care provision given here conceals wide variations in both level and type of provision among different authorities. For example, the number of geriatric beds per 1000 population aged 65 years and over in England varies from 5.8 in the South West Thames region to 8.7 in the Yorkshire region. Similarly, the number of residents catered for or sponsored by local authorities varies enormously from one local authority to another. It is this variation in levels of provision that has enabled researchers to gauge the extent to which pressure in one part of the care system may be associated with demand in another part of the system. For example, a low level of provision in local authority residential Homes (Part III accommodation) was found to be associated with greater sponsorship of elderly people in private and voluntary Homes (Gorbach & Sinclair 1982). Similarly, a high turnover of patients occu-

pying geriatric beds and lower levels of geriatic bed provision was associated with a higher average age of old people in Part III Homes and with increased caseloads for home helps. However, it was suggested that this interrelationship did not necessarily mean that services had been planned in this way but that the relationship derived from transmission of pressure from one part of the system to another (Gorbach & Sinclair 1982).

The discussion document 'A Happier Old Age' (Department of Health and Social Security 1978) noted the large number of hospital beds occupied by elderly people. It was suggested that nursing Homes could cater for physically dependent elderly people who do not require hospital-based resources, and a research project was funded by the DHSS to provide information about the potential clientèle (Wade et al 1983). This research showed that one quarter of the elderly people on community nurse lists and almost one quarter of the residents in Part III Homes had high or very high nursing care requirements and were directly comparable with the majority of elderly patients receiving long-term care in hospital. On the other hand, 11% of long-stay patients in hospital geriatric wards had minimal nursing care requirements. In view of these findings it is not surprising that care staff considered that the needs of almost one quarter of residents in Part III accommodation could be more appropriately catered for in a different environment. Similarly, ward sisters considered that approximately 40% of the long-term care patients could be more appropriately catered for elsewhere, the largest number of single suggestions being for Part III Homes.

Interviews with care staff in this study illustrated the difficulties involved in transferring elderly people from one care setting to another. These interviews also illustrated the lack of collaboration between health and social services. For example, some of the medical consultants suggested that the problem of highly dependent residents in Part III Homes arose because problems which were initially treatable were left until people deteriorated and became more dependent: 'It may be too late to get them fit by the time I am presented with them; they should be referred much sooner.' On the other hand, officers in charge of Part III Homes often complained that they could not gain access to hospital beds: 'If it is somebody that we feel needs geriatric care then we contact the general practitioner, the general practitioner contacts the geriatrician and nine times out of ten they're turned down.' The interviews held with the relatives of people being cared for in Part III Homes reinforce this view. It was exceptional for the residents to have been given a choice of Home. Some people had to wait a very long time before being discharged from hospital to Part III accommodation, and requests for elderly people to be placed in a Home nearer to their relatives were often refused, due to either lack of vacancies or local authority boundaries: 'I'd love to be able to get him nearer but he's not a resident.'

This brief resumé of research clearly illustrates a care system which is under pressure and strongly suggests that the interrelationship between the different parts of the system is due to this pressure, rather than to planned co-ordination. The evidence also suggests that it can be very difficult to transfer elderly people from one care setting to another. The general picture is one of inflexibility and, as far as placement is concerned, it would seem that there is little choice for the consumer.

Yet, the notion of choice can be considered at a different level — that of service delivery. At this level choice is dependent upon organizational factors and is open to manipulation by the people concerned. To what extent do nurses or other care staff safeguard or restrict the control that elderly people have over their own lives?

Interviews with care staff and with the relatives of elderly people being cared for in hospital geriatric units, Part III Homes and private nursing Homes shed some light on this issue. These are examined in the next section.

THE ORGANIZATION OF CARE

Conceptual analysis of the interviews with care staff has been reported elsewhere (Wade 1983). Briefly, four models of care were described. These were derived from the identification of two con-

tinua relating to the organization of care. The first of these ranged from an emphasis on the socio-emotional well-being of the elderly to an emphasis on routine and task completion. The second ranged from an open organization, in which efforts were made to increase the involvement of the elderly with the wider community, to a closed organization wherein contacts with the wider community were restricted.

THE SUPPORTIVE MODEL

This model is characterized by consultation and involvement of elderly people in the care regime. They are recognized as adults and efforts are made to maximize their physical and mental independence. For example:

Maybe a patient has one bad arm, but she can use the other, why take that away from her too? (Ward Sister)

There is thorough involvement of visitors, including relatives, volunteers and children, and a breaking down of barriers between the institution and the wider community:

All my nurses come back, they bring their children, they come home from school and wait here for Mum. They go and see all the patients, sometimes bring a few flowers, a few sweets, sometimes patients give them sweets. The patients know all the nurses' children, but it's home you see (Matron, Private Home).

The residents are encouraged to participate in activities which they see as relevant. For example, one residential Home organized escorts so that the old people could take advantage of late-night shopping facilities.

Suggestions for activities/outings are made by the elderly people themselves, possibly through patient/resident committees.

THE PROTECTIVE MODEL

This model of care is characterized by some degree of choice and consultation, but there is an undue emphasis on safety. Staff decide which activities are suitable for the residents, thus denying them their adult status. For example:

No, I wouldn't let them [go into the garden unaccompanied] because they are responsible to the hospital (Ward Sister).

No, I wouldn't risk kettles or anything (Matron, Private Home).

There is little or no attempt to involve visitors in the care regime:

You know they're very pleased that they don't have to do it [give help in caring] (Warden, Part III Home).

Under this model of care, contact with the wider community is restricted. For example, children may be seen as a source of infection. Diversional activities are provided by staff.

THE CONTROLLED MODEL

Under the controlled model of care the elderly person is subordinate to the care regime. For example:

Most of them want to go fairly early [to bed], because we are dragging them out early (Ward Sister).

Choice is circumscribed by staff:

Yes, we have got a choice of menu, but we choose for them (Ward Sister).

Staff arrange all activities and outings. Although there is open visiting, attitudes towards visitors are related to their possible contribution to routine:

They give them tea or feed them for us (Ward Sister).

THE RESTRAINED MODEL

The restrained model of care operates purely for the convenience of care staff:

Well, of course, you have to appreciate that you have to fit into a certain routine (Ward Sister).

The residents are deprived of choice, there is restricted visiting and little therapeutic input. They are 'batch processed'.

THE VIEWS OF RELATIVES

The above analysis was based on interviews with professionals: those who organize and deliver care.

Although examples of the supportive model of care were seen in all the different settings, interviews with the relatives of 21 heavily dependent hospital patients, 26 heavily dependent elderly people living in Part III Homes, and 26 heavily dependent elderly people in private nursing Homes provided a different perspective. These interviews, which often revealed great perception of the problems inherent in long-term care, are now considered separately for each care setting.

HOSPITAL LONG-TERM CARE

When asked directly about the care given to elderly people, responses from relatives ranged from 'The staff are very kind' to 'The staff are marvellous'. Direct questions gave rise to little criticism and this was limited to comments on cleanliness or the quality of the food. On the other hand, responses to more detailed questions about the care regime were much more discerning.

More than one third of the people interviewed described their elderly relatives as 'withdrawn'. Some attributed this withdrawal to the lack of opportunity to participate in meaningful activities.

She loves the outside, but she never goes out. I can't see why they couldn't push her out in her wheelchair down to the garden.

She hasn't been outside for the last three or four years.

Their brains need stimulating.

She sits and looks out of the window and there's a row of old Victorian terraced houses and she said the other day, 'I sit and look at those houses, I wonder who the people are'. She peoples the houses in her imagination and that passes the day until she falls asleep.

I've never seen her close her eyes and all she can do is just sit and look around. I notice when I'm there she'll watch the nurses, probably she's sitting there and she says in her mind, 'Look at that silly old so and so.'

Approximately one third of patients in hospital long-term care wards had been assessed by staff as having difficulty in hearing or being completely deaf, with a similar proportion as having difficulty in seeing or being completely blind. A further third had speech difficulties. Relatives were sensitive to the problems posed by these sensory impairments:

She's left a lot on her own because she's deaf.

She always has a laugh with me and jokes. They can't communicate with her. I notice when the others are doing therapy she's not.

She can't see but she needs to be talked to and she likes to talk. Sometimes they're forgotten you know, those that can't see.

If she'd had her ears done and a hearing aid then they could have done her glasses. Consequently she's living in a world of her own and she just dwells back on the past.

The problems of withdrawal and the lack of meaningful activities were seen by some people as contributing to the further deterioration of their relatives:

She gradually deteriorated. I'm convinced that if these hospitals had more physiotherapists we wouldn't have so many disabled people.

She deteriorated mentally after going into hospital.

I don't think she knows where she is, which is maybe a good thing.

While they are in their own homes and they are busying about and they have things that interest them they remain mentally and physically active much longer. Once they go into an institution everything is more or less done for them and they sit about and start to deteriorate.

The question of purpose was also brought up by this relative:

Once when we saw her she was sewing bits of leather together. But there is no purpose, is there? It isn't the same as if you had to make yourself a cup of tea. There must be some purpose, I think that is terribly important.

The contrast between the rehabilitation ward and the long-term care ward was noted by one distressed relative who was herself disabled:

The atmosphere there was so different, everyone was alive and visitors were coming. In this ward people sit like zombies. In the first ward she was being nursed, in this ward she is only cared for.

Some of the problems perceived by relatives of the residents were attributed to shortage of staff:

There is not the necessary staff to take them [to the

toilet] and they eventually have to do it where they sit, and I think that really takes away all their self-respect.

It has already been shown that some people saw the mental withdrawal of their elderly relatives as the only means of coping with an environment which was devoid of stimulation. Occasionally, this was taken a step further when staff were seen as contributing to the regression of the residents.

They say you go back to your childhood, don't they? But I think it doesn't help a lot to be called by your first name; it's going back to your childhood for them. They stop being Mrs So and So, they're called like children again.

The sister used to speak to her very sharp when she fell down; she said she'd been a naughty girl.

Approximately one third of the people interviewed stated that the clothes that they had taken in for their relatives had been lost or 'swapped'.

We take her nightdresses and jumpers and that sort of thing and we've never seen them. I suppose somebody else has got them on.

In view of the above comments it should not be surprising that more than one half of the people interviewed said that their elderly relatives were unhappy.

She says, 'I'm fed up I think I'll run away.'

I don't see how anybody could be happy there because they just sit all day. It's a long time just to sit.

He cries because he's parted from his wife. It's sad for both of them.

It breaks their hearts, I think they get worse.

PART III HOMES

When asked directly about the care given to the residents the responses of these relatives were similar to those received from the relatives of elderly people in hospital. There was little criticism. However, more detailed questioning led to some revealing comments:

She has special permission to stay in her room after lunch and for the rest of the day except for meals.

They put him in a high chair with a tray across it

and the trouble is that he can't get out and he gets frustrated.

She keeps talking about her freedom.

One third of those interviewed described their elderly relatives as bored or withdrawn:

She goes to bed at about half past five because she's so bored.

They have a service for them on Sundays and, apart from that, there isn't much else.

I realize they do the best they can but I feel they're all like zombies. They're in the same room, the same chair, they never move. He doesn't speak to a soul.

If they could be given something to do. They could be taken out for a day or a few hours, or if someone came there and, well — tried to talk to her. Life is so boring, isn't it, when you just sit there, you know, the whole day, every day? They just get up to have their meals and they sit down again. I have seen them get up and walk around and immediately they said to them, 'Now sit down on that chair.' Well they're not really doing any harm, just walking around in the corridors aren't they?

The lack of meaningful activities was also pointed out, together with the loss of role:

They wouldn't let her do any work. She thought that she should have hoovered up the carpets and washed the dishes and they wouldn't let her do it.

She used to like to have a little walk in the gardens but there is nobody to take her out.

If they could be given something to do, they could be taken out for a day or a few hours.

When she comes here at weekends she sings and she wipes up. They said to me, 'Well she doesn't do anything here,' but they don't ask her to do anything.

There's an old guy there who can play the piano. Now wouldn't it be a great idea to give him a piano and he can sit there and tinkle away and people can sing. That's all part and parcel of a bit of therapy. It's no good sticking the telly on in a corner.

Make them do something, it doesn't matter how small it is, but make them do something.

The lack of activities was also seen by some of these relatives as contributing to the further deterioration of residents:

I think it's very nice but there's nothing for them to do. I think my mother's deteriorated, they sit there like zombies. You know, the old people just sitting there — they must deteriorate much quicker. The television is always on, nobody watches it.

More than one quarter of people being cared for in Part III Homes were rated as having difficulties in hearing or being completely deaf, one fifth were rated as having difficulty in seeing or were blind, and a little less than one fifth of all residents were dysphasic. The additional problems posed by these sensory deficits were also pointed out by relatives:

She's hard of hearing and of course people can't talk to her. We know how to handle her because she could read our lips you see.

She can't communicate because of deafness and she's a bit blurred in her vision.

The blindness is the greatest single handicap. Whatever she would do she wouldn't be happy.

She's very deaf and she moans at the Home about shouting at her, but it's the walking problem and eyes are the main problem.

Relatives were asked whether the resident had taken personal possessions into the Home.

They can't take furniture of their own, there isn't enough room. They didn't want her to wear any jewellery, watch or anything; it's a temptation to others to lift things.

The problem of pilfering was one which was commented on several times.

She went in there with quite a few bits and pieces of her own and they went missing. She lost a lot of things — cherished possessions.

Clothing, too, was often lost. This was mentioned by one third of those interviewed:

They lose her clothes and they're marked with great big letters and they still get lost. She's a size 44 and they sent her home in a size 36 slip. The other Friday I got really upset because they sent her home in a man's vest.

Less than one third of the people interviewed thought that their elderly relative was happy in the Home and approximately the same number were unsure.

She doesn't complain.

I don't know if she's happy but she doesn't laugh or sing so much.

I think she's happy — every time I go she says, 'When am I going to come out of here?' But basically she's quite happy.

However, more than one third were said to be unhappy:

She's very miserable actually. She says quite openly, 'Please God, take me.'

Absolutely broken-hearted. He's never been away from his sister.

He definitely isn't happy. They try their utmost, but I think it's too impersonal. I think they need a room of their own where they can go on their own and keep their own little things.

PRIVATE NURSING HOMES

The relatives of those being cared for in private nursing Homes were asked about their choice of Home — what did they look for in a Home? One relative who had visited 15 private nursing Homes gave the reasons for her choice:

I chose this one because they don't expect the patient to conform to the Home, they conform the Home to the patient. They don't pressurize her, they let her do exactly what she likes in her own way. She has eccentricities — at 91 we are all going to have them — and they just accept her.

Other relatives stated their priorities:

It's very well run, as the matron says, 'This is their home. You can come and go and there are no rules.'

I think every person has the right to privacy and an individual room where he can have his own bits and pieces around him.

Yet, despite the greater degree of choice some people still complained that their relatives had become withdrawn:

It's painful to go — there's no conversation.

I wish it had a sitting room. I wish it had a proper lift.

I think if you mix with people it keeps you more alert, there's incentive. They are all in their own rooms, they never see each other.

She likes to sit in the sitting room. She likes a bit of life. She's not like the others, she likes to get out. The others don't seem to want to go out.

Sitting rooms were, however, the subject of some criticism.

They sort of all sit round the outside of the room which does seem to me to be a bit austere. If they could divide it up . . .

Yet the privacy afforded by a private room was also valued.

My mother would hate a place where she had to go and talk to people, where they all had to go for meals or something.

One relative took a more positive view of withdrawal:

She's now living in the past and very much happier for it, too, I think.

These relatives also referred to the lack of activities for the residents.

There is nothing for her to do all day.

That's what is so awful about old people's Homes. I've been in three or four and you see these old people just sitting, not doing anything. Oh, it fills me with despair just to see it.

The importance of keeping the residents purposefully occupied was readily perceived. For example, one old lady spent a great deal of time knitting blanket squares:

We can hardly keep her going in wool but her hands have unscrambled as a result.

The problem of sensory deprivation was also noted:

Her sight is very poor. She cannot read. She can barely see the television. She cannot walk. So her world is very limited and she is very bored.

The problems of secondary deterioration were also mentioned:

My mother has gone downhill mentally since she's been there because she hasn't had to think for herself very much.

He doesn't get enough exercise. He is losing the use of his limbs.

I just wish they hadn't allowed Mother to vegetate.

She feels she should be dressed and undressed and of course the reason why they don't do it — if they dress and undress her she'll not do anything. It's terribly important.

One third of those interviewed thought that old people were unhappy in these private Homes. For example:

It's a very caring place and she has got her bits and pieces round her but, I mean, it isn't your home and the company is not exactly exhilarating.

Sometimes she says, 'I wish I was back home,' or, 'I wish I was dead.'

LOSS

These two sets of interviews give us quite different perspectives on the care of elderly people. Interviews with the professionals, which enabled the different models of care to be identified, show quite clearly that, under a supportive care regime, choice can be given to the residents. Equally clearly, supportive care can be given in any setting, but its success depends on the attitudes of care staff.

The interviews with relatives illustrate their concern and, on occasions, their all too apparent despair. Loss of choice was highlighted in interviews with care staff: 'We think it is better to more or less think for them.' However, loss of choice was seen by relatives as one component of loss on a much greater scale. Such loss included:

Loss of clothes — 'They sent her home in a man's vest.'
Loss of possessions — 'She went in there with quite a few bits and pieces of her own and they went missing.'
Loss of privacy — 'It wouldn't take a minute to cover him up.'
Loss of dignity — 'They eventually have to do it where they sit and I think that really takes away all their self-respect.'
Loss of adult status — 'She said she'd been a naughty girl.'
Loss of role — 'They were sewing bits of leather together, but there is no purpose.'
Loss of freedom — 'They put him in a high chair with a tray across it and the trouble is that he can't get out and he gets frustrated.'

Loss of identity — 'They sit there like zombies.'

The loss of independence incurred by elderly people who enter a long-term care facility is often superimposed on the loss which precedes admission. Such loss may include the death of a spouse, friends or relatives, sensory loss and the decline of physical health. Admission in itself can also mean being parted from loved ones: 'He cries because he's parted from his wife. It's sad for both of them.'

COPING AND CONFUSION

Bonar and Maclean (1983) argue that the many crises and losses which occur in old age may contribute to a breakdown. They suggest that psychological defences such as regression and withdrawal may be construed as symptoms of 'senility', whereas if these symptoms were recognized as evidence of coping behaviour, steps could be taken to alleviate the underlying distress. Slater and Lipman (1977) make a similar point:

Staff in homes for old people can readily assume that the expression of confused behaviour by a resident is pathological in origin rather than as signalling efforts to comprehend and/or cope with the experiences of ageing in an institution (p. 523).

One study revealed that 71% of staff working in residential Homes particularly liked working with the 'confused' whereas the lucid and physically able residents were seen by many to be difficult and demanding and provided little in the way of job satisfaction (Evans et al 1981). This same study revealed that a number of residents thought that they were in school.

There is a certain circularity in the designation of residents as 'confused' on the basis of childlike behaviour if, at the same time, staff refer to and admonish them as children, thus reinforcing the behaviour on which they base their 'diagnosis'. The interviews with relatives described above illustrate this very point: 'They say you go back to your childhood, don't they? But I think it doesn't help a lot to be called by your first name; it's going back to your childhood for them.'

Wolanin and Phillips (1981) also suggest that confused behaviours may be positively reinforced and that attempts at control and autonomy may be negatively reinforced. They argue that a patient's credibility is first questioned by staff and later by the patient herself. They suggest that patients are reinforced for withdrawal behaviour. For example, when a patient does not respond, staff give extra attention to draw the patient out. Similarly, patients who indulge in bizarre behaviour are likely to receive extra attention from staff. 'The end result is positive reinforcement for behaviours that are both aberrant and withdrawn.' (p. 21)

SENSORY IMPAIRMENT

In an article on stress and coping, Clarke (1984) suggests that one of the most disagreeable situations known to man is the absence, or a low level, of stimulation. For many elderly people the lack of stimulation in an institutional environment is made worse by sensory impairment and this too was readily perceived by many relatives, some of whom saw withdrawal as one means of coping with an unstimulating environment: 'She peoples the houses in her imagination and that passes the day until she falls asleep.'

Wolanin and Phillips (1981) discuss this problem in great detail, citing the experiments of Bexton et al (1954) and others which have shown that sensory deprivation, sensory overload or sensory distortion in an isolating situation can give rise to profound behavioural changes in normal, healthy, young people. It would seem that there is an optimal range, level and variety of stimulation to maintain awareness.

DEPRESSION AND LONELINESS

The work of Herbst and Humphrey (1980) has demonstrated a strong relationship between deafness and depression, and Clarke (1984) suggests that hospital patients who have little control over the environment may be particularly prone to feelings of depression and helplessness. The interviews described above lead us to believe that considerable proportions of heavily dependent elderly people in all three settings were either unhappy or depressed. This impression is borne out by interviews with the old people themselves; fewer than half of those in hospital or residential Homes who were able to respond to questioning

said that they were happy in their current situation (Wade et al 1983). For example: 'There is no freedom. I get depressed a lot, I've not been out for a year' (Hospital Patient).

The comment which follows was made by an elderly man for whom admission to hospital had meant parting from his wife: 'I'm fed up with sitting in this chair day after day. I've been sitting in this blooming chair since last September. I never go anywhere, sit here all day long. Nobody to talk to. I wish I could go home.' This patient was completely blind and extremely deaf. He was rated 'confused' by the ward sister.

A small pilot study of patient satisfaction reported by Morle (1984) suggests that loneliness may be experienced by the majority of patients, even in a modern geriatric assessment unit. Wolanin and Phillips (1981) argue that the problems of loneliness and lack of meaning are further compounded in long-term care settings where one day may be very like another. Of those who were able to respond, almost one third of old people in residential Homes and long-term care wards said that they were often lonely (Wade et al 1983).

FREEDOM AND PURPOSE

The importance of providing meaningful activity was something which was expressed by many relatives who clearly perceived that inactivity led to apathy, secondary deterioration and, finally, loss of identity.

Diversional activities may be provided by staff but to provide *for* meaningful activity implies making provision for greater participation in the life of the ward or Home. In her book *Rights and Risk* Alison Norman (1980) cites a DHSS study of 124 local authority, private and voluntary Homes in the London area. This survey showed that there were very few Homes in which residents were consulted about the way life was organized. In most of these Homes residents were not encouraged to help with chores or to do things for themselves. Similarly, Brooking (1982) conducted a survey of the practices and opinions of staff, patients and their relatives in 16 wards in two hospitals. Findings indicated only very limited involvement of patients and relatives in the planning and implementation of care.

Evidence is now accumulating to support the view that the attitudes of staff and the way that services are provided may serve to reinforce dependency. For example, Miller (1985) compared task-oriented nursing with individualized nursing care and found that individualized care was associated with lower mortality and a higher rate of discharge from hospital. She reports that patients in traditional wards were significantly more physically dependent and more apathetic. These findings mirror those of the Kent Community Care Project where individualized packages of care were also associated with lower mortality and reduced entry into residential care (Davies & Challis, 1986). See Chapter 29 for further discussion of the Kent Community Care Project.

Bland (1988) maintains that existing services have not been developed to cater to individual needs, that we often fail to offer choices about the services we provide and that older people should be treated as consumers rather than as passive recipients of care. If we accept as Alison Norman suggests, that elderly people should enjoy the liberty granted to other adult citizens — that is, to order their activities, finances and personal affairs — then restrictions should be limited to those which are necessary to provide the level of care they need and to protect the quality of life of others.

This chapter began by focusing on choice and flexibility both with regard to the range and level of provision and at the point of service delivery. Those involved in caring for elderly people have a dual responsibility — as policy makers on the one hand and as carers on the other.

What I can't get across to people — it seems to me that they all talk about the old and young as though they're separate, they're not, they're us. They're us in another 20 years. So what would you like done to you? (Relative).

REFERENCES

Bexton W H, Heron W, Scott R H 1954 Effect of decreased variation in the sensory environment. Canadian Journal of Psychology 8: 70–76

Bland R 1988 Giving the initiative back to the consumer. In: Gordon D S (ed) Independence in old age: issues for planning and practice. June 1988 Aberdeen Group, British Society of Gerontology

Bonar R, MacLean M J 1983 Senility symptoms as a psychological defense. Paper presented at Systed 1983 Conference, Montreal, 15 July

Brooking J I 1982 Patient and family participation in nursing: a survey of opinions and current practices among patients, relatives and nurses. In: Proceedings of the RCN Research Society XIII Annual Conference, University of Durham, p 97–120

Clarke M 1984 Stress and coping: constructs for nursing. Journal of Advanced Nursing 9(1): 3–13

Davies B, Challis D 1986 Matching resources to needs in community care. Gower, Aldershot

Department of health 1988 Health and personal social services statistics for England. HMSO, London

Department of Health and Social Security 1978 A happier old age. HMSO, London

Evans G, Hughes B, Wilkin D, Jolley D 1981 The management of mental and physical impairment in non-specialist residential homes for the elderly. Research Report No 4, Department of Psychiatry and Community Medicine, Manchester University

Fennell G, Phillipson C, Wenger C 1983 The process of ageing: social aspects. In: Elderly people in the community: their service needs. HMSO, London

Gorbach P, Sinclair I 1982 Pressure on health and social services for the elderly. Working Paper, May

Herbst K G, Humphrey C 1980 Hearing impairment and mental state in the elderly living at home. British Medical Journal 28: 903–905

Illsley R 1983 The contribution of research of the development of practice and policy. In: Elderly people in the community: their service needs. HMSO, London

Miller A 1985 Nurse/patient dependency — is it iatrogenic? Journal of Advanced Nursing, 10(1): 63–69

Morle K M F 1984 Patient satisfaction: care of the elderly. Journal of Advanced Nursing 9(1): 71–76

Norman A J 1980 Rights and risk. National Council for the Care of Old People (now Centre for Policy on Ageing), London

Plank D 1978 Old people's homes are not the last refuge. Community Care 202: 16–18

Slater R, Lipman A 1977 Staff assessments of confusion and the situation of confused residents in homes for old people. Gerontologist 17(6): 523–530

Wade B E 1983 Different models of care for the elderly. Nursing Times 79: 12 Occasional Papers 33–36

Wade B E, Sawyer L, Bell J 1983 Dependency with dignity. Occasional Papers on Social Administration No 68. Bedford Square Press, London

Weaver T, Willcocks D, Kellaher L 1985 The business of care: a study of private residential homes for old people. Centre for Environmental and Social Studies in Ageing, Polytechnic of North London, London

Wolanin M O, Phillips L R F 1981 Confusion, prevention and care. Mosby, St Louis

Part 4

Care of elderly people: conclusions

CHAPTER CONTENTS

The impact of an ageing population 531

Women in retirement and old age 534

Men in retirement and old age 537

'Ageism' and 'geriatrics' 538
Louisa: journey into the unknown 540
Fighting prejudice 544

Successful ageing 545

31

The elderly person: the challenge of an aged society

Sally J. Redfern

In this chapter an attempt is made to draw together the earlier discussions concerning the impact of the ageing population in Western societies in general, but particularly in Britain. We highlight some of the experiences that women and men have in being old, victims of discriminatory attitudes and dependent on inadequate services. Finally, and more positively, we discuss some aspects of successful ageing, and what nurses can do to help old people stay healthy.

THE IMPACT OF AN AGEING POPULATION

The demographic trend in all Western industrialized countries is much the same. As discussed by Helen Evers (Chapter 24) the proportion of very old people is rising. There are now over ten million people of pensionable age in the UK, representing 18.2% of the total population. Although the total number of pensioners is not expected to increase very much, by the year 2000 the rise in the over-75 age group will be substantial, and this will be accompanied by a proportional reduction in the fitter 'young elderly', aged 65–74 years (Shegog 1981, Acheson 1982, Age Concern 1989).

The situation in the United States is similar, although the proportion of old people relative to the total population is smaller than in Britain. The 1980 census showed a 27% growth in the 65+ age group since 1970 — an increase from 20 million to 25.5 million people. This represents just over 11% of the total American population, and by the year 2000 it is forecast that this proportion will increase to 13% (Ernst & Glazer-Waldman 1983).

Mortality rates among older people have been falling in Britain, but this does not necessarily mean that health has improved or morbidity decreased (Kalache et al 1988). Kalache and his colleagues revealed the worrying fall of the UK down the life expectancy league table in comparison with other countries (Table 31.1). At the beginning of this century, life expectancy in the UK was amongst the highest of all the countries which kept records. In 1985, England and Wales had fallen below 10 other mainly developed countries for the life expectancy for males at birth, and below 16 countries for females at birth. The positions of Northern Ireland and Scotland were even lower. At age 65, further life expectancy for men was about 13 years for the UK countries, which put them near the bottom of the league table, with only the German Democratic Republic, Poland and Hungary below them with 12 years. Women at age 65 have, on average, 17 more years in England, and 16 more years in Northern Ireland and Scotland, with Eire, Poland, Sri Lanka, the GDR and Hungary falling below Scotland (Kalache et al 1988). Longevity in Japan is particularly high.

Chastening though these league table positions are, the number of extremely old survivors has increased in Britain. Bury (1988) reviewed the literature for England and Wales, and found a dramatic increase in the number of centenarians over the last thirty years: 271 in 1951 rising to 2410 in 1981; a nine-fold increase. Bury thus challenges Fries' argument that the limit of the normal life span is 85 years (Fries & Crapo 1981).

It is becoming increasingly common to hear about the Third Age, as distinct from the First Age, Second Age and perhaps a Fourth Age. Originating in the French universities in the 1970s, 'the Third Age' seems to have entered the English language in the early 1980s with the founding of the first British University of the Third Age (Laslett 1987). Laslett describes the four ages thus: the First Age is an 'era of dependence, socialisation, immaturity and education'; the Second Age is 'an era of independence, maturity, responsibility and earning'; the Third Age is an 'age of personal achievement and fulfilment, . . . the interlude when the goal of the individual life plan is realised'; and the Fourth Age is an 'era of final dependence, decrepitude and death'. The point at which a person moves from one Age to the next is not based on chronological age, although the Third Age often in practice begins, for those who have been employed in paid work, at the end of their earning career at around 65 years of age. The Third Age is an attribute of a population as well as of individuals and can only be experienced in full by those privileged in disposition, freedom and health to do so (Laslett 1987).

Given the association of disability and dependency with increasing age, the consequences of the rise in the very old and most frail are regarded as grave. At least half the expected additional over-85 year olds will need help with bathing, one fifth of those living at home are likely to be housebound, and many will be incontinent (Acheson 1982).

Table 31.1 Life expectancy in selected countries at birth, males and females, 1985. *From Kalache et al (1988).*

Males	(years)	Females	(years)
75.5	Japan	81.6	Japan
73.8	Sweden	80.6	Switzerland
73.8	Switzerland	80.1	France
73.5	Greece	80.0	Canada
73.1	Netherlands	79.9	Netherlands
73.0	Canada	79.9	Sweden
72.6	Spain	78.9	Finland
72.3	Cuba	78.8	Spain
72.2	Australia	78.7	Australia
71.9	FR Germany	78.5	USA
71.9	England and Wales	78.5	FR Germany
71.8	France	78.5	Greece
71.7	Denmark	77.9	Italy
71.3	USA	77.8	Belgium
71.3	Italy	77.8	Austria
71.0	Austria	77.7	Denmark
70.8	Eire	77.6	England and Wales
70.8	Belgium	77.1	Portugal
70.6	Finland	76.5	Northern Ireland
70.3	Northern Ireland	76.3	Scotland
70.2	Portugal	76.3	Eire
70.1	Scotland	75.5	Cuba
69.5	German DR	75.5	Uruguay
68.7	Uruguay	75.4	German DR
68.2	Argentina	75.1	Poland
66.9	Sri Lanka	74.6	Argentina
66.7	Poland	73.3	Hungary
65.3	Hungary	71.9	Sri Lanka

Coupled with other social patterns such as the increasing mobility of younger families, smaller families, more married women doing paid work, and more marital breakdown leading to double the number of old people who live alone and who have no children, the present level of caring services will continue to be stretched to breaking point and beyond.

Although it is important to keep a sense of proportion in that a substantial number of old people have no incapacitating disabilities, nonetheless, the size of the 'crisis' or 'challenge' and the impact on the health services should be assessed. The commonest health and disability problems experienced by very old people are immobility, instability, incontinence, mental impairment, disturbances of hearing and vision, foot troubles and toxic drug effects (Isaacs 1981, Rossiter & Wicks 1982). Reduced mobility leads to a vicious cycle of decreasing social contact, isolation, and inability to keep warm and to prepare food. Mentally frail, demented and depressed elderly people experience greater physical decline and are particularly at risk from malnutrition, burns, falls and other diseases (Rossiter & Wicks 1982).

Even with ill health and disability, old people are the survivors; they have survived in spite of exposure to disease, poor nutrition, defective immunity, and multiple drug taking, which leaves them unfit but does not kill them. The multiple diseases of very old age converge on the four Giants of Geriatrics (Isaacs 1981) — immobility, instability, mental impairment and incontinence. As Isaacs makes clear, these Giants, although not exclusive to the elderly, have four common properties which cause great difficulties for old people: they have multiple causes, they destroy independence, they have no simple treatment, and they need human helpers. They are not inevitable consequences of old age but do require the skills of the specialist. 'Too often they evoke a cry for removal and storage rather than for investigation and treatment' (Isaacs 1981, p. 145).

Population statistics do not emphasize the practical consequences for society of an ageing population. Grimley Evans (in Hodgson 1984) maintains that the British government has based its future policies for health and social services on two fallacies. First, the phenomenon of 'rectangularization', described by Malcolm Johnson in Chapter 1, in which the death rate curve is shifted towards a maximum lifespan. This shift is evident in most industrial countries, and the fallacy is the government's assumption that the shift will also occur in the need for care. This is to say, if life expectancy increases by 10 years, nursing, medical and social services care will be needed 10 years later than at present. There is no evidence for this.

The second fallacy highlighted by Grimley Evans is the assumption that any increase in the care burden can be borne primarily by the community rather than the state. Yet all the evidence indicates that an ageing population generates increased health care needs in general, and there is a huge proportionate increase of old people with conditions requiring skilled nursing care. Grimley Evans predicts that by the twenty-first century, in order merely to maintain present standards, home visits by general practitioners must increase by 9%, district nurse and health visitor visits by 14%, home help by 18%, meals-on-wheels by 23%, and chiropody by 9%. Expert and dedicated 24-hour nursing supervision is needed for demented old people. There is no evidence that dementia itself shortens life, but there is plenty of evidence that lack of care does.

The social context of ageing and retirement reflects negative attitudes. As discussed elsewhere (Chs. 1 and 7) society is still in the early stages of understanding and interpreting old age. It views the 'age explosion' with alarm and regards 'the elderly' as a 'social problem', creating an intolerable economic and social burden. Old age is still seen as a period of 'social redundancy' with an emphasis on the non-productiveness of elders. This stereotype of inevitable physical and mental decline and of elderly people as consumers of excessive amounts of health and social services, even if true of large numbers of old people today, is not an inevitable consequence of survival into very old age. The backgrounds, social and financial status, and environmental and health factors of today's elderly are unique and different from those of the next generation of old people.

Financially, many elderly people are living on

or near the officially defined 'poverty' line. The state pension is the sole source of income for many old people. They are dependent on additional income support, although by no means all who are eligible claim these benefits. This point is made in Chapter 27 by Fiona Ross, who describes the support available in England for old people. Most of their income is spent on necessities like food, fuel and housing, and it is the working-class single women and widows, who have no access to occupational pensions, who are most likely to be below the poverty line. It is women who bear most of the poverty.

WOMEN IN RETIREMENT AND OLD AGE

In many ways ageing is a woman's issue. Of those over 75 years, there are two women to every man and many live alone, a large proportion of these having done so for a long time (Phillipson 1982, and see Ch. 24 of this volume). They are, therefore, very used to being alone and, one would think, are particularly prone to feelings of isolation, loneliness, depression and alienation. Many are on the poverty line and so cannot afford the communication commodities (car, telephone, etc.) which would enable them to be with others more often and be less likely to suffer these negative psychological experiences.

It is not really known what this isolation together with health problems and disabilities means for older women. We know something about the famous exceptions to the old age stereotype (Pablo Picasso, Sybil Thorndyke, Bertrand Russell, Marlene Dietrich, etc.), and about life in institutions for the elderly (see Chapter 29), but we know very little about what the isolated elderly woman living alone does with her time, although Evers (1983) has investigated this. Evers found the commonest response to a question about what they had been doing the day before was 'nothing much' or 'nothing at all'. However, on further questioning, these women had in fact been doing many things, like personal and household tasks, leisure activities and

meeting people. Evers speculates on why such activities were not mentioned, and she offers three explanations of the 'doing nothing much' syndrome. It may reflect a relative reduction in the number and importance of activities with age, or a gloomy outlook on life, or a devaluation of 'women's work', which is not considered worth mentioning. Evers found that the women interviewed could be classified crudely as either 'passive responders' (PR), who seemed to have little control over their lives, or 'active initiators' (AI) who were very much in control and had purpose in life. Ill health and dependency were not, apparently, characteristics exclusive to either group but were represented in both, nor were the groups different according to class, education level, affluence, or contact with surviving children.

Evers has made the link between AI women and 'engagement' and PR women and 'disengagement'. She suggests that AI women had pursued activities in their lives in addition to the traditional work of women as carers, whereas PR women had filled most of their lives with caring activities. The categories are unlikely to be as simple as suggested here, but if confirmed, the implications of Evers' hypothesis are important for health care workers, who should understand the psychological characteristics of women in their care. Otherwise, AI women may resent a loss of control over their lives, and PR women may be unable to respond healthily to enforced independence. Nurses are the workers in the best position to identify such characteristics and to ensure that they and others meet the individual needs of each old woman in their care.

Because they are the survivors, old women are much more likely than old men to spend their final years in an institution. The generally low standards in institutions may be partly a result of there being more women residents. It may reflect external, societal beliefs about the status and rights of elderly women in particular and of women in general (Phillipson 1982).

The effectiveness of future problem-solving and social policy on care of elderly people will depend on whether past and present ageing patterns and needs of women are incorporated into professional and popular perceptions, or are ignored as they are today. Social, professional and legislative systems do not recognize women's needs as a priority or as different from men's (Roebuck 1983). As Roebuck observes, writers on the elderly, be they philosophers, literary writers or gerontologists, from classical Greece to the present, from Aristotle to Shakespeare, write about old age in male terms. Jacques' speech in 'As You Like It' views ageing in terms of the seven ages of man. Writers and politicians continue in this vein even though numerous censuses have confirmed the numerical dominance of old women. They assume that all elderly people either possess male characteristics or are homogeneously sexless.

Elderly women are victims of two stereotypes, one sexist, the other ageist. Even though, as discussed in other chapters in this book (e.g. Chs. 2 and 16), the image of the 'sick and helpless old person' does not apply to most old women or men, the stereotype remains powerful and little is expected of them as a result. They are thought too feeble to have demands made on them. This leads to the self-fulfilling prophecy of asocial functioning, incompetence and dependency (Roebuck 1983). Old people themselves hold these stereotypes and the effect may be disastrous for them because they think they are decrepit burdens to families and to society. They may hate themselves and their contemporaries, and believe that late life can offer nothing useful or interesting.

Roebuck maintains that women are labelled as old sooner than men are, that is, at the menopause. This is the time when women are 'cast off' as old because they can no longer bear children and fulfil the reason for their existence as defined by male-oriented society. In contrast, men at this age may be at the height of their careers. The view that women are old, sick and useless from the menopause to death is not an uncommon one, and this period may be nearly half their lifetime. Negative stereotypes are physically, psychologically and socially damaging to the victims and are extremely difficult to erase because they are rooted in society's deep past. The old people suffer despair and impotence, and the rest of the population ei-

ther ignore the reality or reinforce the negative stereotype. It is not by chance that the negative descriptors which are applied to old age are similar to those often used to describe women, such as lack of vigour or initiative or dynamism, inferior mental capacity, low social status, weakness and economic dependence.

Many writers (e.g. Roebuck 1983) support the view that women have coped better than men with old age. They may have a more diverse social world with friendships outside the family, are more accustomed to widowhood and the need to build new lives without a spouse, and are less used to being looked after. Women are said to be more likely to make and retain strong friendships and so female patterns of life and response to major change are generally more successful than male patterns. Women are, they think, successful survivors and their greater life expectation, which is continuing to increase relative to men's, bears witness to this.

Phillipson (1982) disputes this view and suggests that women have a more difficult time coping with retirement and old age than is suggested. He bases his argument on three factors. First, the position of women in women's studies. Even though women outnumber men after retirement from work, most of the research focuses on the experiences and problems of men in retirement. It is a cause for concern that the feminist literature also puts very little emphasis on older women, who when joining women's groups feel resented as outsiders (Lewis & Butler 1980, Macdonald & Rich 1984). This may, however, disappear as the women's movement grows and its present members become old. In America, elderly women are gaining in political strength, and they have time to be actively involved in consciousness-raising, as Maggie Kuhn has shown with her Gray Panther movement (Kuhn 1980).

Such pressure groups, other than those linked to employment organizations and trades unions, have not yet made much of an impression in the UK, although some are beginning to emerge. For example, the pressure group, Pensioners' Voice (The National Federation of Retirement Pensioners' Association) has over 800 branches in the UK and a few in Canada and South Africa. Its aims are to improve the quality of life for pensioners in general, and, more specifically, to impose pressure on the government for a higher basic state pension.

Another organization, Pensioners' Link, works with local pensioner action committees in London to identify, analyse and take action on issues such as welfare rights, health, education and heating. The British Association of Retired Persons (ARP) is a new national voluntary organization and aims to 'change the whole attitude of people in this country to retirement', and 'to unleash the potential for a tremendous economic, social and political force' (Age Concern 1988). ARP was inspired by the American Association of Retired Persons which now has 29 million members (Age Concern 1988). It will be some time, however, before 'the potential for a tremendous political force' is realized in the UK in comparison, for example, with West Germany where a new political party, the Greys, has been formed. The Greys will fight for parliamentary seats in 1990 on key issues such as pensions, conditions in residential and nursing Homes, sheltered housing and ageism (Age Concern 1989). Malcolm Johnson (Chapter 1) discusses the development of corporate consciousness and action by older people.

Phillipson's second factor relates to women as workers. As unpaid workers women are seen to face less of a crisis in retirement than men do, because they continue to keep active with household chores. On the contrary, Phillipson argues that women's domestic and work responsibilities may create considerable stress in middle and old age. The identity of women as mothers only is outdated because many of those who have children spend a fairly small proportion of their lives caring for them full-time. Even so, the mothering role remains and is extended into women's work, as volunteer carer, nurse, home help, etc., all of which roles concern sick and elderly people. Even though women may try to escape from the caring role when they no longer have dependent children, society limits the work opportunities available and expects them to take on the more nurturing roles. Social policies are, in today's climate of economic restraint, increasing the pressure on women to ac-

cept such roles, especially in the care of elderly relatives, and it is well known that women take on the major burden of caring for old people (see Chs. 24 and 27). Thus, just when a woman feels free to pursue studies or a career, she finds she is tied to yet more dependants, a pressure which is much greater for her than for men. Then, when her parents die, she is faced with caring for an ailing husband.

There has been a large increase since the Second World War of women over the age of 45 years doing paid work, many of whom cope with the dual role of worker and mother/homemaker. The jobs they do are usually poorly paid, unskilled, and auxiliary work which may not carry an occupational pension. Furthermore, social attitudes still regard paid work for women as secondary to their primary homemaker role, and this is reflected in low levels of pay. The Conservative government in the United Kingdom today emphasizes that the woman's place is at home; she should not take jobs away from men, and should care for young and elderly dependants. In other words, she should provide extra domestic labour to compensate for the public services which are cut.

The third factor outlined by Phillipson refers to the implications for later life of female labour under capitalism. Women can experience discrimination at premature retirement when their own careers are sacrificed to care for parents, or for husbands after their retirement. The transition from work to retirement may be extremely stressful for women, especially financially if there is no occupational pension. The full-time homemaker may find that her workload and financial burden have increased with her husband at home all day. Women workers are often more resistant than men to retirement because many have already experienced the isolation of working at home all day with young children, although in some cases, especially the better off, retirement may provide long-sought opportunities for growth and recreation, for both women and men.

In their conversations about old age with elderly women, Ford and Sinclair (1987) confirmed Phillipson's (1982) view. They found that many women have to face enormous changes on retirement, and often alone, especially if they have spent all their lives financially and emotionally dependent on others.

You think that going from school to work is a big thing, but then you've got so much confidence that you sail through it. Retiring is by far the hardest thing I have ever faced (Interviewee in Ford & Sinclair 1987, p. 151).

The women Ford and Sinclair interviewed focused on ensuring that their lives were meaningful and fulfilling. They strove to balance their need for security with the need for independence and self-respect, and some accepted loneliness as preferable to a loss of independence.

The twentieth century has been a period of very rapid modernization in the Western world and women's adaptability to change has been more marked than men's. Women have had to learn to make the most out of scarce or dwindling resources because they tend to bear the major burden of poverty in a period of decline.

Within 'the aged' those most likely to teach us not only how to make the most out of the least but also how to cope successfully with major personal and social changes are women. The future promises to hold challenges very different from the past, but to be no less a time of massive change than the rest of the modern era has been. Perhaps the greatest difference is that the most logical revolutionary leader for the future is that hitherto most unlikely candidate — grandma (Roebuck 1983, p. 264).

MEN IN RETIREMENT AND OLD AGE

This section is much shorter than the previous one on women in retirement and old age. This deliberate bias occurs not because we have less to say about men, but because so much less has been written about elderly women, who are clearly more at risk as a group, as evidenced by the demographic data.

As we have seen, attainment of 'retirement age' is a life event which, for both sexes, is accompanied by many stresses, whatever the quality of the change. There is, however, recent evidence of slightly greater optimism about retirement. In the late 1980s positive views about retirement were often expressed; there was pressure to leave work and create jobs for younger people. This contrasts with the 1950s, when people were encouraged to stay in work and those who were retired were seen as 'a burden' (Fennell et al 1988).

On the other hand, the trend today for early retirement together with an increased life expectancy means that many people spend a third of their lives (20 or 30 years) without paid work. A third of those 'in retirement' are well off and able to enjoy their leisure, cushioned by index-linked occupational pensions. Another third hold less than 1% of pensioner savings and can barely keep going on their only source of income, the state retirement pension. These old people cannot enjoy their old age in the way that those with the means to finance leisure pursuits can (O'Donnell 1988).

Phillipson (1982) has described three main variations in the transition from work to retirement for men. The 'stable withdrawer' prepares for a change in lifestyle and may feel that he has achieved all he can in his work role. The 'unstable withdrawer' may experience retirement as a result of redundancy and perhaps ill health; this may be accompanied by a feeling of having been rejected and discarded, and by dwindling resources. The 'abrupt withdrawer' may experience anxiety before retirement, which interferes with his successful preparation for it. Evidence shows that most men do not prepare for retirement but just let things happen. This clean break from work to non-work is a crisis for most people; it may bring loneliness, and requires adjustment as with any loss. Coupled with a drop in income and perhaps poor health, the main problem may be bewilderment at how to cope with such change, rather than boredom. Social class is important, with middle-class men in professional jobs more likely than working-class men in unskilled jobs to take social roles after retirement. The former may have more skills that can be used in retirement than manual workers.

Even though many men enjoy the sense of freedom and escape from the clock, retirement is not generally seen as a period for growth and self-development. The idea of an active, purposeful retirement is being encouraged, but, as Phillipson argues, it is difficult to see how it can be reconciled with declining income and living standards.

On the one hand, the government promotes retirement as being healthy for the individual (more leisure) and for the state (new job opportunities); yet, on the other, the resources provided for it are small. Retired people feel they are marginal citizens. This low status may not be felt early in retirement but comes later when finances and health decline and contemporaries die.

Phillipson highlights the conflict inherent between work and leisure in a capitalist and bureaucratic society. The opportunities for development of human potential become more and more limited, especially for office and factory workers, yet the expansion of educational, cultural and other activities to fill our leisure time encourages us to realize this potential. Phillipson suggests that improvements would occur if the worker could enter and re-enter the workforce at different times in his career, and spend time on paid educational leave and sabbaticals so that work and education were more closely linked. This would also suit women who need time out from paid work for child-rearing. Also, if workers had more control over the nature and pace of their work, older workers would not become obsolete so quickly and could continue on a part-time basis. Such flexible links between work, education and leisure would make retirement easier, but existing structures are currently too rigid for this to occur on any scale.

'AGEISM' AND 'GERIATRICS'

The term 'ageism' has been introduced into our language much more recently than 'sexism' or 'racism'. It emerged in the United States in the 1960s and became part of UK language fairly recently (Currie 1987). Comfort (1977) popularized the distinction between biological ageing and 'sociogenic ageing' which he defined as the role society imposes on people when they reach a certain chronological age. Ageism refers to prejudice and stereotyping of old age that engenders negative attitudes towards old people such that they are seen in infantile, derogatory or pitying terms

(Norman 1987, Stevenson 1989). Stevenson maintains that 'ageism is pervasive and entrenched in our society'. She contrasts the lack of interest in the 30 and more years following 'retirement' with the numerous developmental stages identified during infancy and childhood that cover a mere 12 years. Norms of development are applied to children but not to old people; over-75 year olds are assumed to be dependent and incapable of development.

Younger people, encouraged by media images, marvel about the capable 'exceptions' to the ageist stereotype: 'Isn't she wonderful, doing that at her age!', with reference to the 70-year-old marathon runner, or the recollections of the centenarian on television. These activities are indeed to be admired, but to single them out for special mention is a form of ageism in that they are seen as so exceptional as to deserve comment.

Most people over 65 years do not feel that they belong to the category 'old' given them by society. They feel the same as they always did 'inside', even though they can see external changes:

I fancy almost everybody who draws near to the beginning of their 70th year must be struck by the oddity of the fact that inside their own skull they are aware of so little difference! I have a notion that elderly people have a tendency to forget the fanciful misconceptions about old age that they had when they were young (John Cowper Powys, *The Art of Growing Old*, quoted in Symonds 1987, p. 10).

Kenneth Andrews shows how much more valuable a person can be in his 70s compared with his 50s, and by implication, how 'old' some people are at 25:

And if anyone asked me if I would like to be 'young' again, I would say no, for I have learned too much to wish to relinquish it.

To my mind I am a far more valuable person today than I was 50 years ago . . . . I have learned so much since I was 70.

We old people . . . should not allow our young people to be impatient with us, to bully us or relegate us. If they do it is because we have not taught them any better — and this is because we have not known our own worth; we have not respected ourselves . . . (Kenneth W Andrews, *Miracle Man*, quoted in Symonds 1987, p. 11).

To combat ageism, nurses would be wise to take Kenneth Andrew's advice and learn from old people how they feel and how they adjust to changes imposed by their physical, social and emotional situation. Thus, nurses should develop the empathy that enables them to step into the old person's shoes and to understand and share that person's experiences. This process is very different from being unduly sympathetic or 'killing with kindness'. Stevenson (1989) identifies the considerable barriers to the development of empathy by younger folk towards old people. First of all, by virtue of not yet being 'old' ourselves, we have not had their experiences. We often do not see them as ordinary human beings with similar responses and reactions; we assume their joys and sorrows to be different from our own. Above all, we assume that no one wants to be old; we do not know what it will feel like and we do not want to know — it is too depressing, we think. We accept the 'tragedy' of old age depicted in King Lear rather than learning from the experts, old people themselves, that old age can be a time of growth, change, joy and fulfilment.

Health professionals who work with elderly people are often more ageist than the general population because they assume that the problems of their patients are common to all old people (Stevenson 1989). A potentially unbearable and pervasive form of ageism practised by nurses and other health workers stems from the belief that old people require only their basic physical needs to be satisfied. All they require is to be warm, comfortable and well fed; social, emotional and spiritual needs are therefore ignored. I remember a sister in a geriatric ward, observing my students in conversation with some of the patients, saying to me, 'There's no point. They don't need talking to. They want to be treated like babies.'

It is, of course, true that a great deal of physical care may be needed, and it is true that mental infirmity may limit a person's capacity, but is this sufficient reason for not making the effort required to relate to the whole person in order to avoid '. . . the stigmatising and depersonalising processes which insult the integrity of the old person'? (Stevenson 1989). The tendency of care staff in long-stay institutions to stereotype the residents,

to attribute incompetence to age, and to exploit their position of unequal power, are aspects of ageism and are discussed also in Chapter 29 of this volume.

The implicitly ageist attitudes of some health professionals who work with elderly people are particularly insidious and subject frail and dependent old people to even more discrimination than they experience simply by virtue of being old. The ageist attitude of these nurses, geriatricians, general practitioners, social workers, therapists and other care staff was termed 'new ageism' by Borkman (1982). He sees 'new ageism' as a more subtle and damaging form of discrimination than ageism because it is held by professionals actually engaged in the care of old people, who ought to employ and promote anti-ageist attitudes. Instead, these professionals pay lip service to the heterogeneity and diversity of old people, but in practice, see them as unhealthy, incapable, unalert, helpless and dependent on services.

This new ageism does not appear to be diminishing to any great extent, at least in the medical profession (Currie 1987). Currie's impressions are confirmed by Maddox and Tillery (1988), who investigated whether old people were portrayed more positively in the professional medical, nursing and health journals of 1986 compared with those published in 1981. They found some evidence of a move away from ageism in the nursing and health journals, but very little change in the medical journals. Maddox and Tillery refer to evidence in the USA of a decrease in negative stereotypes of old people held by nurses who have been educated to a higher level than those with the basic registered nurse qualification. This confirms the impression we have gained in the UK that working with old people is the first choice of many new graduates of nursing who have pursued their education to degree level.

Alison Norman (1984) reminds us of Humpty Dumpty's saying that when he used a word it meant what he chose it to mean. This has been the case with 'geriatrics'. It was coined by Nascher in 1909, from 'geras', meaning old age and 'iatrikos', meaning relating to the physician; it is thus the antithesis of 'paediatrics'. Geriatrics gained acceptance as a new medical specialty but it became corrupted to 'geriatric', meaning an old person, often a confused old person.

Geriatric is a cold, uncreative word. It has no heart. It's fatalistic. And it reeks of mortality. I've learnt that it is possible to have medical training and still not be able to grasp that people old in years are not necessarily senile. Here, this syndrome is taking over — atrophy, apathy, endless, meaningless babble — mental collapse. It's a Pandora's box that holds nothing but distress. Nobody has thought to add any kind of hope. Why? (Ellen Newton 1980, p. 171)

Ellen Newton wrote a moving account of the inadequate care she received in expensive, privately-owned nursing Homes in Australia. Her view of the medical and nursing care she received is summed up here in her chilling definition of 'geriatric'.

We never call a sick child a 'paediatric'. Misuse of language is a serious issue because it creates stereotypes of identity and behaviour which have a powerful effect on those so labelled. Old people are lumped together in a single category to which is attributed the negative characteristics of low social status, non-productivity, physical ill health and imminent brain failure (Norman 1984). This is extremely damaging and hinders efforts to treat the autumn of one's life as a joyful, liberating, peaceful period of psychological growth. Of course the privileged (presidents, archbishops, judges, surgeons) are not so labelled, although they often use the stereotype to refer to others. Alison Norman notes that even the Archbishop of Canterbury, a classical scholar, has described himself as playing 'geriatric tennis', a strictly meaningless term.

LOUISA: JOURNEY INTO THE UNKNOWN

The following moving account of Louisa's, and her family's, experiences of care in a residential Home and in hospital, was written by her daughter, Roberta. The experience occurred in 1988/89 in a town on the south coast of England. At intervals throughout the account we have interjected with a comment to identify the ageist attitudes that we feel were implicitly held by the staff who looked after Louisa. We have chosen to reproduce the whole story here, rather than to truncate it, because it raises many issues of concern from which nurses can learn.

Louisa (her preferred name) is an 83 year old living in a Rest Home where she has been resident for some 10 years. Her rheumatoid arthritis is extensive and there was a particularly virulent attack after her husband died about 15 years ago. She can now do very little for herself and in the past two years her deprivations were accentuated when she gradually became blind. In that time she had been moved into a small, single room and, apart from two or three hourly visits from the care staff and the background sounds from her TV set, she was sightless and alone.

Members of her family visited her from time to time, particularly me, her only daughter. On each visit I took with me a portable tape-recorder and played her favourite music. Louisa has a good natural music sense and still retains what must have been a fine soprano voice. Together we would accompany the recorded pieces with our own renderings. Louisa was also up-to-date with the news and current affairs and seemed to want to discuss them with me on each visit. I concluded that hers was an alert and sharp, if untutored, mind.

I had attempted several times in the past, when she lived in her own home, to get her to accept and try various forms of outside help, even before my father died, which was an uphill battle for me. This finally culminated in her agreeing to be seen by a geriatrician as she steadily and remorselessly deteriorated after her bereavement. She was admitted to a geriatric ward where she was helped to regain some health. After that she was housed by my brother for a while but, on proving to be an excessive burden, was dispatched under great protest to the Rest Home. Since then, realizing her worsening sight, I eventually succeeded in coaxing her, about three years ago, to agree to an eye examination. Unfortunately, just before the appointment she fell during the night whilst trying to use her commode alone. The outcomes were: an indefinite postponement of the eye test, positioning of furniture against her bed so that she could not fall out and the care staff insisting that she use incontinence pads during the night.

Here is an example of ageist attitudes held by the care staff. They insisted on confining Louisa to bed during the night because of their fear of recrimination in the event of an accident. They put greater emphasis on protecting themselves than on allowing Louisa the choice and the right to take a risk. She thus was forced, against her will, to learn to pass urine in the wrong and socially unacceptable place. Her daughter's account continues:

Eventually I felt sufficiently confident about trying again to get her eyes looked at, and she agreed to a domiciliary visit by an ophthalmologist. His opinion was that a cataract operation to her worse eye would be successful, although he felt disinclined to do it in view of her general condition.

Here the opthalmologist conveyed an ageist attitude. He concluded that her 'general condition' contraindicated surgery, although he did not explain to Roberta the exact reasons for his view, nor did he offer referral to a geriatrician who could have checked Louisa's ability to withstand surgery. Many cataract operations are done under local anaesthetic and so the disadvantages of general anaesthesia may not have been a problem. Roberta insisted on more information:

I had to ask the GP for the specialist's address and a copy of the eye report. I spoke with the specialist on several occasions and he struck me as a humane and accommodating person. We agreed to give Louisa plenty of time and support to make her own decision. I was also told that the anaesthetist was familiar with this kind of case and would take the greatest care.

It was before Christmas 1988 when I had these discussions. In the meantime I talked to Louisa about the possible surgery, assured her that she would be allowed to make her own decision, and warned her that there was no guarantee of success. The care staff at the Home encouraged her to think positively about the opportunity, and when I told her it was decision time (February 1989), she gave her consent and emphasized that sight was important to her if she was to live for a further two years or so. I communicated this decision to my brothers, to the eye specialist and to the GP and none raised objections. I expressed concern about using a general anaesthetic with such a frail old lady, and the specialist thought it should be left to make the decision on the day.

We arranged for my sister-in-law, Sonja, who lived locally, to be at the Home on Wednesday, the day of admission, to accompany Louisa to the hospital, and await my arrival from London, where I live and work, later that day. I arrived at the eye ward in the evening to learn that Sonja had taken her to the toilet on her own with great difficulty and that no nursing help had been offered. In fact, the nurses told Sonja that if she could not manage alone, they would have to get porters to help because they could not do it themselves.

Shortly afterwards, the specialist arrived with a junior colleague, who said that they had decided on a general anaesthetic because of Louisa's disability, and they would leave her for an extra day to settle down; she was excitable and her pulse rate was high. Again, I sought and was given reassurances that mother could withstand the general anaesthetic.

Sonja and I were asked to get her into bed ourselves — not an easy task. She asked us for some tea but was told she had missed 'the round'. Sonja then left and I had a sinking feeling that things were going out of control, that Louisa should not be there, and that the situation was irretrievable.

It is difficult to believe that the staff left the relatives to take Louisa to the toilet and get her into bed themselves. The nurses did not see it as their job to attend to the basic needs of a frail old lady. They were clearly not familiar with the needs of old people, even though one would expect old people to frequent eye wards. A detailed nursing assessment of Louisa's problems had not been made and there was no care plan in evidence. The nurses did not know how to care for her, neither did they have any insight into the reasons for and management of her growing excitability, which was clearly a manifestation of her anxiety.

I stayed with Louisa holding her hand and singing with her until 8 p.m. She did eventually get her tea and she managed to eat a little food. Further cardiovascular tests revealed she had begun to settle, and I was told she would be operated on at 10 a.m. the next day after all. I emphasized that Louisa needed help in my absence with the toilet and with eating, and I also checked they had all information about her drugs. I phoned the next day at noon to learn she was still in the theatre, and I was discouraged by the nurse who answered my call from visiting at all that day.

It is clear that Roberta did not trust the nurses to be competent and she felt she had to underline what was needed in order to ensure that minimum care was given. Discouraging her from visiting on the day of the operation demonstrates the nurses' reliance on routines and rituals, and their lack of insight into the value of Roberta's presence to Louisa's recovery.

I visited on the following afternoon to find Louisa out of bed wearing an eye dressing. She was comforted by my presence particularly when the dressing was changed. Sarah, a friend, accompanied me on the next day and we stayed with her until 8 p.m., getting her to drink as much as she would accept. We thought she was recovering well enough from the operation, we played some of her favourite music, and she sang a great deal. It was clear that singing was for her an important way of coping with the stress. The nurses and other patients said that her singing was not a nuisance to them.

I was told that she would be discharged back to the Rest Home on the Monday. I telephoned that day to learn that there were no instructions to discharge her. On the Tuesday Sonja agreed to find out what was happening. Sonja phoned me in London on Tuesday evening to say that Louisa had been discharged, alone, to the Home that afternoon and that the care staff found her in a poor state. She was 'not the same person' who had left them, and was less co-ordinated; the ward sister had told them that Louisa had refused to co-operate in opening her eyes and that she kept singing all the time, thus disturbing the other patients.

Two days later, Sonja and my brother, Richard, phoned me in some distress, because Louisa's GP had seen her earlier that day and thought there might be 'brain damage'; that grandson Jonathan had visited and she did not know him; that Louisa had a few lucid moments and that she had tried to sing a bit but could only produce 'gibberish'. She had lost a lot of weight and looked very old.

I could not believe that Louisa had deteriorated so much, given that she seemed to be recovering when I last saw her. I left straight away for the Home, with Mary, another friend, and we found her in bed and her favourite care assistant was trying to feed her. I flung my arms round Louisa and begged her to return to us and not to give up now we had come this far together. She tried to lift her head and sing a bit, and she was partly coherent, although extremely drowsy. I asked her to press my hand to tell me she understood me, and she clearly did. She volunteered that she was 'poorly'. Later, when we were leaving, she asked me where she was next being taken to. I replied emphasizing that she wasn't going away ever again; that she was staying here with people she trusted and I would see her often. She appeared to understand that.

The failure to provide the necessary discharge information to enable a relative to accompany Louisa to the Home from the hospital, and the lack of understanding by the ward sister of Louisa's behaviour demonstrate to us a clear lack of concern. Louisa did not fit the 'normal' patient role and the nurses were unwilling to respond to her specific needs in a caring way. She had all the 'problems' of a 'geriatric patient' and these were of no interest to nurses specialized in eye care.

Evidence of 'new ageism' is clearly apparent. The assumption of the GP of 'brain damage' was also ageist. He had no evidence for this, not having examined Louisa, and he made no attempt to consider other causes for her confusion (such as a drug reaction or interaction, an infection, dehydration and electrolyte imbalance, malnutrition, or relocation without explanation). It is clear that Louisa had gone through a pathological crisis but she had not suffered irreversible brain damage. It is extremely unlikely that the GP would have come to the same conclusion with a younger patient.

The next day we found her in her chair and noticeably better. She sang a lot although she would drift in and out of awareness and was 'imbecilic' from time to time. She seemed to have lost any memory of the hospital but agreed she had been 'on a journey'. She wanted to drink, but could not feed herself and was still incontinent.

Over the next few days her condition fluctuated. Sometimes she was lucid and aware but at others she was confused, drowsy and did not always respond to my voice, or the care assistants' voices. She seemed to be having difficulty in swallowing and there was a noticeable cough. I was troubled and phoned the GP. He could not tell me if this was a drug reaction, or whether she had an infection or if her electrolyte balance was abnormal. All he could say was, 'Her eyes are alright, but it's her mind', followed by nervous laughter. I expressed shock that she should deteriorate after her initial recovery and asked about getting in a geriatrician. He said he preferred to assess her first, in a day or two. Why not that day?

The care staff in the Home had a good opinion of this GP. They felt that nothing more could be done for Louisa; that they were doing their best; that we must take every day as it comes and be thankful for any small improvement since Louisa was an old lady and was weak before her operation. What counted was her spirit. 'It's happened before with residents going to the hospital. They give up.'

I felt helpless too, and was struck by the ageism of these people. The attitude seemed to be 'what can you expect of an old lady?' My power, such that it was, I knew instinctively resided in my relationship with Louisa. She trusted me: 'I haven't cried for long time. I don't know why. Folks in here think its daft, the way you and I are, but I don't think so, do you? Trouble is I miss you when you've gone.'

She was still confused and didn't appear to realize she'd had an operation. She continued to show some partial recovery of sight but had difficulty keeping her eyes open. I left her feeling very stressed myself and heavy hearted. I feel very uncertain still if Louisa will survive and if she does whether her brain impairment will resolve, and by how much, and whether she will gain much sight after all. I decided that so far it had not been worth it, even if people say I might have regretted not giving her a chance. She and we have paid a big price so far. Why is it so difficult to get information?

The continued ageist attitude of the GP is demonstrated in his assumption of brain damage, his refusal to consider other reasons for Louisa's deterioration or even to assess her thoroughly, and his implicit assumption that nothing more could be done. The care staff in the Home colluded in this. They thought highly of the GP and had little specialist knowledge themselves. Their view was that if anything could have been done it would have been, and the best thing now was to let 'nature' take its course. None of the professionals accepted Roberta's insistence that Louisa's collapse might be treatable and reversible. Nor did they recognize Roberta's key role in Louisa's care and recovery. The healing power of the family tends not to be understood or recognized by health professionals threatened by enquiries which might weaken their power base. In spite of her resistance, Roberta felt that the professionals should know what was happening, and she was beginning to accept the likelihood of brain damage. Her guilt in feeling solely responsible for her mother's deterioration was enormous, and none of the professionals helped her with this. Support for Roberta came from her friends alone.

Sarah and I visited Louisa the next day. Louisa was better, her sight was better and she had no difficulty in recognizing us. She said her body was 'all broken up', and she was unhappy about incontinence, disapproving of the pads. She got us to help her use the commode before we left.

The insistence by the care staff over use of incontinence pads and enforced incontinence was extremely distressing to Louisa, who in fact was continent now, if allowed to be. The staff did not seem willing to try a regime of continence management, finding it easier to change wet pads. They were not concerned about the loss of dignity Louisa experienced.

Later, we learnt that my other brother and his family had visited Louisa in hospital and had found the visit embarrassing and worrying. They hoped I knew what I was doing and remarked on the difference in care between the Home and the hospital. They thought nothing more could be done, Louisa should be allowed to die and they hoped she wouldn't last long; she should not be allowed to go through that experience again.

The burden of feeling solely responsible and the ensuing guilt experienced by Roberta is multiplied extensively by the disapproval expressed by her brother and his family. They colluded with the view of the professionals, leaving Roberta completely alone in believing in the possibility of treatment and cure.

I tried, twice, unsuccessfully to reach the GP. I learnt later that he had visited Louisa and pronounced her better, although all he appears to have done is talk to her and examine her chest. She was pleased to have seen him and could say what he had been wearing. Towards the end of my visit she was flagging again. Some loss of memory persists, including the names of her favourite singers but she was able to recall some recent events. I continue to doubt that she will ever fully recover, or that there will be much gain in sight, or that it had been worth the cost.
The next day Richard and Sonja visited and later phoned me with their evident joy that Louisa was so much improved. She had recognized them instantly.
A week later, there was an order-of-magnitude change in Louisa who did not drift off at all while we were there. There was a marked gain in sight. I wasn't allowed to play music for long since she was much more interested in the horses and their colourful jockeys on TV! She talked in detail about her room, which reminded us that she had never before seen it. Aside from the pressure sores we now learnt she had acquired in hospital, we felt positively elated. It remains now for her to continue to improve and for her eye not to reject the lens. If it does, I can't see us allowing anything but essential intervention. It now looks as if the whole traumatic episode was, after all, worth it. But could better nursing care have prevented much of this trauma? And how far should I have stayed with Louisa throughout the hospitalization? And should she have been discharged sooner? And what price should be paid for visual recovery? Yet . . . she is like a newborn discovering and rediscovering a wonderful world.

The final successful outcome after a long, hard battle for Louisa and her daughter was tremendously rewarding. But it cannot conceal the incalculable psychological stress Roberta suffered, much of which was avoidable. Iatrogenic disease as a result of hospitalization and surgery is clearly evident. Louisa's post-operative acute confusional state was, we suggest, aggravated by poor nutrition, dehydration, a possible chest infection, and adverse reaction to the general anaesthetic. She was given atropine and hyoscine as a premedication which are known to cause post-operative confusion in elderly people (Platzer 1988). The hospital nurses failed to incorporate energetic preventive care that would have circumvented the pressure sores. The Home staff were caring but untrained, and were faced with an old lady in a badly deteriorated state. They provided loving care to Louisa throughout and developed a supportive, respectful attitude to her daughter, but they were in no position to implement an active management regime which could have reversed the decline that started in the hospital.

No credit can be given to the hospital nurses, doctors, or the GP for planned care which would have ensured the best possible outcome and would have prevented well-known complications. The restoration of sight was a medical success, but without the insight and intervention by Roberta and her friends, the outcome would almost certainly have been different. Louisa would have been left to fall into the downward spiral of disability, dependency, helplessness, malnutrition, dehydration, confusion, pressure sores and incontinence and onwards relentlessly towards the inevitable outcome of coma and death.

Louisa's story underlines the importance and value of competent assessment and intervention by knowledgeable doctors and nurses experienced in the care of old people. We submit that the story would have been very different if Louisa had been admitted to an elderly care ward under the care of progressive geriatricians and nurses. The eye surgeon could have performed this cataract operation, preferably under local anaesthetic, and returned Louisa to the elderly care ward so that her eye care could have been integrated with the holistic assessment and care she needed before being discharged to the Home. Follow-up care should have been provided by a district nurse visiting the Home to advise the care staff and to ensure that nursing procedures were implemented to prevent the complications that occurred. The enormous capacity of Louisa's daughter should have been recognized and made an integral part of Louisa's management. Louisa's story illustrates many ageist attitudes that are not uncommon in the care of old people.

FIGHTING PREJUDICE

Ageism can be fought by direct attack, as is the case with racism and sexism, and by encouraging old people to protest against such stereotypes and publicize their creativity and discoveries. This would contribute to a new and wider vocabulary and favourable changes of attitude. Brocklehurst (1984) sees only two ways of remedying the debased 'geriatric's' position and status; by making the practice of geriatrics so excellent and widespread that the term becomes properly understood and respected, or by changing the name. The problem is that no other word fits as correctly. The Americans carefully avoid geriatrics and have adopted gerontology, which is the study of ageing in all living things, and should not refer only to old people, or only to diseases of old people. A gerontologist is thus a scientist and not a clinician. Some geriatric departments have switched to 'clinical gerontology', meaning health care of the elderly, but this is still imprecise. The Anglo-Saxon word 'eld' meaning elderly forms the root of words which convey wisdom as well as age, such as the old term 'alderman' [sic], for an elected councillor in local government in Britain. Some people now advocate the use of the term 'elders' to describe older people because of its positive image of wisdom and experience (for example, Maggie Pearson in Ch. 25). These writers reject the term 'elderly people' because of its recently acquired negative connotations. We should work hard to discard ageist terminology so that words can be used to convey their true meaning.

Brocklehurst suggests using the term 'eld health' in the same way as paediatricians use 'child health'. He prefers, however, the strategy of making geriatrics an excellent specialty and reverting to its real meaning — the medicine of old age.

This is supported by Malcolm Johnson in Chapter 1. Then 'no longer will the adjective "geriatric" be butchered into a noun describing an old man (or old woman)' (Brocklehurst 1984, p. 28, parenthesis added). By the same token, 'geriatric nursing' and 'geriatric nurse' are, strictly, inaccurate, although they are convenient terms to use, as we have seen in a number of chapters in this book. Far better to describe oneself as nursing elderly people, and to teach nurses, other health workers, patients and the public the true meaning of 'geriatrics'.

SUCCESSFUL AGEING

Merton's (1957) notion of the self-fulfilling prophecy, that what we believe will happen we will make happen, applies to so much in social life. It applies in part to the success or failure of the banking system, to education (teachers' expectations of students' examination performance), to sexism and what we expect of women (see Ch. 16), and to ageing and old age. If we expect low quality we will get it. This has been supported by research, particularly in long-term settings for elderly people (Evers 1981a, 1981b, Baker 1983) and is discussed with reference to old people with dementia in Chapter 19.

With the self-fulfilling prophecy in mind, Novak (1983) set out to study 'good ageing' by interviewing 60 active, 'successful', old people in Canada. She wanted to find the healthiest, happiest, most articulate people possible. She justifies this sample bias by arguing that the number in this group will expand and we can learn from them in order to help others. She suggested, 'We need to look at the best ageing has to offer so that we are not doomed by our own expectations to bring about the worst' (p. 232).

The overriding finding from this study was that good age does not come without psychological effort. A clear series of three stages emerged which defined positive development from mid-life to old age, but this pattern was visible only for those who had successfully moved into late life. It was true regardless of ethnic background, sex or income.

All three stages were associated with a realization that ageing should not be denied. People who deny that they are ageing because they want to stay young are less likely to prepare for ageing or to cope successfully with old age. The cost of denial is the shock that one has aged. The first stage is the *challenge*, realizing that change must occur, not denying the fact of ageing and identifying new goals. Then comes the *acceptance*, accepting the challenge that alternative goals are necessary. This transition is not easy and may cause anxiety. It takes courage to age successfully. Finally comes the stage of *affirmation*, when the old person can affirm that she has accepted ageing and is no longer part of the work-oriented hierarchy; she has accepted that she is taking part in a different 'game'. No longer does she strive for high-status rewards but is much more concerned with family and friends. Novak maintains that affirmation is the discovery of the meaning of one's life, and, once discovered, the old person is more likely to help other people. This in itself avoids isolation and meaninglessness to one's life.

Health, social, education and voluntary services can do much to help old people age successfully, but they must first lose their traditional attitudes and assumptions. Jay (1983) observes that for generations it has been assumed that medical advances improve health. Local health initiatives organized by community groups are challenging this assumption, by demystifying medicine, by emphasizing prevention rather than cure, and by educating the public towards a better understanding of the meaning of health and of ways of achieving good health. Community health councils (CHCs), established in England in 1974, were the first real attempt to introduce a line of communication for the public and to encourage community participation. They could be much more influential than they are but they are given very little power to influence the priorities for care and the allocation of funds. As Jay points out, some members of the medical profession, who may feel a threat to their own vested interest, may be hostile towards CHCs, and there has been controversy and uncertainty about their future. They should be developed as an effective consumer voice, not threatened (Batchelor 1984).

Locally-based health projects (such as self-help groups) have had a mixed reception from the medical and nursing professions, who often see them as a threat to their own work. But, on the contrary, these projects have not been set up to compete with conventional services so much as to complement National Health Service provision, and to prevent illness and thereby lighten the burden upon the services. Effective health promotion through prevention rather than treatment has the greatest chance for significantly reducing ill health and mortality in industrialized countries, and it is encouraging to learn that many general practitioners, nurses and health visitors are working closely with community groups to this end, and are enthusiastic about what is being achieved. (See Ch. 23 for discussion of self-care and self-help in old age).

Hospital and community nurses can do much to help old people to become healthy, stay healthy and look after themselves. Old people could remain passive recipients of health care information and services, or they could be encouraged to take an active part in planning and practising preventive health care. They could also be listened to more. Nurses would understand old peoples' beliefs and attitudes better so that they may help them appreciate why some of these views may be incompatible with health. Most elderly people, and unfortunately, many nurses and doctors, believe that health problems of the elderly are due to old age and must be accepted. Understanding this fallacy should be central to any preventive work. Old people and their professional and lay carers can learn that much ill health can be prevented as well as treated.

Exercise benefits everyone, even old and frail people who have chronic diseases. It will increase fitness rather than 'wear out' the body which some old people actually believe. Evidence about good and bad diet has grown enormously, and what constitutes a healthy diet today is very different from that accepted as healthy 40 years ago. Sugar, salt, butter, cream, rich meats, white bread and refined foods used to be the recognized foods of high quality in Britain rather than the unrefined, wholefood, high roughage, low fat diet advocated today (see Chapter 11). It is extremely difficult to change the habits of a lifetime, particularly when there is no obvious sign of ill health (as with high blood pressure or constipation), and when taste buds deteriorate so much that it is tempting to add even more seasonings.

It is not only the old people who need education about healthy living; friends, relatives and health care workers may also hold mistaken beliefs. Often the old person's behaviour will not change without change in attitudes and behaviour of their supporters. Education is available to old people in preretirement groups, Open University courses, old people's clubs and special health courses for the elderly. Nurses have a valuable opportunity to give health care information and advice to individuals in hospital and the community, based on their knowledge of the patient's previous lifestyle. They could exploit the opportunity much more than they do, by a change in their own attitudes and awareness and enhancement of their own skills, particularly skills of communication.

REFERENCES

Acheson E D 1982 The impending crisis of old age: a challenge to ingenuity. Lancet 1: 592–594

Age Concern 1988 Information circular. November, Age Concern England, Mitcham, Surrey

Age Concern 1989 Older people in the United Kingdom. Age Concern England, Mitcham, Surrey

Baker D E 1983 'Care' in the geriatric ward: an account of two styles of nursing. In: Wilson-Barnett J (ed) Nursing research: ten studies in patient care. Wiley, Chichester

Batchelor I 1984 Policies for a crisis? Some aspects of DHSS policies for care of the elderly. Occasional Papers No 1, Nuffield Provincial Hospitals Trust, London

Borkman T 1982 Ageism. In: Kolker A, Ahmed P I (eds) Aging. Elsevier, New York

Brocklehurst J C 1984 What's in a name. New Age 24: 28

Bury M 1988 Arguments about ageing: long life and its consequences. In: Wells N, Freer C (eds) The ageing population: burden or challenge? Macmillan, Basingstoke

Comfort A 1977 A good age. Mitchell Beazley, London

Currie C T 1987 Doctors and ageism. British Medical Journal 295: 19–26

Ernst N S, Glazer-Waldman H R (eds) 1983 The aged patient: a source book for the allied health professional. Year Book Medical Publishers, Chicago

Evers H 1981a Women patients in long-stay geriatric wards. In: Hutter B, Williams G (eds) Controlling women: the normal and the deviant. Croom Helm, London

Evers H 1981b Tender loving care. In: Copp L A (ed) Care of the aging. Recent advances in nursing series, no 2, Churchill Livingstone, Edinburgh

Evers H 1983 Elderly women and disadvantage: perceptions of daily life and support relationships. In: Jerrome D (ed) Ageing in modern society. Croom Helm, London

Fennell G, Phillipson C, Evers H 1988 The sociology of old age. Open University Press, Milton Keynes

Ford J, Sinclair R 1987 Sixty years on: women talk about old age. The Women's Press, London

Fries J F, Crapo L M 1981 Vitality and ageing: implications of the rectangular curve. Freeman, San Francisco

Hodgson J 1984 The age of statistics: in the USSR, US and UK. British Journal of Geriatric Nursing 3(5): 12–15

Isaacs B 1981 Ageing and the doctor. In: Hobman D (ed) The impact of ageing: strategies for care. Croom Helm, London

Jay P 1983 Health for all: a role for the community. Journal of the Royal College of Physicians 17: 2, 93–94

Kalache A, Warnes A M, Hunter D J 1988 Promoting health among elderly people. King Edward's Hospital Fund for London, London

Kuhn M 1980 Grass-roots gray power. In: Fuller M M, Martin C A (eds) The older woman: lavender rose or gray panther. Charles C Thomas, Springfield, Illinois, ch 23

Laslett P 1987 The emergence of the third age. Ageing and Society 7(2): 133–160

Lewis M, Butler R N 1980 Why is women's lib ignoring old women? In: Fuller M M, Martin C A (eds) The older woman: lavender rose or gray panther. Charles C Thomas, Springfield, Illinois, ch 22

Macdonald B, Rich C 1984 Look me in the eye: old women, aging and agism. Spinsters Ink, San Francisco

Maddox M A, Tillery B J 1988 Elderly image seen by health-care professionals. Journal of Gerontological Nursing 14(11): 21–24

Merton R K 1957 Social theory and social structure. Rev edn. Free Press, Illinois

Newton E 1980 This bed my centre. Virago, London

Norman A 1984 Word play. New Age 24: 29

Norman A 1987 Aspects of ageism: a discussion paper. Centre for Policy on Ageing, London

Novak M 1983 Discovering a good life. International Journal of Ageing and Human Development 16: 231–239

O'Donnell M 1988 Whoopie cushions. The Listener, 8 September, 14–15

Phillipson C 1982 Capitalism and the construction of old age. Macmillan, London

Platzer H 1988 A study into the causes of post-operative confusion in the elderly. Unpublished MSc Thesis, King's College, University of London

Roebuck J 1983 Grandma as revolutionary: elderly women and some modern patterns of social change. International Journal of Ageing and Human Development 17: 249–266

Rossiter C, Wicks M 1982 Crisis or challenge? Family care, elderly people and social policy. Study Commission on the Family

Shegog R F A (ed) 1981 The impending crisis of old age: a challenge to ingenuity. Oxford University Press

Stevenson O 1989 Age and vulnerability: a guide to better care. Edward Arnold, London

Symonds A S 1987 Celebrating age: an anthology. Age Concern England, Mitcham, Surrey

CHAPTER CONTENTS

Quality of living 549
Communicating with elderly patients 550
The balance between rights and risk 551
Surgery for old people 556

Quality of dying 560
The patient's right to refuse treatment 561
Care of dying people 563

32

The elderly patient

Sally J. Redfern

In the previous chapter, the discussion focused on the elderly person living in a youth-oriented, industrialized society. In this chapter, we focus on the frail old person who requires continued support in an institutional setting or who needs shorter-term hospital care. The chapter contains two sections, one on the quality of living and the other on the quality of dying. The aim has been to discuss issues, some of which have been raised in earlier chapters, and which require thought and debate by nurses. The choice of issues is based largely on those raised by students, who are profoundly concerned about what they see as the plight of old people who are 'living' and dying in our hospitals and residential Homes, where the opportunity for a fulfilling life or comfortable and peaceful death may not be available to them.

We hope that readers will find these issues sufficiently contentious to want to debate them in their own settings and, in doing so, will examine the quality of care they give to their own patients.

QUALITY OF LIVING

A great deal of research has been published on the quality of life and on nursing care in different settings for old people. In this section, we look at two issues in nursing which have not, on the whole, emerged as high quality aspects of patient care. The first is communicating with elderly patients or clients and the second is the balance between rights and risk in the nursing care of old people. Striking an optimum balance between allowing old people the rights to which any adult is entitled and avoiding unnecessary risk is a theme which runs through the whole chapter and is perhaps the key to successful and high quality nursing. It continues in the discussion of surgery for old people. Two surgical conditions are singled out for discussion because they are so common: the aged hip and vascular problems of the lower limbs, some of which necessitate amputation.

COMMUNICATING WITH ELDERLY PATIENTS

The research published on the amount and quality of communication with elderly patients makes sobering reading. Levels of social interaction between nurses and elderly patients are low, particularly for elderly confused patients, and do not increase when more nurses are on duty (Miller 1978, Wells 1980, Godlove et al 1981, Gilbert 1984; Jill Macleod Clark 1988 and Ch. 4 of this book).

Godlove et al (1981) observed 65 old people in day hospitals, hospital wards, local authority old people's Homes, and day centres in London. Although the staff were aware of the observers, the most consistent finding was that, between 10.00 and 16.00 h, most of the old people spent most of their time doing nothing (70% in hospital wards, 62% in old people's Homes, 54% in day hospitals, and 51% in day centres; Richard 1983). Those who attended day hospitals spent only 18% of their time on rehabilitation and treatment activities, which was less than the time spent on these activities in day centres, whose primary function is to meet social needs. Interaction through conversation or physical contact was lowest in the old people's Homes (3%) and the day centres (5%), and rather more in the hospital wards (11%) and the day hospitals (18%), although nowhere was it very substantial.

Staffing levels did not vary significantly between the settings, and the researchers observed examples of both downright cruelty on the one hand and sensitive staff on the other doing their utmost to retain some dignity and comfort for their patients. The authors suggest that nurses in training should spend time doing similar observations of nurse–patient interaction and should discuss their findings with ward and teaching staff. This could be educational for everyone.

Most of the research in this area has focused on verbal communication. Very little research has been carried out in the UK on the effects of non-verbal communication, particularly touch, between nurses and elderly people. The evidence that does exist, mainly American, demonstrates that the appropriate use of touch by nurses can enhance the patient's well-being and comfort. This is particularly so for those old people who are anxious or dependent, who feel depersonalized, have a low self-esteem, have an altered body image or are dying (Barnett 1972). Our own recent research on nurse–patient touch carried out in institutional settings for elderly people in London showed that most (88%) touch used by nurses was task-defined and 'instrumental'. There was much less (10%) spontaneous, 'expressive' touch unrelated to a nursing procedure. The type of touch the old people received varied between the settings, with significantly more expressive touch occurring in the long-stay elderly care wards (16%) and the day hospital (12%) compared with the acute elderly care wards (6%) and the nursing Home (7%). These findings support earlier research that demonstrated relatively little caring expressive touch by nurses with elderly patients (Le May & Redfern 1987, Redfern 1989).

It is reassuring to see how much attention is now being given to research into interpersonal communication and into teaching communication skills (Macleod Clark 1988). Much of this research and teaching has been located in academic departments and colleges of nursing, and the need for change has been slow to reach wards and community centres. However, things are beginning to change. Nurses who did not have the good fortune to learn about communication skills during their basic training are able to receive training on the job, as is the case at the Oxford Nursing Development Unit (Swaffield 1988). Nurses there participate in video workshops which use material on nurse–patient interactions in the wards, and so the relevance of the exercise is immediately apparent.

It remains the case, however, that many old people continue to experience inadequate care. One such person was a resident of an old people's Home and she had the courage to write about it (Chambers 1982). She maintains that the objectives of care were inadequate, and advocates two steps to catalyze change. First, consumer participation in the way lives are organized, with residents' committees taking an active and influential role. Secondly, a 'listening service', which would enable a resident to discuss anything with a sympathetic listener. This could help sort out problems, prevent loneliness, and enhance feelings of worth. Many residents have the skills and qualities to do this for their companions. It is a tragedy that so many nurses and other care staff do so little.

THE BALANCE BETWEEN RIGHTS AND RISK

We are constantly being told that 'old age is not an illness', but this phrase becomes ambiguous when applied to very old people. It is helpful because it encourages society to adopt positive expectations about ageing and old age and it discourages old people from sinking into a sick role. On the other hand, increasing frailty is inevitable with very old age, and so even if not a 'sickness' in the medical sense, the care it requires is not very different from that needed by people who are sick, dependent or disabled (e.g. the stroke or multiple sclerosis victim). Nurses have the most important role of all health care workers in getting the balance right between fulfilling the nursing needs of old people and ensuring as much independence as possible, and a sense of well-being and purpose in life. Much of the research shows that nurses fail to get the balance right and are more concerned with the risks that independence must carry, than with the rights that old people, like anyone else, have in choosing the way they live.

It is easy for nurses who look after frail, dependent and often ill old people in hospital wards to assume that very little can be done because these are inevitable consequences of old age. These nurses do not often see healthy old people as part

of their work, and so they tend to generalize what they see to all old people. The outcome may be inadvertently to encourage these old people in their care to enter into vicious cycles of disability and dependency, which involve a loss of function and activity in excess of that which can be explained by the undeniable fact of ageing or by the effects of disease (Muir-Gray 1984). The disability cycle starts with the loss of function resulting from disabling disease, which leads to the loss of ability to perform certain actions. The joint stiffness, muscle weakness and loss of confidence which result from typical disease produce further loss of function and an inability to perform more actions. The vicious cycle of dependency makes matters worse. The increasing difficulty an old person has in performing a task means that someone else will probably do it for her. She is less likely to perform it and other activities on subsequent occasions, she will be less involved in decision making, will lose mental and physical fitness and become increasingly dependent and disabled.

When chronic disease is present, it is essential for nurses to promote and sustain exercise in order to prevent loss of fitness, strength and stamina. They should encourage old people to undertake their own personal care and also to keep exercising, such as stretching, walking, dancing, cycling or swimming. One man of 89 years emphasizes how much more stable and mobile he is on a bicycle than on his feet (Clark-Kennedy 1982). The fear of accident so often takes precedence, that nurses, other health workers and relatives at home overprotect the old person and inadvertently assist the vicious cycles. Old people are resourceful and self-reliant if allowed to be. The job of nurses and other health professionals is to work on their disabilities and handicaps so that they do not interfere with that resourcefulness and self-reliance.

No one has complete liberty and freedom of choice, but old people have less than most.

There are ways in which society further restricts this narrowing range of choice by imposing on elderly people forms of care and treatment which are the fruit of social perception, social anxiety, convenience and custom rather than inescapable necessity (Norman 1980, p 3).

This lack of choice, which has been mentioned

in other chapters of this book, (e.g. Chs 2, 7, 29, 30) occurs in all settings. Old people are removed from their homes when they could have remained there with support; they are deprived of dignity in hospitals and old people's Homes, and are not consulted about their care and treatment. Norman (1980) highlights the fundamental need for a change in attitude by society, health and social workers, and old people themselves, away from paternalistic overprotection from risk towards the right to self-determination for each person within the limits of available resources. These sentiments are strongly supported in Chapter 29 of this volume.

Old people in institutions are treated very differently from those outside. Outside, people are permitted to rock climb and hang-glide even though the costs of rescue and disaster are high. Old people at home can live at considerable risk of accidents because of their unsafe environment. But in residential Homes fire precautions have to be so extensive that the increased fees necessary for covering the cost mean that old people cannot afford to live there, or their mobility is reduced because they cannot get through heavy fire doors with a walking-frame. They are not asked how much risk they are prepared to take. The fear of scandal, disaster and litigation takes precedence.

The problem may be even worse for confused old people living at home. Pressure from relatives and neighbours on the police, the welfare services and the primary health care team to remove an old lady from her familiar decrepitude, neglect and squalor to a clean, efficient hospital or residential Home, can be overwhelming for her. There, her confusion, bewilderment and anxiety are likely to increase; she can no longer choose what she does; she becomes restless, disoriented, anorexic and increasingly frail, apathetic, and incontinent; and she knows no one. She is given drugs to calm her down, which increase her confusion and incontinence, and the outcome is a chest infection and death within a few days. This occurs even though she was healthy but dirty when admitted. Or, she may survive at the cost of becoming depersonalized, accepting of loving care and attention by the nurses, being totally dependent with no choice and responsibilities. Skilled nursing and medical care

can keep her alive but at what cost to her quality of life? She might have preferred death.

This is an extreme case, but it does happen. It raises the difficulty of getting the balance right between respecting the rights and wishes of the old lady and those of her neighbours and relatives. It may be right to let her live in squalor and to refuse help if this does not cause danger or inconvenience to her or her neighbours, but the difficulty is knowing what level of inconvenience to the neighbours outweighs an individual's choice to stay at home. Perhaps the answer is to ensure that the health care team in the hospital or residential Home get the balance right between the risk of independence and the risk of institutionalization.

Loss of one's home results in bereavement and produces a grief reaction similar to that which occurs with the loss of a relative. Cognitive ability, physical status, personality factors, and preparing thoroughly for the change are powerful predictors of successful relocation. But it is those who would be the most successful in adapting who are the least likely to need to be moved, because they have their own resources and initiative. Norman (1980) maintains that the evidence suggests more fatal accidents occur in institutions than at home (even allowing for the greater frailty of institutional residents), and so if the main objective is to avoid 'risk', then relocation in an institution may not be the answer.

Most elderly people admitted to hospital for medical treatment recover and return home. But some become longer-term patients because the relatively minor illness has caused a crisis in the system of support at home. It is often the case, except in progressive geriatric units, that a disease is given as the reason for admission rather than that the spouse cannot manage. This means that the real reason may not be the focus of attention and the old person may find it difficult to get fit enough to go home. Or the patient may be detained in hospital because other diseases, which she has lived with for years, are diagnosed. In an acute medical ward, there may not be the facilities, staff or motivation to take time to rehabilitate her, with the result that prolonged rehabilitation in a geriatric unit is necessary before she can go home. The long period away from home may have, in

Norman's (1980) terms, closed up the 'social space', and the outcome may be long-term care and a gradual move towards Muir-Gray's (1984) vicious cycles of disability and dependency. Thus, although hospital admission for old people may be life saving, the dangers must be weighed against the advantages. This problem is increasingly recognized by geriatricians, especially those who do home visits before admission and find out about the patient's circumstances. The wish to keep the old person at home if possible is paramount, and if hospital admission is necessary, the aim is that it should be as short as possible.

Similar problems can occur when old people move to residential Homes. The problems may be worse because in hospital this patient is only in danger of becoming a permanent resident, whereas in a residential Home this is virtually a certainty. It is important that a full medical and social assessment is done before the decision to move into a residential Home is made, irrespective of whether the move is from home or hospital. This will ensure that the move is the right decision for the old person.

Moving to live with a child is also a loss. It may not be successful or not turn out to be permanent, and since the old person will have given up her home, the outcome may be a move to a residential Home or long-stay hospital. If the move to the child's home is permanent, the old person's needs may not be met because of an overprotective, anxious daughter. Norman (1980) points out that much more public education is needed concerning the advantages and disadvantages of an old person moving in with her child's family, and about the potential danger of meeting the child's anxieties and needs rather than the old person's wishes. We need to move towards a system where old people either give up their homes because they want to or, if it is impossible for them or their family to cope at home, are supported by the full range of statutory and voluntary domiciliary services (see Ch. 29).

Nursing old people in hospital

In Chapter 24, Helen Evers discusses the development of geriatric medicine and nursing; in Chapter 29, Sally Redfern focuses on the inadequate care found in hospital wards and nursing and residential Homes; in Chapter 30, Barbara Wade illustrates the lack of choice found in so many long-term settings; and in Chapter 7, Amanda Stokes-Roberts discusses what can be done to enhance well-being of patients and residents in institutions. A generally depressing picture reported in research studies concerning the organization of nursing care emerges. The issue of rights versus risk is particularly relevant to old people in hospital. It is not unusual to see today's hospital wards, particularly long-stay ones, retaining the traditions of the old public hospitals, with rigid lines of authority, housed in a barely disguised workhouse where the patients still carry the stigma of weakness and social incompetence, are seen as recipients of charity and are expected to be obedient, submissive and grateful (Norman 1980). The principles of compulsion and custody continue. Patients are admitted or ordered to hospital, are detained there, and are released. This is the language of custody, not hospitality. Attitudes associated with the Poor Laws continue — relegation, obedience, batch processing and lack of choice (see Ch. 29).

Hospitals need certain rules to achieve their primary aims of healing and rehabilitation, which result inevitably in some loss of autonomy. But, in many long-stay wards, rules inhibit autonomy and work against the goal of rehabilitation. If an old person cannot retain her dignity and autonomy as an individual, she cannot be successful at establishing herself back into the community, nor can she possibly become a purposeful being in a long-stay ward.

Elderly patients in long-stay wards may be subjected to routines and deprived of more choice than that given a two-year-old. In Chapter 28 of this book, Pauline Fielding refers to the routinization and depersonalization of hospital patients. Hospital routines of times for rising and retiring and mealtimes can be extremely rigid and totally different to one's routine at home. Opportunity for choice is often missing. For example, choice of menu: although a choice exists, it is so often the case that the menus are filled in by a nurse or ward clerk (Wade et al 1983). Staff in elderly care wards encourage their patients to dress in day clothes, but so often the patients have no choice, and the dress worn last week may turn up on someone else next week. Clothing should be personal, labelled, attractive, dignified and sufficient. It should include a full complement of underwear, including suspender belts to keep stockings up. It follows that a personal clothing system requires an adequate selection, labelling, laundry, ironing, storage and repair service, which many wards do not have, even though this has been Department of Health policy since 1972 (DHSS 1972). A number of studies have shown the successful outcome of implementing a personal clothing service (see Adams 1984, for a review of the literature).

Control of money is a function most of us take for granted. It is anomalous that pensioners in Britain are required to give up earned benefit in return for long-term medical and nursing care, but the hospital providing the care gets no direct benefit (Norman 1980). In the early 1980s, retirement pensions were reduced by £13.60 per week after an old person with no dependants had been in hospital for eight weeks, and dropped to £6.80 after one year (Smith 1984). The rationale is that the sum taken covers the costs of living at home and these are now met by the National Health Service. But in reality elderly patients forego their income and economic independence and receive no benefit since they 'live' in some of the worst conditions in the health service. In some long-stay wards, patients did not even get the £6.80. Now, the sum is closer to £12 per week, but the problem remains. The administration's fear of theft overrides the old person's need for independence and dignity. Norman (1980) describes one hospital where a clerk visits every patient every two weeks to inform her how much money she owns, and to discuss what she would like to buy. It could be a personal television or radio, a present for relatives, a bottle of brandy, a regular supply of wholemeal bread, or a taxi ride round the town. Why is this not done by more hospitals? It could be a valuable role for volunteers.

Caring for old people is a low status specialty in nursing and it is likely that many nurses working in elderly care wards do so out of convenience rather than a genuine desire to enhance the quality of care for old people. Much of the work is described as dull, 'basic' and unskilled and can be left to untrained nursing students and auxiliaries. 'Real' nursing comprises the high status work of 'dressings, drips and drama' (Evers 1981a) and is not found in long-stay wards. 'Basic' nursing is heavily routinized, and easily conforms to rigid hierarchical control. This acts as a constraint to individualized care and innovation.

In contrast to this view, the pioneers in nursing old people (e.g. Norton 1965) insist that it is this specialty which provides the opportunity for 'real' nursing because the emphasis is on the caring role of the nurse. Sander and Walden (1984) emphasize the challenge of nursing elderly people and the need for nurses in this field to become specialists. Evers (1981a) found that those nurses who preferred to work on elderly care wards did so because of the opportunity they had to care for the 'whole person' rather than a diseased organ, and to get to know the patients and their relatives really well. Yet despite this, care observed by Clarke (1978), Wells (1980), Evers (1981a, 1981b) and Baker (1983) was routinized and task oriented.

Evers (1981b) makes it clear that the predominantly 'warehousing' approach to patient care fails to fulfil the objectives for hospital care of elderly people explicit in various government and other policy documents (e.g. Department of Health and Social Security 1978, 1979, British Geriatrics Society and Royal College of Nursing 1975). She identified four objectives:

1. To make full use of all diagnostic and rehabilitation resources with the aim of discharging patients from hospital as soon as possible
2. To promote patients' physical and psychological independence whilst in hospital
3. To enable patients to engage in purposeful activity whilst in hospital in order to ensure their self-esteem and an optimum quality of life
4. To give patients access to the multidisciplinary team who have specific expertise in the care of the elderly.

The energy found in progressive geriatric units

enables perhaps all the objectives to be fulfilled for the 'acute career' patient, who follows the medical model of diagnosis–treatment–cure–discharge home. This success has been due largely to the initiative of geriatricians, supported by nurses and therapeutic staff. In long-stay wards, however, where geriatricians have not taken the lead, care often falls far short of all these objectives. As the research quoted shows, the factors which produce institutionalization are prevalent (see Ch. 29). Nurses have been slow to take up the challenge of the long-stay patient. Here is a specialty which is crying out for improvement and in which the nurse could take a key role. Where progress has been made the initiative has usually come from someone else — occupational therapists and physiotherapists (Glossop 1983, Clark & Bowling 1989), or clinical psychologists (Woods & Holden 1982), with nurses, until recently, taking very little interest except perhaps in some progressive units for the elderly mentally ill (e.g. Rowden 1983). In recent years, however, nurses have been much more prominent in the development of progressive initiatives in long-stay care. Examples are nurse-led NHS nursing Homes and nursing development units in hospitals (see Ch. 29 of this volume for a further discussion).

Innovative nurses find it very difficult to discuss and implement new ideas unless they are supported by a progressive team which is open to change. Staff in a more traditional, closed environment are likely to feel threatened by innovation, will close ranks, and either force the innovator to conform to their practices or to leave. Achieving change on one's own is close to impossible for the relatively junior ward nurse. There are, however, several strategies that can be used by nurses to achieve success. For example, the nurse might implement her ideas through an understanding doctor, in which case the nursing staff view the idea as a medical instruction and therefore as credible; this approach cannot, however, enhance the emerging professionalism of nursing. Or all the nurses on the ward — the untrained, those in training, and the qualified nurses — could go on a course together so that the ideas for change can be discussed by all of them and they all feel part of the decision-making process. They will be more

likely to have an interest in seeing changes implemented successfully than if they had been excluded. In this case, the ward would have to be closed for a short period, and this could be timed to coincide with a period of ward redecoration.

In defence of those nurses who do attempt to innovate and improve patient care, they sometimes find that it is very difficult to give high quality care or to achieve change because the resources to provide a minimum service are not available. The nurse is in a dilemma if she (or he) cannot provide the care she knows is required. She can take the traditional course of action chosen by many nurses, that is, to make the best of things and keep quiet. Or, she can voice her concerns loudly and agitate for change. It is most rewarding to find increasing numbers of examples where nurses are publicizing the constraints they face in delivering high quality care. Agitation like this is important. Nurses have a professional responsibility to document instances when they are forced to let patients down or when they cannot be the patient's advocate. They should shout about failing the patient rather than respond defensively. The development of peer review, quality circles and standard setting initiatives are expanding throughout the UK (Kitson et al 1988). These initiatives are giving nurses the confidence to act as the patient's advocate.

Relatively little research has been done in the UK to evaluate the quality of patient care, although there have been workload and audit studies to assess the quantity of nursing and the relationship with staff appraisal (Miller 1984). In the current climate of economic stringency, nurses in the UK are under increasing pressure to assure both quality of care and value for money, that is, to provide evidence of cost-effectiveness. The government White Paper, Working for Patients (DH 1989a), and A Strategy for Nursing (DH 1989b) underline the importance of medical audit and quality assurance in health care, and require nurses to become familiar with quality assessment techniques as a target for practice. Following the NHS Review (DH 1989a), regional health authorities were required to have agreed a framework by autumn 1989 for establishing unit-based quality assurance programmes, including specific action plans which should be assessed against predetermined standards so that progress can be monitored (Age Concern 1989). Detailed debate on quality assurance is outside the scope of this volume. For more information the reader is referred to Pearson (1987).

Over the past two decades in the UK, individualized care articulated through the nursing process has been recommended as the method of organizing nursing care, and professional and educational bodies in nursing advocate its widespread use. More recently, the debate has moved on and now encompasses 'primary nursing' as the choice method of organizing nursing care. The reader is referred to Chapter 33 for discussion on primary nursing. The effectiveness of individualized care has been demonstrated in the case of hospitalized elderly people. As discussed in Chapter 29, Miller (1984) found care to be of much higher quality for elderly patients hospitalized for more than one month in individualized care wards than it was for those in task-oriented wards. There was no difference, however, in patient care outcome for short-stay patients who were occupied with intensive medical and therapeutic intervention.

It is clear that individualized, planned nursing care is essential for longer-stay patients because it enhances their quality of life. Miller also counters the persistant cry that individualized care cannot be implemented because of lack of staff. She found that there was no increase in the quantity of nursing given to patients in the nursing process wards except that nurses talked with them more. Thus it is the method of work organization rather than staffing levels which affects outcome for long-stay patients.

Nurses caring for old people in institutions are becoming less medically oriented and less apathetic. They are doing much more to encourage patients to retain their self-respect and their dignity, to avoid depression and the 'learned helplessness' syndrome (Seligman 1975) and to look forward to the future.

SURGERY FOR OLD PEOPLE

A substantial proportion of the beds in surgical wards are occupied by elderly people. Vowles (1979) found in Devon, England, that 30% of sur-

gical patients and more than 50% of all surgical emergency admissions were over 65 years. With increasing numbers of elderly people, the use of resources must be assessed together with the achievements gained in operating on so many old people. Is surgery the treatment of choice? Is it contributing to survival of the unfittest? How much 'heroic' surgery is performed on old people that fails to give them an increased quality of life? Are the patient and her family given an opportunity to take part in the decision to operate?

Selecting an arbitrary age limit for surgery is unethical and unsatisfactory. Many elderly people enjoy a greatly enhanced quality of life after surgery, which is its aim. The surgeon, together with the whole health care team, including patient and relatives, must consider many factors in the decision to operate: the prognosis of disease, the risk of surgery, the chance of cure, the chance of palliation, the patient's will to live, her life expectancy, the presence of other problems, her degree of disability, and the chances of complications developing (Vowles 1979). The surgeon should discuss all the alternatives to surgery with the patient and should help the patient make the final decision. If the patient makes an informed choice and rejects surgery, provided she is judged competent to make that decision, then it should be respected.

Vowles (1979) has identified questions that every surgeon should consider with old people:

Which is likely to be longer, the natural course of the disease or the patient's expectation of life?

Without surgery what will be the patient's quality of life?

What chance has the patient of surviving surgery?

Should the operation be elective and soon, or is it better to leave well alone and risk emergency surgery later?

Should the operation be radical and heroic or modified and palliative?

Assessment for surgery

Assessment should be comprehensive and done by the surgeon and the geriatrician, with support from the knowledge of nurses, health visitor and social worker where possible. Old people admitted to hospital have on average nine separate diagnoses (Vowles 1979) and so the medical and nursing assessment is more difficult than for a younger patient. Other problems may need attention before surgery can be contemplated. Another problem for the doctors is that the usual signs of a diagnosis, or problems post-operatively, may not occur in old people. For example, pain may be absent or vague and difficult to pinpoint; response to fever may be confusion and weakness rather than a raised temperature and abnormal white cell count; a thromboembolism may be 'silent' with no pleural pain or haemoptysis; vomiting may not be obvious but occur as quiet regurgitation and aspiration into the lungs. It may be difficult for an inexperienced doctor to recognize that the patient is very ill, and there is much the vigilant nurse can do to prevent disaster.

The quality of life after surgery

This should be at least as good as before surgery, and preferably better. As with anyone, old people value health over longevity, and palliative surgery which gives a few more high quality years to an 80 year old may be preferable to radical surgery. The British Geriatrics Society's motto, 'Add life to years', is essential for surgeons to remember, particularly when the mortality rate of emergency surgery of old people is double that of elective surgery in this age group (Vowles 1979).

It is essential that the hospital team has knowledge of the patient's home circumstances, suitability of housing, the health of a spouse, etc. and that these are considered with reference to appropriate aftercare. It may be that a follow-up visit is done with the geriatrician or general practitioner (family doctor), and attendence at a day hospital might be an additional help in rehabilitation.

If the surgery was not successful, the question of whether it should have been done will be raised. This is difficult to answer, but Vowles (1979) refers to a study done in the Oxford region of England in which 750 patients over the age of 65 years had elective surgery. The conclusions reached were that, on the whole, patients whose operations had relieved their symptoms lived fuller lives than before the operation, and those whose symptoms were not relieved, or who developed new ones, led more restricted lives. Mortality for the whole group was 8%, usually for non-surgical reasons. The dilemma of whether or not to operate underlines the importance of assessing, preparing and knowing the patient and her family very well before surgery, and ensuring that the patient and family are involved in making the decision.

Mortality and morbidity

Following surgery, mortality is higher for old people compared with younger age groups and this should be taken into account in the decision to operate. Surgical morbidity and mortality tend to be highest for very old patients but these outcomes vary according to the nature of the operation, the ratio of elective to emergency surgery and the patient's condition (Weksler 1985). For very old people, mortality and morbidity are higher after abdominal surgery than for younger people (Palmer et al 1989). Figures like those in Table 32.1 may cause the surgeon who wants to operate at all costs to think twice. However, age should not be the only criterion when assessing surgical risk. The increased mortality for both elective and emergency surgery is related to factors other than age (pneumonia, cardiac complications, malignancy-

Table 32.1 Mortality for abdominal surgery (emergency and elective) by age. *Source: Ziffren and Hartford (1972) quoted by Vowles (1979)*

Abdominal operation	Percentage mortality by age			
	<60	60–69	70–79	80+
Appendicectomy	0.1	3.3	2.7	16.6
Repair of inguinal hernia	0.1	0.2	1.6	3.3
Cholecystectomy	0.8	2.8	5.5	5.4
Partial gastrectomy	3.9	5.0	11.2	19.8
Exploratory laparotomy for inoperable lesion	6.9	9.0	16.6	31.6
Aortic graft	7.5	9.2	16.4	22.2
Closure of wound dehiscence	17.7	15.7	36.3	66.6
Resection/anastomosis of small intestine for obstruction	14.2	13.9	24.3	35.7
Partial colectomy	6.4	6.8	5.4	9.0
Abdominoperineal resection	0.7	4.3	7.6	11.5
Colostomy	5.6	8.1	8.3	14.2

related complications). It is true, though, that old people with heart disease, diabetes or dementia are at greater risk (Mohr 1983).

On the other hand, if the surgeon decides to do as little as is necessary to solve the problem, which is often what is advocated, then the problem may recur when the patient is older and less able to withstand the assault of surgery. When they are carefully and properly assessed, prepared and anaesthetized, and given meticulous post-operative care, most old people can survive any operation (Vowles 1979). Recovery depends mainly on avoiding complications, which old people cannot cope with because they lack the necessary reserves. Weksler (1985) uses the term 'homeostenosis' to describe the loss of physiological reserves which is associated with ageing. Vowles makes clear that the old person experiences more 'loss of elasticity' than the young, which is physical and psychological (e.g. she may give up the struggle) and so knowledge of her state of mind before the operation may be critical to her survival. Nurses caring for aged surgical patients must be involved in the decision to operate and have knowledge of the risk/benefit balance for each patient.

The choice of mode of anaesthesia is important because of the negative effects of general anaesthetics that can occur with elderly patients. These effects include respiratory and cardiac depression, pulmonary aspiration of gastrointestinal contents, and decreased cerebral capacity, which can manifest itself as delirium, apparent dementia and loss of memory (Matteson & McConnell 1988).

A recent British study found a significant relationship between mortality and post-operative confusion of elderly patients, and those who became confused post-operatively spent longer periods in hospital than those who did not become confused (Platzer 1988). Platzer also found a clear relationship between the use of anticholinergic drugs which cross the blood–brain barrier and post-operative confusion. Examples of these drugs are atropine and hyoscine, which are commonly used for premedication before surgery. Platzer recommends the use of glycopyrrolate (Robinul®) as a suitable premedication drug because it does not cross the blood–brain barrier and results less frequently in post-operative confusion.

In view of the major disadvantages of general anaesthesia, regional anaesthesia should be used whenever possible with elderly patients, and probably also with younger patients. Regional anaesthetic techniques include spinal, lumbar or caudal epidural, regional nerve block and local infiltration. These techniques are particularly suited to operations on parts of the body other than the chest and upper abdomen. Examples are hip replacement, fractured neck of femur, operations on the perineum, the lower abdomen and inguinal region, hand surgery, fractured arm and wrist, cataract surgery and dental extractions (Matteson & McConnell 1988).

The aged hip

As populations age there is an increasing incidence of fractured femur, and degenerative and rheumatoid arthritis (Ling 1979). These conditions are not fatal in themselves but their effects on health are severe, causing incessant pain, immobility and a reduced quality of life. The problems are likely to reach epidemic proportions over the next 20 years, and, without adequate planning and resources, many services and professionals will be stretched beyond breaking point (orthopaedic surgeons, geriatricians, nurses, physiotherapists, occupational therapists, psychiatrists, general practitioners, social workers, community services, and the patients' families).

Rheumatoid arthritis strikes 41% of people aged over 65 years, and virtually everyone (96%) over 75 years has osteoarthrosis (Ling 1979) although these figures are not confined to hip disease. Total hip replacement surgery, pioneered in Britain, has made a huge impact on the quality of life of old people because of the pain relief and restoration of function it brings. The benefits for old people of this operation are greater than for almost any other. From the cost-benefit point of view, too, these operations are economic, the cost of treatment being exceeded by the benefits in terms of return to productive work (Ling 1979) and avoiding burden on the services.

Arthritic conditions of the hip appear to be more common for men than women, but the incidence of fractured neck of femur is much higher for elderly women (Table 32.2).

As with arthritis of the hip, the number of frac-

Table 32.2 Incidence of fractured neck of femur by age and sex. *Source: Gallanaugh et al (1976), quoted by Ling (1979).*

		Femoral neck fractures per 1000 population							
Age:	<60	−64	−69	−74	−79	−84	−89	−94	≥95
Men	0.42	0.52	0.70	1.31	2.34	5.13	8.08	14.00	20.00
Women	0.43	1.08	1.58	3.54	6.30	13.03	22.93	32.76	26.15

tured femurs will rise in the next few years, particularly in over-75 year olds, and the increased demand on services will be enormous (Sweatman 1989). Sweatman argues for collaborative schemes in which geriatricians and orthopaedic surgeons work closely together in the treatment of elderly patients requiring orthopaedic surgery. He reviews evidence which demonstrates the effectiveness of closer collaboration: lower bed occupancy, shorter length of stay, lower mortality, shorter waiting lists for elective surgery, fewer patients requiring institutional care, higher discharge rates home, better training for nursing and medical staff, better staff co-operation, improved staff morale and better recruitment.

Emergency admission to hospital is essential for people with fractured femurs, and Ling (1979) suggests how the services might cope. The length of hospital stay could be reduced from the then current average of 22.5 days to 20 days. This requires intensive physiotherapy and nursing resources for rehabilitation to be achieved. Effective hospital-at-home schemes have been set up that enable post-operative care to continue at home and have cut the hospital stay by a week (Pryor et al 1988). Secondly, the available treatment facilities could be increased, which would mean a large injection of funds, which is unlikely in the present economic climate. Thirdly, the number of fractures could be reduced by establishing reasons for and preventing old people from falling, by preventing and treating osteoporosis and osteomalacia, both of which weaken bone, and by reducing long-term drug effects which affect bone density. Osteomalacia is '. . . the defective mineralisation of bone matrix with an excess of uncalcified osteoid' (Medcalf & Woolf 1989). It results from lack of vitamin D and is relatively easy to prevent and treat, with vitamin D and calcium.

Osteoporosis is more difficult. It is '. . . defined as an absolute decrease in the amount of bone leading to fracture after minimal trauma'. (Medcalf & Woolf 1989). Medcalf and Woolf explain that osteoporosis affects postmenopausal women who have likely accelerated bone loss (i.e. those who have had an oophorectomy, or an early menopause, or long distance runners); those with a disease or who are taking drugs which cause osteoporosis (e.g. thyrotoxicosis, Cushing's disease, corticosteroid drugs); and old people. It is uncertain whether osteoporosis is a normal feature of ageing but some loss of bone occurs in all old people of both sexes (Nordin 1985). The most common presenting features are fractures of the vertebrae, the hip, the arm and the wrist. Medcalf and Woolf (1989) identify the following major risk factors for osteoporosis:

Caucasian or Asian
premature menopause
positive family history
leanness
inactivity
nulliparity
smoking
heavy alcohol intake
? low calcium intake
? low fluoride intake

Treatment of osteoporosis is limited since lost bone can only be replaced very slowly (Nordin 1985), but exercise, a dietary intake of 1500 mg/day of calcium, and possibly hormone replacement therapy (HRT), should be encouraged, as well as treating fractures and pain and reducing immobility (Davidson & Woolf 1989).

Prevention is without doubt the most important course of action since the only clinical feature of osteoporosis is its complication, bone fracture (Woolf 1989). Woolf argues that osteoporosis must be prevented during development of the skeleton as well as at the menopause and during later life.

The diet during growth and development should contain adequate calcium and fluoride: exercise ensures maximum peak bone mass, and maintaining female hormone levels with HRT will, together with proper diet and exercise, prevent bone loss. These preventive measures should be directed at those who are at particular risk, and regular checks of skeletal bone mass and women's hormone levels during and after the menopause can identify these individuals. Many hospital doctors and general practitioners who are not specialists in this area exaggerate the side-effects of HRT and do not recommend its use in susceptible women. Although side-effects exist as with all drugs, the risks have lessened with increasing knowledge of types and dosages of HRT. There is no doubt that HRT prevents post-menopausal loss of bone and can reduce fracture rates (Nordin 1985). Nordin also provides evidence for calcium supplementation delaying post-menopausal bone loss because oestrogen deficiency produces an increase in calcium requirement. He recommends low dose oestrogen and a calcium supplement as the most satisfactory regime for preventing osteoporosis in those at risk. If calcium malabsorption exists then vitamin D should also be given. The importance of exercise as a preventive measure is emphasized also in Chapter 23 of this volume.

[T]he causes of osteoporosis are becoming increasingly clear and a defeatist approach to therapy is no longer justified. . . . Enough is now known about bone loss to make the prevention of osteoporosis possible (Nordin 1985, p. 342).

Vascular problems and amputation

Arteriosclerosis increases with age, and is more prevalent for men than women until the menopause, when it equalizes (Vowles & Halliday 1979). It occurs more frequently in tobacco smokers and those with diabetes mellitus or polycythaemia. Improved techniques of diabetic control mean that more diabetics survive into old age, when complications are more common than for young diabetics. In fact, major arterial lesions are no more common for diabetics but, when they do occur, healing is slower and neuropathy and sepsis are more likely. Michael Hobday refers briefly to the care of the diabetic foot in Chapter 9.

Severe intermittent claudication, or pre-gangrene, often requires aortoiliac or femoropopliteal graft surgery. This is major surgery for old people, but it can improve their quality of life substantially. The chances of a graft remaining patent is higher in old than younger people because the occlusive arteriosclerosis is probably no longer progressive.

Unfortunately, the life expectancy of the elderly arteriosclerotic amputee is not good. Seventy-five per cent survive one year, 33% survive five years and have a 50% chance of losing the other leg (Vowles & Halliday 1979). Motivation and psychological strength are essential for these old people. For some, an amputation is another sign of their inability to cope with life, but for others, it is a challenge and the relief of pain is what is important. Talking to other amputees is a great help, together with communal rehabilitation with a specialist physiotherapist. Nurses can do a lot to continue this rehabilitation and to ensure that patients keep in touch with each other. Elderly amputees find artificial limbs difficult to manage, but in expert hands many will achieve independence. For those who cannot, full independence in a wheelchair can increase quality of life a great deal.

Concluding this section on surgery for old people, we have all seen examples where extensive 'heroic' operations have been performed which have not given the patient an increased quality of life. On the other hand, many old people are living happier, pain-free, more independent lives as a result of surgery, and age should never be allowed to become a negative criterion for surgery. Careful assessment, preparation and aftercare by a well-co-ordinated health care team, together with close involvement of the patient and her family at all stages of the process, is the strategy most likely to be successful. An account of a case study where this did not happen can be found in Chapter 31, Louisa's Story.

QUALITY OF DYING

Medicine caters to the biological man, often abandoning the psychological and social one.

Hospitals are antiseptic and impersonal. Pneumonia, formerly the 'old man's friend', is treated with antibiotics. The patient lingers — often in pain. Afraid of litigation, the medical team persists (Humphrey & Wickett 1986, p. 2).

Care of people who are dying is one of the areas which requires much more attention in terms of the quality of care given. Nursing and medical training focuses to a large extent on treating those who will get better, aiming for cure, and so it is no surprise that nurses and doctors working in general settings are ill-equipped and uncertain how to care for the dying person. This section begins with a discussion of the patient's right to refuse treatment, and the complex issue of informed consent. Following this, the focus is on the care of dying people, and some of the lessons to be learned from hospice care are emphasized.

THE PATIENT'S RIGHT TO REFUSE TREATMENT

Advances in medical expertise (resuscitation techniques, life-support systems, etc.) have led to increased public debate on the issue of discontinuing active treatment of a dying or comatose patient, particularly if this is known to be her wish. This is not voluntary euthanasia or assisted suicide, which is a deliberate hastening of death (see Jo Hockley, Chapter 22 of this book).

Consent to treatment is a complex issue and is discussed in some detail by Norman (1980). The Medical Defence Union stipulates that people have a right to refuse treatment, and going ahead without consent could lead to a successful claim for damages. Informed consent cannot be given without sufficient information, and yet we suspect that many elderly patients do not receive such information and so cannot give proper informed consent. There is a mass of evidence that hospital patients want more information and that what they do get is inadequate. They feel their intelligence is underrated and they dislike the exclusion from discussions about them so typical of the ward 'round'. This is even more the case for elderly patients who may be particularly reticent about asking questions and be unable to communicate effectively. On the other hand, some patients say they do not want to know very much; they want

to submit themselves to the doctors' care and take no active part. Nurses can do a lot to check whether this is really what the patient wants.

Lawyers who specialize in ethics maintain that a conscious patient who refuses treatment must have that wish respected whatever her condition, provided she is sufficiently mature and lucid to make that decision (Kennedy 1988). If the patient is not lucid enough, then the decision can be ignored. This is a crucial issue in the care of old people. How many times have we seen a patient fed through a nasogastric tube against her will because she is refusing to eat? Many nurses disagree with the decision because they thought the patient's refusal was made lucidly, which it probably was. Yet later on, the patient has recovered her health and vigour and is now very pleased to be alive. In this case, it was right that she should have been tube fed until able to eat, but does it mean that she cannot have been in a lucid frame of mind when she refused treatment? The definition of lucidity is extremely difficult, particularly for old people who are confused or dying. Doctors are bound to vary in their definition. If our patient above, instead of eventually accepting the nasogastric tube, tries to remove it, is this refusal to co-operate equivalent to refusal to consent to treatment, or is she too confused to make a lucid decision?

The question of lucidity is even harder to answer because many patients will be taking drugs to relieve pain and distress and these may affect their mental competence. The doctor is usually seen to be the final arbiter, but can and should he or she carry that burden alone? It is much more likely that the correct decision is reached for an individual patient after discussion with all those who know the patient well, including the family and friends as well as the patient. In some cases, the doctor may be the least able to make the decision because he or she does not know the patient well enough.

I do not think doctors can be consistent in the respect they owe patients or recognise the real difficulties of negotiating treatment decisions if they do not keep firmly in view that primary responsibility for such decisions belongs to the patient if he is competent (Gormally 1987, p. 186).

The kind of discussion recommended here

would ensure that the patient's values and beliefs are taken into account in the decision-making. In McCullough's (1984) terms, the patient's 'value history' would not be ignored. If the doctor either insists on treatment being given or respects the patient's wishes even if they turn out to be misguided, then in both cases the 'hidden' middle ground is ignored, that is, the material which is based on the patient's value history. It is this which should become the basis for decision-making rather than merely that which the doctor thinks is right for the patient. Such knowledge would enable a decision to be made whether, for example, to treat aggressively or more palliatively, and every decision made would be an individual one. The patient, her family and the primary care team are in the best position to know the patient's value history, and the hospital consultant should make use of their knowledge. It may, however, be necessary for the health professionals to help the family to distinguish between their own wishes and the patient's values.

Making use of the value history is implicit in the idea of 'living wills' or durable powers of attorney which identify a person's wishes about aggressive life-saving treatment in the event of her being unable to make her wishes known (Age Concern, Institute of Gerontology and Centre of Medical Law and Ethics, King's College, London 1988). The living will is a fairly new idea in the UK but is more common in the USA. Between 1976 and 1985, 36 living will laws were enacted in the USA which legally recognized the individual's right to die with dignity (Humphrey & Wickett 1986). Others are not convinced of the need for living wills, believing that, with modern techniques of pain relief and the hospice movement, the prospect of long-drawn-out suffering before death is no longer faced (Hughes 1987). Sadly, this suffering continues to be common today even though the means to avoid it are known; and energetic treatments are given, such as nasogastric or gastrostomy tube feeding, when the patient would have refused these had she been able to express her wishes.

Elaborate and uncomfortable life-sustaining interventions continue to be much more common,

however, in the USA than the UK. Currie (1988) makes a strong attack upon American practice:

The technologies are available, respected and oversold. The same brave combination of technical virtuosity and indifference to cost that once took a handful of United States citizens to the moon serves in health care today to keep tens of thousands of them lingering, dependent and miserable here on earth, with equally questionable benefit. Powerful medico-legal considerations nudge doctors towards doing more rather than less (Currie 1988, p. 297).

Value histories should be considered important in decisions concerning non-terminal treatment, too. It does mean, however, that someone in the health care team must get to know the patient and her family very well and preferably before she becomes ill. The general practitioner is unlikely to be able to devote enough time to this, but it could be an extremely important role for the health visitor in the first instance, and for the district and hospital nurse when the old person becomes a patient. If health professionals would take this albeit complex approach to decision-making, then the principle of self-determination, which is fundamental to the concept of consent would be respected. The idea of the value history is closely related to the importance of the biographical approach to the understanding of ageing, described by Malcolm Johnson in Chapter 1.

Whether or not to instigate an energetic resuscitation procedure with an elderly patient presents a moral dilemma for the nurse. It is not at all clear when or how decisions on this are made. Although most elderly patients who die move into a terminal phase of the illness and gradually deteriorate, the nurse must know how to respond in the event of a sudden collapse. Knowledge of the patient's value history, and the relationship she (or he) has built with the patient over time may enable her to make the 'right' decision, but often there is some kind of policy in the ward. It is not at all clear how the decision is arrived at, but usually it reaches the nurse as an instruction and is made by the doctor without discussion with the ward team. There should be no place for a ward policy on an issue like this which requires a decision specific to an individual patient. The nurse would never be certain that the policy was the right one for an individual case. But if true consultation and co-ordination occurred, as has been advocated earlier, between all members of the health care team, then the dilemma would be unlikely to occur.

The patient's right to refuse treatment is a particularly difficult problem if she is a victim of dementia. Various forms of restraint, such as locked doors, tipped-back geriatric chairs, and tranquillizers may be used as a first rather than last resort in order to control a resistant patient (Jones 1987). The skillful nurse who uses a gentle, questioning approach to discover what the patient wants, and caring, unhurried touch is more likely to calm an agitated and confused patient than any kind of restraint. The Royal College of Nursing (1987) emphasizes the dangers and ethical dilemmas in using restraint with any kind of patient.

Some argue for a patients' 'advocate' who would represent the wishes and rights of the person who is unable to make her preferences known (Age Concern 1989). There is the view, however, that patients' advocates would lead to extensive bureaucracy and rigidity, and involvement of the courts may not necessarily lead to a better decision (Jones 1987). Difficulties would occur if the advocate's view was at odds with the views of either the doctor or the relatives. It would require a determined will and a deep understanding of the patient's wishes for the advocate to persuade a doctor or relative with strong views to change his or her mind.

'"Economic man", unencumbered by morals or emotional ties, would let the demented die' (Jones 1987, p. 66). Many ethical issues confront the health care team caring for victims of dementia. When it comes to choosing the 'right' course of action the doctor should not make the decision alone. He or she is unlikely to know the patient as well as others do, particularly a caring relative, a hospital or nursing Home nurse, a community psychiatric nurse, or a knowledgeable and understanding advocate. Decisions which take account of the views of those people who are most likely to know the patient's wishes will be closest to the 'right' decision. We share Andrews' (1989) view

that nurses should be contributing to public debate about how to treat people who cannot choose for themselves. More research is needed in order to discover what kind of care health professionals are actually giving these people.

CARE OF DYING PEOPLE

Today, most people (70%) in Britain die in an institution, which is in contrast to the position a few generations ago, when home was the commonest place (Ch. 22). Now the trend seems to be moving towards home care with the development of more home management teams specializing in the care of dying patients. This trend parallels the government policy of increasing care in the community, but, since these specialist teams are the initiatives of the hospice movement, there is little evidence that they are reaching most old people who are in the terminal phase of illness. Automatically moving a terminally ill old person into hospital can do immeasurable harm, particularly when 63% of chronically ill people spend more than a year dying (Doyle 1981). Doyle informs us that studies have shown that 60% of patients have at least five symptoms when they die, and they do not tell the doctor about half of these, thinking them too trivial.

So much can be done for dying old people and they deserve the most energetic and skilled nursing care available. Palliative care is therapeutic care. It does not imply withdrawal of therapy, but it is humane rather than technological (Fox 1987). This is the time when patients need more communication with nurses, not less, and the loneliness that many experience is overwhelmingly cruel. The poem written by the old lady of 90 just before her death, which appears in Chapter 22, bears witness to this.

Jo Hockley in Chapter 22 describes the quality of care that hospices give to dying people. So much can be learned from hospice care and using their techniques is surely the aim for all carers of dying people, irrespective of where they are. It is a painful and embarrassing reminder that hospices are necessary because of the inadequate care that most dying people receive in other settings.

Consumers in both general and geriatric hospitals assert that they are too institutionalised, too authoritarian, too rigid in their routines, too threatening in their staff hierarchies. Patients and visitors appreciate the relaxed atmosphere of hospices, the constant availability of staff to talk to them, the intense energy and enthusiasm devoted to symptom relief and the efforts that are made to restore patient dignity. More than anything, they eulogise about the policy of honesty in hospices, the clear explanations, the lack of deceit, the respect for patients who seek genuinely to know the truth, or as much of the truth as they can at that time bear (Doyle 1981, p. 177).

Just as there are specialist nurses in stoma care, infection control, parenteral nutrition and so on, there is a need for specialist nurses working as part of a care team for the dying to bring the principles of hospice care into general and elderly care wards, and to teach their skills to hospital staff. This is now happening in the UK, with increasing numbers of Macmillan nurses and other nurses who are also specialists in the control of symptoms experienced by dying people. Jo Hockley (Chapter 22) is one of these specialist nurses.

Doyle (1981) identifies five prerequisites for adequate terminal care. First, there must be staff adequately trained in terminal care to advise nurses and doctors whose main aim is to cure and rehabilitate, and who therefore have inadequate experience with dying patients. Second, true non-hierarchical teamwork is essential with doctors, nurses, social workers, chaplains, occupational therapists, speech therapists, physiotherapists, patients and relatives. Regular team meetings are important and should be led by the person who best knows the patient, who may not be the doctor. Third, the system of allocating nurses must be sufficiently flexible to allow changes to be made at short notice. Visitors should be allowed complete freedom of access, should be given a space for privacy and solitude, and should be allowed to participate in intimate nursing procedures if they wish. Fourth, an adequate staff support system is essential, so that any member of the team has the opportunity to discuss his or her own emotions, feelings of guilt, isolation, disappointment, failure and inadequacies. Finally, there should be an organized follow-up system for bereaved relatives that is not confined only to the first few weeks

after the death. Research shows that the maximum risk periods are much later, at six weeks, three months, six months and one year. Very few bereaved people receive this kind of attention.

It is not so easy to provide the hospice approach to care of the dying in hospitals which focus on treating disease. With long-stay patients particularly, it may be difficult to identify the terminal phase of life because there may be no acute illness. Furthermore, it may be difficult for nurses to accept impending death and so they keep their 'emotional distance', particularly if they have developed a close bond with the patient over a long period. The nurse may reject the doctor's judgement that the patient is dying.

There is a great need for nurses and doctors to receive training in the care of dying people and to regard it as positive therapeutic care, not as failure. Nurses need emotional support to help them cope with their own feelings about death, and also to be able to provide relatives of the patient with the support needed. Too often, in their own uncertainty, they insist that relatives leave the patient when nursing procedures are performed, when the relatives would prefer to help and the patient wants them to. Relatives feel they cannot protest, or if they do, they are often ignored. As Norman (1980) observes, children are vigorously defended and protected by their parents and by the National Association for the Welfare of Children in Hospital (NAWCH). NAWCH published a Charter for Children in Hospital in 1985 which set out 10 rights for children and their parents. Since then, NAWCH has published its Quality Checklist for Caring for Children in Hospital (1988) and more recently its Quality Review (1989) on setting standards of care for children (Hodges 1989). There is no similar protection for old people in this country. However, with the emphasis on patient choice in the government White Paper, Working for Patients (DH 1989a), the rights of elderly people are being considered more seriously. The association of Community Health Councils for England and Wales has published a Patients' Charter which provides 17 guidelines for good practice (Laurent 1989). The Charter is designed for all adult patients and is particularly appropriate for elderly people in hospital. Laurent refers to two English health authorities, Brighton and Durham, that have developed a Patients' Charter. Durham's Charter is now available at every hospital bedside.

Care of dying people is an area in which nurses should take a key role. They are in a position to get to know the patient and her family well and to help the patient find fulfilment in the final period of her life. Hospices have developed because the care of dying people in institutions is inadequate. Nurses should be taught how to meet the patient's physical needs and above all, her psychological needs. There is very little evidence of a co-ordinated, effective team approach to the care of the dying in most hospitals, although specialist teams have been introduced in some health districts to advise staff on how best to meet the patient's needs. Hospices and their home care counterparts tend to focus on people with cancer, yet it would be wrong if patients had 'good' deaths only in a specialist setting. It would be much more effective to bring the principles of hospice care into all institutions, so that everyone who is close to death feels comfortable, peaceful, close to relatives and friends, and prepared to die.

REFERENCES

Adams S 1984 Clothing in elderly patients in medical and geriatric wards and the relationship of clothing to self-esteem. Undergraduate Dissertation, Department of Nursing Studies, Chelsea College, University of London
Age Concern 1989 Older people in the United Kingdom. Age Concern England, Mitcham, Surrey
Age Concern Institute of Gerontology and Centre of Medical Law and Ethics, King's College London 1988 The living will: consent to treatment at the end of life. Edward Arnold, London
Andrews J 1989 Whose right is it anyway? Nursing Times 85(47): 24
Baker D 1983 'Care' in the geriatric ward: an account of two styles of nursing. In: Wilson-Barnett J (ed) Nursing research: ten studies in patient care. Wiley, Chichester
Barnett K 1972 A theoretical construct of the concepts of touch as they relate to nursing. Nursing Research 21(2): 102–110
British Geriatrics Society and Royal College of Nursing 1975 Improving geriatric care in hospital. Royal College of Nursing, London
Chambers R 1982 How to combat 'doing nothing' — two steps to catalyse change in homes for the elderly. Social Work Service 32 (winter): 51–53

Clark P, Bowling A 1989 Observational study of quality of life in NHS nursing homes and a long-stay ward for the elderly. Ageing and Society 9: 123–148
Clarke M 1978 Getting through the work. In: Dingwall R, McIntosh J (eds) Readings in the sociology of nursing. Churchill Livingstone, Edinburgh
Clark-Kennedy A E 1982 A bicycle is best. Geriatric Medicine 12: 74–77
Currie C T 1988 Life sustaining technologies and the elderly: Americans badly need geriatricians. British Medical Journal 297, 2 July: 3–4
Davidson A and Woolf A D 1989 (4) Osteoporosis: treatment of the established problem. Care of the Elderly 1(5): 215–216
Department of Health 1989a Working for patients: caring for the 1990s. HMSO, London
Department of Health 1989b A strategy for nursing. Department of Health Nursing Division, London
Department of Health and Social Security 1972 Minimum standards in geriatric hospitals and departments. HMSO, London
Department of Health and Social Security 1978 A happier old age. HMSO, London
Department of Health and Social Security 1979 The way forward. HMSO, London
Doyle D 1981 Terminal care of the elderly. In: Kinnaird J, Brotherston J, Williamson J (eds) The provision of care for the elderly. Churchill Livingstone, Edinburgh
Evers H 1981a Women patients in long-stay geriatric wards. In: Hutter B, Williams G (eds) Controlling women: the normal and the deviant. Croom Helm, London
Evers H 1981b Tender loving care. In: Copp L A (ed) Care of the ageing. Recent advances in nursing series, Churchill Livingstone, Edinburgh
Fox R A 1987 Palliative care and aggressive therapy. In: Elford R J (ed) Medical ethics and elderly people. Churchill Livingstone, Edinburgh
Gilbert M 1984 Challenging stereotypes. Nursing Mirror 158(16): 42–43
Glossop E S 1983 Improving quality of life: a case study of a geriatric unit. In: Denham M J (ed) Care of the long stay elderly patient. Croom Helm, London
Godlove C, Richard L, Rodwell G 1981. Time for action: an observation study of elderly people in four different care environments. Social Services Monograph: Research in Practice. Joint Unit for Social Services Research, University of Sheffield
Gormally L 1987 A response to Fox: palliative care and aggressive therapy. In: Elford R J (ed) Medical ethics and elderly people. Churchill Livingstone, Edinburgh
Hodges C 1989 A good deal for kids. Nursing Times 85(47): 22–23
Hughes G J 1987 A response to Jones: problems in senile dementia. In: Elford R J (ed) Medical ethics and elderly people. Churchill Livingstone, Edinburgh
Humphrey D, Wickett A 1986 The right to die: understanding euthanasia. Bodley Head, London
Jones R W 1987 Problems in senile dementia. In: Elford R J (ed) Medical ethics and elderly people. Churchill Livingstone, Edinburgh
Kennedy I 1988 Treat me right: essays in medical law and ethics. Clarendon Press, London
Kitson A, Harvey G, Guzinska M 1988 Nursing quality

assurance directory, 2nd edition, RCN Standards of Care Project, Royal College of Nursing and Kings Fund, London

Laurent C 1989 Patient power. Nursing Times 85(13): 73–74

Le May A C, Redfern S J 1987 A study of non-verbal communication between nurses and elderly patients. In: Fielding P (ed) Research in the nursing care of elderly people. Wiley, Chichester

Ling R S M 1979 Problems of the aged hip. In: Vowles K D J (ed) Surgical problems in the aged. Wright, Bristol

McCullough L B 1984 Medical care for elderly patients with diminished competence: an ethical analysis. Journal of the American Geriatrics Society 32(2): 150–153

Macleod Clark J 1988 Communication: the continuing challenge. Nursing Times 84(23): 24–27

MacGuire J 1989 Primary nursing: a better way to care? Nursing Times 85(46): 50–53.

Matteson M A, McConnell E S 1988 Gerontological nursing in acute care settings. In: Matteson M A, McConnell E S (eds) Gerontological nursing: concepts and practice. W B Saunders, Philadelphia

Medcalf P, Woolf A D 1989 (1) Osteoporosis: the nature of the problem. Care of the Elderly 1(5): 210–211

Miller A F 1978 Evaluation of the care provided for patients with dementia in six hospital wards. Unpublished MSc thesis, University of Manchester

Miller A F 1984 Nursing process and patient care. Nursing Times Occasional Paper. 80(13): 56–58

Mohr D N 1983 Estimation of surgical risk in the elderly: a correlative review. Journal of the Medical Geriatrics Society 31: 99–102

Muir-Gray J A 1984 The prevention of disability and handicap. Nursing Mirror 158(22): 29–30

Nordin B E C 1985 Osteoporosis. In: Exton-Smith A N, Weksler M E (eds) Practical geriatric medicine. Churchill Livingstone, Edinburgh

Norman A J 1980 Rights and risk. National Council for the Care of Old People (now Centre for Policy on Ageing), London

Norton D 1965 Nursing in geriatrics. Gerontologia Clinica 7: 59–60

Palmer C A, Reece-Smith H, Taylor I 1989 Major abdominal surgery in the over eighties. Journal of the Royal Society of Medicine 82: 391–393

Pearson A (ed) 1987 Nursing quality measurement: quality assurance methods for peer review. Wiley, Chichester

Platzer H 1988 A study into the causes of post-operative confusion in the elderly. Unpublished MSc thesis, Kings College, University of London

Pryor G A, Mylers J W, Williams D R R, Anand J K 1988 Team management of the elderly patient with hip fracture. The Lancet 1(8582): 401–403

Redfern S J 1989 Key issues in nursing elderly people. In: Warnes A M (ed) Human ageing and later life: multidisciplinary perspectives. Edward Arnold, London

Richard L 1983 Time for action. Nursing Mirror 156(13): 17–19

Rowden R 1983 A sense of harmony. Nursing Times 79(37): 9–11

Royal College of Nursing 1987 Focus on restraint: guidelines on the use of restraint in the care of elderly people. RCN, London

Sander R, Walden E 1984 So much to learn. Nursing Times 80(32): 50–51

Seligman M E P 1975 Helplessness: on depression, development and death. Freeman, San Francisco

Smith R 1984 Rights guide to non-means-tested social security benefits, 6th edn. Child Poverty Action Group, London

Swaffield L 1988 Communication: tuned in. Nursing Times 84(23): 28–31

Sweatman M 1989 Does formalised orthopaedic–geriatric collaboration work? Geriatric Medicine 19(6): 18–20

Vowles K D J 1979 Surgery for the aged. In: Vowles K D J (ed) Surgical problems in the aged. Wright, Bristol

Vowles K D J, Halliday C E 1979 Vascular problems and the aged amputee. In: Vowles K D J (ed) Surgical problems in the aged. Wright, Bristol

Wade B, Sawyer L, Bell J 1983 Dependency with dignity. Occasional Papers on Social Administration no. 68. Bedford Square Press, London

Wells T 1980 Problems in geriatric nursing care. Churchill Livingstone, Edinburgh

Weskler M E 1985 The evaluation of the elderly patient for surgery. In: Exton-Smith A, Weksler M E (eds) Practical geriatric medicine. Churchill Livingstone, Edinburgh

Woods R T, Holden U P 1982 Reality orientation. In: Isaacs B (ed) Recent advances in geriatric medicine. Churchill Livingstone, Edinburgh

Woolf A D 1989 Osteoporosis: a preventable problem. Care of the Elderly 1(5): 218–219

CHAPTER CONTENTS

The independent nurse practitioner and clinical nurse specialist 567

Individualized care and primary nursing 571
Autonomy and accountability 572

Nurse education 573
Project 2000: the background 575
Project 2000: the strategy 577
The response to Project 2000 579

Conclusion 581

33

The nurse's role in the care of old people

Sally J. Redfern

In this final chapter we move from focusing on the elderly patient, the subject of Chapter 32, to the nurse's role in the care of old people. The development in the UK of the role of independent nurse practitioner and clinical nurse specialist are discussed, followed by an examination of individualized care and primary nursing. Conventional nurse training has not been sufficient to equip nurses for these new roles, nor has it enabled them to assume the accountability that follows from role independence and expansion. We explore recent changes in nurse training, particularly the background and objectives of Project 2000. This is a new strategy for nurse education designed to produce a new kind of nurse, one who is equipped to take on the challenges of the independent and expanded roles envisaged for nurses in the 1990s.

THE INDEPENDENT NURSE PRACTITIONER AND CLINICAL NURSE SPECIALIST

If prevention and health is *everybody's* business, does this necessitate any realignment of position between doctors, patients, nurses, therapists, and other paramedical workers? (Austin 1979, p. 145, emphasis in original)

In the last chapter, it is abundantly clear that, although exciting initiatives have been taken by nurses, a lot more could be done to improve the quality of living and of dying of old people. Nursing has, it seems, on the one hand, encouraged the development of specialist nurses who advise their colleagues and patients on specific areas of nursing (stoma therapists, infection control nurses, incontinence advisers, breast cancer specialists, etc.). Yet, on the other hand, they have given away the fundamental 'basic' nursing care to unqualified students and auxiliaries. The hospital nurse caring for old people is perhaps the nurse who has, to the greatest extent, allowed others to take over nursing care. The geriatrician takes an energetic approach to diagnosis, treatment, rehabilitation, cure and discharge home and requires the specialist skills of the physiotherapist, occupational therapist, speech therapist, dietician and social worker to achieve his or her aim of optimum health for the patient and discharge home. The nurse, however, is everybody's assistant. She (or he) carries out medical instructions and ensures treatments are given, prepares the patient for therapy by the specialist, or delegates someone else to do this. She, typically, does not co-ordinate or continue the work of non-nurse specialists. Her principal role seems to be as a facilitator for others; she reacts to their instructions rather than taking the initative herself.

There is tremendous scope for nurses caring for old people in elderly care, psychiatric and community settings to extend the traditional role of doctor's assistant to that of the independent, autonomous health care practitioner. This requires nurses to develop a sufficient knowledge base to enable them to use their clinical judgement alongside but independent of medical expertise. In certain circumstances, as when nursing patients who are acutely ill, nurses would, of course, defer to doctors when carrying out medical treatments. But the nurse would continue to work towards maintaining and improving the patient's health after completion of the acute treatment, and preferably before illness occurs. As Austin (1979) observed, nursing would become continual rather than episodic and need not be related to a medically oriented setting. Community nurses, especially health visitors, argue that they are giving continual, preventive care as independent practitioners. This is true, but with the exception of those specializing in the care of elderly people, most generic health visitors see child health as their main responsibility (Fitton 1984b, Robertson

1984), and do not see working with old people as so rewarding (see Chapter 26).

Austin (1979) argued for the development of a nurse practitioner who is better suited to the practice of *health* care than the disease-oriented doctor. The impact of bureaucracy and professional territoriality, many believe, has not encouraged health care but has instead promoted a sickness service. The health and well-being of society is more likely to be dependent on factors such as a clean environment, good housing, adequate nutrition, a satisfactory minimum income, physical exercise, stress-alleviating interpersonal relationships and job satisfaction than on medical factors. Austin maintains that the welcome growth of preventive medicine has not been an active effort by the medical profession to promote health, and she sees the need for four changes if the promotion of health is to become a reality: more democratic forms of control, humane organization and management, realistic resource allocation, and changes in the relationships between professionals, and between professionals and their clients or patients.

The health promotion oriented independent nurse practitioner is not uncommon in parts of the United States and Canada and has been a normal feature of developing countries, with their 'barefoot doctors', although these latter practitioners are not usually nurses. The 'geriatric nurse practitioner' in the United States is an independent practitioner, teacher and consultant to hospital and community nurses, and has assumed a role caring for the health of old people, which doctors in that country do not want. The demise of the North American nurse practitioner was forecast by some members of the medical profession (Spitzer in Nursing Mirror 1984) because doctors maintained that they could now cope with the workload which they saw as theirs. But whether the demise will include the geriatric nurse practitioner as well as those working in areas traditionally regarded as the territory of doctors remains to be seen.

In Britain, the independent nurse practitioner is uncommon, but has been successful in the community setting of general practice (Stilwell 1984, 1988). More recently, other nurse practitioners have emerged, for example, in an accident and emergency department (Head 1988) and in district nursing (Andrews 1988). The example described by Head required a nurse with at least five years' post-qualification experience who was able to take responsibility for assessing and dealing with patients requiring minor treatment, for ordering X-rays, and for referring patients to the casualty doctor or to their general practitioners, as appropriate. Head assessed the value of the nurse practitioner and reported approval from the local Community Health Council, support from other health professionals in the department, and satisfaction from patients using the service. The most important benefit was a substantial reduction in waiting time for patients.

In the district nursing example (Andrews 1988), the nurse regards herself not as a nurse practitioner but as a district nurse who has expanded her role to include a wide range of activities considered by others (e.g. Stilwell 1988) to be the province of the nurse practitioner. Andrews sees this expanded role as a goal for all district nurses and not only for the few envisaged in the Cumberlege Report (DHSS 1986). This expanded role requires the nurse to operate as a key worker who prescribes treatment, conducts a regular 'surgery' in the health centre, runs well-woman and well-man clinics, conducts physical examinations, orders pathological investigations, refers patients directly to other agencies, including hospital doctors, provides counselling and advice on prevention of ill health and follows up on people who have been bereaved. 'Far from being the new role of the exclusive few, this could be the aspiration of all' (Andrews 1988, p. 32).

The development of the clinical nurse specialist has made a good deal of progress in the UK over recent years with nurses taking responsibility for clinical practice, educational activities, research and managerial functions with respect to a specific nursing area. Although they do take some clinical responsibility, nurse specialists are more likely to have a consultancy role than the direct practice role of the independent nurse practitioner (Markham 1988). It does seem, however, that some nurses combine clinical specialist and practitioner roles successfully, as in the case of the district nurse described by Andrews (1988). The clinical nurse specialist role described by Markham includes 'direct' and 'indirect' care activities. The direct activities include responsibility for the nurse's own patient caseload, which continues throughout each patient's illness, whether in hospital or community care. Thus, the nurse is responsible for assessment, planning, delivery and evaluation of care of patients and their families, and acts as a role model for other nurses and students. The indirect activities, which help others in their direct care, include teaching, setting clinical standards and policies, evaluating the quality of care and participating in research. A major advantage of these specialist roles is that they are able to combine clinical practice, management and educational aspects of patient care, that are divided into separate and often unco-ordinated roles in traditional nursing.

Until recently, standard nurse training has not equipped nurses for nurse practitioner or clinical nurse specialist roles. Furthermore, continuing education is not yet mandatory for all nurses, which means that their knowledge is not necessarily kept up-to-date. Progress, however, is being made in the UK, although the difficulties involved in establishing a comprehensive, mandatory system are daunting (Morton-Cooper 1989). The growth of degree-level nurse education in universities and polytechnics gives a small proportion of nurses a comprehensive grounding in the biological and social sciences applied to nursing. This comprehensive grounding should start to reach all nursing students as Project 2000 education schemes develop (see below). Research in nursing is increasing, and it is much more common than in the past to find nurses with research degrees working in clinical practice.

Progress in developing nurse practitioner and specialist roles and in improving nurse education has a much longer history in the USA than in this country and, in many ways, the UK has followed the USA's lead. It is of concern, therefore, that the American Medical Association's (AMA) response to the shortage of trained nurses in America is to recommend three new levels of health worker:

an 'assistant registered care technologist' who has had two months' training, a 'basic registered care technologist' with seven months' training and considered to be equivalent to the British enrolled nurse, and an 'advanced registered care technologist' with nine months' training. The AMA maintains that registered nurses would be eligible for entry to this 'advanced' nine month course. All these technologists would be apprentices to doctors, and would be registered by the state medical boards. However, nurses would be responsible for monitoring and supervising their care (Cairns-Berteau 1989). This approach, if followed in this country, would do nothing for the emerging professionalism of nursing, nor would it fit comfortably alongside primary nursing, which is discussed in the next section. It would fragment 'basic' and 'technical' nursing even more than is the case today.

Over the past ten years the Department of Health and Social Security (1981) and the Royal College of Nursing (1981) advocated the development of a professional career structure in clinical nursing. Promotion was to be dependent on acquisition of general and specialist post-basic qualifications, as well as on peer review and experience. These developments would provide nurses with the skills, knowledge and attitudes necessary to take on clinical nurse specialist and independent nurse practitioner roles. Progress in developing a clinical career structure is making headway, and the pay award to nurses together with the restructuring of clinical nurse grades which took place in 1988/89 (DHSS 1988) has contributed to this progress.

It is easier to envisage the successful development of the independent nurse practitioner in the primary care field of community nursing, which is less dominated by medicine than hospital nursing. Much as we would like to see a breakdown in the hospital/community boundary, with the properly educated professional nurse caring for old people in health and illness irrespective of location, the likelihood of this happening seems remote. The possibility is, however, acknowledged in the Project 2000 proposals (see below).

The time is ripe for community nurses to take the initiative and develop their role within the cur-

rent climate of public opinion, which increasingly understands the shortcomings of conventional medicine. The development of public awareness for the need for nutrition and exercise for health, the self-help movement (see Ch. 23), and the rise of alternative therapies have created an ideal environment for nurses to take the lead. Yet community nurses, particularly district nurses, are 'lagging behind the public in utilising and building on innovative approaches and demystifying professional care' (Turton 1984, p. 41).

The nurse who has most contact with old people in the community is the district nurse, and the research evidence suggests that the care district nurses provide is inadequate, especially with respect to health education, counselling and rehabilitation (Turton 1983, 1984; Chapter 27 of this book). They spend most of their time on physical nursing procedures. District nurses see themselves as giving skilled care to people identified as sick, and this does not include preventive care and health promotion, which are regarded as the province of the health visitor, although Fiona Ross (Chapter 27) maintains this is part of the district nurse's role. But, as noted above, health visitors generally restrict their preventive role to child care. As with hospital nurses, this fragmentation of care is compounded by the handing over of 'skilled' aspects of nursing care to non-nurse specialists (physiotherapists, occupational therapists, social workers, etc.), and of 'basic' nursing to untrained nursing auxiliaries, care assistants and home helps. Thus both district and hospital nurses have abdicated their role as providers of comprehensive patient care, except for the few who have taken on the responsibilities of the nurse specialist or practitioner. The emergence of a clinical career structure and the growth of key worker and primary nursing roles (see below) will do much to keep professional nurses in clinical practice and responsible for the delivery of comprehensive care.

The key worker role has been embraced particularly by community psychiatric workers working with elderly mentally ill people as members of the primary care team (see Chapter 19). This primary care team is often exceptionally cohesive, with a community psychiatric nurse, home help, psychogeriatrician, social worker, clinical psychologist and perhaps others, such as an occupational therapist, working closely together. One member takes the role of key worker, depending on the client's needs, and co-ordinates the services required to enable the old person and the family to cope at home. The key worker is the first point of contact for client, family, neighbours and other health and social workers, which ensures proper co-ordination of services and avoids fragmented care. These community psychiatric nurses have developed an independent practitioner role within an integrated and closely co-ordinated multidisciplinary team. Their initiative could be extended to the care of many other old people, particularly those living in the community (Butterworth 1988).

INDIVIDUALIZED CARE AND PRIMARY NURSING

In the USA, the concept of 'the nursing process' has become so well established as the philosophy that informs nursing practice, that discussion about the nursing process has all but ceased, having been replaced by 'primary nursing'. In the UK, discussion on the nursing process continues, but nurses are becoming increasingly familiar with the notion of primary nursing and are ensuring that it is given prominence in debates on nursing issues. An example of this is the invitation to nurses by Wright and Khadim (1989) to participate in a public debate about primary nursing and nursing development units.

Primary nursing is nothing new; rather, it is 'a simple return to the original way of delivering nursing' (Pearson 1988). Pearson and his colleagues describe the development and effectiveness of primary nursing and the introduction of 'nursing beds' in the nursing development units at Burford and Oxford in England (Pearson 1988, Pearson et al 1988). One of Pearson's colleagues at Oxford has demonstrated the value of primary nursing with elderly patients (McMahon 1989). Primary nursing is also a feature of the Tameside nursing development unit in Greater Manchester, England, which caters for elderly people (Wright 1989).

Another study revealed the superiority of primary nursing over team nursing in terms of quality of care and staff satisfaction (Reed 1988). Other research, however, highlights the difficulties of conducting rigorous research which attempts to test the hypothesis that primary nursing is better than team nursing, or patient allocation or task allocation, or whatever (MacGuire 1989). MacGuire found a greater emphasis on interpersonal communication and on helping patients to regain independence on her primary nursing wards compared with the control wards. She recommends that, rather than test the hypothesis that primary nursing is better, more progress would be made if more specific hypotheses were tested; for example, that nursing assessment of new patients is more comprehensive, or that nurses communicate more effectively, or that the incidence of pressure sores is lower in primary nursing wards compared with wards which employ other methods of organizing nursing care.

In the description of primary nursing that follows, we have drawn heavily from Pearson's (1988) work. Primary nursing is a method of organizing care which enables and requires one nurse to be responsible for the care of a patient throughout her stay in hospital. It is a return to the 'case method' approach to nursing which was normal before the 1930s and which continues in community nursing today. The primary nurse is responsible for the care of a caseload of patients throughout the day and night and over seven days per week. She (or he), of course, actually delivers care only during her hours of duty; at other times, care is continued by an associate nurse who follows the primary nurse's care plan. This approach has been accepted in the United States for some 20 years and is only now becoming popular in the UK. The value of primary nursing lies in the ability to facilitate holistic nursing by means of a close therapeutic partnership between nurse and patient.

The method of primary nursing developed at Burford and Oxford enabled nursing to develop there as a healing therapy in its own right with other disciplines supporting nursing. This is the reverse of conventional nursing, which provides a support service to doctors and therapists and which delegates fundamental nursing to untrained students and auxiliaries.

The atmosphere and management of care at Burford and Oxford is informal and patient-centred. Staff do not wear uniforms, visitors are not restricted and can stay overnight, facilities are available for making hot drinks and a bar provides alcoholic and soft drinks. The patient's day is flexible with no waking up or going to sleep times, and the only fixed meals are lunch and dinner.

The primary nurse carries out a holistic nursing assessment and develops a problem-oriented care plan together with the patient. Other members of the multidisciplinary care team contribute to the nurse's care plan, which means that there is just one patient record rather than a separate record for each discipline. The record is kept by the bedside so that it is easily consulted by the patient and the staff. Planning for the patient's discharge is organized by the primary nurse, in close consultation with other members of the multidisciplinary team and also with community nurses.

The management of primary nursing ensures that all nursing is delivered by registered nurses. The primary nurses must have at least two years' post-registration experience and they see themselves as independent nurse practitioners. The caseload each carries is up to eight patients.

Student nurses are always supernumerary, which means that care will continue as planned, with or without students. Support staff consist of non-nurse care assistants and ward co-ordinators who provide administrative assistance. These workers free the nurse to spend her whole time in direct nursing. The care assistants clean the environment, set up and clear away equipment, test urine, etc., as well as assisting the nurse when she (or he) needs help with a patient. There is no need for 'lower-level' nurses such as nursing auxiliaries or support workers who have received training in 'basic' nursing. This method of primary nursing ensures that all nursing care received by the patient is delivered by a registered nurse.

Contrary to what might be expected, Pearson (1988) found that the method of primary nursing adopted in the nursing development units at Burford and Oxford was more cost-effective than conventional care. Staffing and running costs were lower in both units compared with similar units in the health authority. This is because if one nurse is responsible for up to eight patients, then fewer registered nurses are required than are often supplied in areas where a 'mixed' team of nurses is usual. The key is in the addition of the non-nurse assistants, who support the nurses rather than deliver direct care themselves, and who are responsible to the primary nurses. In conventional areas, domestic staff are not accountable to the nurses. The role of the care assistants and the ward co-ordinators in primary nursing is broad, with the result that they and the nurses achieve greater job satisfaction than do staff in conventional units. The patients nursed in the nursing unit had a shorter hospital stay and received a consistently higher quality of nursing than those nursed in conventional hospital units.

Pearson has also found that, after an initial period of high stress for staff, which is inevitable when changes are introduced,

. . . nurses now feel that primary nursing and acting therapeutically are in fact less stressful than practising in a traditional style which demands detachment, conformity to routines, and a clouding of the opportunity to be responsible for one's own work (Pearson 1988, p. 145).

The developments at Burford, Oxford, Tameside and other nursing development units which are being set up throughout the UK are exciting and show the challenge of and scope for nurse-initiated change in the care of old people. We are sufficiently optimistic to believe that initiatives like these will spread and professional nurses will regain their responsibility for the delivery of comprehensive patient care. In a recent paper, Salvage (1990) reviews the effectiveness of primary nursing and nursing development units and identifies the complex issues in what she calls the 'New Nursing' movement.

AUTONOMY AND ACCOUNTABILITY

The move towards autonomous nurse practitioners is implicit within a context of primary nursing in which *expansion* of the nursing role is favoured over a more task-oriented *extension* of the role

(Vaughan 1989). As Vaughan makes clear, extending the nurse's role has been advocated by the medical profession, and usually refers to the acquisition of technical skills such as venepuncture, taking ECGs or setting up intravenous infusions. Extended roles also include nurse research assistants in medical research and some nurse practitioners. These roles are often considered to consist of more highly valued and advanced skills compared with those required for giving high-quality care to elderly people.

Vaughan describes the expanded nursing role as a very different concept, and one which values the skills required to give high quality care to 'low tech' groups such as old people:

This [expanded nursing] recognises the true value of nursing as a separate therapeutic activity in its own right . . . [I]t explores nursing as a service to patients, helping them to reach predefined health-related goals . . . [I]t challenges nurses to develop their understanding of human nature, of feeling, as well as physiologically being, well. It recognises the need of people to learn through their own experiences and requires expertise in both interaction and teaching as well as in the more traditional functions of acting on behalf of others (Vaughan 1989, p. 55).

Expansion need not preclude extension, but the trend has tended to be towards extension, which, as Vaughan observes, is likely to result in nursing's dependence on other professions and the control of health care and resources by a single profession, medicine.

It seems that if the dependent extended path is followed alone there is a risk that the 'artistry' of nursing, the caring component, may be lost in the rush to gain new skills, and that reductionism and compartmentalisation of care will be perpetuated (Vaughan, ibid).

Role expansion offers quite the reverse: the opportunity for a role independent of yet complementary to other health care workers. It requires nurses to retrieve nursing from those to whom they have given it away, that is, from social workers, physiotherapists, occupational therapists and untrained assistants.

If we continue to extend into delegated technical functions with a consequent splitting off of fragments of care, then what we used to know as nursing will be lost for ever (Vaughan, ibid).

Primary nursing is an important component of autonomous expanded nursing practice in which accountability is an essential requirement. A recent document on accountability, published by the UKCC (1989), makes very clear that silent compliance is no longer acceptable if quality has been contravened. The report requires nurses to become assertive and to speak up when they witness unacceptable care. If they do not, they could face disciplinary action themselves. This is a new requirement for nursing and is essential if role expansion and primary nursing are to flourish.

NURSE EDUCATION

A substantial part of a nurse's formative experience is gained in hospital and a significant contribution to learning is made during the ward round. Consultants will agonize over the finer points of a medical diagnosis. The social worker gives an analysis of social circumstances; the psychologist presents a battery of mental tests; the physiotherapist or occupational therapist presents a report on functioning and progress. If pushed, the nurse says 'slept well', 'up and about' or 'appears a bit anxious' (Butterworth 1988, p. 38).

Some people hold the view that nursing management and education are responsible for the lack of nurse initiative. For example, Turton (1984) maintains that the characteristics valued by nurses in authority are obedience and conformity to current practice rather than independence and initiative. Turton maintains that the conventional hospital-based, treatment-of-disease oriented nurse training does not prepare district nurses to be flexible and responsive to social and technological change, to be leaders and co-ordinators of care at patient, family, team, local and national levels, and to be the patient's advocate. Turton is critical of the criteria used for selecting students into nurse training, which value conformity and competence in convergent thinking (seeking single solutions to problems) rather than the non-conformist creativity of the divergent thinker; this is a trend that continues (Wondrak 1989). Turton describes an educational model based on holistic medicine which could be used as the basis for the district nurse training curriculum:

Emphasis would be placed on understanding the factors that make the individual vulnerable to disease — the complex interplay of body, mind and spirit, and/or a recognition and deployment of the skills of the 'pharmacopoeia of people' available to aid the patient and his carer. The role of the district nurse as a health educator in its broadest sense is equally important — not as a didactic teacher, but as a facilitator, enabling patients and carers to co-operate actively in sharing information and maximising their self-healing potential in a more egalitarian relationship with the health professionals (p. 42).

If district nurse training were to develop along these lines, then the argument for a single community nurse for the elderly, rather than the present fragmentation between the district nurse and health visitor, may gain support. In spite of their preference for children, health visitors see their unique skills as essential in the care of old people (Fitton 1984a, 1984b, and Chapter 26 of this book. But, since district nursing focuses almost entirely on old people (see Chapter 27) and since most health visitors' priority is with children and their families, then combining district nurse and health visitor training into a curriculum for educating a generalist community nurse for the elderly would surely be a wise move. Such a move has its supporters (e.g. Batchelor 1984), and Nuttall (1984) had predicted this would occur within five years.

Nuttall's prediction has not yet come true, but a shared training among community nurses, health visitors, social workers and general practitioners has been advocated (Butterworth 1988). Initiatives are developing. For example, King's College, London University runs a Bachelor of Science degree in Community Nursing for registered nurses. The graduates are registered as district nurses and health visitors although the two qualifications retain a separate identity.

There is plenty of evidence in the literature that basic and post-basic education of nurses in Britain and in other countries has been inadequate (Cox 1983, World Health Organization 1983, Hall 1984a). Concern was so great in England that the Royal College of Nursing set up a Commission on Nursing Education in April 1984 to examine the whole field of nurse education and training and to make recommendations. This Commission led to publication of the Judge Report (RCN 1985), which had an important role in the development of Project 2000 (see below).

If we look at the definition of nursing given by the World Health Organization, it is clear that nursing is seen in terms of health promotion as well as caring for the sick and dying:

Nursing is a fundamental human activity and in its organised form a discrete health discipline. Its primary responsibility is to assist individuals and groups (families/communities) to optimise function throughout the lifespan as well as to care during acute and protracted illness and disability. It also makes social contributions maintaining, promoting and protecting health, caring for the sick and providing rehabilitation. It is concerned with the psychosomatic and psychosocial aspects of life as these affect health, illness and dying (WHO 1983, p. 31, emphasis in original).

If health for all is to be achieved by the year 2000, then nursing education and practice must move away from an emphasis on hospital-based disease-oriented care. The World Health Organization stipulates that basic curricula for nurse education should include theories of human development and ageing, self-care, health promotion and community health, as well as of the development of disease, disability and social dysfunction, and specific treatments and rehabilitation.

A vision of the nurse of the future, provided by Hall (1984a, 1984b) underlines the need for change in basic nurse education. She outlined 12 features of this future nurse:

- She would focus on health rather than ill health and recognize her role as a health educator.
- She would operate as a member of a true team, recognizing her own unique role and that of the other professionals.
- She would work with individuals and their families in attaining and promoting health.

- She would have a comprehensive knowledge base and be able to initiate and direct her own subsequent learning.
- She would be competent in relevant nursing skills, including those of communication.
- She would be analytical and critical without being defensive, and be able to conceptualize.
- She would be able to apply and adapt general principles to particular situations.
- She would make use of research.
- She would recognize both the art and science of nursing.
- She would understand the need for continuing education to maintain her competence, and the value of higher education for new and extended roles.
- She would accept the responsibility of professional accountability and understand its implications.
- She would be committed to a standard of professional conduct based on ethical principles.

Hall firmly believed that nursing students should cease to be part of the National Health Service labour force and that the proportion of nurses educated to degree level should increase. If newly qualified nurses possessed the qualities outlined by Hall, then those who specialized in the care of old people would be in an ideal position to develop their knowledge and skills through further education and research, and to take the lead in improving the standards of health care for elderly people. Many people, including Hall, recommend that nurse teachers should be graduates. This recommendation has been endorsed by the United Kingdom Central Council, which is the statutory body for nurse, midwifery and health visiting education (UKCC 1986). It has been recommended that there should be an increase in joint appointments between teaching and research, between research and practice, and between teaching and practice. The arguments for joint teaching–practice posts are appealing because teaching would occur in clinical areas. But, in the present structure in the United Kingdom, teachers could not take a full-time clinical load and carry respon-

sibility for student and post-basic teaching and research. This role would be easier for the independent nurse practitioner or clinical nurse specialist, who would not, however, carry full-time clinical responsibility.

PROJECT 2000: THE BACKGROUND

Project 2000 was the outcome of the work of the Project Group set up by the United Kingdom Central Council for Nursing, Midwifery and Health Visiting (UKCC). Its aim was 'to establish and improve standards of training and professional conduct for nurses midwives and health visitors' (UKCC 1986, p. 3). The Project 2000 report (UKCC 1986) sets out the background to the proposals, the deficiencies in the current system of nurse training, and the proposed structure for nurse education for the future.

The background to the proposals is described as arising from several sources. The Briggs Report (Committee on Nursing 1972) had recommended a plan of education which would lead to a certification stage, a registration stage, and the opportunity for higher certificates in different specialties. In the 14 years between Briggs and Project 2000 the NHS was reorganized twice; health care started looking towards health promotion, community care, and targeting priority care groups; and the economic recession deepened, with profound effects on health and welfare provision. Nursing education developments during that time included a greater emphasis on continuing education, the development of degree courses in educational institutions, the promotion of community psychiatric nursing and the widening of the nurse training syllabus. Clinical nursing developments included the introduction of the nursing process and nursing models, an increase in clinical research, and the development of the notion of primary nursing. Particularly significant to the development of Project 2000 was the increasing frustration and mounting pressure to improve nurse training which led the Royal College of Nursing to set up its Commission on Nurse Education (the Judge Report, RCN 1985).

The educational deficiencies in current nurse

training are described in the Project 2000 report. Students are employed as workers and contribute about 20% of the staffing establishment in hospital wards, with the result that their service contribution takes precedence over their educational needs. Concern has been constantly raised about the inadequate teaching students receive in the wards, their disillusionment, and the lack of confidence and defensiveness of teachers, both in the school and the ward. Student wastage rates are described as high, although at 15–20% of initial intake over three years, this is lower than it was in the mid-1970s. However, on top of the drop-out figure is an additional 15–20% who fail to pass the examinations, leaving only 65% of entrants to nurse training who achieve registration. Nurse teachers face a constant grind of repeated teaching to what was until recently up to six student intakes per year. The teachers have no time for updating their teaching, for research or professional development, and their teaching plans are frequently compromised in order to ensure that wards are adequately staffed. Whilst students are needed as pairs of hands to get the work done, educational improvement cannot occur. Another educational deficiency is that the current system of nurse training, with the exception of degree courses in universities and polytechnics, isolates the students and teachers from education generally.

In addition to these educational deficiencies, Project 2000 identifies service disadvantages emanating from the current system of nurse training. Partly as a result of implementation of the European Economic Community (EEC) Directives, the range of clinical experience required in all education programmes has expanded so that allocation difficulties and bottlenecks arise (particularly in specialist areas such as children's wards, maternity wards, operating theatres and accident and emergency departments). Furthermore, the criteria for designating wards and units as suitable clinical learning areas have tightened, with the result that fewer wards than previously are accepted for student placements. The result is a continuous conflict between service and education, with the service managers trying to keep wards staffed and teachers trying to meet education needs. The fact that education is taking place in a National Health

Service which is required to reduce costs has compounded the conflict. It is not unusual for wards to close, or to change their use, or for patient admissions to be halted, or for temporary agency nurses and unqualified staff to make up the shortfall in student labour. A staff mix with a high proportion of unqualified and temporary staff leads to fragmented care and reliance on a task allocation approach. An inevitable outcome is withdrawal of approval of nurse training schemes, which occurred in some London hospitals where these difficulties were particularly serious.

Additional problems are an unacceptable wastage and turnover of qualified nurses, which some researchers link to the reliance on student labour. The student labour system, which relies on 'constant replacement' in that a new cohort of trainees replaces the one that has completed the course, is cheap but

inefficient, ineffective, unjust and in severe need of overhaul. Both educationally, and in terms of service delivery, we believe that the present pattern is on a collision course (UKCC 1986, p. 12).

Student labour and constant replacement require a substantial number of 18-year-old school leavers to enter nurse training each year. However, the reduction in the birthrate in the UK between 1964 and 1976, which has become known as nursing's 'demographic timebomb', has meant that the number of 18-year-old recruits is not at all sufficient in the late 1980s and early 1990s. Much more effort is required in recruiting a workforce which does not rely on student labour and which can be retained. Particularly important is facilitating the return of women to nursing after a career break, and attracting new kinds of recruits such as more men, graduates, the unemployed and those taking early retirement. The present system is extremely wasteful of resources, with high student wastage, low retention of staff, little effort in encouraging leavers to return, and qualified nurses no longer doing real nursing.

The need for change in nurse training stems not only from the educational and service deficiencies summarized here. The Project 2000 report also points to the changing health needs in our society and to other changes affecting the National Health Service. There is no doubt that since the inception of the NHS in 1948 personal health and social conditions have improved. More people have comfortable living conditions and access to a comprehensive education. Working conditions have improved, and women are healthier and are producing fewer children, more of whom survive. Tuberculosis and other infective diseases can be successfully treated, and it is accidents, cancers and circulatory diseases that are today's killers. Anxiety and depression are the most frequent reasons given for visiting a general practitioner, after nasopharyngitis, particularly for women; and child morbidity from eczema, asthma, accidental injury, diabetes and obesity has risen. Most important is the increase in social class inequalities in levels of health and access to services, made clear in the Black Report (Townsend & Davidson 1982). The Project 2000 report concludes that

it is overwhelmingly clear that the people most in need are not getting the most resources with our present patterns of delivery of care (UKCC 1986, p. 15).

The evidence suggests that the need for health care will increase. The population is ageing and there are increasing numbers of people surviving into and facing the frailty of extreme old age. Changes in households and their composition mean that there are more single parents, more people living alone, complex kin networks resulting from divorce and remarriage, more women taking on the dual role of working at home and at work, and increasing relative poverty for disadvantaged groups, many of whom are old people.

The Project 2000 report sees health care in the next decades as focusing on three themes. First, the targeting of services for client groups such as old people, mentally ill and mentally handicapped people, and children. Second, an emphasis on health promotion, disease prevention, primary health care and care in the community. Third, the plan to rationalize and reduce the proportion of the health service budget devoted to acute hospital services, together with an emphasis on cost-effectiveness.

With reference to health service provision for elderly people, the emphasis is on keeping them at home with the necessary services, and providing energetic treatment and rehabilitation in hospital so that they can return home. Home care requires adequate respite care for relatives, night sitters, regular surveillance and proper support for terminal care at home. Plans for long-stay care vary across the country. Nurse-led nursing Homes are advocated by some, whilst others see long-stay care as a social services responsibility (see Chapter 29). More day care and small residential units are planned for elderly people suffering from dementia (Chapter 19).

PROJECT 2000 : THE STRATEGY

The educational deficiencies, the service problems, the changing health needs and the health care provision described in the Project 2000 report and summarized above provide the background for an educational strategy identified by Project 2000. Extremely important is the need to orientate nursing education towards community care. The report emphasizes care in the home, the assessment of health care needs, and the promotion of self-care and independence. Experience of hospital care continues to be important, of course, but initial training, Project 2000 argues, should be community based. Acute hospital nursing will become the preserve of the specialist nurse, the report predicts.

A second theme identified in the Project 2000 report is the need to prepare future nurses to contribute effectively to the planning, assessment and development of services. They must be better informed about the planning process, about information systems and about policy debates that influence health care provision. They need training in evaluating their own practice and skills to argue effectively for specific services.

The third theme identified is the importance of implementing an educational strategy which enables the professional nurse of the future to cope with uncertainty. We live in the midst of rapid change, and the future nurse must be able to adapt with confidence to changing health care needs. Project 2000's authors are convinced that the old 'once and for all' training should be replaced by a sound common foundation course, followed by units of learning arranged as a series of building blocks that match perceived need. The product of this education is regarded as a new kind of nurse who is

. . . a mature and confident practitioner, willing to accept responsibility, able to think analytically and flexibly, able to recognise a need for further preparation and willing to engage in self development (UKCC 1986, p. 33).

Project 2000 envisages two levels of nurse. At the point of registration, at the end of the three-year programme, the 'registered practitioner' will be

. . . competent to assess the need for care, to provide that care, to monitor and evaluate care and to do all this in a range of institutional and non-institutional settings (UKCC 1986, p. 40).

Thus the registered practitioner is regarded as not just a 'doer' but a 'knowledgeable doer' who can practise as an independent practitioner and be accountable for actions taken.

Senior to the registered practitioner will be different kinds of 'specialist practitioner', who will continue to have responsibility for direct care and will be able to advise and support the registered practitioner. Project 2000 envisages a range of specialist practitioner roles in hospital and the community. Some will be disease linked, some will have particular competence in specific nursing areas and others will be specialists in health promotion. They will maintain a caseload but will also have a teaching and in some cases, a management function. Examples of specialist practitioners in health promotion include health visitors, occupational health nurses and school nurses. Specialist practitioners in clinical specialties will become team leaders working with a team of registered practitioners. Present charge nurses, ward sisters and district nurses belong to this group. Project 2000 envisages that the specialist practitioner will require further education, but detailed plans for their preparation are not included in the report.

A third level of worker envisaged by Project 2000 is the 'aide', who will assist and be directly supervised and monitored by the registered practitioner. The aide, recently more often given the title of 'support worker', would have some training specific to the work setting and would have the

opportunity to move into professional preparation provided the entry requirements were met.

Project 2000 proposes a three-year preparation consisting of a Common Foundation Programme (CFP) for all students, followed by preparation, before registration, into the adult, mental illness, mental handicap, child and midwifery branches of nursing. Since publication of Project 2000, midwives have argued against midwifery being a branch, preferring it to continue as either a post-registration training or a direct-entry programme, or both. The Common Foundation Programme focuses on health rather than illness and exposes students to a wide range of community as well as hospital settings. Project 2000 sees the CFP as spanning about two years, with the branch programme lasting one year, although flexibility in length is possible. The main difference between Project 2000 and existing programmes for the different parts of the register that exist today is the much greater emphasis on community placements. The Project 2000 registered practitioner will have had much less exposure to hospital practice than the RGN of today. Instead, she (or he) will have a much wider knowledge of caring and support services in the community, which is essential to preparing a practitioner who can meet today's health needs.

After much debate, the Project 2000 committee decided against proposing a branch in care of elderly people. They acknowledged the priority given to the elderly in terms of policy and the growing need suggested by demographic changes but they were concerned about the arbitrary and possibly harmful effects of defining 'the elderly' as a group, coupled with the likely difficulty of recruiting students to a specialist branch. Project 2000 thus opted for an initial acquaintance with elderly people incorporated as an essential part of the CFP, followed by integrating care of elderly people into the branch programmes. Post-registration programmes for practitioners working with elderly people was wiser in the current climate, it was thought, than creating a separate branch.

Nurses choosing to specialize in the care of elderly people will, therefore, have completed the adult or the mental illness branch. We are delighted to see, in the Project 2000 proposals, the explicit intention to integrate the work of the hospital and the community nurse. Continuity of care is not facilitated by the strict division between hospital and community nursing and nurses need knowledge of the range of settings in which elderly people are cared for. Hospital nursing activities are increasingly moving into the home, 'and it is not inconceivable that this nurse might in her training, *and perhaps even in her practice,* move across settings with her client' (UKCC 1986, p. 49, emphasis added). With supernumerary status, the continuity of care of old people by students across settings is achievable. The likelihood of this occurring within the registered nurse's practice is more difficult to envisage, in view of the continuing distinction between hospital and community nursing, but now that the possibility has been made explicit, it has a chance of becoming reality.

Project 2000 recommends that education beyond registration level should be 'coherent, comprehensive and cost-effective'. It should provide consolidation in the immediate post-registration period and should include opportunities for regular updating of knowledge and skills. Also, it should provide a range of specialist courses which would include shared learning with other disciplines. Health visiting, district nursing, community psychiatric nursing and community mental handicap nursing are seen as appropriate qualifications for specialist practitioners. In hospital, a recognized preparation will be required for the clinical specialist caring for critically ill patients. Hospitals will be increasingly caring for acutely ill people and the registered practitioner will need support from a specialist. Some of the specialist practitioners in hospital will manage the ward or unit and also have a teaching and clinical role. The Project 2000 report maintains that present ward sisters and charge nurses will welcome the opportunity and the need for additional preparation for their role.

Fundamental to the introduction of Project 2000 is the requirement that students should be supernumerary to the ward or community staffing establishment. This does not mean that they will not gain experience by looking after patients. Students will not be part of the workforce but will look after patients and clients under supervision. This change will enable students to be self-directive in their learning and to explore areas of knowledge and skill individually. Clinical teaching will help students to integrate health care principles and theoretical issues into their practice and will encourage them to review research-based literature.

No longer employees, students will receive bursaries or grants which are likely to be more than the education grant but less than the current student salary. Project 2000 also proposed that hospital schools of nursing should be grouped into larger colleges and linked, where appropriate, to existing colleges, polytechnics and universities, so that more facilities and expertise are available. Library facilities would increase and opportunities for research and collaboration with other disciplines would be facilitated. This merging and grouping of colleges is now taking place. Project 2000 also recommended that in future all teachers should be educated to first degree level.

THE RESPONSE TO PROJECT 2000

The UKCC published Project 2000 in 1986 and presented its proposals to government health ministers in February 1987. The government approved in principle many of the proposals put forward, but inevitably, there were strings attached (Salvage 1988). Approval was given for an 18-month rather than a two-year Common Foundation Programme, followed by 18-month branch programmes in adult, child, mentally ill and mentally handicapped nursing; to supernumerary student status; to non-means-tested student bursaries; to cessation of enrolled nurse training; to the introduction of the support worker; and to consideration of midwifery as a direct entry course (Lampada 1988). The government recommended further discussion on widening the entry gate into nurse education, on the role and function of the specialist practitioner, on shared learning with other professions, on community nurse education, and on introducing credits for degree courses.

The strings attached involve the role of the support worker. The government sees a generic health care assistant in this role, rather than a nursing support worker who would be entirely under nursing control. Nurses welcome the government's commitment to continue to plan, deliver and monitor nursing care but they fear loss of control over the support worker. This is a justifiable concern, given the evidence for the contribution of the nurse-controlled support worker to the success of primary nursing (Pearson 1988). There is great concern that the support worker may become a lower-level nurse if the expected three-month training for support workers becomes a two-year course, a possibility that is denied by the Department of Health and the UKCC (Fardell 1989). Fardell remains unconvinced of government assurances, however. She reports the outcome of a DoH workshop, which identified four grades of future nurse: the registered nurse with three years of training, the enrolled nurse with two years, the 'senior' support worker, also with two years of training, and the auxiliary. It is clear that substantial confusion remains, and since primary nursing has been shown to be highly cost-effective by employing untrained nurse helpers (Pearson 1988), then it would be unwise and unnecessarily expensive to give substantial training and lower-level nurse status to the support worker.

Another 'string' is the government's intention to discontinue enrolled nurse training on condition that the entry gate into nursing is widened. Many nurses have voiced their concern that relaxing the entrance requirements will lower nursing standards (e.g. Kratz 1988), although others see it as a sensible response to recruitment difficulties and do not regard high academic qualifications as an essential requirement for professional nursing (Orr 1988, Salvage 1988).

Other reactions within the nursing profession to Project 2000 indicate an understandable uncertainty surrounding any change (Fardell 1988, Gaze 1988, Swaffield 1988, Turner & Dickson 1988). For example, there are concerns that supernumerary student status will result in insufficient clinical practice and culture shock on qualifying. There are concerns that loss of the student labour force will leave wards so understaffed that nursing will

be delegated to untrained support workers. The costs of Project 2000 are considered by some to be so high as to make it unworkable. The actual costs have been estimated by Bosanquet (1988), who argues that, although costs will rise in the short term, they will drop in the longer term as the benefits from a better-trained, more stable staff take effect. Bosanquet maintains, even so, that the costs estimated compare reasonably with those for other educational courses.

One of the most serious concerns is that voiced by Salvage (1988). She maintains that the government is prepared to end enrolled nurse training so that it can introduce a variety of assistants trained to different levels of competency. These people may not be educationally or managerially accountable to nurses. In the context of the financial cutbacks to the health service, and the Prime Minister's NHS review, Salvage forsees a continuing, but different, two-tier nursing system. The Project 2000 graduates will be a small, highly educated elite. Those who choose to work either in 'the government-bolstered private sector' or in the protected acute specialty of the NHS, will work as nurse practitioners. This leaves those who work in non-acute areas spending all their time not as nurses but as supervisors of large numbers of support workers. The workload may not allow them to operate as key workers or primary nurses.

Robinson (1988) is concerned that 'high-tech' nurses employed in intensive therapy units, operating theatres and paediatric wards will be seen as having 'additional expertise', and therefore warranting a higher salary, than those working in the 'low-tech' areas of mental illness and mental handicap nursing and elderly care. It follows that 'real nursing' may be seen in the future as high-tech nursing and low-tech nursing will be given away to the social services, as is implicit in the Audit Commission (1986) and the Griffiths proposals (1988); this would perpetuate the medical view of nurses as doctors' assistants. It is of vital importance that highly educated nurses, that is, those Robinson refers to as the nursing elite, retain and promote holistic nursing and 'basic' care.

Following acceptance by the government of Project 2000 in principle, 13 demonstration sites were set up in 1989 in new nursing colleges across the country. The Nursing Times is following students and staff in two of these colleges throughout the three-year course in order to document their experiences and expectations (Nursing Times 1989). It remains to be seen whether the graduate of Project 2000 will receive an education that is sufficient to match the 12 features of the future nurse described by Hall (1984b) and outlined above.

CONCLUSION

In this chapter we have looked briefly at the developing role of the nurse, particulary that of the nurse practitioner and the clinical nurse specialist, and at the emerging popularity of primary nursing. The quest for improving the quality of nursing makes the climate right for nurses to take the initiative in promoting change and improvements in care. This is not easy for most nurses. They have not, on the whole, been given a sufficiently comprehensive education, nor are they accustomed to initiating change. The style of working, at least in hospital nursing, is such that they are expected to be fully exposed on the job for the whole of their working time. Traditionally, nurses do not choose, nor are they given time, to absent themselves for reading, thinking and writing. Other health care workers (doctors, therapists, managers, teachers) are visitors to the ward and can work more independently. They can more easily introduce changes in their care.

The chapter continued with a description of the changes that are occurring in the UK in nurse education. Project 2000 is the strategy that has been recommended as the means of bringing nurse education up-to-date. The first Project 2000 schemes started in 13 demonstration sites in 1989, and so we must wait some time before we will know whether the improvements predicted have occurred. Project 2000 aims to produce a new nurse, an independent, accountable practitioner who can meet the health needs of society in the 1990s and beyond. The new practitioner who specializes in the care of elderly people will increasingly focus on primary health care and care in the community,

as well as on health promotion and disease prevention. Care in hospital will remain important and necessary, but as a short-term and integral component, rather than a separate feature, of the old person's care in the community. The changes envisaged for basic and continuing nurse education will produce nurses who will examine their own practices, and who will investigate nursing questions themselves. In so doing, nurses can only improve the quality of care and with it the quality of life for old people.

REFERENCES

Andrews S 1988 An expert in practice. Nursing Times 84(26): 31–32

The Audit Commission for Local Authorities in England and Wales 1986 Making a reality of community care. HMSO, London

Austin R 1979 Practising health care: the nurse practitioner. In: Atkinson P, Dingwall R, Murcott A (eds) Prospects for the national health. Croom Helm, London

Batchelor I 1984 Policies for a crisis? Some aspects of DHSS policies for care of the elderly. Occasional Papers No 1, Nuffield Provincial Hospitals Trust, Oxford

Bosanquet N 1988 What will it cost? Nursing Times 84(31): 34

Butterworth T 1988 Breaking the boundaries. Nursing Times 84(47): 36–39

Cairns-Berteau M 1989 The doctor's apprentice. Nursing Times 85(7): 21

Committee on Nursing 1972 Report of the Committee on Nursing. (Briggs Report), HMSO, Cmnd 5115, London

Cox C 1983 Mightier than an army. Nursing Mirror 156: 15 Nurse Education Conference Report, vi–vii

Department of Health and Social Security 1981 Professional development in clinical nursing — the 1980s. DHSS, London

Department of Health and Social Security 1986 Neighbourhood nursing: a focus for care. Report of the community nursing review (Chairman: Julia Cumberlege). HMSO, London

Department of Health and Social Security 1988 Clinical grading structure for nurses, midwives and health visitors. DHSS EL (88), London

Fardell J 1988 The supernumerary student. Nursing Times 84(32): 32–33

Fardell J 1989 Short cut or short change? Nursing Times 85(7): 30–31

Fitton J M 1984a Health visiting the elderly: nurse managers' views — 1. Nursing Times Occasional Paper 80(10): 59–61

Fitton J M 1984b Health visiting the elderly: nurse managers' views — 2. Nursing Times Occasional Paper 80(11): 67–69

Gaze H 1988 For better or worse? Nursing Times 84(38): 48–49

Griffiths R 1988 Community care: agenda for action. HMSO, London

Hall C 1984a A springboard to the future. Nursing Mirror 158(4): 39–41

Hall C 1984b A time for vision. Nursing Mirror 158(3): 32–35

Head S 1988 Nurse practitioners: the new pioneers. Nursing Times 84(26): 26–28

Kratz C 1988 Widening the entry gate: the case against. Nursing Times 84(31): 33

Lampada 1988 Congress hails Moores acceptance of Project 2000. Lampada 15: May/June, 1

MacGuire J 1989 Primary nursing: a better way to care? Nursing Times 85(46): 50–53

McMahon R 1989 Primary nursing: one to one. Nursing Times 85(2): 39–40

Markham G 1988 Special cases. Nursing Times 84 (26): 29–30

Morton-Cooper A 1989 Refreshing news. Nursing Times 85(50): 18

Nursing Mirror 1984 The nurse practitioner. (Editorial) Nursing Mirror 158(1): 21

Nursing Times 1989 Project 2000: starting with a bonus. Nursing Times 85(37): 28–31

Nuttall P 1984 Shape of things to come? Nursing Times 80(1): 8–10

Orr J 1988 Widening the entry gate: the case for. Nursing Times 84(31): 32

Pearson A (ed) Primary nursing: nursing in the Burford and Oxford nursing development units. Croom Helm, London

Pearson A, Durand I, Punton S 1988 The feasibility and effectiveness of nursing beds. Nursing Times 84(47) Occasional Paper (9): 48–50

Reed J A 1988 A comparison of nurse-related behaviour, philosophy of care and job satisfaction in team and primary nursing. Journal of Advanced Nursing 13: 385–395

Robertson C 1984 Old people in the community 1. Health visitors and preventive care. Nursing Times 80(34): 29–31

Robinson J 1988 Elitism in nursing. Nursing Times 84(40): 50–51

Royal College of Nursing 1981 A structure for nursing. RCN, London

Royal College of Nursing 1985 The education of nurses: a new dispensation. Commission on Nursing Education (The Judge Report), RCN, London

Salvage J 1988 Brighton breezes. Nursing Times 84(24): 22

Salvage J 1990 The theory and practice of the 'New Nursing'. Nursing Times Occasional Paper 86(4): 42–45

Stilwell B 1984 The nurse in practice. Nursing Mirror 158(21): 17

Stilwell B 1988 Nurse practitioners: their place in the NHS. Kings Fund Centre, London

Swaffield L 1988 The new face of nursing. Nursing Times 84(31): 27–29

Townsend P, Davidson N (eds) 1982 Inequalities in health: the Black Report. Penguin, Harmondsworth

Turner T, Dickson N 1988 Project 2000: a new dawn for nursing? Nursing Times 84(22): 12–13

Turton P 1983 Health education and the district nurse. Nursing Times Community Outlook 79(32): 222–229

Turton P 1984 Nurses working in the community. Nursing Times 80(22): 40–42

United Kingdom Central Council for Nursing, Midwifery and Health Visiting 1986 Project 2000: a new preparation for practice. UKCC, London

United Kingdom Central Council 1989 Exercising accountability. UKCC, London

Vaughan B 1989 Autonomy and accountability. Nursing Times 85(3): 54–55

Wondrak R 1989 A uniform bunch. Nursing Times 85 (22): 58–59

World Health Organization 1983 Medicosocial work and nursing: the changing needs. EURO Reports and Studies 79. WHO Regional Office for Europe, Copenhagen

Wright S 1989 Defining the nursing development unit. Nursing Standard 4 (7): 29–31

Wright S, Khadim N 1989 Primary nursing — your questions answered. Nursing Standard 4(7): 32

Index

AARP, 14
Abdominal surgery
  mortality, 557
Abuse, 459–460
  by carer, 459
Accountability, 572–573
'Active initiators', 534
Activities, 107–111
  maintaining, 99–100
  of daily living, 491–492
  score, 492
Activity
  in COAD, 168
  meaningful, 527
Activity theory, 31
Activity Nurses, 108–109
Adjustment
  to change, 30–34
Adult status
  loss of, 526
Advocate, patient's, 563
Affective states, 342
Afferent mechanisms, 123
AFFOR (All faiths for one race), 474
Aftercare, 473–474
Age, old
  biology, 4–5
  meaning, 3–4
  pathology model, 6–7
  research on, 5–15
Age Concern, 100, 103, 474, 495
Age stratification theory, 32
'Age Well', 100
Age Well Forum, 457
Ageing
  animal models, 41
  biology of human, 39–63
  cultural stereotype, 21
  demographic trend, 531–534
  'error theories', 57
  experience, 21
  'normal', 39–40
  physiological changes, 40
  population impact, 531–547
  prejudice, 544–545
  preprogrammed, 57
  process, 39–40

psychology, 19–34
social context, 531
study of human, 41–42
successful, 545–546
theories, 56–60
'Ageing brain hypothesis', 347
Ageism, 15, 293, 294, 355–356,
    538–544
  stereotypes, 535
Agitation
  in depression, 349
Aids and equipment
  in community nursing, 472–473
  lifting, 491
Air
  sufficient intake, 164–165
Air wave system mattresses, 232
Alcohol, 384–385
  increases heat loss, 205–206
  with meal, 395
Alcoholism
  and malnutrition, 174
Aldosterone, 48
Alternate pressure mattress, 232
Alveolar
  dilatation, 158
  hypoventilation, 255
Alzheimer's disease, 52, 291, 314–321
  causes, 320–321
  gait in, 119
  'old — old', 320, 324
  'young — old', 320, 324
Alzheimer's Disease Society, 475
American Association of Retired
    Persons, see AARP
Amputation, 560
  mobility, 122
Anaemias, 175–176
  pressure sores and, 227
Anaesthesia
  choice of mode, 558
Analgesics
  for dying, 395
Anorexia, 175
  affects sleep, 251
  and pain, 278

in dying, 395
Antibodies
  decrease with age, 47
Antioxidants
  effect on lifespan, 59
Anxiety
  affects sleep, 251–252
  with breathing problems, 166
Aphasia, 75
Apnoea, sleep, 254–255
Appendicitis
  pain in, 277
Appetite
  loss, 180–181
  in depression, 348–349
Aram House, 474
Arcus senilis, 53
Art therapy, 109
Arteriosclerosis, 560
Arthritic conditions, 121–122
Arthritis
  self help groups, 408–410
Ascorbic acid, 46
Assessment, 299–304
  by district nurse, 467–468
  during short stay care, 509
  in hospital, 491–492
  prompt list, 299
  scales of mobility, 130–131
Association of Retired Persons, 536
Asthma, 254
'At risk' registers, 453
'Attachment'
  of district nurse, 466
Attendance Allowance, 478
Auditory orientating reflex, 53
Auto-antibodies
  increase with age, 47
Autonomic dysfunction, 52
Autonomy for nurse practitioners,
    572–573

B cells, 47
Backwards shuffle from fall, 136
Balance, 131

and falls, 123–124
in ageing, 53
managing poor, 135
Baldness, 54
Baltimore Longitudinal Study
of Ageing, see BLSA
Basal metabolic rate, 205
Batch treatment
of patients in institutions, 501
Baths in hospitals, 489
Beds, 490
areas in hospitals, 487–489
for hemiplegics, 132–133
geriatric numbers, 520
incontinence pads, 195
positioning in, 228
times, 331
Behaviour
effects of pain, 278
Behaviour therapists
nurses as, 360
Behavioural
determination model, 325
disorders
in dementia, 323–324
in depression, 350–351
reducing, 336–337
Behind the Ear hearing aids, 85–86
Bereavement, 33, 460
counselling, 352–353, 358
depression, 9
caused by loss of home, 552
of relatives, 564
Biodressings
for pressure sores, 238
Biography
importance, 8–10, 562
Black elderly people, 474
care of, 437–447
Black Elderly Project, 474
Bladder
atonic, 192–193
care, 186
dysfunction, 191–193
training, 194
Blind, 100
registration, 97–98
Blood pressure
changes in ageing, 51–52
higher in winter, 206–207
BLSA, 41
'Blue bloaters', 255
Bobath
method, 121, 132, 141
stand, 138–139
Bocosan ★
mouth cleansing, 224
Body types,
susceptible to pressure sores, 226
Bone
in ageing, 55, 116–117
Bowel
care, 186, 189–190

disorders, 177–178
Braden scale, 230
Braille, 97
Brain weight, 51
Breast tissue
atrophy, 56
Breathing, 157–169
Breathlessness
in dying, 395–396
Briggs Report, 575
British Geriatrics Society, 425, 431
Broca's aphasia, 75
'Brompton cocktail', 395
Bronchitis, 9, 159
Bronchoconstriction, 165–166
Bronchodilating drugs, 165
Bronchopneumonia
cause of confusion, 311
Budget
and malnutrition, 173
schemes for heating, 212
Bulbs, electric, 96
Bursitis, 151

Calcium, 46, 54, 177
Calluses, 148–150
CAPE, 35
Carbohydrate intolerance, 49
Carbon dioxide, 157
Cardiac output, 44, 117
Cardiovascular
disease and sex, 267
system, 44, 50–51
response to
stimuli, 52
Care
assistants, in residential homes, 506
lack of, shortens life, 533
models, 521–522
organisation, 521–522
planning by district nurse, 468–470
process, 305–306
staff, ageist attitudes, 540
Carers, 398, 419–421, 456, 500
informal, 479–480
stress, 324
Carib Housing Association, 474
Caring for People, 420
Cartilage
in ageing, 55
Cataract, 93–94
Catheters
incontinence, 195–196
Cell cultures
in ageing studies, 41
Cell mediated immunity, 47
Central mechanisms, 123
Central nervous system
depressants, 252–253
stimulants, 253
Centre for Health and
Retirement Education, 100

Cerebral blood flow, 51
decreases with age, 52
Chairs, 118
hemiplegics sitting in 133–134
in hospitals, 490
incontinence pads for, 195
Change
adjustment, 33–34
related to ageing, 20–30, 40
Charitable organisations, 423
Chemical damage
in dementia, 320
Chest infection
care plan, 160–164
Chilblains, 151–152
Child proof drug containers, 383
*Children in Hospital,
National Association for Welfare*, 564
Chiropody
need for, 147–148
service, 154
Choice, 104–112, 503–506, 519–528
lack of, 552, 553
Chromosome damage
in dementia, 320
Chronic obstructive airways disease,
see COAD
Chronically Sick and Disabled
Persons Act 1970, 87, 475
Cilia
loss in ageing, 50
Circadian rhythm
and sleep, 243–244, 248–249, 257
disordered, 252
Cities
growing old in, 457–458
Civil rights, 15
Clifton Assessment Procedures
for the Elderly,
see CAPE
Climatic
factors in ageing, 102–104
Clinical nurse specialist, 569–571, 578, 581
Clinical Nursing Unit, 514
Clitoris, orgasm, 265
Clothing, 331, 553–554
as insulation, 202
expressing sexuality, 213, 269–270
lost in Homes, 524, 526
to minimise skin discomfort,
222–223
warm, 211
Clubs, old peoples', 10
COAD, 166–167
Coffee, 251
Cognitive
abilities, 22–23
behaviour therapy, 358–360
problems, 313, 322
in depression, 349–350
Cohorts, 10–12
effect, 41

Cold
  effects on elderly, 206–207
Colour
  in design, 96
Committee for Safety of Medicines, 387
Common Foundation Programme, 578
Communication, 105–106, 549–551
  as counselling, 357
  between professionals, 473
  elements of, 67–68
  improving, 83–84
  in assessing mobility, 125–126
  international, 68
  needs of elderly, 68–70
  non verbal, 68–69
  paralinguistic, 68
  problems, 70–77
    in confusion, 313–314
    in dementia, 324, 328–329
  skills, 68–70
  verbal, 68
  with elderly, 67–77
Community care
  current policy, 480
Community Care Centre, 473
Community Care Scheme, 510–511
Community Health Councils, 543
Community hospitals, 473
Community nursing service, 305, 420,
    465–483, 570
  psychiatric nurses, 475
  see also District Nurse
Concentration
  poor in confusion, 313
Confidence, 44
Confused
  living at home, 552
  residents in Homes, 506, 526, 552
Confusional states, 291–292, 309–339
  causes, 311–314
  chronic, 314–315
  in dying, 397
  identified problems, 313
  nursing care, 315–317
  physiological needs, 315–316
  post operative, 558
  prevention, 315
Connective tissue
  in ageing, 55
Consciousness
  clouding, 313
    due to air lack, 165
Constipation, 46, 177–178, 189–190
  in COAD, 167
  in dying, 396
Continence, 185
  advise on, 196–197
  promotion, 193–489
Continuity theory, 32
Contrast
  in design, 96
Controlled model of care, 52

Cooking, 102–103
Co-ordination, 131
Coping behaviour, 526
Coronary ateriosclerosis, 43–44
Corporate consciousness, 13–14
Corns, 148
  plasters, 153
Corticosteroids, 165–166
Cortisol
  secretion, 48
Cough
  in dying, 395–396
Cough reflex, 158, 165
Counselling
  by district nurse, 470–471
  in depression, 354–357
Cramps, 255
Crime
  prevention, 459
Cross linking in macromolecules
  ageing theories, 58
Crossroads Care Attendant Scheme, 456
Cruelty, 550
Crystallized intelligence, 22
Cultural
  factors in nutrition, 174–175
  factors in retirement, 101–102
  packages, 438
  stereotype of ageing, 20–21, 30
Cumberlege Review, 466

Day care, 476
Day centres, 476, 509
  for ethnic minorities, 444
Day hospitals, 473
Day space in hospitals, 488
Deafness, 71–72, 79–90, 100
  communication in, 71–72
  consequences, 88–89
  prevalence, 81–82
  sensorineural, 84
  social theories of ageing, 82–83
  stigma, 79–81
Death, 391–401
  causes in elderly, 392
  coming to terms with, 33–34
  fear of, 31
  natural, 392
  place of, 393
  sudden, 392
Death rate curve, 533
Debriding agents
  pressure sores, 235–236
Debt
  fear of, 211
Deconditioning, 45
Decubitus ulcers
  see Pressure sores
Defaecation, 186–191
  assessment, 188–189
Degeneration

age related, 4
Dehydration, 175
Delusions, 72
Dementia, 291, 295, 306–339, 533
  causes, 318
  classification, 317–318
  deafness confused with, 80
  depression and, 345
  ethical issues, 563
  malnutrition and, 173
  multi infarct, 321–322
  nursing management, 326–332
Demographic trends, 418–421
Dental services, 182
Dentition
  and malnutrition, 174
Dependency, 419, 551
  cycle, 553
Depersonalisation, 501
  in hospital, 495, 552
Depression, 20–26, 292, 341–371, 527
  and malnutrition, 173
  and pain, 278
  bereavement, 9
  control, 365
  definition, 342–343
  drug therapy, 360–361
  ECT, 362–363
  explanations, 343–347
  intervention, 366
  nursing care, 354–360
  outlook, 365–366
  physical illness associated with, 344
  prevention, 351–354
  social causation, 346–347
Despair, 31
Detrusor instability, 191–192
Deviance theory, 32
Dexamethasone Supression Test, 364
Dextranomer beads, 236
Diabetes, 97
  and sexuality, 267–268
  footcare in, 153
  peripheral nerve pathology, 149
Diabetic retinopathy, 95
Diet, 388
  and demented patients, 332
  and malnutrition, 173
  healthy, 546
  high fibre, 189–190
  history, 179
  special, 181
Dietary
  allowances recommended, 46
  effect on sleep, 251
  requirements, 167, 172
Digitalis
  causing confusional states, 310
Dignity, 328–330
  loss of, 526
Digoxin, 310
Dihydroepiandrosterone, 48
Dining environment, 180

in hospitals, 488
Disability
  and malnutrition, 173
  cycle, 553
  early detection, 460
Disabled Living Foundation, 97
Discharge planning, 473
Disengagement theory, 30–31
Disorientation, 73, 334–335
  in confusion, 313
  in dementia, 322
Displacements (falls), 124
Disposable soma theory
  of ageing, 59–60
District nurse, 466–472, 569–570
  carer support, 480
  decision making, 471
  innovators in care, 481–482
  role, 467–471
  specialisation, 481
  training, 574
DNA
  ageing theory, 58
Domestic tasks, 105
Domiciliary
  care assistant, 476
  services, for ethnic minorities, 444
Down's syndrome
  features similar to ageing, 57
Dressing, 105
Dressings
  for pressure sores, 236–238
Drinking, 105, 171–183
Drug industry, 387–389
Drug Surveillance Research Unit, 387
Drugs
  absorption ability, 376–377
  acute confusional state, 310
  adverse reactions, 379–380
  antidepressants, 360–362
  compliance, 380–382
  district nurse and, 471–472
  distribution, 377–378
  elderly and, 373–389
  excretion, 378–379
  for dementia, 322
  for Parkinson's disease, 310
  history, 385–386
  hoarding, 375
  malnutrition and, 174
  metabolism, 378
  overprescribing, 505
  pressure sores and, 28
  receptor sensitivity, 379
  response, changes with age, 376
  sexuality and, 268–269
  sleep disorders and, 252–253
  symptomatic relief, 374
  therapeutic, 374
Duke studies of ageing, 41
Dying, 391–401
  care of, 563–565
  emotional reactions to, 397–398

quality of, 560–565
Dysarthria, 74
Dysphasia, 75

Ear
  changes in ageing, 52–53
  hearing aids, 84–86
Eating, 105, 171–183, 331–332, 489
  habits affect sleep, 251
Economic
  factors in ageing, 104
Efferent mechanisms, 124
Ego integrity, 31
Elderly At Risk
  record cards, 453, 454–455
Elderly people
  challenge of ageing society, 531–547
Elders, 437–447
Eldership
  recolonisation, 14–15
Electric blankets, 211, 213
Electrolyte balance, 43
Elimination, 185–198
Emotional
  distress, alleviating, 316–317
  problems, 313, 323
  support in health care, 412
  well being, 292–294
Emphysema
  tobacco smoke's role, 159
Endocrine system, 48–50, 52
Endogenous depression, 343
Endorphins, 274
Energy
  intake, 46, 172
  loss of, in depression, 349
Environment
  change causes confusion, 312
  misinterpretation, 313
Environmental
  causes of sleep disturbance, 250–252
  factors in ageing, 103–104
  temperature, 204
'Environmental docility hypothesis',
    501
Equipment
  in community nursing, 472–473
Erythema ab igne, 153
Ethics, 561
Ethnic minorities
  care of, 437–447, 474
  in cities, 458
  major diseases, 442–443
  mental health in, 443
Euthanasia, 400–401
Everyday Living Skills Inventory, 301
Exchange theory, 32
Excreta
  ability to hold, 187–188
Exercise, 109, 284, 546, 551
  in depression, 363, 364
  in health maintenance, 61

stimulates bowel muscle, 178
  training, 117
EXIT, 400
Expectoration, 165
Eye
  changes in ageing, 53

Faecal incontinence, 191
Falls, 122–124
  getting up from, 136
  prevention, 125
Family
  expectations of hospital
    discharge, 473–474
  involvement, 36
  networks, 441
Fear
  in confusion, 313
Femur, fractured, 141–142, 206,
    559–560
'Festinating gait', 120
Fibroblasts
  replication in humans, 57
First Age, 532
Flatlet, residential, 510
Fleeces, 233–234
Fluid
  balance, 43
  intake
    in COAD, 167
Fluid intelligence, 22
Fluorescent tube lighting, 96
Foam dressings
  for pressure sores, 237
Folic acid
  deficiency, 176
Food, 213
  energy, 172
  in COAD, 167
  refusal, 350
Foot
  care, 147, 155
  deformity, 151
  infections, 150–151
  ulceration, 149–150
Fostering schemes, 10
Fourth Age, 532
Free radical, 60
  theory of ageing, 58–59
Freedom, 527
  loss of, 526
Friendship, 269
Function
  assessment, 104–107, 127
Functional
  assessment, 491–492
  reserve, 43–44, 45–56
Furniture
  in residential homes, 327

Gait, 119–120, 131, 148

pathological, 120–124
Games
  as therapy, 109
Gangrene, 151
Gardening, 102, 109
Gastrectomy, 176
Gastritis, atrophic, 46
Gastrointestinal
  function, 52
  tract, 45–47
Gate theory of pain, 274
General practitioners
  old peoples' use of, 465
Generalizability problems, 28–30
Generations, 10–12
  sociological, 10–12
Genitourinary diseases
  and sexuality, 268
Geriatric
  medicine, 424–429
    admissions policy, 486
    contemporary, 427–429
    ethos, 494
    organisation, 424–429
    relationship with nursing,
      432–434, 508
    speciality, 424–427
  nursing, 429–434, 485–495, 508–509
    low status, 554
    origins, 429
    relationship with medicine,
      432–433
    research based, 429–432
  services
    age related, 427–428
    integrated, 426–427
    organisational solutions, 433–434
    residual, 427
  ward
    death in, 393
Geriatrics, 15, 538–544
  Giants of, 533
Gerontology, MSc in, 517
Glaucoma, 94–95, 97
Global
  aphasia, 75
  dysphasia, 75
Glucose tolerance test, 49–50
Government
  policy on elderly, 422–424
Grants
  for insulation, 212
Greenfield Report, 387
Grey Panthers, 9–10, 14, 413, 535
Grey Party, 536
Grief, 358
Griffiths report, 499, 510, 517
Grooming, 105
Group work
  with demented, 333–334
'Growing Younger Program', 410
Growth hormone
  secretion, 48

Hachinski score, 322
Hair
  greying, 53–54
Hallucinations, 72, 316, 349
Hallux valgus, 148, 151
'Happier Old Age', 520
Hastings approach
  fractured femur, 142
Health, 12–13
  and disease in the elderly, 60–62
  care, preventive, 546, 568
  education, 387–388, 546
  factors influencing, 39
  for all, 574
  in old age, 405–415
  service, 34–35
Health centres, 466–467
Health visitors, 449–463, 570
  alternatives, 456–457
  process, 460
'Healthy Lifestyles for Seniors', 410
Hearing, 52–53, 79–90
  aids, 71–72, 84–86
  loss
    assessment, 83
    recognising, 71–72
    rehabilitation, 83–84
Heart
  changes in ageing, 50–51
  failure, 167
Heat loss, 202
Heating, 207, 212–213
  cost, 206, 211–212
Hemiplegia
  gait in, 121
  left sided, 75–76
  loss of muscle tone, 129–130
  positioning patient, 132–136
  right sided, 74–75
Herbalism, 385
Heredity
  part played in ageing, 57
'Heterosexual living space', 266
Hip, aged, 558–560
Hoists, 491
Holidays, 332–333
Holistic approach, 295
Home
  assessment, treatment strategy, 426
  conditions, assessment, 106
  death in, 394
  hazards to mobility, 118
Home help, 10, 182, 475–476
Homeostasis, 116, 203
  maintenance in elderly, 42–45
Homes, residential
  Part III, 498, 520–521
  relatives views, 523–525
Homes for incurables, 393
Homosexuality, 266
Horlicks *, 251
Hormone levels
  factors influencing, 48

Hospices, 399
  death in, 393, 563, 565
  movement, 36
Hospital
  admission, 365
    affects sleep, 250
  continuity care in, 507–509, 511
  discharge, 386–387, 426, 493–494
    rehabilitation, 137
  nursing the old in, 485–495, 553–556
Hospital-at-home scheme, 481
Hotel concept
  of residential care, 498
Housework, 102
Housing, 418–419, 440, 477
  heating standards, 210
  in cities, 457
Housing Benefit, 478
Howell, Trevor
  pioneer of geriatric Medicine, 425
'Human growth and development
    studies', 7
Humoral immunity, 47
Hydration
  importance in pyrexia, 165
Hydrocolloid dressings
  for pressure sores, 238
Hydrogels
  for pressure sores, 238
Hydrogen peroxide
  mouth cleansing, 224
Hyperkeratotic lesions, 148, 149
Hypersomnolence, 256
Hypochlorite solutions, 236
'Hypokinetic disease', 117
Hypothermia, 199–201, 331
  care of patient, 214–217
  detection, 213–214
  prevention, 211–213
  signs of symptoms, 211, 215
Hypothyroidism, 48, 205
  affects sexuality, 267

Iatrogenic disease, 509
Identity
  loss of, 526
Ignorance
  and malnutrition, 173
Illness
  affects sexuality, 267
  sleep, 253–256
  depression in, 344–346
Immobility
  assessing, 124–125
  contribution to pressure sores, 227
  management, 124–139
  prevalence, 115–116
Immune system, 47–50
Immunocompetence
  decline with ageing, 47
Inactivity
  in demented patients, 332

Income, 418–419
  expectations in retirement, 13
  support, 478, 534
Incontinence, 185–186, 187, 326, 350
  aids, 194–196
  and pressure sores, 227
  community services, 196
  in dying, 396–397
  in management of intractable,
    194–196
Independence
  in ethnic elders, 442
  loss of, 526
Independent Living Fund, 196, 478
Individuality, 36, 328–330
Individualized care, 528
'Induced dependency hypothesis', 502
Influenza
  vaccinations, 159
Informed consent, 561
Innovation
  by nurses, 555
Insight
  lack of, in dementia, 323
Insoles, 151
Insomnia
  in dying, 396
Institutional living, 103–104, 107, 118
Institutionalisation
  of Home staff, 503
Institutions
  characteristics, 500–502
  numbers in, 498
Insulin insensitivity
  in ageing, 49
Interaction
  with demented, 328–329
Interdisciplinary care, 35–36
Intelligence, 21–23
  crystallized, 22
  fluid, 22
  tests, 24
Interests
  maintaining, 99–100
Intervertebral discs
  degeneration, 127–128
Invalid Care Allowance, 478
Inverse Care Law, 452
Iron, 46
  deficiency, 175
Irish
  elderly, 458
Isolation, 356
  affects sleep, 248

Kent Community Care Project, 510,
  512
Kidneys
  blood flow, 51
Kings Fund Centre, 515
Knoll scale, 229

Labelling theory, 32
Lambeth Community Care Centre, 515
Language
  problems, 440
Lavatory
  ability to reach, 187
Laxatives, 190
'Learned helplessness', 104, 502, 556
Learning skills, 7, 23–24
Leg movements
  sleep related, 225
Lesbians, 266
Liaison health visitors, 457
Life
  expectancy, 530
  history interviewing, 7–8
  review, 111–112
  satisfaction, 289
Lifespan, 19
'Lifespan' studies, 7
Lifestyle, 4
  health correlated with, 12
  in institutions, 501
  influencing ageing process, 41, 42
  skin disorders and, 223
Lifting, 491
  old people, 137–139
  techniques, 231
Lighting, 327
  in hospitals, 489–490
  standards for elderly, 95–97
Limbs
  assessment in elderly, 128–130
Lip-reading, 71
Lipofuscin accumulation
  in ageing, 57
'Listening service', 557
Liver, 46
Living
  activities, 44
  quality, 549–560
  skills, 301
'Living will', 400, 562
Local Authority Social
  Services Act, 422
Lockers
  in hospitals, 490
Loeb Centre for Nursing
  and Rehabilitation, 514
Loneliness, 260, 505, 527
  predisposes to malnutrition, 173
Long stay
  patients, maintenance treatment,
    136–137
  settings
    care in, 497–518
    choice, 519–528
    flexibility, 519–528
    quality of, 502–507
Longevity
  upper limit, 4
Longitudinal
  studies of ageing, 41–42

Lorgnette, electric
  as hearing aid, 86–87
Loss, 526–528
Louisa's story, 541–543, 561
Low back pain
  in nurses, 137
Lucidity
  definition, 561
Lung
  changes in ageing, 50, 158
  expansion, 165

Macmillan nurses, 564
Macular degeneration, 94
Malabsorption, 174
Malnutrition, 46, 171–183
  predisposes to hypothermia, 206
    to pressure sores, 227
Maltreatment in Homes, 503
Massage, 228, 284
  in hemiplegia, 129
Masturbation, 265, 266
Mattresses
  recommended, 233
Meals, 331–332
  choice, 553
Meals on Wheels, 10, 213, 476
Medical consultants
  contractual responsibility, 513
Medicare, 14
Memory, 23–24
  aids, for drug administration,
    382–383
  dysfunction in pain, 278
  function, 7
  impairment in dementia, 322
  impairment, 20
    and hearing aids, 71
Men
  in old age, 537–538
  in retirement, 537–538
Menopause, 55–56, 62, 265, 266
Mental disorders
  organic, 310
Mental health
  assessment, 301
  in ethnic minorities, 443
  problems, 289–307
Mentally ill
  elderly people, 474–475
Menu planning, 179–180
Methodological issues
  in ageing research, 27–30
Micturition, 186–188, 191–196
  assessment, 192
'Mid-life crises', 21
MIND, 475
Mobility, 104, 115–145
  aids, 136
  assessment scales, 130–131
  factors affecting, 117–120
  foot problems and, 148

in ethnic elders, 442
  necessary to reach lavatory, 187
Money, 212
  control, 332
Mood
  in depression, 348
Moon
  type for blind, 97
Morphine
  in pain relief, 284
Motivation, 44
  key to mobility, 126
Mourning, 33
  encouragemant of active, 36
Mouth care, 223–224
  in dying, 395
'Mucociliary escalator', 50
Multidisciplinary
  care in Homes, 513
  care in hospital, 493
  teamwork, 294–295
Multiple pathway model, 324–326
Muscle strength
  assessment, 128–129
  imbalance, 132
  in ageing, 44, 116–117
Muscular excitability
  in confusion, 314
Musculoskeletal disease
  and sexuality, 267
Music therapy, 109
Myocardial infarction, 207
  and pain, 276–277
Myoclonus
  nocturnal, 255

Narcolepsy, 255
Nasogastric feeding, 179, 181
National Advisory Committee
  of Nutrition Education, 180
National Assistance Act, 422
National Council of Senior
  Citizens, see NCSC
National Health Service Act, 422
Nausea
  in dying, 395, 396
NCSC, 14
Nebulizer, 165–166
Neck
  problems in elderly, 127–128
Negative thoughts, 349
Neighbourhood
  care groups, 478
  nursing, 466–467
Nerve conduction velocity
  in ageing, 44, 52
Nervous system
  changes in ageing, 51–52
  diseases
    affect sexuality, 267
    sleep, 254
'Neurasthenia', 252

Neurofibrillary tangles
  in normal brains, 52
Neurological disease
  pressure sores and, 227
Neuromuscular facilitation, 141
Neuronal loss
  in ageing, 51–52
Neurotransmitters
  changes in ageing, 52
  defects, 319
Niacin, 46
Night
  nursing staff, 251
Nightclothes
  in hospital, 495
'Nightingale' ward
  noise levels in, 250
Nightmares, 255
Noise
  effects on sleep, 250–251
Noradrenaline
  plasma levels in ageing, 52
'Normalization', 329
Norton scales, 216, 229–230
NRTA, 14
Numerical rating scale
  for pain, 280–282
Nurse
  education, 573–575, 577–579
    in long stay care, 575–576
  future, 574–575
  levels, Project 2000, 578
  practitioner, 567–571, 578, 581
Nurses
  educators in sexuality, 269–270
  key workers in care team,
    305
  role in care of old people, 567–581
Nursing
  career structure, 570
  definition, 574
  entrance requirements, 580
  student
    labour wastage, 576
Nursing Development Units, 431,
    515, 571
  Burford, 431, 571–572
  Oxford, 431, 550, 571–572
  Tameside, 572
Nursing homes, 423, 511–515
  death in, 394
  NHS, 511–513
  private, 499, 503
  relatives views, 525–526
Nursing process, 305–306, 571
Nutrition
  and immunity, 47–48
  education, 182
  influencing ageing process, 41
  maintaining body function, 45–47
  requirements, 174
  services in community, 181–182
  status, assessment, 179

Nutritional supplements
  reduce illness duration, 48

Occupation
  effect on mobility, 126
Occupational therapy, 107, 109, 475
  in immobility, 125
Oedema
  in hemiplegia, 129
  in hypothermia, 214
Oestrogen
  cream, 270
  deficiency, in osteoporosis, 54
Old Age Pensions Act, 421–422
Oliguria, 167
Onychogryphosis, 148, 152–153
Ophthalmic opticians, 97
Orem's self care model, 164
Orientation signs, 327
Orthodox sleep, 244–245
Orthopaedic units, 141–142
Osteoarthritis, 121–122
Osteomalacia, 177
Osteoporosis, 44, 46, 55, 62, 177,
    559–560
Out of hours
  nursing service, 481
Outings, 332–333
Overprescribing, 375
Oxygen, 157
  administration, 166–167
    in COAD
  continuous, during sleep, 255
  normal values, 166
  transport capacity, 117

Pads and pants, 194–195
Pain, 273–287
  acute, 274
  assessment, 280
  chronic, 274
  control in dying, 394–395
  in the old, 275
  misconceptions, 279–280
  nature, 274–275
  pharmacological approaches, 283–284
  relief, 131, 278–280
  scales, 280–282
  sensitivity, 54
  sensory dimensions, 275–276
Pain charts, 282
Paradoxical sleep, 244–245
Paranoid states, 292
Parasomnias, 255
Parasympathetic nervous system, 52
Parathyroid hormone, 55
Parkinsonism, 52, 70, 178, 376, 383
  drugs for, 310
  gait in, 120–121
Paronychia, 151
'Passive responders', 534

Paternalistic practices
  amongst welfare workers, 15
Patient, elderly, 549–566
Patient's Charter, 564–565
Peer Health Counselling, 412–413
Peer review, 555
Pegasus* air wave system, 232
Penile sheath
  for incontinence, 194–195
Penis
  impaired erection, 52, 265–266
  scleritic changes, 56
Pensioner's Link, 536
Pensioner's Voice, 535
Peptic ulcer
  pain in, 277
Perception, 24–25
Personal
  contacts, maintaining, 328
  hygiene, 105
  possessions
    in Homes, 524
    in Hospitals, 36, 495
Personality
  change, 323
  integration, 7
  stereotype, 25–27
Pes cavus, 151
Pethidine*, 284
Pets, 110, 111
Phosphorus, 46
Physical
  deterioration
    in dementia, 324
    in depression, 363
  examination, 301
  fitness
    maintains mobility, 116–117,
      119–120
  problems, 314–315
Physiological changes
  in ageing, 40
Physiotherapy, 125
Place
  perception, 73
Plamtar fasciitis, 152
Poor Laws, 421–422
Possessions
  loss of, 526
Postural hypotension, 43, 52, 62
Presbyopia, 53, 97
Prescribing patterns, 374–376
Pressure
  sensitivity, 54
  ulcers on feet, 149
Pressure sores, 54, 224–239
  assessment, 234
  classification, 225–226
  cost, 225
  in dying, 396
  location, 225–226
  management, 234–238
  pathology, 239

prevalence, 225
preventing, 231–234
risk factors, 228–230
team, 239
Preventive care, 449–450
  by district nurse, 469–470
Primary
  health care team, 466, 570–571
  nursing, 556, 571–572
Privacy, 270, 487, 501
  loss of, 526
Private sector
  residential care, 423
Problem oriented records, 304
Problem solving, 24
Progeria
  features similar to ageing, 57
Project 2000, 567, 569, 574, 575–580
  response to 579–580
Proprioceptor system, 53
Prostatectomy
  and sexuality, 268
Prostate gland, 56
  enlargement, 192
Protease activity
  and smoking, 159
Protective model
  of care, 521–522
Proteolytic enzymes, 236
Pruritis, 222, 223
Psychiatric disorders
  affect sleep, 253–254
  in elderly, 291–292
Psychogeriatrics, 425
Psychology
  of ageing, 19–34
Psychological
  disorder, 293
  factors
    in retirement, 101
    pressure sores and, 227
  function, 34–35
Psychomotor retardation
  in depression, 349
Psychosocial factors
  causal factors in confusion,
    312
  in sexual behaviour, 266–267
Public transport, 103, 118
Pulmonary function
  alteration with age, 158
Purpose, 527
Pyrexia, 207–208
  care of patient, 217
  pressure sores and, 227

Quadiceps contraction
  reduces with age, 45
Quality
  assurance, 555–556
  circles, 555
  of life after surgery, 557

Questionnaire
  geriatric assessment, 452

'Race-track' ward
  noise levels in, 250
Radiation
  life shortening, 59
Radio, 102
Reactive depression, 343
Reality orientation, 111–112, 334–335
'Recall' package, 358
Rectangular curve, 4–5
Rectangularisation, 531
Reflexes, 52, 123–124
Rehabilitation
  in hospital, 492–493
Relatives
  in care of dying, 398
  moving in with, 553
  views in long term care, 522–523
Relatives' Groups, 328
Relaxation, 284
Religious
  factors
    in ageing, 101–102
    in nutrition, 174–175
Relocation
  effect on mortality, 498
Reminiscence, 32, 36, 111–112, 180
  therapy, 355–356, 358
Renin, 48
Reproductive system
  in ageing, 56
Rescue chair, 136, 137
Residential
  environment, 326–327
  homes, 509–511
    for dementing people, 326–330
    psychological characteristics,
      500–501
    staff/patient interaction, 327
  places, fewer in UK, 499, 507
  provision, 498–500
    private, 499, 503
    state, 499, 503
Residents, in homes
  turnover, 506
  what they experience, 505–507
  what they want, 504–505
Restrained model of care, 522
Resolution therapy, 336
Respiratory system, 44–45, 50–51
  ageing, 158
  disorders and sexuality, 267
Rest, 243–261
  in COAD, 168
'Restless leg' syndrome, 255
Restlessness
  in confusion, 314
  in dying, 397
Restraint, 563
Resuscitation dilemma, 562

Retirement, 12–13, 20, 26, 33, 99
  ages, 6
  early, 15
  in France, 14–15
  in U.S.A, 14
  men, 537–538
  preparations for, 101
  social context, 533
  women, 536
Retirement Pension, 478
Rheumatoid arthritis, 121–122, 126
Riboflavin, 46
Rights, 551–553
'Rigidity' in old age, 26
Risk, 553
  taking, 552
Role
  changes in ageing, 20–21
  loss of, 526
Roll and crawl from fall, 136
'Routine geriatric' nursing, 430–431
Royal National Institute for
  the Blind, 98
Royal National Institute for
  the Deaf, 87

Safety, 330
Schizophrenia, 292, 310
  affects sleep, 253–254
Screening
  for health problems, 295–296
Scurvy, 176
Second Age, 530
Secretions
  removal of dust, 165
Security, 330
Sedatives
  tolerance to, 252–253
'Self-actualisation', 32
Self care, 405–415
  neglect, 314
  promotion, 337–338
Self determination, 552
Self-esteem, 44
Self-fulfilling prophecy, 545–546
Self-help, 407–409, 570
  groups, in ethnic minorities, 441–445
  organisations, 408, 479
  pressure groups, 408
  support systems, 408
Self-medication, 383–385
  hazards, 384
'Senile emphysema', 158
Senile plaques
  in normal brains, 52
Sensation
  loss in feet, 153
Sensory
  deprivation, 72–73
  dimensions of pain, 275–277
  impairment, 527
  input, reduced, 131–132, 206

Sex
  can be good for you, 265
  differences in ageing, 25
  drive, loss in depression, 349
  in old age, 102, 264
  therapist, 270
Sexist
  stereotypes, 535
Sexual function, 196
Sexuality, 263–271
  double discrimination, 264–265
  physiological aspects, 265–266
Share the Care Scheme, 456
Shivering, 203, 205–206
Shoes
  badly fitting, 148
  for the elderly, 134–135, 151
Shopping, 102, 103
Short-stay residential care, 509
Shoulder
  dislocation in hemiplegia, 129
  lift, 138
Sick
  care of the elderly, 417–435
Sight, 91–98
  assessment, 92–93
  assumptions about, 91
  disabilities, 92–98
    prevalence, 92
Size
  enhancement in poor vision, 97
Skills training, 360
Skin
  ailments, 130
  assessment, 221–222
  changes in ageing, 53–54, 221
  hygiene, 227–228
  lesions, common in old, 222
    stigma, 223
  maintaining healthy, 221–241
  nursing management, 222–223
  protection, 222–223
Sleep, 243–261
  and waking confusion, 72
  assessment, 256–260
  cycles, 246–247
  deprivation, 249, 363
  disturbances, 349, 363
  in COAD, 168
  length, 246–247
  normal adult, 244–245
  problems, 247–256
  questionnaires, 258–259
  REM, 253
  stages, 244–245
  types, 245
Sleep apnoea, 254–255
'Sleep latency', 247
Sleep walking, 255
Slumberland Vaperon*
  patient support system, 233
Smell sense
  deterioration in ageing, 53, 174

Smoking, 39, 40, 388
  in lung disease, 159
Social
  factors,
    in temperature control, 210–211
  problems, 313–314, 321–322
  services, 106–107, 196
  surveys, 6–7
  withdrawal in depression, 350
'Social deprivation syndrome', 346
Social Fund, 478
Social interaction
  between nurses and patients, 550
Social Problem Solving, 360
Social security benefits, 477–478
  low take up by ethnic minorities,
    440
Social Services
  personal, 475
Socks, 153
Sodium bicarbonate
  mouth cleansing, 224
Solitude, 168
Somatic complaints
  in depression, 348
Somnolence, 254
Spastic hemiplegia, 126
Spasticity
  treatment, 131
Speech
  difficulty in understanding, 52
  impairment, 73–74, 80–81
Speech therapy
  in stroke patients, 77
Sperm production
  in old age, 56
Sphincter
  incompetent, 192
Staff attitudes
  to disabled patients, 329–330
Staff/residents interaction
  in institutions, 501
Standard setting initiatives, 555
Standing, 137
Standing Committee for Ethnic
  Minority Senior Citizens, 446
Stereotype
  of old age, 20–21
Stimulants
  non drug, 384–385, 386
Stimulation
  lack of, 527
Stockings, 153
Strategy for Nursing, 555
Stress
  in Home staff, 503
  mortality associated with, 49
  response, 51, 116
Stroke, 207
  communication
    difficulties, 74–77
  guidelines, 76
  rehabilitation, 140–141

severity ratings, 139–140
therapy, 141
units, 139–141
Suicide, 366–368, 392–393
Sunlight
prevents osteomalacia, 177
Support systems
bedsores and, 228, 232
Supportive model of care, 521
Surgery
assessment, 556–557
for old people, 550, 556–560
Surveillance programme
health, 451–453
Swallowing problems, 178–179
Sweating, 203–204
Sympatho-adrenal system, 49
Symbolic interactionism, 32

T3, 48
T cells, 47
Tagging systems, 330
Talking Book Service, 97, 98
Task oriented care, 528
Taste sense
deterioration in ageing, 53, 174
Teaching Nursing Home, 516
Team approach, 555
in geriatric medicine, 493
in terminal care, 564
Tear production
diminished in ageing, 53
Teeth, 395
Television, 102
Temperature
low body, 199–201, 209–211
maintaining body, 199–218, 222
measuring, 208–209
raised, 207–208
care of patient with, 217
room, 210
sensitivity, 54
Tenosynovitis, 151
Terminal care, 564–565
Thermography
detecting pressure sore risk, 230
Thermoregulation
age changes, 52, 205–206
normal, 204–205
physiological aspects, 201–206
Thiamine, 46
Third age conception, 15, 532
Thorax
changes in ageing, 50
Thymic hormones
decrease with age, 47
Thymus gland, 47
Thyroid, 48
Time
factors in retirement, 100
perception, 73
Toenails, 148

care of, 152–153
Toes
deformed, 151
Toilet
facilities in hospitals, 489
management, 105, 193–194
neglect, 314
skills, 188
Toileting, 338
Touch
as communication, 67, 70, 550
sensitivity, 54
Transcutaneous electrical nerve stimulation, 284
Transient ischaemic attacks, 52, 56
Treatment
right to refuse, 561–563
sexuality and, 268–269
Trunk
problems in elderly, 128
Tube feeding, 178, 181
'Turning clock', 231
Turning devices, 233

Ultrasound
detecting pressure sore risk, 230
Urinary
incontinence, 52
output in COAD, 167
tract infection, 193
Uterus
in ageing, 56

Vaginal
changes, 56, 270
orgasm, 265
Validation techniques, 36, 336
Value history, 562
Vascular problems, 560
Vasomotor tone, 204–205
Vegan diets, 176
Verbal rating scale
for pain, 280
Vestibular system, 53
Violence, 458–460
domestic, 408
inside home, 458–459
outside home, 459–460
Vision
changes in ageing, 53
causes, 93–95
impairment
and communication, 70–71
seeking help, 97
testing, 92–93
Visual analogue scale
for pain, 282
Vitamin A, 46
Vitamin B complex
deficiency, 174

Vitamin B12
deficiency, 176
Vitamin C, 46, 59
deficiency, 176–177
Vitamin D, 55–56
deficiency, 177
Vitamin E, 59
Volunteers
in residential homes, 328
Voluntary organisations, 423
Voluntary Sector
as carers, 478–480
Vomiting
in dying, 396

Wagner report, 499, 503, 504, 507, 510
'Wandering', 330
WAIS, 21–23
Walking, 11
as transport, 118
'manner of', 119–120
with aids, 135–136
Walking sticks, 134–135
Wards
multi-purpose, 486
single-purpose, 486–487
Warren, Marjory
pioneer of geriatric medicine, 424–425, 485
Warts
digital, 150–151
plantar, 150–151
Waterbeds, 223
Waterlow scales, 216, 230
Wechster Adult Intelligence Scale
see WAIS
Weight, 179
loss in depression, 348–349
monitoring, 332
Well Elderly Program, 410
Wernicke's aphasia, 75
Wheelchair
mobility, 122
Women
as workers, 536
in old age, 534–537
in retirement, 534–537
live longer than men, 418, 534
Women's Movement
and the elderly, 535
Work, 12–13
Working for Patients, 420, 555, 564
Wound dressings
pressure sores, 236–238
Wound healing
in elderly, 54–55, 237
in pressure sores, 235
'Wrinkle'
cause, 54